Hazardous and
Toxic Materials

Second Edition

HAZARDOUS AND TOXIC MATERIALS
Safe Handling and Disposal
Second Edition

Edited by Howard H. Fawcett, P.E.
President, Fawcett Consultations

WILEY

A Wiley-Interscience Publication
JOHN WILEY & SONS
New York   Chichester   Brisbane   Toronto   Singapore

Library of Congress Cataloging in Publication Data

Hazardous and toxic materials: safe handling and disposal/edited by
  Howard H. Fawcett.—2nd ed.
      p.   cm.
  "A Wiley/Interscience publication."
  Rev. ed. of: Hazardous and toxic materials/Howard E. Fawcett.
1st ed. ©1984.
    ISBN 0-471-62729-1
    1. Hazardous wastes—United States—Safety measures. 2. Poisons-
-Safety measures.   I. Fawcett, Howard H.
TD811.5.H384 1988   87-34084
363.1'79—dc19   CIP

Printed in the United States of America

10 9 8 7 6 5 4 3

This book is dedicated to a bright future,
as personified by my grandchildren:
Erik Howard Fawcett (born October 22, 1984) and
Kirstin Beatrice Fawcett (born March 4, 1987)

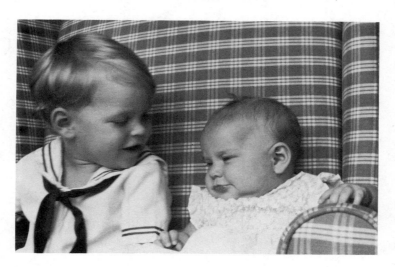

Contributors

Audrey Armour, Ph.D.
York University
Faculty of Environmental Studies
Lumbers Bldg., 4700 Keele St.
North York, Ontario, M3J 1P3 Canada

J. C. Astro
Deputy Head
Dangerous Goods Section
Directorate-General of Transport
Ministry of Transport and Public Works
Postbus 20901, 2500 EX The Hague
Netherlands

James M. Brown, J.D.
Professor
National Law Center
The George Washington University
Washington, DC 20052

Howard H. Fawcett, P.E.
President
Fawcett Consultations
P.O. Box 9444, Wheaton, MD 20906

Ralph W. Fawcett, M.D., Ph.D.
Medical Associate
Fawcett Consultations
P.O. Box 9444, Wheaton, MD 20906

Massod Ghassemi, Ph.D., P.E.
Director, Solid and Hazardous Waste Management Programs
URS Consultants, Inc.
Long Beach, CA 90802

Susan Goddard, M.S.
P.O. Box 1787
Alvin, TX 77512

Roy W. Hann, Jr., Ph.D., P.E.
Professor of Civil Engineering and Research Scientist
Department of Civil Engineering
Environmental Engineering Division
Texas A&M University
College Station, TX 77840

Pamela Harris, M.P.H.
Occupational Health Specialist
Browning-Ferris Industries
8119 Wood Downe Lane
Houston, TX 77040

Ronald D. Hill, P.E.
Land Pollution Control Division
Hazardous Waste Engineering Research Laboratory
U.S. Environmental Protection Agency
Cincinnati, OH 45268

D. Jack Kilian, M.D.
Corporate Medical Director
Browning Ferris Industries
Adjunct Professor of Occupational Medicine
Department of Preventive Medicine and Community Health
The University of Texas Medical Branch
Galveston, TX 77550

Henry Lau, Ph.D.
TSCA Technical Data Center, East Tower
U.S. Environmental Protection Agency
Washington, DC 20460

Edward C. Norman, Ph.D.
Vice-President
National Foam System, Inc.
150 Gordon Drive
Lionville, PA 19353

J. Van der Schaaf
SAVE Consulting Scientists
Deventerspraat Str. 37
7311 LT Apeldoorn
Netherlands

Elizabeth K. Weisburger, Ph.D.
Assistant Director for Chemical Carcinogenesis
National Cancer Institute
National Institutes of Health
Bethesda, MD 20892

Preface

The growing awareness and uneasiness of the public sector about hazardous and toxic chemicals and related materials has created a strong determination by legislators at national, state, and local levels to attempt to control these chemicals by laws and regulations. Since the publication of the first edition of this volume in August 1984, we have seen a tide of legislation and enforcement reflecting this public concern. In this volume we continue to document new developments and to provide sensible, balanced information that will be useful to the makers, users, and disposers of chemicals, which includes nearly every person on planet Earth today. This volume combines the wisdom of several experts in various fields, all presenting a positive viewpoint that hazardous and toxic chemicals and related materials can be controlled and disposed of without adverse effects on people, the environment, or future generations. If we have managed to bring a little order out of the widespread confusion, this effort will not have been in vain.

Wheaton, Md

Acknowledgments

A book, much like a jigsaw puzzle, is the sum of many pieces which, when assembled, present an image. Of the many who assisted greatly in our efforts these individuals are noted with sincere appreciation:

My two sons, Ralph Willard and Harry Allen, have given me encouragement since the demise of my wife, Ruth. George Proper, Jr., Loudonville, N.Y., continues a 30-year interchange of information that documents the leading role of fire services in emergency planning and response to hazardous chemicals. The American Chemical Society library staff, especially Ms. H. Adams, Henry Saxe, and Dr. Maureen Matkovich, have been very responsive to my frequent requests for assistance. Mike Heylin, editor of *Chemical and Engineering News,* has afforded me a unique overview of the passing parade by allowing me to review the safety letters to the editor. Dr. Dan Marsick of the OSHA Technical Data Center has always responded to my requests promptly and accurately. Dr. R. Cothern of the EPA supplied much background data on radon-222 and its implications, as did Nucleonics Lecturn Associates. Henry Lau, in addition to contributing Chapter 7, has always been a valuable source of information regarding TSCA. Marjorie Fawcett, RN, of Dayton, Ohio, kindly escorted me to the scene of the Miamisburg derailment and is a most enthusiastic data source. Jessie Nash of Memphis, Tennessee, helped me find and explore the Hollywood and Frasier (Tennessee) hazardous waste sites. Harry Allen and I narrowly avoided arrest for our zeal in wanting to see the Stringfellow acid pit in California, and Mrs. Penny Newman supplied additional data on this continuing environmental tragedy. Harry Wray, undisputed expert and dean of ASTM flash-point, gave us his insight into this important technique. Henry Morton, of 3M Engineering Services, submitted his wisdom on fire and explosion control. Phillip Wingate and his wife Sue entertained me at a delicious planked shad dinner to confirm without question that the shad had returned (Chapter 14). Leslie Bretherick of the United Kingdom has been a frequent inspiration as well as a dependable resource on chemical compatability. Professor Warner Stumm and his associates were most courteous when I visited them in Switzerland, and the excellent input provided by the staff of Sandoz, Inc., resulted in Chapter 23.

Ambassador Kohl of the Indian Embassy in Washington provided much valuable data regarding the Bhopal tragedy. Jack Leach and Richard Shaff of the National Institutes of Health and Safety, have been helpful over many years. Dr. Elizabeth Weissburger (Chapter 9) has extended much insight into chemical carcinogens, mutagens, and teratogens. Professor Gary Bennett, co-editor of the *Journal of Hazardous Materials,* has provided many valuable viewpoints. John Moran and his staff at the NIOSH Laboratory in Morgantown, West Virginia, assisted greatly in the preparation of Chapter 12. Aldo Osti, a dedicated safety professional, suggested we include home chemistry (Chapter 15). The vital contributions of Thomas Sinderson, M.D., and his associate, Sunny Fagley, RN, in helping me maintain my essential heartbeat, is gratefully acknowledged. James Smith, editor at the Interscience Division of Wiley, and Melinda Wirkus of Cobb-Dunlop Publisher Services were instrumental in bringing together these many pages into what we hope is a useful volume. Thanks.

To the sage words of Dr. Madame Curie

> Nothing in Life is to be Feared;
> It is only to be Understood

we add: Happy Landings and a sunny future.

Contents

Appendices

Acronyms and Abbreviations

APCA	Air Pollution Control Association (U.S.)
AAIH	American Academy of Industrial Hygiene (U.S.)
AAOM	American Academy of Occupational Medicine (U.S.)
AAOHN	American Association of Occupational Health Nurses (U.S.)
ABC	Always Be Careful (with chemicals) (universal)
ACGIH	American Conference of Governmental Industrial Hygienists (U.S.)
ACS	American Chemical Society (U.S.)
AIChE	American Institute of Chemical Engineers (U.S.)
ADI	Acceptable daily intake
AIHA	American Industrial Hygiene Association (U.S.)
AMA	American Medical Association (U.S.)
ANSI	American National Standards Institute (U.S.)
APHA	American Public Health Association (U.S.)
API	American Petroleum Institute (U.S.)
ASB	Asbestos Information Bureau (Canada)
ASSE	American Society of Safety Engineers (U.S.)
ASTM	American Society for Testing and Materials (U.S.)
AXE	Alpha Chi Sigma, Professional Chemical Fraternity (U.S.)
BNA	Bureau of National Affairs (U.S.)
BOHN	British Occupational Hygiene Society (U.K.)
BSC	British Safety Council (U.K.)
C&EN	Chemical and Engineering News (U.S.)
CATLINE	National Library of Medicine current catalogue (U.S.)

CAG	Cancer Assessment Group, U.S.E.P.A. (U.S.)
CBC	Circulating bed combustor (U.S.)
CEPP	Chemical Emergency Preparededness Program
CERT	Chemical Emergency Response Team
CFR	Code of Federal Regulations (Laws) (U.S.)
CGA	Compressed Gas Association (U.S.)
CHEMTREC	Chemical Transportation Emergency Response Center (CMA) (800-424-9300); for Alaska & Hawaii, (202)483-7616) (U.S.)
CIA	Chemical Industry Association (U.K.)
CIIT	Chemical Industry Institute of Toxicology (U.S.)
CMA	Chemical Manufacturers Association (U.S.)
CPSC	Consumer Product Safety Commission (U.S.)
CRACK	An addictive drug, controlled substance (U.S.)
CSMA	Chemical Specialties Manufacturers Association (U.S.)
DCHAS	Division of Chemical Health and Safety, American Chemical Society (U.S.)
DOA	Department of Agriculture (U.S.)
DOD	Department of Defense (U.S.)
DOE	Department of Energy (U.S.)
DOL	Department of Labor (includes OSHA) (U.S.)
DOT	Department of Transportation (U.S.)
EPA	Environmental Protection Agency (U.S.)
FDA	Food and Drug Administration (U.S.)
FEMA	Federal Emergency Management Agency (U.S.)
FM	Factory Mutuals (insurance) (U.S.)
FNRC	Federal National Response Center (reporting of spills or releases) (800-424-8802) (U.S.)
FR	Federal Register (publication of laws) (U.S.)
GPO	Government Printing Office (U.S.)
GRATEFUL MED	A medical computerized data base by the National Library of Medicine (U.S.)
HEW	Department of Health and Education (no longer known by that name) (U.S.)
HHS	Department of Health and Human Services (U.S.)
HIT	Hazard Information Transmission (a service of CMA) (U.S.)
HPS	Health Physics Society (U.S.)

HSELINE	Health and Safety Executive Laboratory Hazard Bulletin (U.K.)
HTH	A brand of calcium hypochlorite
HW&HM	Hazardous Waste and Hazardous Materials (Mary Ann Liebert, Inc.) (journal) (U.S.)
IARC	International Agency for Research on Cancer (France)
ICWU	International Chemical Workers Union—AFL-CIO (U.S. and Canada)
ICO	International Consultative Organization (maritime) (London)
IChE	Institution of Chemical Engineers (U.K.)
IHF	Industrial Hygiene Foundation (U.S.)
ILO	International Labour Organization (not a labor union) (Geneva, Switzerland)
IOM	Institute of Medicine, National Academy of Sciences (U.S.)
JOHM	Journal of Hazardous Materials (Elsevier, Netherlands)
LEPC	Local emergency planning commission under Title III of P.L. 99-499 (U.S.)
LORAD	Low-level radioactive (waste)
MSDS	Material Safety Data Sheet (an OSHA requirement) U.S.
NAS	National Academy of Sciences (U.S.)
NAE	National Academy of Engineering (a division of NAS) (U.S.)
NAPAP	National Acid Precipitation Assessment Program (U.S.)
NBS	National Bureau of Standards (U.S.)
NFPA	National Fire Protection Association (U.S.)
NPL	National Priority List for Superfund (SARA), EPA (U.S.)
NRC	National Research Council, NAS (U.S.)
NTIS	National Technical Information Service (U.S.)
OCAW	Oil, Chemical and Atomic Workers—AFL-CIO (U.S.)
OHM/TADS	Oil and Hazardous Materials, Technical Assistance Data System (EPA) (U.S.)
OS&H	Occupational Safety and Health (journal) (U.S.)
OSHA	Occupational Safety and Health Agency, Department of Labor (U.S.)
PACT	Powder-activated carbon technology (U.S.)

PBB	Polybrominated biphenyl
PCB	Polychlorinated biphenyl
PE	Professional Engineer; also Pollution Engineering (journal) (U.S.)
PEL	Permissible exposure limit (OSHA) (U.S.)
ppb	Parts per billion
ppm	Parts per million
ppt	Parts per trillion
RCRA	Resources Conservation and Recovery Act (U.S.)
RSoC	Royal Society of Chemistry (U.K.)
RTECS	Registry of Toxic Effects of Chemical Substances (U.S.)
RTK	Right-to-Know (OSHA Hazard Communication Regulation) U.S.
SARA	Superfund Amendments and Reauthorization Act, 1986 (U.S.)
SERA	State Emergency Response Authority (see Title III of P.L. 99-499, 1986) (U.S.)
SGPT	Liver enzyme test
SFM	State Fire Marshal (U.S.)
SITE	Superfund Innovative Technology Evaluation (U.S.)
SOT	Society of Toxicology (U.S.)
STEL	Short-term exposure limit (ACGIH) (U.S.)
TLV	Threshold limit value (ACGIGH) (U.S.)
TSCA	Toxic Substance Control Act, P.L. 94-469 (U.S.)
TTDU	Transportable thermal destruction treatment unit
TWA	Time-weighted average (ACGIH) (U.S.)
UFFI	Urea formaldehyde foam insulation
U.L.	Underwriters Laboratories (a testing and listing organization) (U.S.)
VOC	Volatile organic compounds

Hazardous and Toxic Materials

Second Edition

1

The ABCs of Chemical Safety

Howard H. Fawcett

Erik Howard Fawcett, age 30 months, is busily engaged in many activities, but few are as important as learning what keys on the computer correspond to certain letters of the alphabet. As we watch this "learning" process, we recognize that this is only the beginning of a lifetime search for deeper meanings.

Erik's experiences have an analogy in our learning about chemicals and chemically related materials. No one letter of the alphabet can be a sentence; it takes a combination of letters to produce understanding. In chemical health and safety, if we are truly to have a concept of the need for control and management of chemicals, we must know more than one or two "constants"—our view must be much broader, and excursions into areas of knowledge foreign to our previous training and interest must be explored. A few of these will be outlined below. For details, consult other sections of this or related texts, printouts, or even the daily news media—print and TV.

A is for *awareness*. Unlike the ostrich, we cannot afford to put our heads in the sands of know-it-all land. We must be willing to learn, and to accept new knowledge and information as it becomes available. No matter how extensive our training is in a specialized area of chemistry, engineering, physics, or biology, new information is continually appearing in journals and reports that should be added to our stockpile of wisdom. For many chemicals, this knowledge has arrived surrounded by media sensationalism—such as the mercury poisonings reports from Japan, which led to a greater awareness of mercury poisoning; the asbestos issue, which was first known and publicized in London in 1899 but deliberately ignored in large measure until the 1960s; and ammonium nitrate's explosive potential, adequately demonstrated at Oppau, Germany, in 1923 but reconfirmed with the loss of hundreds of lives and millions of dollars worth of damage at Texas City in 1947. More recently of course, were the Bhopal, India, tragedy that resulted when the accidental release of a known toxic material caused the 1747 deaths and many

1

thousands of injuries, and the Chernobyl nuclear power plant incident, where a chemical explosion tore apart containment, resulting in a release of radioactive material that caused serious contamination over thousands of miles. The Hazard Communication Rule of the U.S. Occupational Safety and Health Agency (OSHA), which became effective May 25, 1986 (see 29 CFR Part 1910.1200), with its requirement for precautionary labeling and availability of material safety data sheets (MSDSs), if properly implemented may be helpful in creating awareness, but the knowledge base on which the MSDSs are prepared is not always complete or accurate. In any event, we must keep our minds open to new knowledge, from whatever the source and whether or not it is in our personal interest, for truth ultimately will prevail.

B suggests *biological effects*. The effects of chemicals on living organisms are highly variable, depending in large measure on the exposure level, duration of exposure, and ability of the "host" to tolerate or eliminate the substances. This introduces the concept of toxicity (too much, too fast) and brings us to the reality of both acute (short-term) and chronic (long-term) effects. Some exposures, such as low-level exposure to carbon monoxide in a bus or automobile, for example, are reversible if fresh clean air is available to neutralize the carboxymethhemoglobin. On the other hand, some chemicals, such as benzene, asbestos, carbon tetrachloride, and vinyl chloride monomer (to cite only a few from the known list of chemicals with subtle effects that surface only months or years after exposure), apparently linger in the body and become a problem long afterward. For details, see Chapters 7–9 on toxicity and references cited on toxicity, carcinogenicity, teratogenicity, and mutagenicity. Such considerations are no longer debatable; ample scientific evidence is now available to give serious pause to anyone handling, using, or disposing of chemicals or mixtures.

C suggests *chemical reactions*. Many reactions are relatively simple and safe, such as the titration of a dilute acid with a dilute alkali, but many about which we know (and undoubtledly thousands about which we have limited information) are capable of either highly exothermic action, or run-a-way. Precautions that have been developed for safe operation should be carefully adhered to; it is never wise to push conditions, such as temperature, concentrations, or reaction times, beyond the limits imposed by the original work on the reaction. Even relatively common household chemicals can produce unfortunate results; the instability of calcium hypochlorite (widely used in water treatment, as in swimming pools), when challanged by a variety of substances, including acids, cigarettes, and nitromethane, either will ignite or evolve highly irritating or toxic gases, such as chlorine and dichlorine monoxide. Before undertaking a reaction with which one is not completely familiar, a search of the literature, combined with a check in National Fire Protection 491-M (Hazardous Chemical Reactions) and the *Handbook of Reactive Chemical Hazards* (fourth edition, by Leslie Bretherick, Butterworth, 1985) is clearly preferable to rediscovering hazardous chemical reactions.

D reminds us of *disposal*. The day when every chemical or waste could be flushed down the drain has long passed, even for relatively small amounts of materials. If the present drive toward "cradle-to-grave" control and management of chemicals is to continue and be successful, as much thought has to be given to chemicals before they are ordered and used as to after this occurs. Although so-called small-scale generators may be exempt from many provisions of the U.S. Environmental Protection Agency (EPA) hazardous-waste-management systems, that hardly gives permission for anyone to be careless with chemicals. Even a few grams of a pesticide or herbicide used in home gardening when being disposed of in a public waste collection can cause injury to the personnel handling the disposal. We must learn to think *disposal,* just as we have learned to appreciate the *benefits* of chemicals.

E reminds us of *energy.* In the true sense, chemicals represent energy, and hence respond to both its input and withdrawal. The fire triangle—in which a flammable material in the proper state of vaporization or dust, in air or some other oxidizer (such as oxygen, chlorine, fluorine, bromine, or iodine, or compounds containing these, such as $KClO_3$ or $NaClO_4$)—may be perfectly stable until a source of ignition (usually a spark or electrical discharge) sets the material into action, resulting in either a fire or an explosion, depending on the conditions and concentrations. One more element is needed to sustain a fire, namely, sufficient heat transfer to ensure that the reaction will continue as a chain. It is interesting that we tend to discuss toxicity alone without noting that most chemicals, especially gases and liquids, are *both toxic and flammable or combustible* to some degree. To ensure that at least some ignition sources will not ignite materials, the National Electrical Code provides for classification of various degrees of explosionproof equipment, so designed and built that any internal pressure will not be transmitted to the outside. Electric refrigerators, telephones, lighting, portable radios, and other devices that might produce a spark are thus made "intrinsically safe" so that they will not be an ignition source, even in a potentially flammable or explosive atmosphere.

In recent times, much discussion has ensued as to the relative hazard created by certain building and home materials of plastic origin, where fires may decompose or pyrolyze them. A recent publication of a committee of the National Research Council (NRC), *Fire & Smoke* (National Academy Press, 1986), concluded that our present knowledge of test methods is incomplete, and that, although burning plastics, pesticides, and other substances may be a problem, especially to fire and police personnel and the occupants of homes, it is still too early to legislate definite regulations or test procedures. Fire personnel have become very conscious of the problems in recent years: in Long Beach Calif., the department faced a potential hazardous materials incident when a fire in a storage building set 14 different kinds of toxic chemicals ablaze (see *American Fire Journal,* pp. 32–35, Feb. 1986) and fire fighters in Westbrook, Maine, let a town store burn to the ground because it contained 7756 pounds plus 670 gallons of pesticides and herbicides. The fire was considered too hazardous for control or extinguishment (see *Fire Command,* pp. 40–42, Oct. 1985). It is now recognized that a well-trained response team on site to make the initial survey of the problem, and, if possible, to control or contain the fire, is very useful, and this is especially valuable during night and off-days emergencies. The local fire department must be aware of the type of property, and know where updated factual information can be obtained, preferably even before arrival on the scene. Publications of the National Fire Protection Association (NFPA) and fire insurance companies, as well as state and local departments, should be consulted for details.

F reminds us of *fire,* humankind's friend and enemy.

As noted under "**E**", fires do not just happen; they are the result of a combination of forces and circumstances, any one of which can be controlled with significant results. Most chemicals either burn or decompose in a fire; even relatively "fire-proof" materials such as iron can burn, if in the proper physical state. In the real world, most fires result from a failure to recognize that certain fundamentals must be observed. For example, on November 1, 1985, at a large plant in New York State, a chemist on the midnight-to-8 A.M. shift was transferring a known flammable liquid from one container to another. Although both company and OSHA regulations require that the two metal containers be grounded to each other and the chemist wear protective clothing and face protection, this was not done. The resulting flash fire burned the man seriously enough that he died a few days later. The company was fined $650 each on two counts—failure to bond and failure to require the chemist to wear adequate protection; however, the second fine was appealed. Failure of the human element is not an uncommon component of accidents, especially at 3 A.M.

A 10-minute video tape highlighting the analogy between Erik's quest for knowledge and the ABCs of chemical safety was presented at the Denver spring meeting of the American Chemical Society, April 7, 1987, by Fawcett Consultations, P.O. Box 9444, Wheaton, MD 20906.

2
Cliches

Howard H. Fawcett

Every human activity, including chemistry and chemical control and their corresponding management, has its background of experiences, which through the years have been reduced and oversimplified into generalizations. This is frequently referred to as "building on experience," and constitutes a learning experience of great value if properly utilized. However, half-truths and incomplete ideas are sometimes venerated in the process, without scientific justification. Time-honored phrases creep into conversations as accepted and ironclad truths, often producing a serious negative effect on progressive informed enlightened thinking. For example, consider the following.

SAFETY FIRST

This supposedly inspiring slogan was first adopted by a major steel company over 70 years ago, and had a specific meaning at that time. The phrase was widely publicized, and was helpful to the then-infant safety movement (the National Safety Council was organized by electrical engineers in 1912). Unfortunately, *safety never was and never will be the first consideration in any entreprenurial operation* (be it academic, commercial, or legal); the operation or activity is the important *first*, and all other factors are secondary. This fact does not degrade safety—it simply places safety and health management where they rightfully belong as essential aids to those who are performing the actual operations. One company rephrased the slogan to "Production with Safety," which gave due credit to the necessary role that safety and health play in any operation, since it involves the essential human/operational interface.

The phrase "Safety first" has caused considerable fundamental misunderstanding and distrust of what sincere and dedicated safety and health professionals are trying to achieve, and probably has set the safety and health movement back rather than advanced it, due to a misunderstanding of its motive and its value to the operations. The prime focus will always be on the production or maintenance of a product line or a service that can be sold at a profit. Thus, economics is really first, but this does not imply that safety and health (especially in the control of chemical exposures and ultimate disposal) does not have a very vital and important input. To ignore that input is to court economic, as well as legal and public relations, disaster, especially in today's world.

THE UNIONS WILL NOT GO ALONG WITH MANAGEMENT IN THIS

When this phrase surfaces in a conversation, examine the operation carefully, as well as the union and its officers. Often you will find a serious misunderstanding based on incomplete communications—the old "them-versus-us" dialog. Safety and health are far too important for misunderstanding to be encouraged. Actually all responsible union leaders are deeply concerned about the safety and health of their members. This is especially true of the two unions that represent the majority of oil, chemical, and atomic energy workers, as well as the American Management Association, which fully understands that good health and safety contribute to good management and favorable economics.

ALL ACCIDENTS ARE PREVENTABLE

Academically this may be a true, but abstract, statement; in reality, it is false for the real world and for real people doing real jobs. Each of us brings many variables into the equation of human activity—that, in reality, it is not actually 100 percent possible either to predict or to prevent all injuries. This does not minimize the fact that most accidents can be prevented, if we are willing to apply the knowledge, the techniques, and the training at all levels, from top management down to the workers. However, until the concept of perfection in safety and health (which we have yet to achieve in any other activity involving humans interacting with systems or organizations) is achieved, it will not be possible to prevent or completely control all possible situations as the variables and combinations are overwhelming.

The data bases on many chemicals are far from complete; in spite of the OSHA Hazard Communication Rule requiring informational labels and MSDS, many of the seven million chemicals listed by *Chemical Abstract'*, in addition to the thousands of mixtures in daily commerce, have not been studied for their effects on humans or the environment. Therefore, we must be realistic, and prepare for all possible contingencies, whose consequences we can *reduce* with proper emergency planning.

MOST ACCIDENTS ARE DUE TO CARELESSNESS

This widely quoted phrase is true or false, depending on how one defines "carelessness." If we mean that the whole accident-prevention system, from top management through the environment to the human factor, has been less than successful, and hence complete, it is probably true. Unfortunately, as usually applied, it is intended to pass judgment on a specific act or on persons performing an act. As Trevor A. Kletz, writing in *What Went Wrong?* (Gulf Publishing Co., Houston and London, 1985), notes, although the accidents of the past made vivid impressions at the time and usually set in motion a series of actions to prevent a recurrence, the fact is that people leave or retire from a company, and the newer, less experienced personnel feel that it could not happen again. In fact, however, it often does. People will do (1) what they have to do, or (2) what they are told to do, or (3) what they feel like doing at the time. If this complex system of human variables includes ignorance, indifference, incompetence, misunderstanding, rebellion, emotional instability, or hostility at any particular instant, the results can be less than desired. This is especially true of people who work on rotating shifts: the *internal* human clock is not calibrated to the clock on the wall, especially during the midnight-to-8 A.M. shift. In spite of all this, most accidents (perhaps more than 90 percent) can be prevented or controlled, *if* we are willing to apply knowledge, understanding, proper procedures, and training at all levels. In this world of several hundred languages and dialects, not every person can comprehend completely the full and complete meaning of words, whether oral or written. In the United States alone, over 20 million persons are classified as "functionally illiterate," suggesting that our training and education systems at all levels, through that of Ph.D., M.D., and LL.D, is less than adequate to meet today's needs. However, until the goal of perfection in safety and health is achieved, a goal that has escaped our grasp in other phases of human activities, we should realize that, while accidents can be controlled or prevented, they cannot be completely repealed from the human scene. In the meantime, contingency plans must be in place and operational.

WE HAVE POLICY AND HAVE ALWAYS DONE IT THIS WAY

In a era of rapid and fundamental changes in the social, technical, and business world, the policy may well be out of date, unless it has been carefully and intelligently reviewed very recently. Old policies may well be a deterrent to realistic modern accident prevention. Policies are guides to be used and applied with understanding and intelligence; they are never an inflexible rule abstracted from the infinite wisdom.

THE FOREMAN IS RESPONSIBLE FOR SAFETY

While the foreman, like any other front-line director or leader, is close to the point where safety and health (or the lack of them) become most obvious, this phrase is a residue from days when the job description of a foreman was far different than it is today. As a part of the management team, he or she should be directly involved in and responsible for all the common objectives of the operations. To single him or her out solely as responsible for safety and health is a gross oversimplification that is unrealistic. Likewise, unless "interest" and "responsibility" (real or imagined) are backed up by other staff members and management, so that the unsafe acts, practices, and equipment he or she reports that need attention beyond his or her time and talents to perform, are promptly considered, the foreman's interest in safety and health will tend to become "lip service," and hence less than effective.

IF WE LISTENED TO OUR MEDICAL STAFF, OUR SAFETY RECORD WOULD REALLY BE POOR

In theory, the accident-prevention personnel (safety, fire prevention, industrial hygiene, health physics, and the medical staff) should share the same objectives and approaches. The goal should be to achieve a high level of on-the-job effectiveness. In fact, safety and medical personnel occasionally work at cross-purposes. The occupational health nurse is often in the middle of the cross-fire. To expect the nurse to be completely neutral or objective is to overlook the basic orientation of his or her prime concern for human life. In many cases, the safety engineer is too preoccupied with his or her "safety record," statistics on the number of accidents and lost-time days complicated by compensation or insurance costs, to realize that the medical staff, while more directly involved in the personal aspect, is also dedicated to keeping people well, free from common ills as well as occupational disease, and restoring them to their normal, productive work as soon as possible. Part-time or guided work should be kept at an absolute minimum since it tends to be degrading. Until this gulf of mistrust and misunderstanding is bridged, and both medical and safety staff personnel respect their true mutual objectives, the safety effort will continue to be less than effective. It might be noted that 25 percent of occupational health nurses also do the "safety" work in their operations. (See "Credibility Gap: Some Concerns Fudge Their Safety Records to Cut Insurance Costs," *Wall Street Journal,* pp. 1, 28, Dec. 2, 1986.)

WE HAVE DONE THIS OPERATION A THOUSAND TIMES AND IT NEVER WENT BAD BEFORE

While this phrase may be true in the particular context used, it indicates a complete lack of understanding of the probability of an accident and the variables that create them. It is possible to observe unsafe acts and sloppy operations that do not result in injury, which might have been fatal if even a very minor change had taken place. For instance, a 4-foot by 10-foot metal fragment from a steel tank car, $5/8$ inch thick and weighing nearly half a ton, traveled almost three-quarters of a mile and landed 6 feet from the front porch of an occupied house, and still had sufficient energy to sever a gas pipe 3 feet underground. No injuries resulted. However, minor changes in the trajectory could have caused a crash landing on the house, with possibly fatal results. System safety analysis, which has evolved from the analysis of highly complex systems such as aircraft, space vehicles, and oceanographic devices and their missions, encourages a detailed piece-by-piece analysis of the system, and then assignment of some overall safety and reliability standards. For example, see W. H. Hallenbeck and K. M. Cunningham, *Quantitative Risk Assessment for Environmental and Occupational Health* (Lewis Publishers, Chelsea, Mich., 1986.)

SELF-PRESERVATION IS THE FIRST LAW OF NATURE: OUR PEOPLE DO NOT WANT TO GET HURT OR KILLED

As the causes of unaccountable accidents and suicides become more clearly defined, the pattern emerges that at least some accidents and deaths have a high component of self-inflicted pain or the urge to "end it all in a moment of glory," no matter how unpleasant this thought may be. In fact, self-preservation is quite far down on the list of motivations as human beings will tolerate almost impossible situations and conditions if they see no alternative; it is only when hopelessness overpowers that the easy way out is taken.

I WEAR CONTACT LENSES: THEY PROTECT MY EYES

Contact lenses are *not* eye protectors—dusts or liquids from splashes or other conditions in close contact with the eye are a serious potential hazard where chemical irritants or chemicals dangerous to the eye are handled. Severe injuries have resulted from the inability of the worker or nurse to remove the contact lens quickly for a flushing with water and other treatment. Metal-working operations, where grinding, chipping, and other particle-producing tasks are involved, also constitute a serious hazard due to the possibility of particles lodging under the contact lens. Quality eye protective devices, recommended by the American National Standards Institute (ANSI) and endorsed by OSHA for the exposures involved, should always be used in the laboratory or at the work station, and contact lenses preferably left at home. Prescription safety glasses, goggles, or other approved safety shield or protector should be worn.

Cliches and time-worn phrases, often with misleading or false implications, have no place in a vigorous chemical health and safety effort. Most (even if not all) accidents can be prevented, or their effects minimized, if we apply existing knowledge, and admit to our human condition.

3

Effective Presentation: The Key to Successful Hazard Communication

Howard H. Fawcett

As a result of the recent OSHA Hazard Communication regulation, in addition to the requirements of PL 99-499 that communities and the public, upon request, must be properly informed as to the identity and potential hazards of chemicals and other hazardous materials in plants and laboratories, the old axioms "tell them anything" and "don't tell them it is dangerous" no longer will be accepted, either by society or by the courts. Stiff fines are possible if the revelations are not complete and truthful.

Although others, including the American Chemical Society (ACS), the American Institute of Chemical Engineers (AIChE), the National Safety Council (NSC), the National Fire Protection Association (NFPA), the Health Physics Society (HPS), the American Institute of Chemists (AIC), have taken actions in this direction, this chapter will stress the human considerations we feel are essential for a truly effective and satisfactory hazard-communication program.

The true objective of any such program is not merely legal or moral, but is to bridge the gap between two minds: that of the "teacher" and that of the "student" or listener. The mechanisms such as warning labels, MSDSs, and informational meetings, either with employees or public groups, are only means to an end— namely, the effective transport of that knowledge, similar to a journey across a bridge over the river of ignorance or incomplete information to a safe arrival on the shore of knowledge, and hence safer conduct.

As Henri Poincaré noted: "A collection of facts is no more a science than a heap of stones is a house." A carefully planned education program is essential if the spirit, as well as the legal and moral aspects, of hazard communication is to be achieved. The "stones" of information must be properly prepared and presented. The reaction of the student, immediately and over the long haul, is the only criterion as to whether or not *communication* has actually occurred, and has been accepted by the student. Words and slides, or even videos, are not adequate by themselves.

Chemical hazard control, or chemical health and safety, is not usually a subject of overriding concern to most persons, even to those who handle and dispose of hazardous substances. The cliches "no dirt, no work, no paycheck," heard often in the past, especially in "smokestack industry," and "it smells, but so what, we have a job" near chemical, petrochemical, or pulp and paper mills, are still in the backs of many minds. A recent survey of salaried employees suggests that the most important work-related information for them concerns benefits, pay, the future of the company and their role in it, how to improve work performance, and how the employee's work fits into the total picture, in that order. Safety, health, and environmental concerns on the job were not mentioned as important. However, another recent opinion poll suggests that, at least in research and development laboratories, the safety and health picture is of considerable gravity. In this context, it may be noted that today not all personnel are overly enthusiastic about loyalty to their jobs or to the company. To add concerns about hazards, without telling them why or what is in it for them may not be wise at this time.

We realize that we are surrounded by hazards, some of which we cannot control personally. The recent survey showing that one in four tractor-trailers on the highways were found to be "rigged" for "disaster" hardly speaks well for our daily movements, especially when many of these trucks contain hazardous materials. The smoking issue is one that also deserves much attention, but at least we have a personal choice in this matter.

We live at a certain rhythm in time, at a certain level of size, time, and space; beyond certain limits, events in the outer (real) world (including health and safety) are not directly appreciable by the ordinary channels of sense, although a symbolic picture of them may be presented to us by the intellect. Therefore, to communicate effectively, we must break through that "out-of-this-world" layer and stress the reality, even though to the purist it may be a painful and unrealistic idea.

To achieve that symbolic picture in the context of hazard communication, we suggest the use of four "As."

ATTENTION

Every student, as noted above, has many thoughts on his or her mind, which may partially or totally block out a hazard warning. Chemists, engineers, and even physicians have been trained to recognize that chemicals are building blocks to life itself, as well as to our culture. Unless we can appeal to the "student" on a bsis of personal or financial relevance, or perhaps company loyalty ("unless it is good for the company, I'm against it" syndrome), perhaps some simple demonstrations should be included as part of the presentation in order to gain attention.

If flammability is of interest, fill a flint lighter with a typical flammable liquid and demonstrate how a simple spark can ignite the material. This is an introduction to the whole subject of flammables and combustibles and their control.

If reactivity is of interest, a few drops of acetone (such as nail polish remover) or methyl ethyl ketone on a small quanity of anhydrous chromium trioxide will attract attention.

If toxicity is the issue, exposure of one or two animals (small white mice are ideal, and are usually available in any biology department) in a large glass dessicator or glass cake holder, using a few drops of a common substance from the plant or laboratory (such as benzene or carbon tetrachloride, on filter paper), will usually be effective in demonstrating the acute effects of common chemicals as the animals change their behavior.

If dust hazards are at issue, a few grams of the plant dust from a filter or dust collector placed in a nylon hose and shaken over a candle will suggest the concerns for dusty atmospheres. If available, a "dust explosion gallery" developed by the U.S. Bureau of Mines may be useful.

To increase awareness of odors, prepare in advance filter papers with a drop of the material in question, seal the papers in envelops, and distribute them to with appropriate remarks as to the utility and limitations of odors in hazard control. Some utility companies, including the Washington (D.C.) Gas and Light Company, include such cards with their mailings to make their customers aware of the odor of mercaptans used to safeguard against undetected leaks in the distribution of natural gas.

The teacher should take care in all such demonstrations, using as little material as possible, and carefully explaining to the students what is being done and why.

If demonstrations are not practical, consider a short video or movie, slides, or posters, and invite the highest-level manager or professor available to the presentation; the presence of a higher authority always increases interest and adds credibility to the session. The teacher should encourage questions; if answers are not immediately available, the questions should be written down and the student should be sent a written response within a reasonable length of time.

ADVANTAGES

Companies and academic institutions take action when a favorable cost/benefit ratio or risk assessment has been demonstrated and the legal or moral responsibility is high. Safety education, long considered an expendable overhead, is slowly being recognized as an effective loss-prevention tool, as well as a legal requirement. The favorable public image that such education creates for the company or laboratory cannot be evaluated in dollars, but is very real. Chemists and engineers can be motivated if they realize that health and safety knowledge, in practice, gives assurance that no excessive exposures or personal contacts with hazardous materials or substances have disrupted the day's work, and that the use of proper practices and protective measures and equipment increases or ensures productivity. Even "No Smoking" signs, increasingly common in offices, laboratories, plants, and public places, are an important protective device whose effect may be highly significant, as well as legally important. The increased use of the NFPA 704-M hazard marking system, along with the now-recognized radiation-hazard symbol, is more important than ever as a method of informing both employees and the public of potential hazards. Even a small fire or explosion may produce significant loss, and perhaps long-lasting contamination, such as the combustion/pyrolysis of polychlorinated biphenyl (PCBs) to produce dioxin (see Chapter 10). All PCB-containing electrical devices must be phased out of buildings by 1990.

While a few chemists and engineers continue to demonstrate little or no sensitivity concerning their moral responsibility, most have a reasonable or high sense of their stewardship. Health and safety knowledge may be an important adjunct to technical information and other data, as well as a legal asset highly useful in tort suits involving personal liability.

ACTIVATION

By reducing hazard information to simple statements, and by presenting it in clear, understandable language or by other modes (including demonstrations, videos, movies, slides, or even a computer screen), the message is more likely to be favorably received. The use of graphs to present flammable limits and the occasional introduction of humor in the form of cartoons are desirable to hold the audience's attention. If the "rules" can be reduced to easy-to-use form, such as the safety index used by Virginia public schools, the National Institutes of Health (NIH) guide to hazardous-waste disposal, or, as noted, the NFPA 704-M system, the more likely it is that the information will be actually used.

While English is specified in the United States and England as the appropriate language for hazard communication, a significant number of persons in both countries today do not relate to English as their native tongue. In addition, more Americans have limited education than we like to admit, and those who are functionally illiterate cannot be expected to grasp the meaning of highly technical or relatively uncommon words. As noted in Chapter 5, to expect a Polish immigrant with little knowledge of English to work with cyanide solutions and be provided with minimal or no instructions as to precautions is hardly to be commended on a cost/benefit basis. The simpler and more effective the labels, MSDSs, and instructions for processes and practices, the more likely it is that they will be received and observed. The use of international signs and warnings should be considered, even if not legally required at this time.

ACTION

To test the student's reaction, a short quiz or test may be useful. This test should relate to the real world in which the student will work. For example: "What steps do you take if 10 percent hydrofluoric acid is spilled on your hand or in your eyes?" "Why are 'No Smoking' signs posted in the receiving area?" "What action do you take if you suddenly become conscious of a strange odor?" "In case someone shouts 'fire,' what do *you* personally do?"

We must admit that our knowledge of hazards is incomplete, and that eternal vigilance is a requisite to chemical health and safety. In evaluating our hazard-control program, perhaps the rating scheme should include the three elements of the popular television program, PUTTIN' ON THE HITS: *originality* (are we as innovative in hazard control as we are in finding better and more effective ways or procedures to produce?); *appearance* (proper protection, procedures, and good housekeeping even when superiors and visitors are not present); and *lip synch* (can we easily recite the hazards and their controls—as well as transform them into real hazard control?). If so, "Puttin' on the Chemical Safety Hits" may be the outstanding program of the year, and will receive high ratings in terms of human conservation and economic and legal input.

SUGGESTED READINGS

29 CFR 1910.1200, "Hazard Communcation: OSHA Instruction CPL 2-2," Aug. 5, 1985, Office of Health Compliance Assistance, U.S. Department of Labor.

PL 99-499, Oct. 17, 1986, "Superfund Amendments and Reauthorization Act of 1986" (note especially "Title III—Emergency Planning and Community Right-to-Know").

Federal Register, Friday Dec. 19, 1986, 29 CFR Part 1910, "Hazardous Waste Operation and Emergency Response; Interim Final Rule," OSHA.

"Chemical Emergency Preparedness Program, Interim Guidance," 9223.0-1A U.S. Environmental Protection Agency, Washington, D.C. 20460 (Nov. 1986).

Rae Tyson, "1 in 4 Tractor-Trailers Rigged for Disaster," *USA Today,* March 24, 1987, pp. 1A, 6A

4

Emergency Planning and Community Right-to-Know

Howard H. Fawcett

Emergency planning for responding to chemical and other emergencies involving hazardous materials has long been a goal of everyone who has studied without bias the human/chemical/environmental interface. Planning has been achieved to some degree by communities and companies, but not until the passage of PL 99-499, and its signing by President Reagan on October 17, 1986, was it recognized as a national objective.

Title III of the PL 99-499 specifically directs itself to this goal, and attempts to bring about a closer understanding among the companies, transporters, users, and the community, down to the citizen level. (Titles I and II of this Act are oriented to the provisions relating primarily to response and liability involving the waste sites designated as national priority and to the cleanup of leaking underground storage tanks, while Title IV deals with radon gas and indoor-air-quality research.)

Since the Title III laws will more directly affect chemists, engineers, and executives of organizations that manufacture, handle, transport, or dispose of hazardous chemicals on a daily basis, its effect is of most direct interest to day-by-day operating personnel, and to the emergency personnel who must respond to chemical spills, fires, explosions, and other incidents.

The law attempts to organize and coordinate on a state-by-state basis the planning necessary to assist emergency services in order to respond to community needs more adequately and more intelligently. Undoubtedly, the Bhopal, India, tragedy, followed by the Chernobyl nuclear accident, the Institute W. Va., release of toxic materials (in spite of considerable attention to the problem), and the Miamisburg, Ohio, train derailment, which necessitated the evacuation of 32,000 people to escape the fumes of white phosphorous from a burning tank car, all contributed to

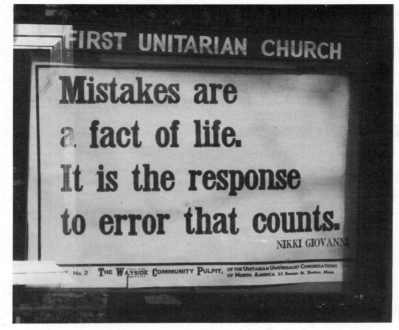

Figure 4.1

making Congress aware of the problem. To illustrate that the problem of emergency response is both real and timely, a United Press report to the *Washington Post* (March 29, 1987, page A11) describes how a fire fighter suffered a fatal heart attack and 33 others suffered injuries at a warehouse fire in Miami, when water (still the only extinguishing agent the fire services have in abundant amounts) reacted violently with chlorosulfonic acid, producing a large mushroom cloud as they fought the blaze by directing streams of water into the building. Had the responders been informed of the potential for this reaction, they would have been more alert to the danger involved.

Under the new law, state commissions were appointed by each state governor by April 17, 1987, to be called "emergency response commissions." The law provides that each governor may designate as the state commission one or more existing emergency response organizations that are state sponsored or appointed. The governor shall, to the extent practicable, appoint persons to the commission who have technical expertise in the emergency response field. The state commission will then appoint local emergency planning committees, and will supervise and coordinate the activities of such committees. The state commission will establish proceedings for receiving and processing requests from the public for information on chemicals and related materials. Local emergency planning committees were appointed by July 19, 1987, for each of a state's district.

Each local committee will have, as a minimum, representatives from each of the

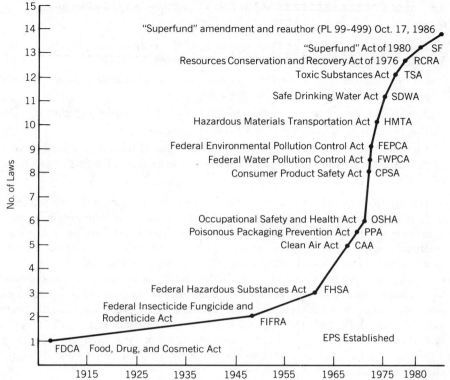

Figure 4.2. Chronology of major federal laws concerning chemicals.

following: elected state and local officials; law enforcement, civil defense, fire fighting, first aid, health, local environmental, and community groups; and owners and operators of facilities subject to the requirements of the subtitle. The committee will appoint a chairperson and will establish rules by which the committee will function. Such rules shall include provisions for a public notification plan, public comments, response to such comments by the committee, and distribution of the emergency plan. The local emergency planning committee will establish procedures for receiving and processing requests from the public for information under section 324, including tier II information under section 312. Section 324 indicates that each emergency response plan described in section 311(a)(2) and requiring, under OSHA, an MSDS (material safety data sheet), the chemical name or common name of each chemical, and any hazardous component (except if classified information or trade secrets exclusion can be justified as provided under the law in section 322) shall be made available to the public. Tier II information, referred to above, relates to an inventory form that provides the following additional information for each hazardous chemical present at the facility, but only upon request and in accordance with subsection (e) (available to state commissions, local committees, fire departments, other state and local officials, and any person who formally requests it):

The chemical name or the common name of the chemical as provided on the MSDS;

An estimate (in ranges) of the maximum amount of the hazardous chemical present at the facility during the preceding year;

A brief description of the manner of storage of the hazardous chemical;

The location at the facility of the hazardous chemical;

An indication of whether the owner elects to withhold from disclosure information as to the location of a specific hazardous chemical as classified or as a trade secret.

Tier II information should be available to state commissions, local committees, and fire departments on request, and, on request, to the state commission or local emergency planning committee, to local officials. Tier II information that a state emergency response commission or local committee has in its possession shall be made available to a person making a request under section 324. If the state or local committee does not have such information, it can ask the facility owner or operator for the information with respect to a hazardous chemical a facility has stored in an amount in excess of 10,000 pounds at any time during the preceding calendar year, and make such information available to the person making the request, according to section 324. A state emergency response commission or local emergency planning committee shall respond to a request for tier II information no later than 45 days after the date of receipt of the request.

Upon request to an owner or operator of a facility that files an inventory form by the fire department with jurisdiction over the facility, the owner or operator of the facility shall allow the fire department to conduct an on-site inspection of the facility and shall provide to the fire department specific location information on hazardous chemicals at the facility.

The law defines in some detail the toxic substances subject to the reporting by owners and operators of facilities that have 10 or more full-time employees and that are in Standard Industrial Classification Codes 20–39 (as in effect on July 1, 1985) and that manufactured, processed, or otherwise used a toxic chemical listed as follows:

Chemicals on the list in Committee Print Number 99–169 of the Senate Committee on Environment and Public Works, titled "Toxic Chemicals Subject to Section 313 of the Emergency Planning and Community Right-to-Know Act of 1986" plus any chemical the Administrator may add (or delete) if there is sufficient evidence to establish:

(A) The chemical is known to cause or can reasonably be anticipated to cause significant adverse acute human health effects at concentration levels that are reasonably likely to exist beyond facility site boundaries as a result of continuous, or frequently recurring, release;

(B) The chemical is known to cause or can reasonably anticipated to cause in humans—

      (i)   cancer or teratogenic effects, or
      (ii) serious or irreversible—
           (I)   Reproductive dysfunctions,
           (II)   neurological disorders,
           (III)   heritable genetic mutations, or
           (IV)   other chronic health effects.
(C) The chemical is known to cause or can reasonably be anticipated to cause, because of—
      (i)   its toxicity,
      (ii) its toxicity and persistence in the environment,
      (iii) its toxicity and tendency to bioaccumulation in the environment,
      a significant adverse effect on the environment of sufficient seriousness, in the judgment of the Administrator, to warrant reporting. The number of chemicals on the list described above may constitute in the aggregate no more than 25 percent of the total number of chemicals on the list.

The Administrator is also enpowered to delete a chemical if he or she determines there is not sufficient evidence to establish any of the criteria described above.

A uniform toxic chemical release form for facilities covered by the law was to have been published no later than June 1, 1987; if the form was not published, the owners and operators of facilities were to provide the information required by June 1, 1987, by mail, as outlined in the law.

As with any law or regulation, the implementation of Title II, which is intended to protect the public from releases or other deviations into the public sector of chemicals deemed hazardous to health or the environment, will be no more effective than the sincerity and dedication of the personnel who are appointed, as well as the degree of cooperation with the owners and operators of facilities that handle, process, transport, or dispose of such substances. Reliance on lists of chemicals, which may or may not contain materials with unusual properties that make them subject to the listings but are of little real hazard, as well as the MSDSs required under OSHA (data sheets that are known to be less than accurate and complete, and may be misleading in some cases), is probably the only route available under the American system. Apparently the United States did not consider the approach the Health and Safety Executive of England would have used to attact the problem of chemical releases by requiring the owners and operators to develop a truly local comprehensive plan based on the specific information the facility certainly has on hand, and to place the responsibility on the facility rather than on state commissions or local committees.

One could also be concerned about how the state and local groups are to digest and codify the large volume of reports, inventories, and other details without a large expenditure (always a major concern) for competent staff members who have a working knowledge of the chemicals involved and can spot errors of commission and omission in the paperwork. Even if the information is computerized, the problem of selecting the proper key words for retrieval in emergency situations is real, unless full-time, 24-hour staff members are available, as with the CHEM-TREC and HIT programs of the Chemical Manufacturers Association (CMA).

The fire services, which are really the instrument of on-scene movement of the emergency response, are still, with few exceptions, inadequately trained in chemical emergencies. No mention is made in PL 99-499 of the necessity for posting areas or buildings with updated information, such as with the NFPA 704-M marking system, to give on-scene warnings of flammability, health hazards, and chemical reactivity, as well as water compatibility or incompatibility, and other unusual conditions that may be encountered, such as radiation or infectious-disease agents. Exactly how the police and other personnel should be coordinated with the fire services in this context is not clear. Really extensive and thorough training and orientation are needed to bring industry, academic, and governmental resources into play in the national interest.

One specific example of emergency planning that is operational and includes much of the basic elements discussed is the NIH Division of Safety Chemical Emergency Response Plan, dated April 1985, by Richard E. Shaff of the NIH in Bethesda, Md. This facility covers a large area, with many buildings and literally hundreds of laboratories concerned with studies of diseases and related aspects of knowledge dedicated to public health. In these buildings literally thousands of chemicals are used by the large staff in various ways.

The NIH Chemical Emergency Response Team (CERT) is a specialized team of knowledgeable and experienced personnel, trained and equipped to manage all types of chemical emergencies. The CERT is *not* a first-response entity; rather the team is summoned only after an initial evaluation has been made and it has been determined that additional specialized assistance is required. Nonhazardous situations are handled through normal operating procedures. The CERT may be requested by the NIH fire department or the on-site coordinator (in the case of fires, explosions, or hazardous-chemical spills) or the Environmental Protection Branch, subsequent to notification by the Chemical Waste Disposal Contract, in matters regarding the removal of reactive chemicals from the workplace. The CERT mission does not usurp the responsibility of the fire department officer-in-charge in the management of the emergency scene. For the removal of potentially reactive chemicals, the CERT, once notified, is responsible for the removal and transportation of the material to a safe location. The CERT does not, in any way, interfere with the authority of the project officer over the Chemical Waste Disposal Contract.

The Chemical Emergency Response Team performs the following services:

1. Provides advice, guidance, and other assistance, as necessary, to the fire department and all other responding personnel in the assessment, containment, and cleanup of chemical spills in incidents in which additional technical assistance is required.

2. Responds, under the provision of the ORS (Office of Research Service) Emergency Response Plan (Code Safety), to the scenes of fires and/or explosions where chemicals may be present; to assess the chemical and toxicological hazards, recommend control procedures and personal protective equipment requirements to the fire department and others (e.g., maintenance, housekeeping security personnel, BID [Bureau Institute Division] managent, etc.), and provide guidance and direction in the decontamination of personnel and facilities.

3. Evaluates potentially explosive or otherwise reactive chemicals to determine by what method, and when and by whom, these chemicals may be safely removed from the facility; the necessity for area/building evacuation; and protective equipment requirements for personnel involved in the removal. The CERT may elect to utilize existing contract support or others as necessary, or may choose to effect the removal itself. If the CERT determines that the material may not be safely stored on the reservation or that transportation of the chemical may present undue risks, it will then utilize appropriate inactivation or destruction methods to eliminate the hazard.

4. Provides training to other Division of Safety components, security personnel, housekeeping staff, maintenance personnel, and others who may be required to respond to emergency situations in which hazardous chemicals may be involved.

5. Maintains adequate reference materials, individual personal protective equipment, and any specialized apparatus necessary to fulfill the responsibilities of the CERT.

6. Prepares detailed reports of incidents requiring CERT involvement, participates in critiques of the events, and assists the Occupational Safety and Health (OSHB) staff in the development and implementation of measures designed to prevent similar incidents from recurring.

Travel, leave, and other activities are coordinated to ensure that two team members are available each working day. Furthermore, the CERT is responsible for after-hours response as well. A CERT call list is available for distribution to appropriate offices.

TEAM MEMBERSHIP

A CERT member must conduct critical evaluations under extreme conditions and be able to make quick, accurate decisions that may affect the lives of those responding to the emergencies, as well as the building occupants. Expensive scientific equipment, ongoing research, the facility itself, and the environment may also be compromised. It is, therefore, extremely important that personnel considered for this function be carefully selected and trained prior to membership. In general, individuals designed to serve on the CERT should have experience in handling toxic and reactive chemicals, familiarity with appropriate reference materials, and experience in the management of emergencies on the NIH reservation. The following areas of knowledge and experience are considered to be essential for an employee to be qualified to serve on the CERT.

Knowledge and understanding of organic and inorganic chemistry, with particular appreciation of the chemical and physical properties (e.g., flammability, corrosivity, reactivity, etc.) of hazardous chemical compounds.

Knowledge of toxicology, especially a familiarity with appropriate reference materials and data bases and the ability to interpret the data in order adequately to evaluate situations involving potential exposures to toxic chemical compounds, and understand the uses and limitations of personal protective equipment in order to protect all responders from the hazards involved in the emergency.

Training and experience in engineering control measures and knowledge of the capabilities and limitations of the facilities at the NIH (e.g., ventilation systems, plumbing systems, containment devices, etc.).

Familiarity with laboratory equipment and operations in order appropriately to evaluate the inherent hazards these operations or equipment may present in an emergency.

Experience in managing emergency situations at the NIH and the ability to communicate effectively in terms of providing advice, guidance, and direction to emergency response personnel, the scientific community, support personnel, and BID directorate-level officials.

Adequate physical condition to be able to utilize specialized personal protective equipment (e.g., positive-pressure self-contained breathing apparatus) and be physically able to work under emergency conditions.

Knowledge and experience in methods and procedures for decontaminating personnel, equipment, and facilities following potential chemical contamination.

The team leader is responsible for the administrative functions of the CERT and serves as the principal liaison. Specifically, the duties are as follows:

1. Serves as the primary responder and resource person, thus providing maximum continuity to the effort.
2. Develops standard operating procedures for specific compounds and situations.
3. Maintains the records, reports, and other files relevant to CERT activities.
4. Plans and conducts periodic training sessions, drills, and other exercises necessary for effective operations of the team.
5. Conducts "postmortem" examinations of all incidents that either involved or should have involved a CERT response.
6. Coordinates the purchase and/or design and fabrication of specialized equipment and assures access to all materials and supplies necessary for the CERT function.
7. Serves as primary spokesperson for the team.

CERT RESPONSE

The typical CERT response involves two team members, one at the scene of the emergency and the second remaining in the office to relay technical information from reference sources as necessary. Each CERT member is provided a "grab bag" containing individual personal protective equipment to be carried to the scene. In addition to these devices, the team utilizes fire department equipment as needed. The CERT has been instructed in the use of the NIH fire department positive-pressure, self-contained breathing apparatus.

FIRES/EXPLOSIONS/SPILLS

When called to the scene of fires, explosions, or spills, the CERT representative first reports to the fire department officer-in-charge to gain whatever information is available at the time. The emergency area is then evaluated as quickly as possible, utilizing fire department positive-pressure, self-contained breathing apparatus as necessary. Chemical and toxicological hazards (e.g., release of toxic materials, spread of contamination, reactive/explosive chemicals, damaged or pressurized containers as a result of exposure to water or heat) are assessed.

The CERT member advises the fire department on the necessity for area/building evacuation, shutdown of utilities, ventilation, and sealing off areas of the building. Methods for the containment and removal of affected chemicals are determined. The CERT ensures that all personnel needed for the operation (e.g., maintenance, housekeeping, and contract personnel, as well as NIH and Montgomery County (Maryland) fire fighters) are aware of the potential hazards and are appropriately protected. Furthermore, if personnel and/or equipment decontamination is required, the CERT provides the necessary guidance and directions to those involved. If injured or exposed persons are transported to the OMS or to outside medical facilities, the CERT is prepared to provide information on the chemicals involved and decontamination strategies as necessary. Finally, the CERT ensures that all affected areas have been sufficiently cleaned and/or decontaminated prior to the readmittance of personnel. To achieve this, the team may require bulk or environmental samples to be taken prior to reoccupancy. The Environmental Protection Branch is immediately notified any time the chemicals involved may be relased into the environment or whenever disposal of these materials is required. Similarly, if potentially radioactive materials are involved, the Radiation Safety Branch is promptly contacted.

REMOVAL OF POTENTIALLY EXPLOSIVE OR REACTIVE CHEMICALS

The CERT response to potentially explosive or otherwise reactive compounds is typically initiated by the Environmental Protection Branch (through the Chemical Waste Disposal Contractor) or by Safety Operations Section personnel who may be alerted to the problem through their respective NIH personnel. The CERT must be immediately notified whenever a chemical is encountered by the on-site Chemical Waste Disposal Contractor that may be beyond that person's capabilities and before any additional support (contract or otherwise) is contacted to assist in the removal operation.

The CERT representative promptly responds to the location of the material, together with the Environmental Protection Branch Chemical Waste Disposal Contract project officer. The project officer may elect to designate someone else to respond; however, this designee must have full contractual authority over the contract operation. The CERT evaluates the hazard potential and then determines the necessity for sealing off areas of the building and/or the evacuation of adjacent areas, corridors, or the building itself. The team consults with and advises BID officials, the fire department, and security personnel in this regard. The CERT representative then determines by what methods, and by whom, when, and to what location, the reactive/explosive material may be safely removed. Before removal, however, the CERT ensures that the group selected to effect the removal is knowledgeable, capable, appropriately equipped, and suitably protected against the hazards involved. Other considerations include whether removal will be during or after normal working hours, the route of transport through the building and across the reservation, special equipment requirements, and immediate removal from the NIH versus storage of the material in either Building 26 (chemical waste storage facility) or the explosive bunker in Building 21 or other suitable locations. Once the material has been transported to the designated storage area, the emergency is over and the CERT responsibilities end. The Environmental Protection Branch handles the chemical disposal through normal contractual channels, requesting advice from the Technical Assistance Section if desired. The CERT then convenes a postmortem review of the incident so that any suggestions to improve the response can be addressed.

TRAINING

Because of the CERT member's technical expertise and experience in the management of chemical emergencies, little formal training is required. Commercial courses are continually evaluated and will be requested if any are found to be beneficial. The team has been trained in the use of positive-pressure, self-contained breathing apparatus and other fire department equipment that may be utilized in emergency situations. Periodic refresher sessions are regularly provided. Furthermore, as specialized equipment is obtained by the team, each member is instructed in its use and limitations prior to the equipment's being placed in service. Team members are also provided with training in accessing computerized data bases for chemical and toxicological information retrieval.

Drills simulating chemical emergencies that involve the CERT response are a regularly scheduled part of the team agenda. After such events, members of the team critically evaluate the CERT portion of the response in detail.

Training for the fire department and various support functions (e.g., security, housekeeping, maintenance) is provided by the CERT, with additional support of other OSHB members as necessary.

An updated roster of the personnel, with both their office and home telephone numbers or other contact (such as radio), is a part of the CERT documentation.

From the above it is clear that the control and management of chemical emergencies require highly specialized personnel, properly trained and equipped, backed up by service personnel who will carry out the mechanics of the operations, and by a management that believes that human life and health should be the primary concern. Many of the items in the CERT document are clearly translatable to other real-world facilities.

PL 99-499 required the appointment of a facility representative who will participate in the emergency planning process.

Releases of both CEPP (EPA's name for the Chemical Emergency Preparedness Interim Guidance list) and CERCLA reportable-quantity (RQ) chemicals must be reported on an emergency basis. The threshold releases that trigger the notification requirements are either the RQ amount or an interim level in excess of 1 pound until EPA sets notification quantities. The provision identifies what information is required to be included with the notification in section 304.

Section 305, Emergency Training and Review of Emergency Systems, authorizes EPA and other appropriate agencies carrying out existing programs to provide emergency training, with special emphasis on hazardous chemicals. The Federal Emergency Management Agency (FEMA) is to be appropriated money for making grants to state and local governments and universities to improve emergency response preparedness, in addition to the training programs at its academy in Emmitsburg, Md. The "Hazardous Materials Emergency Planning Guide" is being published by the National Response Team (NRT), and is designed to assist local communities in planning for hazardous materials incidents. It replaces FEMA's "Planning Guide and Checklist for Hazardous Materials Contingency Plans" (FEMA-10), as well as the general portions of the EPA's "Chemical Emergency Preparedness Program Interim Guidance." EPA publishes separately the final CEPP technical materials, including site-specific guidance, criteria for identifying acutely toxic chemicals, chemical profiles, and a list of acutely toxic chemicals. The new guide also references portions of the Department of Transportation's "Report on Lessons Learned from State and Local Experience in Accident Prevention and Response Planning for Hazardous Materials Transportation and Community Teamwork: Working Together to Promote Hazardous Materials Transportation Safety," in addition to health, medical, natural resources, and related concerns. The new guide is available by writing to: Proposed Hazardous Materials Emergency Planning Guide, P.O. Box 70274, Washington, DC 20024.

From the above it should be obvious that a new approach is being attempted to protect the public, the workers, and the environment from imprudent operations involving chemicals. If the PL 99-499 is actually implemented in detail (as Congress intended), a considerable improvement in chemical health and safety should result. We can only hope that the persons involved will have the wisdom to put human concerns over politics and legal loopholes.

SUBSTANCES AND FACILITIES COVERED AND NOTIFICATION

A substance is subject to the requirements of the law if the substance is on the list of extremely hazardous substances, which is the list that was published on November 17, 1986, by the EPA Administrator in the "Chemical Emergency Preparedness Program Interim Guidance."

This list includes an interim final regulation establishing a threshold planning quantity for each substance on the list. The list may be revised from time to time. Any revisions to the list shall take into account the toxicity, reactivity, volatility, dispersibility, combustibility, or flammability of a substance. "Toxicity," as used here, shall include any short- or long-term health effect that may result from a short-term exposure to the material. (See Appendix B.)

FACILITIES COVERED

A facility is subject to the requirements of the law if a substance on the list referred to is present at the facility in an amount in excess of the threshold planning quantity established for each substance.

By May 17, 1987, the owner or operator of each facility covered shall have notified the emergency response commission for have the state in which the facility is located that the facility is subject to the requirements of the law. Thereafter, if a substance on the list of extremely hazardous substances becomes present at the facility in excess of the threshold planning quantity established, or there is a revision of the list in excess of the threshold planning quantity established for the substance, the facility shall notify the state emergency response committee within 60 days that such acquisition or revision is now subject to the requirements of the law.

The state commission shall notify the administrator of facilities subject to the law by notifying the administrator of each facility of each notification received from a facility under this law, and each faculty designated by the governor or state emergency response commission under the law.

SUGGESTED READING

Anon., "EPA Issues Sixth NPL Update; 64 New Sites Brings Total to 951," *Hazardous Materials Control Research Institute Newsletter*, March 1987, pp. 1, 2.

J. Newton, SARA Title III—An Overview of the Right-to-Know Act, *Pollution Engineering*, Sept. 1987, 66–73

5

Legal, Cost/Benefit, and Ethical Aspects

Howard H. Fawcett

The most obvious and time-tested motivation for the control of chemicals and related materials is economic. This point is often overlooked, as we argue that entreprenurial activity should have no restraints; that the *bottom line* is the only determining factor to be considered. However, to flout moral obligations and responsibilities, and to discount completely the value of human life with its attendent input to the morale and life blood of any organization or activity, is to be unrealistic.

PROFESSIONAL ETHICS

Many "professions" are aware of the moral responsibility to those served. Formal codes of ethics have been developed by and for the ACS, the AIChE, the American Bar Association, the British and American medical societies, and others.

The Society of Toxicology in the United States recently conducted an unsolicited and unremunerated survey of 1682 of its members, 20 percent of whom replied. In reporting on the ethical issues in toxicology (obviously of interest to chemists and engineers), the term "ethics" was used to signify nothing more than a set of rules of behavior, since there are many types of ethical rules. The following examples of ethical rules were suggested.

Interpersonal:
   "Golden rule"/categorical imperative
   Honesty is the best policy.
On the job:
   Do an honest day's work.
   Don't rock the boat.

Societal:
   Patriotism
   Obey the laws.
Professional:
   Use best data available.
   Be objective.

Four situations were postulated and described, and the members were asked to react to real-world situations where judgment was required as to a course of action. The conclusion of the study was that, although toxicologists exhibit a great deal of respect for formal bureaucratic lines of authority, even a few nonconformists could precipitate serious dialog within the institution if they judged the suggested course of action to be opposed to ethical standards. One of the criteria for a professional is that he or she is expected to exercise independent judgment based on a data base of technical knowledge.[1]

HEALTH AND SAFETY PRODUCTIVITY VERSUS THE LAW

In the past, the impression surfaced that health and safety were nonproductive expenses, which could be reduced, or at least minimized, by lip service to health and safety with no real commitment by management or supervision. When a serious incident occurred as a result of an accident, injury, fatality, fire, explosion, disruption of production or research, or unfavorable public relations, a temporary "damage control" effort would be instituted, and eventually the incident would be largely forgotten. However, in recent years, especially with the strong interest of the legal profession in following the various activities and regulations promulgated by such agencies as OSHA, National Institute for Occupational Safety and Health (NIOSH), EPA, the Food and Drug Administration (FDA), Consumer Product Safety Commission (CSPC), Department of Energy, and Department of Defense, a new attitude has developed on the part of the public, as well as of employees and employers. A recent example is the efforts of some members of the legal profession to encourage persons who were exposed to asbestos to file claims if it can be shown their health was damaged.[2]

LAW: AN ESSENTIAL ELEMENT

Since the legal aspects of health and safety regulations and compliance with the letter as well as the spirit of the laws, are important factors in the modern world, a fundamental awareness of the legal system, with its implications, is an essential element in the data base even of chemists and engineers who have no direct legal responsibilities. Fortunately, books are readily available for a quick scan of important elements of laws that relate to the real world.[3]

THE VALUE OF HUMAN LIFE

Unfortunately, these references give no real indication of what price tag is placed on a human life. A recent judgment against a major safety-conscious chemical company involving a worker who died of leukemia after, as the jury found, he had been exposed to benzene, in spite of company claims that benzene does not cause the type of leukemia involved, raised the value of one life to $1 million in punitive damages and $8 million in actual damages.[4] Over the years, the value placed on a life, in terms of the dollars spent for prevention, has varied widely according to agency and source. For example, see Table 5.1.

In another evaluation,[4b] the value of a life as determined by three federal agencies has been reported as:

Environmental Protection Agency	$400,000 or more
Federal Aviation Administration	$650,083
Occupational Safety and Health Administration	$3,500,000

OSHA estimates that it will cost employers about $24 million annually to meet the reduced standards on benzene exposures, covering about 240,000 workers.[4c]

FINES FOR NONCOMPLIANCE

An indirect measure of the value of life according to the OSHA viewpoint is noted in the largest fines OSHA proposed against companies during the past decade for violations of various occupational safety and health regulations, as shown in Table 5.2.

Other government agencies have the power to levy fines for noncompliance with regulations. For example, the EPA issued a civil complaint assessing a $4.3 million penalty against BASF Corporation and its Inmont Division, charging that Inmont imported seven new chemical substances into the United States without the 90-day advance notice required by law. The notice is mandated so that the agency can

TABLE 5.1. Value of Human Life

Agency or Activity	Dollars Spent per-Human Life Saved*
National Highway Traffic Safety	240,000
Consumer Product Safety Commission (lawn mowers)	1,000,000
Kidney transplants	72,000
Railroad crossings	100,000
Ejection from airplane	4,500,000
Coke-oven emissions	158,000,000
Acrylonitrile exposures	624,976,000

* Calculated in 1982 dollars.[4a]

TABLE 5.2 Proposed Fines

Year	Company	Amount of Proposed Fine*
1987	Bath Iron Works	$4,200,000
1986	Union Carbide Corp.	$1,377,300
1979	Newport News Shipbuilding and Dry Dock Co.	786,190
1980	Inland Steel Co.	523,500
1980	Weirton Steel Division	462,300
1982	Wheeling Pittburgh Steel Corp.	367,000
1979	Berwick Forge and Fabricating	366,800
1979	General Dynamics Electric Boat	213,740
1978	Texaco, Inc.	207,500
1978	U.S. Steel Corp.	206,600
1979	Bethlehem Steel	193,800

* Note that some of these fines were later reduced.[4d]

evaluate chemicals' potential for harm to health or the environment. EPA alleged that Inmont also failed to give prior notice that it was distributing four other new chemicals. The penalty, which can be appealed, is the largest ever assessed under the Toxic Substances Control Act.[5]

EPA also takes legal action against companies for alleged lack of full disclosure of information. A company was recently indicted by a federal grand jury for making false statements to the EPA during a 1982 investigation of the cause of industrial contamination of two municipal wells in Woburn, Mass. The EPA alleged that the "company concealed from the EPA" that solvents and other wastes were being poured into the ground behind the plant. Each of the two felony counts is punishable by a $10,000 fine, according to the Justice Department.[6]

In another case, a large metals company agreed to pay a $127,500 fine for dumping waste into Hurricane Creek in Arkansas during 1983–85.[7]

In still another case, on October 22, 1986, a federal judge in Miami imposed criminal fines against a development and management firm of a private residential report community located in North Key Largo, Fla. The defendant and two of its officers were found guilty of criminally violating the Clean Water Act and endangering the ecosystem of the coral reefs and marine life of the nearby offshore John Pennekamp State Park, which attracts more than 500,000 visitors a year. The company was ordered to pay $600,000 for willfully and negligently discharging raw or improperly treated sewage from the resort community into a channel flowing into the ocean waters of the Florida Keys. The sewage was discharged through a sewage bypass pipe unknown to state and federal environmental authorities. On July 31, the corporation pled guilty to 40 counts, and its vice-president and utilities director each pled guilty to one count. The vice-president was fined $5000 and the utilities director $2000. Both were placed on one-year probation. As part of the plea agreement, the firm agreed to pay the state of Florida a $60,000 penalty.[8]

In another case, the EPA issued an administrative civil complaint, with an assessed penalty of $1.46 million, against a Long Beach, Calif., concern for failure to submit completed studies, as required by the Toxic Substances Control Act. Section 8(d) of the Act requires submission to EPA of health and safety studies of any chemical substance deemed potentially toxic, and applies to studies by manufacturers, processors, or distributors of such chemicals, even when there are negative results. The studies in question were in the form of aggregated air-monitoring data evaluated for worker safety exposure, and were to be made known to EPA in 1982.[9]

IMPROPER DISPOSAL AND SUBSTITUTION CAN BE COSTLY

Disposal of chemicals is also watched closely by the EPA; proposed penalties of $125,550 were imposed against an Idaho company for allegedly violating the Toxic Substances Control Act in the handling of PCB wastes at a Grand View, Ida., facility. The complaints include improper burial, spills, removal, tank repairs, and storage. Two previous PCB violations were resolved in 1983 and 1984 with the company agreeing to pay fines totaling $47,750.[10]

International activity in hazardous substances can sometimes turn into unfortunate activities. Two major national and international hazardous-waste shippers and chemical brokers each received a 13-year sentence, the longest sentence ever imposed in any state or federal case involving hazardous substances. On July 28, 1986, the two men and their companies, located in Mount Vernon, N.Y., were sentenced in the U.S. District Court in White Plains on charges that included wire fraud, mail fraud, making a false claim against the United States, obstruction of justice, and conspiracy. The men allegedly substituted cheap hazardous chemicals for commercial-grade chemicals ordered from them by the country of Zimbabwe. After conviction on 106 counts, EPA also submitted information to the court on the improper storage or abandonment of hazardous wastes in various areas along the East Coast (many of which have required cleanup actions under the federal Superfund hazardous-waste-site program), which implicated the two men. As a result, the judge concluded that the men were a danger to the community, revoked bail, and ordered the unusually long sentences. The companies also were fined $250,000 each.[11]

A TRAGIC MISTAKE OF IDENTITY

A simple mistake, in which contents of bags of polybromthated biphenyl (PBB) were accidentally mixed with cattle-food supplement, resulted in serious financial, as well as human, costs. In addition to the thousands of animals destroyed to prevent further contamination, and the possibility that many people in Michigan will retain the PBB in their system for years, the firm involved agreed to pay $38.5 million for the cleanup following the 1973 incident in St. Louis, Mich.[12]

MENTAL HEALTH IS NOT JUST MENTAL

Mental health also has high financial aspects. An $850,000 jury award in San Francisco Superior Court has challenged a critical cost-containment technique in the private health insurance industry. In Hughes vs. Blue Cross, a jury decided that Blue Cross behaved improperly in denying insurance coverage for a patient's psychiatric hospitalization after a retrospective review. In addition to awarding the plaintiff $150,000 in compensatory damages, the jury also awarded $700,000 in punitive damages to underscore the fact that Blue Cross had not acted in good faith.[13]

It is small wonder that the National Academy of Engineering recently noted that collisions are taking place among engineers, other scientists, and physicians versus lawyers.[14]

States also have the power and ability to levy fines. For example, in Ohio, the Dayton Power and Light Co. agreed to pay $100,000 to the state for air pollution violations in 1983 and 1984, as well as to monitor continuously and report monthly air pollution outputs at the plant and to install a sophisticated monitoring system, consisting of two monitoring stations, near the plant to measure emissions.[15]

In Maryland a rigging and hauling company, which, along with the Potomac Electric Power Co., had been part of a yearlong grand jury investigation into allegations of illegal disposal of PCB, was fined $75,000 for PCB pollution of a nearby stream in Beltsville Industrial Park.[16]

ROLE OF THE MEDIA IN PUBLIC AWARENESS

The news media (both print and electronic) have, in their zeal to cover the news, often sensationalized the reports of environmental releases, starting with Rachel Carson's book *Silent Spring,* the drama of the Love Canal toxic waste discoveries, and the Times Beach (dioxin) discovery. The reports of the harmful effects of chemicals, food additives, and pesticides, and the mutagenic and teratogenic fears of certain chemicals and distrust engendered by the Bhopal, India, accident, the Chernobyl nuclear contamination, and the five-day fire in a white-phosphorous-containing railroad tank car at Miamisburg, Ohio, on July 6, 1986, that forced the evacuation of nearly 30,000 persons, have gained for the chemical and related industries a less than favorable image. Books that attempt to put all this in perspective or to excuse certain aspects (such as E. M. Whelan's *Toxic Terror,* 1985, or E. Efron's *The Apocalyptics: Cancer and the Big Lie,* 1984) undoubtedly have served a useful function. However, they must be carefully reviewed in an unemotional, detached, scientific manner as they neutralize certain points that have contributed to the uneasiness about our ability to understand and control the hazards of chemicals and related projects. A better perspective on the part of the writers would be helpful, both to the public and to the industry. Still, it must be noted that chemistry is not the main interest of most people, and it is true that emotions regarding chemicals are often more heated than the facts justify.

Mike Heylin, Chemical and Engineering News, in an editorial in his publication, notes that, in spite of the problems, about 84 percent of the public agrees that chemistry has produced more desirable than undesirable results, whereas only 10 percent disagree, based on findings of a public opinion survey conducted for the ACS by Cambridge Reports. The high public regard for chemistry and chemists (and presumably chemical engineers) apparently persists even when problems with chemicals are at issue. For instance, when asked which group is most to blame when such problems are identified, only 7 percent of respondents to last fall's survey chose "chemists." This was down from 10 percent in 1980. The public is apparently considerably more likely to blame government regulators than chemists for problems with chemicals. In that survey, 20 percent of respondents chose regulators as being primarily responsible, second only to manufacturers at 46 percent, and well ahead of chemists at 7 percent. With regard to the health-related problem, those blaming regulators numbered 27 percent, compared with 9 percent pinning the primary responsibility on the chemist. As Heylin concludes, these findings give cause for concern and are thought provoking.[17]

THE LAW IS NOT SUPERSONIC

When legal actions are taken, the course of justice may be very time consuming. The longest jury trial in history ended 44 months after it began, after 182 witnesses, 6,000 exhibits, and more than 100,000 transcript pages. At issue was whether 65 residents of Sturgeon, Mo., were harmed when 19,000 gallons of wood-preserving chemicals spilled from a rail car in the center of the town on January 10, 1979. The chemicals contained minute traces of dioxin (TCDD) (see pages 107–119). None of the victims appeared visibly ill. At the time of the accident, a "powerful stench" hung over the town. Monsanto Lawyer David F. Snively felt that the claims were "utterly without merit. These people were not hurt."[18]

WHEN THINGS GO WRONG

The tendency suddenly to "discover" the need for further research into health and safety is not uniquely chemical. For example, after every coal mine disaster, a new wave of dedication sweeps the mining community, but all too often is forgotten as economic pressures prevail.[19] In a similar manner, the operation of American railroads, with which we have had a century and a half of experience (mostly favorable in spite of occasional derailments), is suddenly under renewed scrutiny following the Amtrak-Conrail accident near Baltimore, Md. on January 4, 1987, when three Conrail locomotives crashed into an Amtrak passenger train, resulting in 16 deaths and 75 injuries. Investigators are focusing on "survivability" issues to determine whether the interior design of the cars contributed to injuries, as well as on the role that track signals, inoperable warnings, and possible illegal alcohol and/or drug use and excessive attention to television sports by the train crew, along with the absence of automatic braking devices on Conrail locomotives, may have contributed to the tragedy.[20]

Midair collisions of aircraft are hardly a new hazard, yet after every incident an investigation produces detailed suggestions, which are often only partly implemented.[21a,b] Recommendations of the National Transportation Safety Board—an independent agency that investigates all serious transportation accidents—are often ignored by the regulatory agencies and by the Congress. Known and well-tested advances, such as antijackknifing control devices for large tractor-trailers and tank trucks (which have a long history of serious jackknifing accidents), have been resisted for decades although the savings in lives and disruption of traffic on main highways would far outweigh their relatively small weight and cost.[22] Years of tests have shown air bags in passenger automobiles to be effective in mitigating injuries in accidents, but their use, even today, is limited.[23]

The recent emphasis on hazard communication, or right-to-know, at the federal (OSHA), state, and local levels has brought many of these concerns into focus, as both employees and employers face up to the real world. PL 99-499 is beginning to affect employers by requiring them to provide information on hazardous substances used in the workplace to communities about them in the same way that they are already required to notify their employees under the OSHA Hazard Communication Regulation. The success of these laws and requirements largely relies on the communication of truthful and complete data.[24] Even in academic circles, the importance of hazard communication and Title III of PL 99-499, iterated by state and local regulations, should not be underemphasized. As hazards and their control become better understood, overall safety and health for workers and for the community should improve, even in academic circles. Economics alone may be an incentive; significant liability should give pause to any responsible manager or student of chemical health and safety. Consider the Karen Silkwood accident in 1974[25] or the class-action cases pending with 5000 homeholders over alleged exposure to toxic chemicals in the Stringfellow acid pit, which have seriously affected the value of formerly highly desirable homes and properties in a wide area near the dump site in Glen Avon, Calif.[25a] (See Figures 5.1A, B.)

RIPS IN THE GOLDEN PARACHUTES

Criminal convictions of three officers of a silver-reclamation plant in a Chicago suburb in which cyanide was used and handled without proper identification, precautions, or labeling, resulting in the documented death of a Polish immigrant who read and spoke little English, suggest that golden parachutes may not be the only exit route for executives who ignore or actually reject chemical hazards.[26]

In another case, on September 15, 1986, a federal judge in Orlando, Fla., sentenced Arthur J. Greer to five years in prison (with four years and six months suspended), levied a $23,000 fine, and added five years' probation to include 1000 hours of community service, for falsifying records associated with the disposal of hazardous waste. Greer and his company attempted to collect payment from other

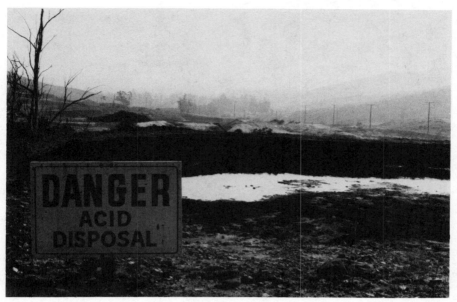

Figure 5.1A. Overall view of disposal site near Glen Avon, CA. Problem was first recognized in 1969.

firms and from the Florida Department of Environmental Regulation for hazardous-waste treatment, storage, and disposal that were never undertaken. Greer also falsified the results of tests performed to identify hazardous waste, and labeled drums containing hazardous waste as "dirt." The conviction came as a result of work by EPA's criminal-enforcement investigators, who have had a growing impact on violations of environmental laws.[27]

EPA also is able to take legal action that can result in serious disruption of executives' lives. On December 1, 1986, Rad Services, Inc., a Pennsylvania corporation, and two of its corporate officers were sentenced in Bowling Green, Ky., for criminal violations of RCRA, the federal hazardous-waste management and disposal law. The charges arose over the illegal storage in a Bowling Green warehouse of hundreds of tons (47 truckloads) of toxic lead and cadmium emission-control dust, which the company had arranged to have transported and abandoned at strip mines in Kentucky and Tennessee. Although advised by its own waste-management division of the legal methods for handling this waste, the company hired a "midnight dumper" for $60,000 to dispose of the waste illegally. Bills of lading were then falsified to make it appear that the waste had been legitimately transported and disposed of out of the state. Executive vice-president Arthur Scuillo and George Gary, the head of the Rad Chemicals Division, each was sentenced to two years in jail, a $10,000 fine, and two years' probation, including 200 hours of community service. Scuillo pled guilty on October 20 to charges of conspiracy to violate RCRA and of unlawfully disposing of waste, and was ordered to serve six months of his jail term. Gary pled guilty to conspiracy to violate RCRA

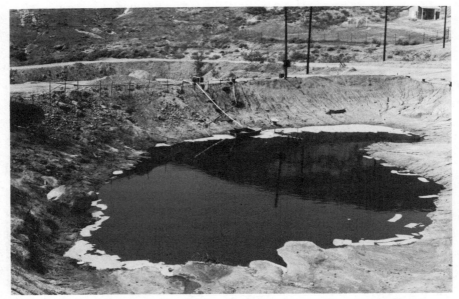

Figure 5.1B. Closeup of Stringfellow acid pit in 1978. The liquid has since been partially neutralized and covered, but leachate remains a serious problem in 1988. (Photos courtesy Ms. P. Newman.)

and was ordered to serve 30 days of his jail sentence. The company was fined $75,000 for unlawful storage of hazardous wastes. The midnight dumper, James Hedrick, was sentenced in March 1985 to a year and a day in jail, and, in an unrelated case, a corporate officer of a second firm that had utilized Hedrick's services was prosecuted and sentenced to a six-month jail term.

REDUCTION IN THE STAFF

In the past few years, there has been a determined effort by many companies to reduce the workforce as an economy measure, or so-called "cutting the fat," by offering early retirement to employees. From the short-range, end-of-the-year-report view, this is useful, but in the longer haul, when the experience and expertise of more experienced personnel are needed but no longer available, the early retirement program may be less than wise.[27]

WHAT DO HEALTH, SAFETY, AND ENVIRONMENTAL PROGRAMS COST?

Unfortunately, a data base upon which to project a truly meaningful and effective cost of accidents does not really exist. We do know that fires, explosions, accidents, health impairment (including cancer), and other situations have many indirect aspects—such as lower employee morale, increased insurance premiums, unrest and discontent among the 27 percent of industry that have labor unions, and adverse effects on the shareholders' trust in their investment. The time necessary to manage and supervise the investigation or to study accidents is another aspect, as are the salaries of the safety, fire protection, industrial hygiene, health physics, occupational medicine, nursing, and environmental compliance staffs. Time for "accident prevention" in the form of meetings and other presentations to employees may run into large increments, to say nothing of the engineering, maintenance, and program expenses associated with running a clean shop. The more obvious out-of-pocket expenses for such items as protective equipment (eye, face, head, respiratory, feet, and body), the disposal, cleaning, and maintenance of the equipment, welding hoods, ventilation, and waste packaging and disposal can be measured but their real-world value and benefit are seldom fully monitored or appreciated.

The successful manager, supervisor, or professor must therefore strike a balance between the losses from an inadequate program and the gains of an effective loss-prevention effort, with little firm data as a guide. Cost/benefit analyses should be carried out in sufficient detail to permit management to budget a reasonable amount to health, safety, and fire prevention in the interests of a well-run and -administered operation, as well as for the boost in productivity and morale that can be expected from a sincere protection and environmental compliance program.[28]

It does little good to point fingers at safety and health. In reply to a charge that accidents such as those in Bhopal and Chernobyl are the results of willful actions by engineers, Theodore Rockwell, PE, writing in the *Washington Post* (Jan. 24, 1987, page A21), replied to another writer who felt that engineers (and presumably chemists and other professionals) have no feelings. Rockwell noted that a major industrial accident costs money, ruins reputations, and is an unmitigated loss to all concerned (except for the lawyers). He feels it is nonsense to argue that anyone would knowingly increase the chance of an accident.

The previous writer had implied that engineers make quantitative decisions on how safe a product is to be, balancing safety against cost. It seldom works that way. Design features are evaluated on how they will affect reliability and safety, and the final design is always believed (at the time) to be safe.

However, Rockwell went on, accidents do happen. A well-engineered system may fail because of operator error, field changes, or poor maintenance. Management may override engineers' warnings (e.g., Challenger). But the most important factor is that too many technical decisions are made by fiscal people who are seldom technically knowledgeable and who measure everything in dollars. This is bad on two counts: the cheapest item is often unsatisfactory, and when maintenance and other expenses are considered, the cheaper item may be the more expensive. This includes saving the cost of the time of employees who devote careful attention to the overall safe operation of a process or program.

Consider the case of many purchasing agents, each trying for a "best buy" on different sets of valves for a large power plant. Some if these valves cost hundreds of thousands of dollars and are large, complex machines. At best, all the valves will work, but the plant ends up with scores of different kinds of valves, each with a different maintenance manual, spare-parts system, and training program, none interchangeable. I know from experience that this is not only a source of confusion, errors, and accidents, but also a serious cost burden.

Concern has been expressed that "powerful engineering elites would have license to make their own rules" and would "wield such power as to invite unprecedented visitations of technological horrors." On the contrary, our lack of technically knowledgeable people in places of power is a national disgrace. Congress, the state houses, and the boardrooms of American businesses are nearly devoid of engineers. In fact, it is the financial managers rather than the engineers who "have already seized the reins."

It is easy to blame other persons or institutions for our problems. We say our poor health is the result of industrial pollution, food additives, and poor doctors, not our own choice of cigarettes, junk food, alcohol, and lack of exercise. We let Ralph Nader tell us that auto companies chose "profits over safety" when they fought seat belts, yet we know that seat belts are sold at a profit. We curse the airlines for crowding the coach seats, yet we choose the lower prices that the crowding makes possible. We forget that food preservatives were developed to reduce sickness and death from food poisoning, not as an evil scheme to make money at the expense of public safety.

Rockwell concludes there is no such thing as absolute safety. Public health officials estimate that 50 children suffer permanent brain damage each year from pertussis vaccine, which is required by law. But it is believed that more would die without vaccination. Similarly, a power plant or a bridge or a dam may cause deaths, but these structures are built to meet a public need, expressed through city and state councils and public referendums. It is irresponsible to blame others for these deaths and injuries. It is a responsibility we must all share. After all, we all share the benefits.

THE PSYCHIATRIC BY-PRODUCT

In recent times, as prevention of conventional injury has reduced the claims in that regard, psychiatric industrial disability compensation claims now surpass all other industrial disability claims; while other claims were falling by 10 percent, psychiatric claims were soaring by more than 100 percent, according to the Centers for Disease Control (CDC). During the annual meeting of the American Academy of Psychiatry and the Law, Dr. Robert C. Larsen noted that workers in service occupations filed three times as many stress-injury claims as did workers doing physical labor. Dr. David B. London said that 15 percent of the 100,000 worker's compensation claims filed in 1985 were stress related. Dr. John M. Henderson found that among more than 450 claims of psychic trauma over five years, 75 percent of the personal-injury cases and 80 percent of the worker's compensation cases were manufactured, were fictitious, or involved malingering.

The CDC reported that when workers are asked the causes of psychic complaints, they cite repetitive, deadly dull, machine-paced, demeaning duties, and they fault their supervisors. Whatever these working conditions are like, they are less onerous overall than were those of the 19th century; lung-mincing coal mines; hand-amputating unshielded machines; stuffy, dim sweatshops; and bosses who were paternalistic martinets.

At first glance, the cynic can observe that some Americans have become overwhelmed by life—even though that life meets the most abundant and pervasively shared living standards of any country in human experience. The very chemicals that have contributed to our "better life" are now suspected of evil. Firm data on troubled workers as individuals are scanty. Studies of psychiatric failure in the workplace tend to focus on workers' complaints and what they call *work stress,* rather than on the workers themselves. The studies do not correlate specific worker personality type with differing patterns of worker failure and varying nuances of work milieu, or how the workers' past responses to past stresses (or exposures) relate to their present responses to present stresses. They do not show how workers who fail compare and contrast with bench mates who cope. It would be useful to discover just which psychological traits enable a worker to tolerate stresses that crush comrades without those traits so that we could improve current inadequate treatment programs. Dr. Henderson warns that many workers stop work for reasons other than overwhelmingly noxious (or hazardous) job ambience. They are *not disabled* by the job; the job gives them a *pretext* for complaint. They are seeking socioeconomic profit, not a return to work. The experience of having a minor injury or of having seen hurt (or exposed) co-workers compensated has revealed to them both beguiling escape hatches from tedium and doors to personal gain. When others involved in the disability compensation process, such as orthopedists, lawyers, and judges, read the reports and hear psychiatric testimony, they infer that psychiatrists abet claimants who are raiding the economic system.

Disability claimants tend to be heavily loaded with psychopathology; the need is for psychiatrists to contribute to their evaluation. Just as chemists must be meticulous in seeking the truth about chemicals and their interface with living systems, including humans, the psychiatrists, other medical personnel, the claimant, and the consumers of goods and services all must take a factual look at their obligations and responsibilities, both to the claimant and to the economic system.[29]

All this must not be construed to mean that chemical exposures are not real hazards. Dr. Ruth Lilis has noted that neurotoxicity induced by repeated exposure to organic solvents is real, and is not confined to industrial or agricultural workers. Dr. Lilis presents strong evidence linking long-term solvent exposure with chronic, irreversible neurotoxic effects, according to data from epidemiologic studies. Neurophysiologic testing, brain imaging, and cerebral blood flow studies have demonstrated that cerebral and cerebellar atrophy occur in individuals with severe solvent-induced encephalopathy. These tend to be people who have deliberately inhaled or sniffed the solvents, a practice that has reached epidemic proportions in some areas.

Occupational exposure never reaches such intensity, but the number of people who are exposed to toxic chemicals (including alcohols, ketones, ethers, and aliphatic, aromatic, and halogenated hydrocarbons) is increasing because the chemicals are found in more and more household products and materials for arts, crafts, and hobbies. Symptoms of repeated exposure tend to be nonspecific. The majority of experts agree, however, that certain core sympotoms are almost always present: a basic change in personality, developing over time and affecting intellect, emotional balance, energy, and motivation; fatigability; memory impairment; difficulty in concentration; loss of initiative; and depression. Often associated with these symptoms are emotional lability, irritability, headaches, sleep disturbances, and paresthesia. In the majority of cases, these symptoms are mild, but they appear sometimes to be irreversible, even after the individual has been removed from exposure to the solvent.[30] Dr. Lilis has not yet studied the combined occupational–recreational exposures to solvents, another aspect that is worthy of investigation.

A more common, but possibly even more serious, economic loss to employees and employers involves the question of smoking. There is a growing conviction that smoking is both a personal and an occupational hazard of great importance. Figures hardly tell the story, but one accounting is that an estimated 1000 smokers die each day in the United States as a result of this habit, and recent evidence suggests that nonsmokers are also dying from (or at least are endangered by) exposure to second-hand smoke. Ventilation in confined areas, such as airplane cabins, has been shown to be totally inadequate to remove the smoke.[31] The time that smokers take away from their bench or desk while smoking in unobserved areas has not been recognized in numbers. The potentiating effect of cigarette smoke on additional insults from other materials inhaled is slowly being appreciated. There is no question but that the habit is very difficult to control; the writer actually found cigarettes and matches carefully hidden in operating areas of plants involving high explosive materials so that, when no observers were present, the workers could have a quick smoke, with complete disregard for their own lives and for the lives of others in the plant. One carelessly discarded cigarette could have destroyed many millions in investment, to say nothing of the lives that would have been lost.

The mundane spill problems, which sooner or later every chemical and petrochemical operation encounters, are also of economic interest. In a recent action, a major oil company was fined $6000 for the accident and $46,000 in cleanup costs after a oil spill of about 100,000 gallons that contaminated a California sewage-treatment facility and caused it to be shut down. The oil could have mixed with the pure oxygen located in the second stage of the facility and have caused an explosion. The company's own cleanup costs were about $250,000 in addition to another fine of about $80,000 by the California Regional Water Quality Control Board.[32] In another incident, in Ohio, an oil company agreed to a $762,500 penalty to settle charges, brought by the Justice Department on behalf of EPA, of discharging excessive pollutants into a river from a refinery, in violation of the Clean Water Act.[33]

Accident and injury records have never been high on the list of concerns that many consider important, but the accuracy of such records should be beyond question if prudent action is to be taken in prevention. If safety records are "fudged" or inaccurate, serious problems may be overlooked that could, and often do, prevent adequate health and safety control measures from being implemented.[34]

Another management concern that is receiving increasing attention is the control of reproductive hazards. While private policies have concentrated on removing women from risk, these broad-based policies can infringe on women's employment rights and may not protect the reproductive health of men, according to Prof. Lindsey V. Kayman of Boston University Medical Center. Professor Kayman has listed the following elements of a comprehensive reproductive-hazard-limitation program.

Reproductive Hazards Committee: The formation of a reproductive hazards committee should be structured to include persons with knowledge of the workings of the institution and technical expertise in many areas. The committee will participate in the development of the policy and should ensure that the policy is feasible, is ethical, and does not contain any illegal provisions.

Designation of Current Potential Parents: Special precautions may be necessary for employees who are attempting to conceive as well as for pregnant employees (who form a separate category). Since designation of current potential parents may invade an employee's right to privacy, status of "current potential parent" should be a voluntary reporting procedure.

Designation of Reproductive Toxins: Designating materials as reproductive toxins involves identifying materials that are being used and then evaluating them as causing reproductive impairment or birth defects. In states with right-to-know laws, many medical institutions have performed chemical inventories of laboratories, patient-care areas, and other departments where chemicals are being used.

Control Measures for Reproductive Toxins: Whenever feasible, less toxic material will be substituted for reproductive toxins. When substitution is not possible, all exposures to reproductive toxins will be kept as low as reasonably achievable (ALARA). This will involve the use of engineering controls such as laboratory fume hoods or local exhaust ventilation, good work practices, and personal protective equipment, and, in some cases, respirators. Medical removal protection may be necessary when substitution of a less toxic material is not possible, or it is not possible to determine whether achievable exposure levels are adequate to prevent reproductive harm to exposed employees or their unborn children.

Protection of Employees' Future Reproductive Health: A policy focusing only on current potential parents does not protect employees who are planning to have offspring in the future. Since safe exposure limits cannot be defined at this time, a prudent course is to use engineering and administrative controls to keep exposures to reproductive toxins as low as reasonably achievable.

Employee Awareness: Programs to promote employee awareness are invaluable in assuring voluntary cooperation. Employees must know where they can receive information and obtain status as current potential parents. Counseling should be provided for all employees who have questions.

REAL ESTATE AND HOUSING VALUES

The value of property that developers have constructed on former toxic-waste-disposal sites is another indication of growing concern regarding chemicals. Under PL 99-499, any party having a contractual relationship with an owner of a toxic-waste site would be liable. The law stipulates that land deeds would be considered contracts and that any lender having a management relationship with an owner of a toxic-waste site also could be found liable. This has forced developers of land to examine new sites for possible undetected hazardous wastes, possibly disposed years before with no records. The monitoring of homes and offices for radon-222 is also of growing concern, as is the monitoring of asbestos in older homes and offices.[35]

REFERENCES

1. D. A. Bronstein, "Some Ethical Issues in Toxicology," *Fundamental & Appl. Toxicol.,* **7,** No. 4, 525–534 (Nov. 1986).

2. B. Richards and B. Meier, "Widening Horizons: Lawyers Lead Hunt for New Group of Asbestos Victims with Offers of Free X-rays, Attorneys Solicit Seamen, Tire Workers and Others: Just Chasing Ambulances?" *Wall St. J,* 1, 24, (Feb. 18, 1987); S. S. Chissick and R. Derricott, *Asbestos: Properties, Applications and Hazards,* vol. 2, Wiley-Interscience, Chichester and New York, (1983), vol. 2, (1979).

3. West Publishing Co., P.O. Box 3526, St. Paul, MN 55101, publishes paperback books on professional responsibility, environmental law, contracts, worker's compensation and employee protection, torts—injuries to persons and property, and insurance law. Additional legal references are available from the American Bar Association, 750 N. Lake Shore Drive, Chicago, IL 60611, phone (312) 988-5000.

4. S. Kilman, "Monsanto Told to Pay Award," *Wall St. J.,* 13, (Dec. 15, 1986). Note also on same page, "Manville Hearing Delayed by a U.S. Appeals Court, concerning 1982 action for filing under Chapter 11 after thousands of asbestos-related claims were filed against the company. (See also reference 2.)

4a. E. Schrage, P. Engel, "The Decision Maker's Dilemma," *Sciences,* **22,** No. 6, 26–31 (Aug.–Sept. 1982).

4b. Anon., *U.S. News & World Rep.* 58 (Sept. 16, 1986).

4c. A. R. Karr, "U.S. Tightens Benzene Rule for Workplace, Allowed Level of Exposure for Carcinogen Is Cut 90 percent under OSHA Order," *Wall St. J.,* 24 (Sept. 2, 1987).

4d. Anon., *Washington Post,* A17 (Apr. 4, 1986).

5. *Wall St. J.,* 30 (Jan. 2, 1987).

6. *Wall St. J.,* 10 (Jan. 29, 1987).

7. *Environmental News,* USEPA, 2, 3 (Oct. 20–27, 1986).

8. *Environmental News,* USEPA, 3 (Oct. 20–27, 1986).

9. *Environmental News,* USEPA, 3, 4 (Oct. 20–27, 1986).

10. *Environmental News,* USEPA 4, 5 (Aug. 4, 1986).

11. *Environmental News,* USEPA, 4, 5 (Aug. 4, 1986).

12. *Environmental News,* USEPA, 3 (July 8, 1986); see also E. Chen, *PBB: An American Tragedy,* Prentice-Hall, New York, 1979.

13. J. L. Schwart, "Jury Awards $850,000 Over Retrospective Review," *Psychiatric Times*, **III,** No. 9, 1, 23 (Sept. 1986).

14. Anon., " 'Collisions' Are Taking Place Between Engineers and Lawyers," *News Report,* National Research Council, Nov. 1986, pp. 22–24.

15. *Dayton (Ohio) Daily News,* 1 (Dec. 24, 1986).

16. *Washington Post,* 31, 34 (April 26, 1986),.

17. M. Heylin, Editorial, "The Public View of Chemists," *C&EN* 5 (Jan. 19, 1987).

18. P. B., Gray, "Endless Trial: Dioxin Damage Suit Ties Up Courthouse and Angers Judiciary," *Wall St. J.,* 1, 24 (Jan. 13, 1987); see also "Monsanto Punished as 44-Month Trial Ends," *C&EN,* 5 (Nov. 2, 1987). The award of $16.3 million doubtlessly will be appealed.

19. C. Seltzer. *Fire in the Hole: Miners and Managers in the American Coal Industry,* The University Press of Kentucky, Lexington, 1987. On Dec. 26, 1986, the *Wall Street Journal,* p. 1, quoted Tass to the effect that a concentration of methane exploded in a coal mine in the Ukraine, 575 miles from Moscow, and several miners were killed.

20. L. McGinley, and D., Machalarba, "Wide Review of Railroad Safety Expected in Aftermath of Amtrak-Conrail Disaster," *Wall St. J.,* 27 (Jan. 12, 1987); J., Lancaster, "U.S. May Toughen Train Safety Rules, Drug Policy Questions Raised," *Washington Post,* A1, A12 (Jan. 19, 1987).

21. "Movement for New Union for Controllers Takes Off," *Washington Post,* A10, 11 (Feb. 8, 1987); Anon. "Plea to FAA, Spend More Money on Air Traffic Safety," *USA Today,* 1 (Aug. 28–30, 1987).

22. U.S. Patent 2,838,325, 2,822,188, and 3,082,019 K-W New Safety Jackknife Device (Canadian Patent 639546). For details contact S. J. Begin, 414 Bedford St., Schenectady, NY 12308, or Nelson R. Carter, 1500 College Parkway, 61A, Fort Myers, FL 33907.

23. "About Air Bags," 3rd ed., 13 pp., 1985, and "Myths and Facts About Air Cushions," 10 pp., 1984, Insurance Institute for Highway Safety, 600 New Hampshire Ave., Suite 300, Washington, DC 20037.

24. Chemical Hazard Communication, OSHA 3084, U.S. Dept. of Labor Occupational Safety and Health Agency, Washington, D.C., 1986; note also Title III, Emergency Planning and Community Right-to-Know, in PL 99-499 (Superfund Amendments and Reauthorization Act of 1986); see also *Hazardous Materials: Right-to-Know News,* biweekly, Thompson Publishing Group, 1725 K St., N.W. Suite 200, Washington, DC 20006; "Informing Workers of Chemical Hazards: The OSHA Hazard Communication Standard," prepared by the Task Force on Occupational Health and Safety, American Chemical Society, 14 pages, April 1985; "Right-to-Know," a new BNA special report and documentary film, two presentations exploring federal and state right-to-know requirements and controversies, 1986, Bureau of National Affairs, Inc., 1231 25th St., N.W., Washington, DC 20037; H. H. Fawcett, *The OSHA Communication Standard or "Right-to-Know,"* vol. 63, pp. A70–A703, March 1986, and H. H. Fawcett, "Safety: What Do We Really Mean?," *J. Chem. Ed.,* **58,** No. 2, A45–A48 (1981).

25. Silkwood vs. Kerr-McGee Corp., CA 10, No. 79-1894, settled for $1.38 million for dismissing all claims against company, August 22, 1986. Incident occurred in 1974.

25a. M., Weisskopf, "Toxic-Waste Site Awash in Misjudgment: Deadly Chemicals Seep Into Town's Water Supply Despite Superfund," *Washington Post,* A1, A18 (Nov. 16, 1986); "America's Toxic Tremors," *Newsweek,* 18–19 (Aug. 26, 1985). Note also "Hazardous Waste: EPA Has Made Limited Progress in Determining Wastes to Be Regulated," report to the Chairman, Subcommittee on Commerce, Transportation and Tourism, Committee on Energy and Commerce, House of Representatives, U.S. General Accounting Office, GAO/RCED-87-27, 56 pp., Dec. 1986.

26. State of Illinois vs. Steven O'Neill, Charles Kirschbaum, and David Rodriquez et al. (Circuit Court of Cook County, Ill., No. 83 C 11091, cited in Bureau of National Affairs Report, July 4, 1985, p. 76; see also "Workplace Murder Conviction May Spur Similar Prosecutions," *C&EN,* 24–24 (July 8, 1985).

27. R. E., Winter, "Trying to Streamline, Some Firms May Hurt Long-Term Prospects," *Wall St. J.,* 1,

10 (Jan. 8, 1987). see also "Cost-Benefit Analysis and Environmental Regulations: Politics, Ethics, and Methods," 196 pp., Conservation Foundation, 1717 Massachusetts Ave., Washington, DC 20036, 1983.

28. Book review, "Moral Dealing for Managers," *Wall St. J.*, 5 (Dec. 26, 1986).

29. W. F. Sheeley, "As Workplace Becomes Safer, Claims of Psychic Injury Are Soaring," *Clin. Psychiat. News*, **15**, No. 1, 1, 31 (1987).

30. Anon., *Clin. Psychiat. News*, **15,** No. 1, 30 (1987); see also "Inhalant Deaths Rare, But Continuing Problem," *Dayton (Ohio) Daily News*, 1, 12 (Aug. 16, 1986).

31. R. H., Shipley, "Smoking-Reduction Programs Help Businesses Snuff Out Health Problems," *Occupational Health & Safety*, **56,** No. 1, 73–78, (1987); see also videos: *Business Look at Smoking: the $50 Billlion Cigarette* and *Air We Breathe,* Smoke Free Environments, 1137 Xerxes Ave S., Minneapolis, MN 55405; "Behavior Modification in the Workplace: Behavior Modification Key to Fewer Accidents," *Focus,* **2,** Issue 1, p. 1, ITS Industrial Training Systems Corp., 20 West Stow Rd., Marlton, NJ 08053; I., Molotsky, "Surgeon General, Citing Risks, Urges Smoke-Free Workplace," *N.Y. Times,* A22 (Dec. 17, 1986), and A. L. Otten, "Sharpest Attack Yet on Passive Smoking Issued in New Study by Surgeon General," 8 (Dec. 17, 1986, N. A. Adler, "End Air Pollution in Airplanes," *Wall St. J.,* 22 (Jan. 30, 1987).

Additional smoking-cessation resources include: *A Decision Maker's Guide to Reducing Smoking at the Worksite,* 1985, Office on Smoking and Health, Parklawn Building, 5600 Fishers Lane, Rockville, MD 20851; *Creating Your Company Policy,* 1985, American Lung Association local chapters or National Headquarters, American Lung Association, 1740 Broadway, New York, NY 10019; "Quit Smart Stop Smoking Kit," 1986, JB Press, P.O. Box 4843-H, Duke Station, Durham, NC 27706; *Freedom from Smoking in 20 Days* and *A Lifetime of Freedom 1980,* American Lung Association; *see* also video *Secondhand Smoke,* Pyramid Film & Video, Box 1948, Santa Monica, CA 90406-1048; S. Walton, "Other People's Smoke May Be Risky for You," News Report, National Research Council **XXXVII**, No. 1, 8–11, (Dec. 1986–Jan. 1987).

32. Anon., Company Pays Fines for Calif. Spill, *Occupational Safety and Health*, **56**, No. 1, 10 (1987).

33. Press Advisory, USEPA, Office of Public Affairs, 1, (July 7, 1986).

34. B. Burrough, S. H. Lubove, "Some Concerns Fudge Their Safety Records to Cut Insurance Costs," *Wall St. J.*, 1, 28 (Dec. 2, 1986) see also Anon. "Chrysler to Pay Record Penalty in OSHA Case," *Wall St. J.*, 7 (Feb. 2, 1987).

35. Anon., "Toxic Waste Poses Problems for Developers," *Washington Post*, E1, E4 (Feb. 22, 1987); see also S. Hankin, "Fear Dims Appeal of Old Offices," *Washington Post*, E1, E6, (Aug. 9, 1986), and M. Yancy, "U.S. Orders Tenfold Reduction in Worker Asbestos Exposure: OHSA Action Expected to Lower Death Toll," *Washington Post*, AS, (June 14, 1987), and W. Swallow, "Building Owners May Face Costly New Asbestos Rules; Pressure Grows to Remove Carcinogen," *Washington Post*, E1, (March 7, 1987) Anon., "Asbestos Suit Settled for $130 Million," *Occupational Health & Safety*, 9 (May 1986).

SUGGESTED READINGS

Legal and Regulatory

M. Abramowitz, "OSHA to Enforce AIDS Safety Rules: Health Facilities Can Be Fined if They Do Not Protect Workers," *Washington Post*, A12 (July 23, 1987).

D. Akst, "Waste Management Unit, 2 Other Firms Are Charged in California Antitrust Case," *Wall St. J.*, 16 (June 10, 1987).

M. Allen, "U.S. Companies Pay Increasing Attention to Destroying Files: The Ethics of Shredding," *Wall St. J.*, 1, 10 (Sept. 2, 1987).

American Chemical Society, "Informing Workers of Chemical Hazards: The OSHA Hazard Communication Standard, Task Force on Occupational Health and Safety," ACS, Washington, D.C., 14 pp. (April 1985).

American Law Institute–American Bar Asssociation Course of Study, Amrican Law Institute, 4025 Chestnut St., Philadelphia, PA 19104.

Anon., "Businessmen Convicted of Polluting Arkansas Dairy Products, Waterways with Carcinogenic Pesticide Heptachlor," Press Advisory, May 25, 1987, EPA, Washington, D.C.

Anon., "EPA Hit for Not Banning Chlordane Outright," *C&EN,* 6 (Aug. 31, 1987).

Anon., "First Criminal Conviction Under Safe Drinking Water Act," Press Advisory, May 25, 1987, EPA, Washington, D.C.

Anon., "Chemical Safety: Industry Dealing With Tighter Rules, *C&EN,* 4, 5 (Feb. 9, 1987).

Anon., "Court Rules Standards to Be Based on Health," *C&EN,* 6 (Aug. 3, 1987).

Anon., "Hazardous Materials: Right-to-Know News," biweekly, Thompson Publishing Group, Washington, D.C.

Anon., "New Requirements Governing Work in Confined Spaces on Vessels," *Industrial Hygiene News Rep., 29,* No. 10, 4 (Oct. 1986).

Anon., Southwest Air to Pay Fine of $402,000 Levied by U.S.," *Wall St. J.,* 4 (Feb. 11, 1987).

Anon., "Survey of State Ground-Water Quality Protection Legislation," 1985, available from Office to Ground-Water Protection (WH-550G), EPA, 401 M. St., Washington, DC.

Anon., "Syntex Agribusiness Is Named in Lawsuit in Dioxin Exposure," *Wall St. J.,* 14 (Feb. 11, 1987).

Anon., "Workplace Health Rules: OSHA Fines Chrysler Record Amount," *C&EN,* 4 (July 13, 1987).

Anon., "OSHA Proposes Expanded Hazard Communication Standard," *Occupational Health & Safety,* 22–23 (March 1987).

P. Brodeur, *Outrageous Misconduct: The Asbestos Industry on Trial,* Pantheon Books, New York, 1985.

M. W. Browne, "Chemists Suicide Rate Soars All Out of Proporation." *Dayton (Ohio) Daily News and Journal Herald,* 20 (Sept. 7, 1987).

W. A. Burgess, *Recognition of Health Hazards in Industry: A Review of Materials and Processes,* 275 pp., Wiley-Interscience, New York, 1981.

M. Casey, "U.S. E.P.A. Seeking $4.7 Million in Penalties from Four Refining Companies for Violations of the Lead phase-down regulations, May 26, 1987, *Environmental News,* EPA, Washington, D.C.

K. B. Clansky, *Chemical Guide to the OSHA Hazard Communication Standard, The Suspect Chemicals Sourcebook,* Roytech Publications, Burlingame, Calif., 1987.

G. D. Clayton and F. E. Clayton (eds.), *Patty's Industrial Hygiene and Toxicology,* 3rd ed., in five volumes, (approx. 6000 pp.), Wiley-Interscience, New York, 1978–1987.

J. F. DiMento, *Environmental Law and American Business,* Plenum Press, New York, 1986.

Editorial, "Inexorable Laws and the Ecosystem," *Science,* 3 (July 1987); see also Editorial, "Ice Minus and Job Minus," *Science,* 761 (May 15, 1987).

J. R. Emshwiller and E. White, "As Air Traffic Rises, So Does Difficulty of Tracking It All," *Wall St. J.,* 11, 20 (June 4, 1987).

H. H. Fawcett, "The OSHA Communication Standard or 'Right-to-Know,' " *J. Chem. Ed.,* **63,** A70–73 (March 1986).

H. H. Fawcett, "Safety: What Do We Really Mean?," *J. Chem. Ed.,* **58,**, No. 2, A45–48 (1981).

H. H. Fawcett, "An American View (of regulations)," pp. 585–598, in *Hazards in the Chemical Laboratory,* 4th ed., edited by L. Bretherick, Royal Society of Chemistry, London, 1986.

C. R. Goerth, "Legal Services Packages Benefit Workers and Employers," *Occupational Health & Safety,* 18 (May 1986).

P. B. Gray, "Under Fire: Regulators, the Courts, and Clients Bear Down on Lawyers, *Wall St. J.,* 17 (Aug. 21, 1987).

D. Hanson, "Academic Labs Face Compliance with Emergency Planning Rules," *C&EN,* 19–20 (May 18, 1987).

A. Heier, Registration of Pesticide EPN Voluntarily Cancelled, *EPA Press Advisory,* July 6, 1987, 1, 2, Environmental Protection Agency, Washington, DC 20460.

A. Heier, "Registrants of Captafol Pesticide Voluntarily Cancel Products, *EPA Press Advisory,* 2, 3, (July 6, 1987), Environmental Protection Agency, Washington, DC 20460.

E. Holtzman, "States Step in Where OSHA Fails to Tread," *Wall St. J.,* 36 (March 31, 1987).

C. Jendras, "U.S. E.P.A. Proposed $685,000 in Fines Against Nine Companies in New England for Violating Federal Regulations Designed to Protect People from Exposure to Toxic PCBs Released During Fires of PCB Electrical Equipment in Commercial Buildings, *Environmental News,* (May 26, 1987,) Environmental Protection Agency, New England Regional Office, Boston, Mass.

A. R. Karr, "OSHA Expands Scope of Requirement for Warnings of Hazardous Substances," *Wall St. J.,* 8 (Aug. 20, 1987).

A. R. Karr, "U.S. Tightens Benzene Rule for Workplace," *Wall St. J.,* 24 (Sept. 2, 1987).

A. R. Karr, "U.S. Proposes $2.6 Million Fine Against IBP," *Wall St. J.,* 1, 10 (July 22, 1987).

E. Marshall, "Woburn Case May Spark Explosion of Lawsuits," *Science,* 418–420 (Oct. 24, 1986).

R. K. Miller, "OSHA Compliance Strategies Decisions on Cost Benefit Analysis, *Occupational Health & Safety,* 18–22 (Apr. 1979).

K. Murphy, "Court Orders 13 Firms to Finance $100 M Mopup of Hazardous Wastes," *Wall St. J.,* 1 (June 8, 1987).

D. L. Ormond, Landfill, Incinerate or Recycle? What About Plastics in Municipal Solid Wastes, *Chem. Processing,* Oct. 1987, 8–12.

C. Rice, "EPA Announces Major Revisions of the National Clean Air Standards for Particulate Matter, Changing the Focus from Larger, Total Particles to Smaller, Inhalable Particles More Damaging to Human Health," *Environmental News,* EPA, 2–5 (June 3, 1987).

B. Richards, "Waste Management Faces More Inquiries," *Wall St. J.,* 6 (Sept. 28, 1987).

W. A. Rodgers, Jr., *"Environmental Law: Air and Water,* in two volumes, 1393 pp. West, St. Paul, Minn., 1986.

V. Royster, " 'Regulation' Isn't a Dirty Word," *Wall St. J.,* 32 (Sept. 9, 1987).

B. Siegel, "EPA Policy Choices, 'Managing' Risks: Sense and Science," *L.A. Times,* 1, 26, 27 (July 5, 1987).

E. Sussman, "Construction of Heavily Polluting Sites in 14 Municipalities to Be Barred by EPA," *Wall St. J.,* 36 (June 30, 1987).

R. E. Taylor, "EPA Plans to Require the Replacement of Many Storage Tanks Within 10 Years," *Wall St. J.,* 4 (Apr. 3, 1987).

C. Trost, "Shell Oil Is Cited by Labor Agency on Job-Safety Data," Wall St. J., 4 (Dec. 24, 1986) [$244,960 fine proposed)].

E. Thome, "Trade in Human Tissue Needs Regulation," *Wall St. J.,* 16 (Aug. 19, 1987).

W. K. Viscusi, "The Impact of Occupational Safety and Health Regulation," *Bell J. Eco.,* **10,** No. 1, 117–114, (Spring 1979).

R. K. Willard, "The Liability Crisis: The Government's Viewpoint," *Consulting Eng.,* **67,** No. 1, 36–38 (July 1986).

F. J. Weigert, "Ignorace No Excuse," *C&EN,* 3 (Aug. 31, 1987).

J. L. Wood, "Right-to-Know Laws: Maintaining Compliance," *Occupational Health & Safety,* 20–29 (March 1987).

Professional Ethics and Morals

R. Cahn, *An Environmental Agenda for the Future,* 155 pp., Island Press, Washington, D.C., 1986.

D. Chenoweth, "Personalized Incentives Influence Acceptance of Worksite Health Programs," *Occupational Health & Safety,* 39 (Nov. 1986).

T. D. Morgan and R. D. Rotunda, *Problems and Materials on Professional Responsibility,* 482 pp., The Foundation Press, Mineola, N.Y., 1984.

E. H. Morreim, "Physicians Face New Ethical Binds," *Wall St. J.,* 26 (Sept. 24, 1987).

R. Rhodes, *The Making of the Atomic Bomb,* 886 pp., Simon & Schuster, New York, 1987 (review in *Science,* 974–975 (May 22, 1987).

Health and Safety Aspects

Anon., "The Provisions of the Basic Safety Standards for Radiation Protection Relevant to the Protection of Workers Against Ionizing Radiation," *Occupational Health & Safety,* 23 (May 1985).

Anon., Is Your Job Dangerous to Your Health?" *U.S. News & World Rep.,* 39–42 (Feb. 1979).

N. A. Ashford, "Worker Health and Safety: An Area of Conflict," *Mgt. Rev.,* 52–57 (Feb. 1976).

AIChE, *International Symposium on Preventing Major Chemical Accidents,* 1018 pp., American Institute of Chemical Engineers, New York, 1987.

W. W. Allison, *"Profitable Risk Control—The Winning Edge,* American Society of Safety Engineers, Des Plains, Ill., 1986.

Anon., "New Requirements Governing Work in Confined Spaces on Vessels," *Ind. Hyg. News Rep.,* **29,** No. 10 (Oct. 1986).

Anon., *National Safety News,* monthly publication, National Safety Council, 444 N. Michigan Ave., Chicago, IL 60611.

G.R.C. Atherley, *Occupational Health and Safety Concepts: Chemical and Processing Hazards,* 408 pp., Applied Science Publishers, Ltd., Barking, Essex, England, 1978.

L. Bretherick, *Handbook of Reactive Chemical Hazards,* 3rd ed., 1852 pp., Butterworths, London, Boston, 1985.

D. Chenoweth, "Companies Use Rewards, Incentives to Promote Health and Safety," *Occupational Health & Safety,* 74–77 (Apr. 1987).

H. H. Fawcett and W. S. Wood (eds.,), *Safety and Accident Prevention in Chemical Operations,* 2nd ed., 910 pp., Wiley-Interscience, New York, 1982.

F. Forscher, "Understanding Risks," *Hazard Prevention,* **22,** No. 4, 26–28 (July/Aug. 1986).

C. F. Fuhrmann, Prescriptions, *"OTC* Drugs Affect Worker Performance Safety," *Occupational Health & Safety,* **55,** No. 12, 60–66 (Dec. 1986); see also *Drug Evaluations,* 6th ed., 1654 pp., American Medical Association, Chicago; M. Waldholz, "Prescription Drug Maker's Ad Stirs Debate Over Marketing to Public," *Wall St. J.* 35 (Sept. 22, 1987).

C. L. Gilmore, *Accident Prevention and Loss Control,* American Management Association, New York, 1986.

D. S. Gloss and M. G. Wardle, *Introduction to Safety Engineering,* John Wiley, New York, 1984.

J. V. Grimaldi, *Safety Management,* 5th ed., Irwin Press, Homewood, Ill., 1987.

C. R. DeReamer, *Modern Safety Practices,* 3rd ed., Wiley, New York, 1987.

A. W. Hayes, *Principles and Methods of Toxicology,* student ed., 750 pp., Raven Press, New York, 1984.

L. H. Keith and D. B. Walters, *Compendium of Safety Data Sheets for Research and Industrial Chemicals,* five vol., (approx. 3000 pp.), VCH Publishers, Deerfield Beach, Fla. 1985–1988.

W. Hammer, *Occupational Safety Management and Engineering,* 3rd ed., Prentice-Hall, Englewood Cliffs, N.J., 1985.

W. M. Kizer, *The Healthy Workplace: A Blueprint for Corporate Action,* 187 pp., Wiley, New York, 1987.

H. S. Kemp, "Process Safety—A Commitment?" *Chem. Eng. Prog.,* 46–7 (May 1987).

R. D. Kennedy, "Management and Safety," *C&EN,* 3 (Aug. 3, 1987).

J. E. Katzel, "Putting Personal Computers to Work in the Plant," *Plant Eng.* 40–45 (Apr. 24, 1986).

M. Krikorian, "Elements of a Plant Safety Program," *Plant Eng.*, 79–81 (May 22, 1986).

J. Lederiq, *The Nuclear Age,* 414 pp., Sodel, 1986, Publication by LeChene and distributed by Hachette, New York.

O. A. Martinez et al., "Damage to and Replacement of an Ammonia Storage Tank Foundation," *Plant/Operations Prog.,* **6,** No. 3, 129–141 (July 1987).

NAS-NRC, *Environmental Tobacco Smoke: Measuring Exposures and Assessing Health Effects,* 337 pp., National Academy Press, Washington, D.C., 1986.

D. Nelkin and M. S. Brown, *Workers at Risk: Voices from the Workplace,* 220 pp., University of Chicago Press, Chicago and London, 1984.

A. C. Nixon, *Professional Employee Protection, C&EN,* 3 (Apr. 21, 1986).

L. N. Marks, "OHN (Occupational Health Nurse) Can Provide Listening Ear Dealing with Employee's Problems," *Occupational Health & Safety,* 45–47 (May 1986).

G. D. Clayton and F. E. Clayton (eds.), *Patty's Industrial Hygiene and Toxicology,,* 3rd ed., in five vols., (approx. 6000 pp.), 1978–1987.

D. A. Pipitone, *Safe Storage of Laboratory Chemicals,* 280 pp., Wiley-Interscience, New York, 1984.

R. W. Prugh, "Guidelines for Vapor Release Mitigation," *Plant/Operations Prog.,* **6,** No. 3, 171–174 (66 ref.) July 1987).

G. O. Sofoluwe, "Occupational Health and Economic Development in African Countries," *Arch. Environ. Health,* 165–168 (Apr. 1973).

L. J. West, *Alcoholism and Related Problems: Issues for the American Public,* Prentice-Hall, Englewood Cliffs, N.J., 1984.

R. Sass, "Occupational Health and Saffety Contradictions and Conventional Wisdom," *Labour Gazette (U.K.),* 157–161 (Apr. 1977).

R. S. Smith, "Feasibility of an Injury Tax Approach to Occupational Safety," *Law & Contemporary Problems,* 730–744 (Summer–Autumn 1974). 1974

L. Slote, *Handbook of Occupational Safety and Health,* 744 pp., Wiley-Interscience, New York, 1987.

V. Steiner, "Assessing the Safety Climate of a Plant Yields Long-Term Benefits," *Plant Eng.,* 26–29 (Apri. 23, 1987).

W. E. Tarrants, *The Measurement of Safety Performance,* Garland STPM Press, New York, 1981.

R. J. Thomas, "A Proper Computer Program Can Enhance Health, Safety Practices," *Occupational Health & Safety,* 20–24 (May 1986).

H. G. Wittington, "Strengthening the Web and Net of Human Resource Conservation," *Occupational Health & Safety,* **52,** No. 9, 25–30 (Sept. 1983).

6
Fires and Explosions

Howard H. Fawcett

Fire is probably the oldest known chemical reaction, but the uncertainty and incompleteness of our understanding of this elementary force is only vaguely appreciated even today. This is true especially when one tries to relate materials to fire losses, deaths, and escape times, as well as to response to hazardous materials of unknown or incompletely known properties.

The nature and potential of the risk introduced by fire where chemicals and related materials are involved are still little appreciated outside fire-protection circles.

The potential for fire, explosion, decomposition, or pyrolysis is still not fully known for most materials and mixtures. Many chemical materials will burn or decompose; the redeeming feature is that all factors that are required to be present before a fire or explosion can occur are not usually there at the same time. On the other hand, *human failure,* such as puncturing an aerosol can to release a pesticide in an apartment house and thus releasing the propane propellant near an ignition source, has led to serious consequences and, in this case, losses amounting to approximately $300,000.[1]

In handling, reacting to, and disposing of flammable or combustible materials, either in processes or in waste, there are fundamentals involved that should be appreciated. In the United States, standards for such handling and storage have evolved from NFPA 30, and such standards are usually adopted by individual states.[2]

Housing and areas of other human exposure should be evaluated in terms of the degree of hazard and the quantity of materials encountered. Dr. Pape of ILO rates the relative fire hazards of flammable substances in increasing order: solids, liquids, liquefied gases, pressurized gases, and pressurized liquefied gases/superheated liquids. For assessment purposes, he suggests that people within a flame envelope may be assumed to be killed whereas those exposed to very intense radiant heat may be injured or killed if they cannot escape. People must be able to escape in a few seconds. A level of heat that allows many seconds to elapse between the onset of pain and the onset of injury is unlikely to be hazardous. The British Health and Safety Executive uses a level of 300 kilojoules per square meter exposure from a brief intense event as a criterion above which human exposure would be discouraged, but a lower level might be used for very vulnerable populations (such as elderly people). Dr. Pape, in discussing the effects of explosions produced by delayed ignition of flammable gas clouds or large accidental detonation of solids such as ammonium nitrate or sodium chlorate, noted that the consequences are assessed by comparison with the effects of standard TNT explosions, using a "TNT equivalent model." England uses 14-kPa overpressure as a criterion for advising against the construction of new housing.[3]

For disposal purposes, the Resources Conservation and Recovery Act (RCRA) definitions use the term "ignitability," which means:

1. For liquids, as a material having a flash point less than 60°C (140°F) by specified methods.
2. For nonliquids, as a material capable of ignition under normal conditions of spontaneous and sustained combustion;
3. For an ignitable compressed gas, per Department of Transportation regulations, and/or
4. For an oxidizer, per Department of Transportation regulations. The EPA hazard code for ignitability is "I" with EPA hazardous-waste number D001.

In addition to ignitability, another very important consideration from a fire and explosion viewpoint is "reactivity." The EPA defines this characteristic in terms of:

Normally unstable—reacts violently.

Reacts violently with water.

Forms explosive mixtures with water.

When mixed with water, generates toxic gases, vapors, or fumes.

Contains cyanide or sulfide and generates toxic gases, vapors, or fumes at a pH between 2 and 12.5.

Capable of detonation if heated in confinement or subjected to strong initiating source.

Capable of detonation at standard temperature and pressure.

Listed by Department of Transportation as class A or class B explosive.

Reactive materials have been assigned the EPA hazardous-waste number D003.

Regardless of the terms used, the fundamentals of ignition must be understood by prudent persons who handle or dispose of chemicals. Even then, care must taken at all times; if, as occurred on November 1, 1985, a chemist transferred a flammable liquid from one container to another at 3:00 A.M., we cannot ignore the necessity for electric bonding (British usage: "earthing") between the two metal containers. The resulting flash fire from the static ignition produced fatal consequences.

It must never be forgotten that fire is combustion or oxidation at a rate fast enough to produce heat, and usually light. The speed of the reaction differs widely between "smoldering" and "detonation."

For a fire to be sustained, four essentials, or "legs," are necessary:

1. A fuel (solid, liquid, or gas in a proper degree of dispersion or subdivision).
2. Oxygen or other oxidizers (such as the halogens and nitrogen oxides).
3. An ignition source (usually a flame, spark, or hot element).
4. A chain reaction, which permits the energy of combustion to be transferred to product additional available fuel.

Since many hazardous wastes are liquids, or are easily liquefied or volatized, the classification as outlined by the NFPA 321 may be of interest.

FLAMMABLE LIQUIDS

Class IA is defined as having a flash point below 73°F (22.8°C) and a boiling point below 100°F (37.8°C).

Class IB is defined as having a flash point below 73°F (22.8°C) and a boiling point at or above 100°F (37.8°C).

Class IC is defined as having a flash point at or above 73 F (22.8°C) and below 100°F (37.8°C). (Figure 6.1 illustrates the real world definitions when more than one commodity is carried; Figure 6.2 how placards hardly protect.

COMBUSTIBLE LIQUIDS

Class II is defined as having a flash point at or above 100°F (37.8°C) and below 140°F (60°C).

Class IIIA is defined as having a flash point at or above 140°F (60°C) and below 200°F (93.4°C).

Class IIIB is defined as having a flash point at or above 200°F (93.4°C).

Flash point, the temperature at which the vapors directly over the surface of a liquid will flash or ignite, can be determined by several procedures and forms of apparatus, as specified by the standards and practices of the American Society for Testing and Materials (ASTM). Fire point, sometimes referred to, is usually a few degrees higher than the flash point, and is the temperature at which the flash fire will continue to burn. (For a more complete understanding of these tests and procedures, the reader should refer to the publications of the NFPA, Batterymarch Park, Quincy, MA 02269.)

Harry A. Wray, chair emeritus of the ASTM Coordinating Committee on Flash Point, has contributed the following background information on various attempts to standardize on flash-point methods and determinations.

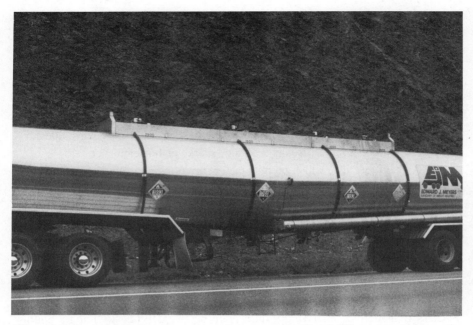

Figure 6.1. Road tank truck may carry more than one commodity of different hazard classes; the "real-world confusion" is understandable.

The flash point of a liquid is one of the properties that defines its flammability, and thus its hazard characteristics. Among the other properties that are useful in this respect are the lower and upper flammable limits (LFL/UFL) and the autoignition temperature (AIT).

One of the important functions of flash point is to define classes of flammable liquids for use in governmental regulations. In the late 19th century, a rash of house fires in England and the United States was attributed to the adulteration of the kerosene used for light and heat. Petroleum light ends (gasoline) were used to extend the kerosene. These fires resulted in a demand for regulations together with the necessary methods to control the sale of kerosene. Flash-point methods and apparatus were developed to determine the extent of the adulteration. The first method to be developed was the open-cup test, in which a liquid was heated in an open vessel and the minimum temperature determined at which the vapor of the liquid would ignite when a small flame was passed over the liquid's surface. Shortly thereafter, England established by law the Abel closed-cup method for control of flammable liquids. In the United States, open-cup methods continued to be used by federal agencies until the early 1970s. Meanwhile, the NFPA adopted for its Code 30 closed-cup methods to classify liquids as flammable and combustible.

Upon passage of the Occupational Safety and Health Act in 1970, the OSHA included in its regulations controlling the use of flammable liquids in the workplace the NFPA's Classification System. Thus OSHA became the first U.S. regulatory

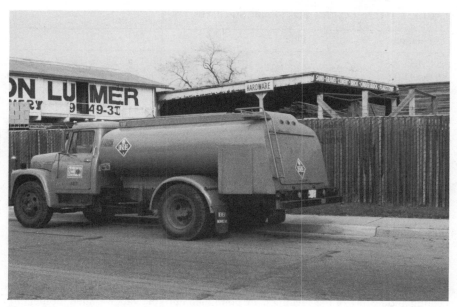

Figure 6.2. Gasoline truck parked near lumber yard, where fire potential is high. Truck belongs to county government.

agency to adopt closed-cup methods for the control of flammable liquids. In 1976, the U.S. Department of Transportation adopted the use of the closed-cup method in its regulations. Following the establishment of the EPA, closed-cup methods were permitted and are now required in regulations for solid waste. Finally, in 1986, the U.S. Consumer Products Safety Commission established a closed-cup method to become effective in 1987 to regulate the labeling of consumer products.

The open-cup methods continue to be specified to a minor extent in some U.S. regulations. In addition, the Cleveland open-cup method is used extensively throughout the world to determine the flash point of high-flash-point materials, such as oils, coal tar, and asphalt products.

At the present time, the major open-cup methods are those using the Cleveland open cup and the Tag open-cup apparatus. The closed-cup methods use the following equipment: (1) the Abel closed-cup apparatus, (2) the Tag closed-cup tester, (3) the Pensky-Martens closed-cup apparatus, and (4) the Setaflash (rapid tester) closed-cup apparatus. The French test, using the Luchaine apparatus, is employed in a number of countries. Table 6.1 lists the present U.S. flash-point methods with their ASTM designations and titles.

Flash point is now defined as follows: the lowest temperature corrected to a pressure of 760 mmHg (101.3 kPa or 1013 mbar), at which the application of an ignition source causes the vapor of a specimen to ignite.

In each of the standard flash-point methods, except for the Setaflash method, the liquid is heated in a cup at a specified rate with or without stirring. At specified

TABLE 6.1 U.S. (ASTM) Flash-Point Standards

Designation	Title
ASTM D-56	Test Method for Flash Point by Tag Closed Tester
ASTM D-92	Test Method for Flash and Fire Points by Cleveland Open Cup
ASTM-D-93	Test Method for Flash Point by Pensky-Martens Closed Tester
ASTM-D-1310	Test Method for Flash and Fire Points of Liquids by Tag Open Cup Apparatus
ASTM-D-3278	Test Method for Flash Point by Setaflash Closed Tester
ASTM-D-3934	Test Method for Flash/No Flash Test Equilibrium Method by a Closed Cup Apparatus
ASTM-D-3941	Test Method for Flash Point by the Equilibrium Method with a Closed Cup Apparatus

temperature intervals, a small flame is passed either over the open cup filled with the liquid specimen or into the vapor space above the liquid in a closed cup. This heating and testing of the specimen are continued until the vapor ignited momentarily and a flame spreads across the surface of the liquid.

In the flash/no-flash Setaflash method, the specimen is heated to a specified temperature, such as a classification temperature in a government regulation or in a product specification, and held there for one minute. The test flame is then inserted into the vapor space to determine whether or not it will flash. If the actual flash point is desired, an estimated flash point is used as the specified temperature. Depending on whether the material flashes or not, a new specimen is tested at a higher or lower temperature. This is continued with new speciments until the flash point is determined to the nearest 0.5°C (1°F).

These Setaflash methods are considered equilibrium methods as they test the material when the temperature of the vapor above the liquid is at approximate equilibrium with the liquid in the cup and is the same throughout the liquid. Equilibrium conditions assure a more accurate flash point than that obtained with the other standard methods. In order to approach equilibrium conditions using present standard cups, such as the Tag closed cup, the International Standards Organization (ISO) has developed two methods, of which the ASTM counterparts are ASTM D-3934 and ASTM D-3941.

To define further the hazards of mixtures of liquids that may have a closed-cup flash point in the flammable range but will not sustain combustion, ASTM has developed two additional methods: ASTM 4206, Standard Test Method for Sustained Burning of Liquid Mixtures by the Setaflash Apparatus (Open Cup), and ASTM D-4207, Standard Test Method for Sustained Buring of Low Viscosity Liquid Mixtures by the Wick Test.

While U.S. agencies have not established regulations using these methods, England has been using the Setaflash sustained burning test since 1972 to control mixtures.

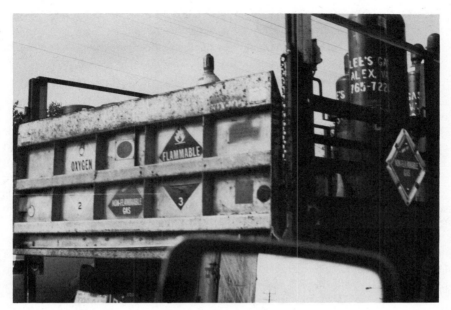

Figure 6.3. Meaningless confusion when truck carries several gases. Placards tend to conflict rather than help.

One of the most interesting developments in the Regulations on the Transportation of Hazardous Goods, including flammable liquids, is the issuance of the "Transport of Dangerous Goods, Recommendations of the United Nations Committee of Experts on the Transportation of Dangerous Goods." These recommendations do not have the effect of regulations, but international regulatory bodies, such as the International Civil Aviation Organization and the International Maritime Organization, have adopted these recommendations as their regulations for their mode of transportation. They also have been adopted by many nations. The Department of Transportation has permitted the transshipment of dangerous goods through the United States to other countries by air or sea under these international rules.

In cooperation with the Dept. of Transportation and the UN Group of Experts on Explosives, the Bureau of Mines has been conducting research on the development of tests designed to determine whether a substance has explosive properties. These tests are currently under consideration for international standardization, and are called the Bureau of Mines Gap Test and Internal Ignition Test. The Bureau of Mines has proposed that these tests are suitable to determine the properties described in 40 CFR 261, Subpart C, "Characteristics of Hazardous Waste," in particular, paragraphs 261.23(a)(6) and (7), "Characteristic of Reactivity," which defines a solid waste as having the characteristics of reactivity if it has, among others, any of the following properties. It is:

(a)(6) Capable of detonation or explosive reaction if subjected to a strong initiation source, or if heated under confinement;

(a)(7) Readily capable of detonation or explosive decomposition or reaction at standard temperature and pressure.

The EPA has tentatively adopted the tests as suitable for evaluating the explosive reactivity of solid wastes. This report provides descriptions and procedures for these two tests.

The Bureau of Mines also conducts testing on new explosives and recommends classifications to the Department of Transportation as detailed in 49 CFR, part 173.86 (b). This testing satisfies the requirements of 40 CFR, part 263.23 (a)(8), which states that a solid waste must be considered hazardous if it is a forbidden explosive, a Class A explosive, or a Class B explosive. Further information on this subject may be obtained from John N. Murphy, Research Director, Pittsburgh Research Center, (412) 675-6602, or Richard Mainiero, (412) 675-6636.

Also refer to Transport of Dangerous Goods (a Compilation of the Recommendations Prepared by the United Nations Committee of Experts on the Transport of Dangerous Goods), "International Regulations Publishing and Distributing Organization, Chicago, Ill. 1981.[3]

Metal dusts are also an important hazard, as noted in Table 6.2.

Air, which is the usual oxidant in most fires, supports combustion readily but at a controlled rate. When the oxygen percentage in air is increased even a few percent, the rate of burning increases radically, and great danger can be encountered. Other oxidizing agents include chlorine, fluorine, ozone, nitrogen oxides, the interhalogens (such as ClF_3 and other substances containing oxygen, including $KMnO_4$, $K_2Cr_2O_7$), the chlorates, perchloric acid, and the perchlorates. All may be found in waste sites, alone or in combinations.

The third aspect of liquid or gas flammability—namely, the necessity for the liquid or gas to be either in a mist or within the "flammable" range (sometimes referred to as the "explosive" range)—is the salvation in many situations since, unless the lower flammable limit is present in air, ignition and burning are not possible. For materials that are highly volatile, such as the ethers, acetone, benzene, and naphthas, the lower flammable limit (known as LFL) is present over the surface under normal conditions. The application of an ignition source of sufficient energy, plus the ambient air, then supplies all the essentials for a fire, which, once the chain reaction occurs, is self-sustaining. If, on the other hand, the conditions are "too rich" to burn, by the substance being above the "upper flammable limit" (or UFL), fire is not possible, but becomes very real when the vapor or gas is diluted to within the flammable range (which can easily occur from air movements or other agitation).

For some substances, such as diborane, ethylene oxide, and hydrogen, the flammable range is wide, while for other substances, such as toluene and motor-fuel-grade commercial gasoline, the range may be only a few percent. (Figure 6.4 presents typical values for flammable ranges of common chemicals.)

For additional values, consult the publications of the NFPA; Appendix 1, pp. 865–875 of *Safety and Accident Prevention in Chemical Operations,* 2nd ed.,

TABLE 6.2 Metal-Dust Explosions

	U.S. Sieve No.
Aluminum, atomized, MD 101, jet atomized	90%—200
Aluminum, atomized MD 101, cold air atomized	96%—200
Aluminum, atomized, MD 101	96%—200
Aluminum, atomized R 120	96%—200
Aluminum, atomized, AA 101	85%—325
Aluminum, atomized, AA 140	100%—325
Aluminum, atomized	100%—400
Aluminum, grained	80%—200
Aluminum, stamped, AA 322, 2.75% stearic acid	95%—325
Aluminum, stamped, AA 522, 1.0% oleic acid	97%—325
Aluminum, stamped, AA 408, 3.0% stearic acid	99%—325
Aluminum, stamped, AA 422	100%—325
Aluminum, stamped, AA 422 4.25 stearic acid	100%—325
Aluminum-cobalt, 60% Al-40% Co	89%—325
Aluminum-copper, 50% Al-50% Cu	100%—325
Aluminum-nickel, 58% Al-42% Ni	84%—325
Aluminum-nickel, 50% Al-50% Ni	88%—325
Antimony, MD 101	100%—200
Boron, amorphous, 85% B	100%—400
Calcium silicide	71%—200
Chromium, electrolytic, milled	100%—325
Iron, carbon reduced, 100A	61%—200
Iron, carbon reduced, 300A	94%—200
Iron, carbon reduced, 300A plus C	100%—200
Iron, carbonyl	99%—270
Iron, electrolytic, annealed	100%—325
Iron, hydrogen reduced	100%—325
Iron, sponge, unannealed	100%—200
Ferrochromium, high carbon, 69% Cr	95%—325
Ferromanganese, medium carbon, 83% Mn	100%—325
Ferrosilicon, 83% Si	100%—200
Ferrosilicon, 85% Si	100%—200
Ferrosilicon, 88% Si	92%—325
Ferrosilicon 94% Si	100%—200
Ferrotitanium, low carbon, 19% Ti	85%—325
Ferrovanadium, crucible grade, 40% V	92%—325
Magnesium, atomized, grade 3	21%—200
Magnesium, atomized, grade 5	100%—200
Magnesium, milled, grade C	1%—200
Magnesium, milled, grade A	15%—200
Magnesium, milled, grade B	87%—200
Magnesium, milled	92%—200
Magnesium, milled, grade B	93%—200
Magnesium, stamped, grade A	20%—200
Magnesium, stamped, grade B	93%—200

TABLE 6.2 *(Continued)*

	U.S. Sieve No.
Magnesium-aluminum (50% Mg-50% Al)	82%—200
Magnesium-aluminum (Dow metal)	100%—325
Manganese, electrolytic	100%—200
Manganese	93%—200
Silicon, milled, 98% Si	100%—200
Silicon, milled	86%—270
Tin, atomized	97%—270
Thorium, 99% Th	100%—400
Thorium hydride, 98% Th	100%—400
Titanium, 97% Ti	100%—200
Titanium, 96% Ti	100%—325
Titanium, copper coated, 88% Ti-7%Cu	100%—325
Titanium hydride, 97% Ti	100%—325
Titanium hydride, 95% Ti	96%—325
Titanium, plant dust, 85% metallic material	90%—200
Uranium	100%—325
Uranium hydride	100%—400
Vanadium, 86% V	100%—200
Zinc, 91% Zn	100%—200
Zinc, technical grade, 95% Zn	100%—200
Zinc	99%—270
Zinc, 97% Zn	95%—325
Zinc, 96% Zn	99%—325
Zirconium, 97% Zr	100%—325
Zirconium, 99% Zr	100%—325
Zirconium, copper-coated, 91%Zr-4%Cu	100%—325
Zirconium hydride, 94% Zr	96%—325
Zirconium hydride, 97% Zr	100%—325
Zircaloy, mechanically attrited	65%—200
Zircaloy, hydride-dehydrided	100%—200

Source: J. Negy, H. G. Dorsett, and Murray Jacobson, *Preventing Ignition of Dust Dispersions by Inerting,* Bureau of Mines, R.I.; See also B. L. Bronson, "Precautions Needed to Prevent Aluminum Dust Explosions," *Occupational Health & Safety,* 39–43 (Sept. 1986).

edited by H. H. Fawcett, Wiley-Interscience, New York, 1982; publications of the U.S. Bureau of Mines; local insurance carriers, such as Factory Mutuals or the Factory Insurance Association; local or state fire marshal's office; the MSDSs required under the OSHA Hazard Communication Rule, or right-to-know laws; or the supplier.

If any hint or suspicion exists that a flammable gas or vapor is present or being evolved, a survey with a portable gas detector is in order. Most fire departments have these devices and will lend them or make surveys on request. The recom-

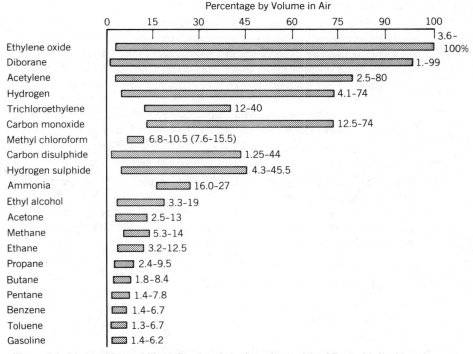

Figure 6.4. Limits of flammability define the relative hazard potentials of flammable liquids and gases.

mendations of the National Safety Council Chemical Section "Safety and Health Information Sheet" (CHM 83-1, Aug. 1983) should be useful.

"The information sheet discusses the two basic types of instruments—aspirated or nonaspirated (diffusion). Aspiration can be manual, using a squeeze bulb, or can use an electric pump. Some nonaspirated types have the capability for aspiration as an added feature. The detector is usually a catalytic element that is part of a Wheatstone bridge electrical circuit. The gas to be tested is brought to the detector by aspiration or diffusion, depending upon the type of instrument. If the gas is flammable, it will react with the catalytic element, producing a change in the electrical resistance, which will then produce a deflection in the instrument meter. The meter reads in percentages of the lower flammable limit (or LFL). The instrument is calibrated with a known flammable gas, such as methane. It should be recalibrated on a schedule, such as once or twice a month, to detect changes in the instrument which could give inaccurate results.

"To use the instrument, the following steps are recommended:

"1. Read and understand the instrument manufacturer's instructions.

"2. Be certain the instrument has been recently recalibrated or within the scheduled time for recalibration.

"3. "Zero" the instrument in clean (uncontaminated) air.

"4. Size up the sampling job by asking such questions as: What flammables are likely to be present? How can a representative sample of the atmosphere be obtained? It must be appreciated that most vapors are heavier than air and tend to 'pocket' or seek lower areas. This is especially true when investigating tanks and other enclosed spaces (See T. A. Kletz, 'Hazards in Chemical Systems Maintenance: Permits,' pp 807–836, and "Safe Handling of Flammable and Combustible Materials," pp. 339–356 in *Safety and Accident Prevention in Chemical Operations,* 2nd ed., edited by H. H. Fawcett and W. S. Wood, Wiley-Interscience, New York, 1982.)

"5. If ventilation is in use, sample with it both off and on,

"6. Watch the instrument meter at all times during the sampling, since a rich mixture may cause a momentary positive reading that may then drop back to zero as the oxygen inside the meter is consumed. Unless the instrument operator saw this momentary meter deflection, he or she might assume incorrectly that the atmosphere was safe.

"Some pitfalls to avoid include "real-world aspects":

"1. Failing to recalibrate an instrument on a scheduled basis with records to back up the recalibration.

"2. Failing to obtain a representative sample of the atmosphere.

"3. Sampling an atmosphere that would damage the instrument or detector, such as atmospheres containing acid, lead, or silicones.

"4. Permitting liquid or condensate to enter the instrument or contact the detector. This can result in inaccurate readings or seriously damage the detector. Sampling close to a liquid surface, sampling an atmosphere containing steam, or sampling a hot atmosphere containing condensable vapors is to be avoided.

"The following must be considered if results are to be properly interpreted. since the instrument is calibrated on a known flammable gas, other flammable gases and vapors with different molecular weights can often give significantly different readings. Consequently, unless the flammable gas in the atmosphere being sampled is the same as the calibration gas, the meter reading may not be correct. The meter reading can also be very sensitive to how the instrument is operated. Thus, meter readings should be regarded only as estimates, and should be repeated several times to ensure better and more accurate readings. For additional precautions where "hot work" or confined-space entry work is involved, the recommendations of persons skilled in the use of such instruments should be taken very seriously. In general, if readings above 10 percent of the LFL are obtained, hot work or tank or vessel entry would be very unwise, if not dangerous.

"It should be noted that some detectors for flammable materials also may be recalibrated for use as industrial hygiene survey instruments, with a different range on the meter. Most reputable instrument manufacturers can recommend the particular instrument most suitable to the applications that may be anticipated."

In addition to the "hot wire" type of instrument described above, thermal conductivity, diffusion rate, specific gravity, and infrared spectrum instruments are coming into use, and may find applications in surveys and investigations.

The growing use of plastic containers, which are much less costly than approved metal "safety cans," introduces another problem in control not previously noted. When safety cans, with their all-metal construction, and frequently with a flame arrester (a metal screen that prevents flame flash either into or from the can), were standard, considerable security was present. When exposed to fire, of course, the plastic containers tend to soften or melt, releasing the contents into the fire. When disposed of in a landfill, plastic containers are more likely to puncture from careless handling. The self-closing top on metal safety cans also acts as an additional safeguard. As a minimum, plastic containers can be surrounded by a metal can or other metal shielding to protect them from accidental puncture.

SELF-IGNITION

3M Engineering Analyst, Ltd., 103 N. 4th Avenue, St. Charles, IL 60174-2017, notes that self-ignition is also possible even in the absence of a conventional ignition source. Fire originates from one of two thermodynamic situations involving heat energy: (1) the application of heat energy from outside the mass of material, or (2) self-heating of a material by its own inherent energy, leading to ignition. Whenever a material absorbs or generates heat energy at a rate faster than the energy can be dissipated to the surrounding atmosphere, heat will accumulate within the material and ignition will occur.

Spontaneous combustion (ignition) involves contaminated materials and materials subjected to bacterial action. Autoignition is an ignition that occurs by application of heat to a material without the application of open flame or spark. Self-ignition, on the other hand, involves clean, dry, uncontaminated materials. A self-ignition reaction is always recognized by a cavity near the center of a pile of material.

The initiation of combustion or explosion of a fuel and oxidizer is described as the ignition process. Because of the large variation in the combustion characteristics of fuels and oxidizers, and the variations in ambient conditions, the ignition process will assume a variety of formms. The ignition reaction is a complex process involving chain reactions that cannot be briefly explained. Each step in the chain reaction is dependent upon completion of the previous step in the chain for completion of the combustion process.

Two main factors are necessary for self-ignition to occur. The material must be sufficiently porous to permit oxygen to permeate the mass. When ignition takes place, the material must produce a rigid char that will support the weight of the mass. Other considerations that affect the possibility of self-heating and self-ignition are the ambient atmospheric temperature, the length of time the mass is exposed to the self-heating conditions, and the size of the mass.

Ventilation of the material must be adequate to allow for penetration of oxygen to the area where self-heating is found. Without oxygen, no ignition or combustion will occur. Too much ventilation will allow the heat generated to be rapidly dissipated to the surrounding mass and then to the atmosphere, thus preventing accumulation of heat within the mass of material.

When ignition takes place, the material begins to produce char and to liberate heat. If the char is rigid, the integrity of the mass is retained and smoldering combustion can continue. If the char is not rigid, the mass of material may collapse on itself and smother the combustion reaction by excluding oxygen from the combustion zone.

The rate of heat transfer is determined by the difference in temperature between the hot body and the cooler body. The greater the difference in temperature between the two bodies, the greater will be the rate of heat transfer. Therefore, the cooler the air mass surrounding the self-heating material, the greater will be the rate of heat transfer from the material to the surrounding atmosphere. This lessens the possibility of self-heating leading to self-ignition.

The length of time a material is exposed to conditions that would allow self-heating is critical. Self-heating reactions may take months to reach ignition of the material. Usually, a material must be exposed to the self-heating phenomenon for an extended time before ignition occurs.

The self-ignition phenomenon is usually associated with large masses of material such as coal piles, sawdust heaps, cotton bales, cordage, or stacks of petroleum-based insulation materials. A smaller mass may self-heat and ignite under favorable conditions. Ignition occurs deep within the mass at the geometric center where the effects of self-heating are the greatest. Smoldering combustion develops at the point of the greatest heat concentration and propagates slowly outward to the surface of the mass, where flaming combustion develops. (March 1987, used by permission of H. S. Morton, P. E.)

Unsupported compressed gas cylinders represent a serious explosion/fire hazard (Figure 6.5).

Open-pit burning was the commonly accepted disposal method for waste solvents and other common wastes until about 1960, when the importance of air pollution controls began to be noted in state and local ordinances. For many locations, the pits were used both to evaporate liquids and as a training ground for local fire brigades to practice extinguishment and control. Such open-pit burning has been outlawed by the Clean Air Act and other laws.

In view of the deemphasis on landfills, especially for liquid wastes, it is hoped that more attention will be given to the design and construction of incinerators on site, which will eliminate the costly transport and handling problems encountered at present.

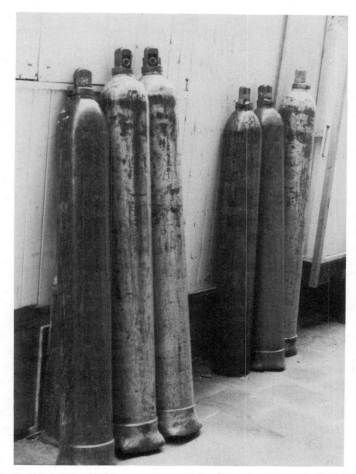

Figure 6.5. Careless handling of acetylene and oxygen cylinders at a construction site in The Nether-lands, April 1987, suggests the potential explosion/fire danger is still not widely appreciated. (Photo by H. Fawcett.)

RIGHT-TO-KNOW

The extreme importance of knowing what exactly is involved in any emergency, including fires, spills, or human exposures, so that intelligent and prompt action can be taken, has now been recognized not only by the OSHA Hazard Communication Regulation[4] but by several state laws as well. Included in the items required for compliance in the MSDSs are the flammable limits, the extinguishing agents recommended, and other data that will aid in control of the materials. In some states, the owner or manager of the establishment is required to file a list of these hazardous materials with the local fire department so the responders will have updated information immediately available on which to base intelligent and prompt action. Expanded use and applications of the NFPA 704-M Hazard Information Marking (which makes visible to emergency personnel on first approach at least the degree and severity of the potential danger they face with respect to fire, health risk, reactivity, and radioactivity, and whether or not the contents are water compatabile) would be a very significant addition to the safeguards for life and property.[5] (See also Chapter 4, Title III.)

RESPONSE TO CHEMICAL AND RELATED EMERGENCIES

Over the years, fire departments have evolved procedures and equipment designed and dedicated to "ordinary" or "normal" hazards. The introduction of thousands of chemicals, either alone or in mixtures and compounds, into the workplace, the home, the highways, the railroads, pipelines, waterways, and air and sea transport has created the necessity for a much expanded awareness of the necessity for proper and adequate training and a knowledge base for emergency response personnel, as well as for normal operations. Fire personnel must be alerted to the potential dangers both to themselves and to the general public. Taking cues from, among many, the 1976 Seveso, Italy, catastrophe, where a white aerosol cloud carried a reaction mixture of trichlorophenol and other chemicals including TCDD, that contaminated an area of approximately 320 hectares, the 1984 Bhopal, India, release of a chemical pesticide reaction product; the 1986 Chernobyl, Russia, nuclear reactor explosion that released radioactive fallout over most of the northern hemisphere, and the 1986 Miamisburg, Ohio train derailment where the delay in communications doubtlessly played a factor in the control of the white phosphorous fire, it is now recognized that state and local emergency planning committees must take an active role in chemically related problems. The recent action of the federal government, in which the emergency planning was included as part of the reauthorized Superfund 1986, involves extensive requirements for industry to report on routine releases of hazardous substances to the environment, and must also provide local governments with information about the chemicals kept on-site and their health hazards. Unfortunately, no financial aid was extended to local groups to implement this planning. As Barbara Sonnengerg of the Memphis City Council and chair of the National Hazardous Materials Transportation Advisory Committee has said: "This leaves local governments being asked to do one more thing, among many things, that Washington wants done without the assistance of federal funds."

In most communities, the planning will be by ad hoc organizations with minimal staff of their own or staff on loan from some other community agency. It has been noted that most local governments are not very well prepared for hazardous-materials incidents and need financial help for planning and training. The effect is that if an incident occurs in their jurisdiction, owing to their inadequate training the response can be mishandled, resulting in a serious problem. The cost of training is a significant factor, particularly in smaller communities. Tuition for a course in handling train derailments at the American Association of Railroads' training facility is $600 per person, which, when coupled with the cost of transportation and room and board, is more than $1000 and most fire departments do not have budgets that can accommodate many training activities of that magnitude. Another aspect is that the local government is paying to protect its citizens from a risk from which they derive no benefit. Chief Mulligan of Fort Collins, Colo., estimates that 25 percent of the hazardous materials passing through Colorado pass through Fort Collins, and yet only 3 percent originate or are destined for there. The result is that Fort Collins has to prepare itself for an emergency response to deal with materials benefiting other communities, not its citizens.

Because of the interstate nature of hazardous-material shipments, the problem is a national one, needing a national perspective and national assistance for local responders.[6] It should be noted that the problem also is international, since the safe movement of dangerous goods (hazardous materials) by waterways and the sea is also important, especially to ports on the inland waterways, oceans, and gulfs. The Ninth International Symposium on the Transport and Handling of Dangerous Goods by Sea and Inland Waterways was held April 13–17, 1987, in Rotterdam, the Netherlands; its proceedings reflect the international concerns in chemical hazard control in water transport.[7]

Already much progress has been made in the training process on a local level. Fire fighters in the Rockland County Fire Training Center in New York recently learned a new meaning for the term "hands-on training," when they practiced their strategies by utilizing a tabletop simulation that featured scaled-down models of structures and apparatus. Giving fire fighters a panoramic view of a community and its hazards at a glance, the simulation presents a variety of fire-fighting challengers in a minimum of space. Sponsored jointly by the center and the County Fire Chiefs' Association, and coordinated by George Proper, Jr., of Proper Fire Tech Associates, the tabletop simulation training seminar was one in a series of daylong presentations offered at the center to supplement the skills of local instructors and to upgrade the level of suppression services. As Proper notes, the spatial relationships developed by the training remind us that fire fighting is a three-dimensional process. The hazards portrayed include an occupied hotel, a rural dairy farm, a petroleum-storage facility, a shopping mall lacking hydrants, and tractor-trailers transporting hazardous materials.[8]

Progress is also being made in understanding the control measures for hazardous-material spills. Some 1000 gallons of hydrofluoric acid was spilled in a test at the Nevada Test Site to evaluate spills of this material, and the vapors were monitored to trace the movement of the cloud. These tests, the first of a series at a Department of Energy facility, will give user companies a real-life simulation of how far a cloud could travel before diluting to a harmless concentration. Such information could be used in new plant design and development of emergency management procedures, and was funded by Amoco Corporation.[9]

Another bright spot in the darkness of emergency control is the recent announcement by the National Chemical Response and Information Center of the Hazard Information Transmission (HIT) program, which was developed for fire and police departments. This permits the transmission of hard-copy report to aid the first responder in making a positive identification, by allowing a direct comparison of the information at the scene to the report. The electronic transmission should speed the relay of emergency information because it will not have to be relayed through a dispatcher. The report, prepared promptly in response to a request by phone, is generated in the CHEMTREC computer. It is transmitted to the receiving site via telephone lines, where it is captured by modem and printer and/or personal computer.[10]

Other data bases are becoming available on a commercial basis. Listed in the following are a few of the recently announced chemical data bases for computer software:

CHEMTRAK integrated software chemical information data, Information Dimensions, Inc.
655 Metro Place South, Dublin, OH 43017-1396
(614) 761-8083 or -7300
(mainframe, minis)

BRS Information Technologies
1200 Route 7, Latham, NY 12110
(518) 783-1161
(on-line service)

Carlton Industries, Inc.
P.O. Box 280, LaGrange, TX 78945
(800) 231-5988
(various systems)

Chem Service, Inc.
660 Tower Lane, P.O. Box 3108,
West Chester, PA 19381-3108
(215) 692-3026
(MSDS PC version 3.0 12/20/86 on double-sided 360K diskette for use on IBM PC compatible system using MS-DOS or PC-DOS version 2.0 or later)

Clough Management Services, Mitimite Software Division
P.O. Box 625, Rouses Point, NY 12979-0625
(518) 298-4350
(various systems)

CIS User Support, Computer Sciences Corp.
6565 Arlington Boulevard, Falls Church, VA 22046
800-368-3432
(on-line services)

Healthcare Services, Occupational Health Management Program
Control Data Corp., P. O. Box 0, Minneapolis, MN 55440
(612) 853-7777
(mainframe)

Digital Equipment Corp., Medical Systems Group
Two Iron Way, P.O. Box 1003, Marlboro, MA 01752
(617) 467-2369
(various systems)

ERM Computer Services, Inc.
999 West Chester Pike, West Chester, PA 19382
(215) 696-9110
(micro)

Fisher Scientific
711 Forbes Avenue, Pittsburgh, PA 15219
(412) 562-8468
(micro)

Flow General, Inc.
7655 Old Springhouse Road, McLean, VA 22102
(703) 893-5915
(time sharing, various systems)

Genium Publishing Corp.
1145 Catalyn Street, Schenectady, NY 12303-1836
(518) 377-8854
(micro)

Hawkwa Group, Inc.
P.O. Box 321, Mundelein, IL 60060
(312) 949-8488
(micro)

Hazox Data Systems, Inc.
15066 Los Gatos-Almeden Road, Los Gatos, CA 95030
(408) 559-0303
(micro)

ICI Information Consultants, Inc.
1133 15th Street, N.W., Suite 300, Washington, DC 20005
(202) 822-5200
(on-line service)

Icotech
Route 202, Raritan, NJ 08869
(201) 685-3400
(time sharing)

Marcom Group, Ltd
no. 4 Denny Road, Suite 22, Wilmington, DE 19809
(302) 764-3400
(micro)

National Safety Council
444 N. Michigan Avenue, Chicago, IL 60611
(312) 527-4800
(micro)

NUS Corp.
Park West Two, Cliff Mine Road, Pittsburgh, PA 15275
(412) 788-1080
(micro)

Occupational Health Services, Inc.
400 Plaza Drive, Secaucus, NJ 07094
(201) 865-7500
(various systems)

OSHA-Soft Corp.
31 Industrial Park Drive, P.O. Box 337-P, Concord, NH 03301
(603) 228-3610
(micro)

Pro-Am Safety, Inc.
4943 Route 8, Gibsonia, PA 15044
(412) 443-0410
(micro)

Questel
1625 Eye Street, N.W., Suite 818, Washington, DC 20006
(202) 296-1604
(on-line service)

Radian Corp.
8501 Mo-Pac Boulevard, P.O. Box 9948, Austin, TX 78766
(512) 454-4797
(micro)

Resource Consultants, Inc.
P.O. Box 1848, Brentwood, TN 37027
(615) 373-5040
(micro)

Safer Emergency Systems, Inc.
5700 Corsa Avenue, Westlake Village, CA 91362
(818) 707-2777
(micro)

Safety Sciences, Inc.
7586 Trade Street, San Diego, CA 92121
(619) 578-8400
(various systems)

Stewart-Todd Associates, Inc.
1016 West Ninth Avenue, King of Prussia, PA 19406
(215) 687-2030
(mainframe)

Sun Information Services
280 King of Prussia Road, Radnor, PA 19087
(215) 293-8235
(mainframe)

U N Z and CO.
Department BM-SPI, 190 Baldwin Avenue, Jersey City, NJ 07306
(201) 795-1200
(various systems)

Van Nostrand Reinhold Co.
115 Fifth Ave., New York, NY 10003
(212) 254-3232
(micro)

Because combustion, the chemical process of oxidation, continues to be a major hazard, the following scorecard produced by the New York State Department of Education, the New York State Office of Fire Prevention and Control, the New York State Association of Fire Chiefs, and the New York Yankees should be more widely appreciated:

FIRE SAFETY SCORECARD

To Stay Safe at Home We Have:

Yes	No	Posted emergency numbers on our phone or other well-known locations
Yes	No	Properly installed and maintained smoke detectors
Yes	No	Developed our home escape plan
Yes	No	Regularly practiced Exit Drills in the Home (EDITH)
Yes	No	Looked for and corrected common fire hazards
Yes	No	Learned to stop, drop and roll
Yes	No	Properly installed and maintained one or more fire extinguishers
Yes	No	Looked for two ways out on our way into theatres, stores or restaurants, or while staying at hotels
Yes	No	Discussed fire safety with our local firefighters or teachers
Yes	No	Installed residential sprinklers

As noted in Table 6.3, a significant number of chemicals and/or chemical mixtures are fully recognized as explosive.

TABLE 6.3. Unusually Hazardous or Explosive Materials

The following chemicals and mixtures have been known, either alone or in combinations, to prepare or cause explosions:

Acetylene (ethyne), a colorless gas, flammable limits 2.5 to 80 percent by volume in air, $HC{\equiv}CH$

Aluminum dust, Al

Ammonium dichromate, $(NH_4)_2Cr_2O_7$

Ammonium perchlorate, $NH_4 ClO_4$

Calcium carbide CaC_2

Carbon disulfide CS_2

Glycerine (glycerol) $CH_2OH\ CHOH\ CH_2OH$ used in pharmaceuticals as well as nitro-glycerine

TABLE 6.3. (*Continued*)

Hydrazine, also UDMH, H_2NNH_2
Hydrogen peroxide (in higher concentrations) H_2O_2
Magnesium Mg (ribbon or powder)
Nitric acid, HNO_3
Oxygen, O_2
Perchloric acid, $HClO_4$
Phosphorus P_4 (white ignites in air, red burns easily when ignited)
Potassium chlorate, $KClO_3$
Potassium nitrate (saltpeter), KNO_3
Potassium perchlorate, $KClO_4$
Potassium permanganate, $KMnO_4$
Sodium, Na (metal); lithium, Li; potassium, K; rubidium, Rb
Sodium-potassium alloy, (NaK) (water-reactive to produce hydrogen gas)
Sodium hydroxide (caustic soda or lye), NaOH
NaOH and KOH react with Al, liberating hydrogen
Sulfur, S (brimstone), produces SO_2 when ignited
Sulfuric acid H_2SO_4

Explosive Mixtures

Bangor: six parts KNO_3, 3 parts Al dust, 1 part S
Berge's blasting powder: 1 part $KClO_3$, 0.1 part $KCrO_3$, 0.45 part sugar, 0.9 part beeswax (if molasses or honey is substituted for sugar, the mixture is called morlex)
Black powder: 15% carbon, 75% KNO_3, 10% S
Chlorate-sulfur mixtures, catalyzed with MnO_2
Match heads (especially strike-anywhere matches)
Perchlorate mixtures with organics or aluminum dusts
Zinc-sulfur mixtures (2 parts Zn, 1 part S)

High Explosives

Ammonium nitrate, NH_4NO_3
Nitrogen triiodide contact explosives (very unstable), NI_3
Lead styphnate (or lead trinitroresorcinate), $PbC_6HN_3O_8$
Mercury fulminate, Hg
Nitrocellulose (or cellulose nitrate), $(C_6H_7N_3O_{11})n$
Nitroglycerine or glyceryl nitrate, $C_3H_5N_3O_9$
Nitroguanidine, C $H_4N_4O_2$
Pentaerythritol tetranitrate PETN, $C_5H_8N_4O_{12}$
Picric acid or trinitrophenol, $C_6H_3N_3O_7$
Tetranitromethane or tetan, $C(NO_2)_4$ (mixtures with nitrobenzene, 1- or 4-nitrotoluene, 1, 3-dinitrobenzene or 1-nitronaphthalene are high explosive of high sensitivity and detonation velocities. Mixtures of tetranitromethane with nitrobenzene are spark-detonable. Tetranitromethane with ferrocene under various conditions leads to violent explosions. With hydrocarbons, a sensitive highly explosive mixture results.)
Tetryl, $C_7H_5O_8N_5$
Trinitrotoluene or TNT, $C_6H_3(NO_2)_3$

Source: R. Meyer, *Explosives,* 2nd ed., Verlag-Chemie, Weinheim-Deerfield Beach, Fla., 1981; see also L. Bretherick, *Handbook of Reactive Chemical Hazards,* 3rd ed., Butterworths, London and Boston, 1985, and NFPA 491-M, *Reactive Chemical Hazards,* National Fire Protection Association, Quincy, Mass., 1985; L. Bretherick, "Reactive Chemical Hazards," Chap. 5, pp. 63–79, and "Hazardous Chemicals," Chap. 8, pp. 141–556, in *Hazards in the Chemical Laboratory,* edited by L. Bretherick, 4th ed., Royal Society of Chemistry, London, 1986.

It is fully appreciated this list is not complete; the reader is urged to consult the references cited, as well as the NFPA, the Institute of Makers of Explosives, the U.S. Bureau of Mines, and the local authorities, including the local and state fire commissioners, to ascertain the exact status of knowledge and any local or state regulations that may apply, before making or conducting experiments in chemicals or mixtures known to be unstable. A complete literature search, including use of the several on-line systems now available, as well as consultation with persons who have proven expertise in the field of explosives, is clearly indicated.

REFERENCES

1. "Pesticide Ignites 2-Alarm Condo Fire in Silver Spring," *Washington Post*, DS (Jan. 8, 1987).
2. National Fire Protection Association, Quincy, Mass.
3. ILO in cooperation with the Ministry of Labor, Government of India, International Programme for the Improvement of Working Conditions, and Emvironment (PIACT), *Asian Regional Workshop, Major Hazards and their Control in Industry*, Bombay, Nov. 4–8 1985, *Proceedings*, International Labour Office, Geneva, Switzerland, PIACT/1985/3
3a. R. J. Mainiero and J. E. Hay, "Bureau of Mines Internal Ignition and Gap Tests," Internal Report No. 4521, U.S. Dept. of the Interior, Bureau of Mines, Pittsburgh, Pa. Apr. 1985, 11 pp.
4. *Federal Register*, **48,** No. 228, 53280–532348 (Nov. 25, 1983) (29 CFR Part 1910.1200, Hazard Communication, Final Rule (effective May 28, 1986).
5. NFPA 704-M, *Identification of Hazards*, National Fire Protection Association, Quincy, Mass.
6. *American City & County*, 12 (Sept. 1986).
7. For details contact TD9, Stichtig TDG-9, Congresbureau-VVV Rotterdam, Stadhuisplein 19, 3012 AR Rotterdam, The Netherlands.
8. *Firehouse*, 24 (June 1986). For details contact George Proper, Jr., 27 Pheasant Ridge Lane, Loudonville, NY 12211.
9. Anon., *Plant/Operations Prog.*, **5,** No. 4, 4 (Oct. 1986).
10. Contact CHEMTREC, R. J. Chezem, Manager, Chemical Manufacturers Association, 2501 M St., N.W., Washington, DC 20037. In a transportation emergency, call (toll-free) 1-800-424-9300.

SUGGESTED READINGS

Anon., *Aluminum Alkyls, Texas Alkyls*, Stauffer Chemical Co., Westport Conn., 71 pp., 1987

Anon., "New 'Sniffer' Finds Explosives," *Wall St. J.*, 33 (July 21, 1987).

Anon., *OSHA Requirements Affecting Fire Departments*, two-page bibliography 1986; see also *Selected Materials on Incident Command*, seven-page bibliography, 1987, New York State Academy of Fire Science, Montour Falls, N.Y.

Anon., *Current Intelligent Bulletin* (CIB) #47, 4-4' methyldianiline (MDA), revised, 23 pp. DHHS (NIOSH) 86–115, 1986; "Requests for Assistance in Preventing Fatalities Due to Fires and Explosions in Oxygen-Limiting Silos," six pp., DHHS (NIOSH) 86–118, 1986; National Institute for Occupational Safety and Health, Cincinnati, Ohio.

Anon., "Protective Layers on Laboratory Glassware," *Sichere Chemiearbeit*, **38** (8), 93 (Aug. 1986). For details contact Firma BUCHI, Laboratoriums-Technik, GmbH, Postfach 11 54, 7332, Eislingen/Fils, West Germany.

V. Babrauskas, "The Cone Calorimeter: A Versatile Bench-Scale Tool for the Evaluation of Fire Properties," nine pages, National Bureau of Standards, Washington, D.C., 1986

P. J. Brennan and W. F. Donnelly, *Fire Protection Handbook Study Guide:* based on the *Fire Protection Handbook,* 16th ed., 404 pp., Top It Publishing, New York, 1986.

L. Bretherick, "Azide—Halosolvent Hazards, *Chem. Ind. (London),* No. 21, 729 (Nov. 3, 1986).

F. Bouissou, *Nitrogen Blanketing for the Prevention of Explosions in Centrifuges,* HSE transl. Apr.–June 1986 (HSE/LIS Translation Service, Harpur Hill, Buxton, Derbyshire SK 17 9JN, England; order HSE 11402).

CPSC, "CPSC (Consumer Product Safety Commission) Warns of Gas Hazard," *Siren,* **3,** No. 3, 3 (1987) (published by New York State Dept. of State, Office of Fire Prevention and Control, Albany, N.Y. (CPSC hotline number is 800-638-CPSC).

L. E. Calonius, "Anglicans Debate God's Purpose in Fire at York's Cathedral," *Wall St. J.* 1, 13 (Aug. 21, 1984).

R. L. Craig, *Training and Development Handbook: A Guide to Human Resource Development,* 3rd ed., 878 pp. McGraw-Hill, New York, 1987

C. J. Dahn et al., "Contribution of Low-Level Flammable Vapour Concentrations to Dust Explosion output," *Plant/Operations Prog.,* **5,** No. 1, 57–64 (Jan. 1986).

T. E. Drabek, *Human System Responses to Disaster: An Inventory of Sociological Findings,* Springer-Verlag, New York, 1986.

H. H. Fawcett and W. S. Wood (eds.), *Safety and Accident Prevention in Chemical Operations,* 2nd ed., 910 pp., Wiley-Interscience, New York, 1982.

FEMA, EENET Local Receive Site Coordination Guide, "Information Management: Avoiding the Disaster," 14 pp., Aug. 19, 1987; note also residency programs in Incident Command, Advanced Incident Command, Fire/Arson Detection, Chemistry of Hazardous Materials, Hazardous Materials Tactical Considerations, Planning for a Hazardous Materials Incident, and Emergency Medical Services; Federal Emergency Management Agency, National Emergency Training Center, Emmitsburg, Md.

FEMA-DOT Hazmat Planning Exchange, available on (800) 756-3667; data accessible by modem into personal computer by calling (312) 972-3275.

Firemen's Association of the State of New York, *Informational Bulletin,* "Outside Assistance: Identifying and Managing Resources Needed in Incident Command," 12 pp., 27 Pleasant Ridge Drive, Loudonville, NY 12211, 1986.

D. Fromm and W. Rall, "Fire at Semi-Lean Pump by Reverse Motion," *Plant/Operations Prog.,* **6,** No. 3, 162–164 (Mar. 1987).

J. R. Hughes, *Storage and Handling of Petroleum Liquids,* 3rd rev. ed., 332 pp., Wiley-Interscience, New York, 1987.

Z. Kister and T. C. Hower, Jr., "Unusual Operating Histories of Gas Processing and Olefins Plant Columns," *Plant/Operations Prog.,* **6,** No. 3, 151–161 (July 1987).

T. J. Klem, "Explosion in Cold Storage Kills Fire Fighter," *Plant/Operations Prog.,* **5,** No. 1 (Jan. 1986).

G. Kolata, "U.S. Leads World in Fire Deaths; Experts Blame Ignorance of Population, and Look to Computers as an Answer," *Washington Post Health Supplement,* 10 (Feb. 3, 1987).

H. Kunreuther and E. V. Ley, "The Risk Analysis Controversy: An Institutional Perspective," *Proc. Summer Study,* Laxenburg, Austria, June 22–62, 1981, Springer-Verlag, New York, 1986

B. C. Levin, "Toxicological Effects of the Interactions of Fire Gases," 12 pp., National Bureau of Standards, Washington, D.C., 1986.

B. J. McCaffrey, "Momentum Diffusion Flame Characteristics and the Effects of Water Spray on Gas Well Blowout Fires, 65 pp., National Bureau of Standard, Washington, D.C., 1986

H. S. Morton, "Explosion Sounds," 3M Engineering Analyst, Ltd., 103 North 4th Ave., St. Charles, IL 60174-2017.

J. Morris, *The Library Disaster Preparedness Handbook,* 129 pp., American Library Association, 1986.

D. Moss, "Explosions Ignite Safety Issue, Bans on Fireworks," *USA Today,* 1 (June 30, 1987).

NFPA, *Fire Protection Handbook,* 16th ed., National Fire Protection Association, Quincy, Mass., 1987.

M. A. Nettleton, *Gaseous Detonations: Their Nature, Causes, and Control,* 250 pp., Chapman & Hall, New York, 1987.

D. D. Perrin and W.L.F. Aarmarego, "Silver Nitrate—Ethanol Explosion," *Chem. Br. (Australia),* **22,** No. 12, 1084 (Dec. 1986).

RISC, Rotterdam International Safety Centre booklet, Europaweg 930, 3199 LC Maasvlakte (Rotterdam), The Netherlands.

RSOC, *Chemical Hazards in Industry,* monthly or on-line; also *Laboratory Hazards Bulletin,* monthly or on-line, Information Services, Royal Society of Chemistry, The University, Nottingham NG7 2RD, England.

R. Schierdug, "Computerized Monitoring System Controls Build-up of Combustible Hydrogen," *Chem. Proc.,* 70–73 (Sept. 1987).

J. F. Straitz III, "Flare Technology Safety," *Chem. Eng. Prog.* 53–62 (July 1987).

P. B. Willis, "Sulphur Trioxide," *C&EN,* **64,** No. 38, 2 (Sept. 22, 1986).

L. A. Zuccarelli, "Care Recommended with Sand Extinguishers," *Occupational Health & Safety,* 57 (Nov. 1986).

7

The Toxic Substances Control Act of 1976 (PL 94-469)

Henry P. Lau

The Toxic Substances Control Act (TSCA), which became effective January 1, 1977, charged the EPA with the responsibility to protect human health and the environment from unreasonable risks of injury from toxic chemicals. Over the past decade, programs have been established under TSCA to gather information about the toxicity of particular chemicals and the extent to which people and the environment are exposed to them, to assess whether these chemicals pose any unreasonable risks to human health and the environment, and to formulate appropriate regulatory control actions after weighing the potential risks of the chemicals against their intended benefits to the nation's economic and social well-being.

Before discussing the major provisions of the act and their applications, it may be useful to review the findings of the Congress and the policy of the United States.

Findings. The Congress finds that:

1. Human beings and the environment are being exposed each year to a large number of chemical substances and mixtures.
2. Among the many chemical substances and mixtures that are constantly being developed and produced, there are some whose manufacture, processing, distribution in commerce, use, or disposal may present an unreasonable risk of injury to health or the environment.
3. The effective regulation of interstate commerce in such chemical substances and mixtures also necessitates the regulation of intrastate commerce in such chemical substances and mixtures.

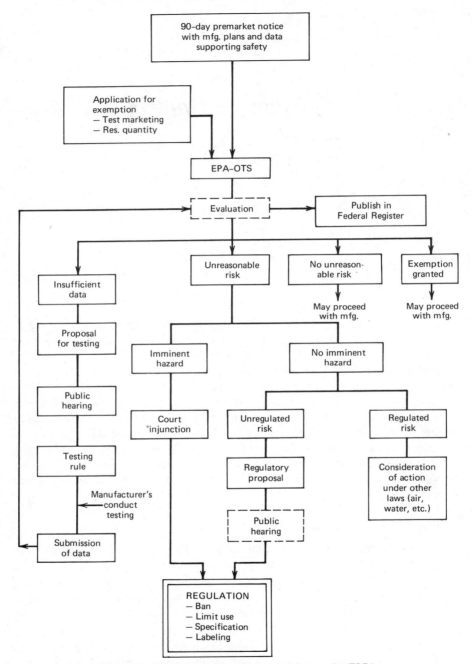

Figure 7.1. Regulatory scheme for new products under TSCA.

Policy. It is the policy of the United States that:

1. Adequate data should be developed with respect to the effect of chemical substances and mixtures on health and the environment and the development of such data should be the responsibility of those who manufacture and those who process such chemical substances and mixtures.

2. Adequate authority should exist to regulate chemical substances and mixtures that present an unreasonable risk of injury to health or to the environment, and to take action with respect to chemical substances and mixtures that are imminent hazards.

3. Authority over chemical substances and mixtures should be exercised in such a manner as not to impede unduly or create unnecessary economic barriers to technological innovation while fulfilling the primary purpose of this act to assure that such innovation and commerce in such chemical substances and mixtures do not present an unreasonable risk of injury to health or the environment.

The authority of TSCA covers all chemical substances, except those that are specifically excluded or exempted, whose manufacture, importation, processing, or distribution for commercial purposes in the United States has taken place since January 1, 1975. The act specifically required EPA to identify, compile, keep current, and publish a list of chemicals existing in commerce during the period January 1, 1975, through December 31, 1977. In accordance with this requirement, the Inventory Reporting Regulation (40 CFR Part 710) (Code of Federal Regulations) was promulgated. Data were reported on nearly 60,000 chemicals, and were used by EPA to compile the TSCA Chemical Substances Inventory. The purpose of this inventory was to define what chemicals are existing in the commerce of the United States. The inventory, however, is not a list of toxic chemicals since toxicity was not a criterion in determining which chemicals should be included.

The act requires the EPA to order animal testing of any chemical or mixture for which data and experience are insufficient, and which are relevant to a determination that the manufacture, distribution in commerce, processing, use, or disposal of each substance or mixture, or any combination of such activities, do or do not present an unreasonable risk of injury to health or the environment. The standards to be prescribed for the testing of health and environmental effects will include carcinogenesis, mutagenesis, teratogenesis, behavioral disorders, cumulative or synergistic effects, and any other effect that may pose an unreasonable risk of injury to human health or the environment. Among characteristics to be considered are persistence (how long the material will still be active before it is degraded or otherwise converted to a biologically inactive form), acute toxicity (high dose over short time), subacute toxicity (produces effects but not fatal), and chronic toxicity (low-level doses over long periods).

Essentially, the law applies to all new chemical substances, and to new uses of existing substances. Notification and test data must be submitted 90 days before the manufacture or significant new use is begun. If the data are acceptable to the EPA, clearance will be given, otherwise the EPA may request additional evidence or prohibit or limit production and use. The EPA will compile and keep current a list of chemical substances it finds unacceptable.

Polychlorinated biphenyls (PCBs) are specifically considered in the Act, with provision for new regulations for disposal of PCBs, and "clear and adequate" instructions in the marking or labeling. Inasmuch as the main uses of PCBs were as a heat-transfer agent and as the main dielectric insulating fluids in electrical transformers, capacitors, and ballasts for fluorescent lamps (manufactured before 1972), PCBs are very widespread. In a fire, as in the Binghamton State Office Building (see page 115), pyrolysis and decomposition can cause serious problems of toxic smoke and residues that are very difficult to decontaminate. All indoor electrical transformers containing PCBs are to be removed by 1990. Services are available to replace or "retrofit" the PCBs with other fluids, such as the services of the General Electric Company, #2-525, 1 River Road, Schenectady, NY 12345.

In enacting TSCA, the Congress intended that the term "chemical substance" be somewhat narrowly defined so as not to overlap with the coverage of other environmental legislations. Therefore, for the purpose of TSCA, chemical substance does *not* include, among other things, any mixture (chemical components of mixtures are, however, included), pesticide, food, food additive, drug, or cosmetic. Furthermore, the Inventory Reporting Regulations specifically exempt, among other things, impurities, by-products, and chemicals manufactured only in small quantities (as defined by rule) solely for purposes of scientific experimentation or analysis, or chemical research, analysis, or product development. Chemicals that are manufactured for the purpose of test marketing, however, are not exempt even if they are produced in small quantities.

Over the past decade, several TSCA programs were developed, implemented, and refined. EPA promulgated a wide range of regulations to gather information from industry or to control the proliferation of chemicals that were found to be hazardous. These regulations include the Inventory Reporting Rule, the Pre-manufacture Notification Reporting Rule, the PCB rules, the chemical testing rules, the "significant new use" rules, and the health and safety data reporting rule, as well as other information-collection and control-action rules.

In 1986, EPA began developing a Comprehensive Assessment Information Rule to consolidate into a model rule a wide range of reporting provisions and questions on selected existing chemicals. Reporting requirements for a particular chemical can be specified from a list of standard questions, and individual chemicals can be added to the rule as the need for information arises. An Inventory Update Rule was also promulgated to collect current production and plant-site information on certain chemicals reported for the inventory.

In response to the chemical tragedy that took place in Bhopal, India, EPA issued a comprehensive air toxic strategy, and prepared criteria and guidance for local communities for evaluating and responding to accidental releases. A list of substances was announced by the agency.

Recognizing the emerging need for controlling the potential proliferation of commercial products of biotechnology, EPA issued a policy statement describing how TSCA would be applied to these products. This statement was published in a joint *Federal Register* notice with the White House Office of Science and Technology Policy, the FDA, and the U.S. Department of Agriculture.

The control of toxic chemicals should always be based on a careful consideration of two important factors, namely, toxicity and exposure level. If a chemical is found to be sufficiently toxic and has a relatively high level of exposure, that chemical would generally be a good candidate for review under TSCA. This would ensure that substances that have the greatest potential of inducing harm to health and the environment be kept under close scrutiny of the law.

8
Toxicity, or Biological Action

Howard H. Fawcett

Although the word "toxicity" is often equated with "poison," such an over-simplification may lead to false impressions. In fact, the biological systems of humans and animals can tolerate considerable abuse from foreign substances, but when the exposure is excessive, damage takes place—which may be mild, serious, short term, chronic, or even fatal, depending on the substances involved, and their toxicity, mode of action, concentration, and duration. We note the above to put in perspective the real need for a more complete understanding of toxicity, and the limitations of our knowledge concerning its effect on living organisms.

It has long been known that some substances are more hazardous than others; the alchemists of the Dark Ages were often involved in studies that would aid in converting base metals into more precious ones (lead into gold, for example), and in the process often used such substances as mercury, zinc, antimony, roots and flowers of plants, and related materials that today we know to be toxic. In recent years, the screening of materials for toxic effects before releasing them for wide-spread use has become a legal, as well as a moral, obligation, as consumer groups and various agencies, such as the FDA, the CPSC, NIOSH, OSHA, Department of Transportation, EPA, Department of Defense, Department of Agriculture, National Cancer Institute (NCI), and others attempt to guide the ultimate user or contact person from adverse exposures. Major chemical companies, including Dow, Du Pont, Carbide, and Monsanto, and, more recently, the petrochemical industry through its trade organizations the American Petroleum Institute, the Industrial Hygiene Foundation, and the Chemical Industry Institute of Toxicology, all have made major contributions to our understanding of toxicity problems when they have arisen. Recently, attention has been given to smoke, pyrolysis products, and combustion toxicity of many materials, from wood to synthetics, in an attempt to understand more completely the potential materials have for presenting difficulties, if misused or misapplied. Even an element that is absolutely essential to human life—namely, oxygen—is toxic under conditions of prolonged inhalation at elevated pressures, such as in scuba diving for extended periods below 32 feet (9.76 meters). Several elements essential to life in low concentrations, such as zinc, copper, magnesium, selenium, and arsenic, are injurious in higher concentrations. Hence simply to label a substance "toxic" or "nontoxic" without specifying details is hardly in order. Until the "dose" of the material has actually entered the body and reached critical organs by one or more routes, including inhalation, ingestion, and skin absorption, abstract discussions of toxicity are of limited significance in the real world.

As we have noted previously, writers such as E. M. Whelan in *Toxic Terror* have attempted to put into perspective many aspects of the current concern about toxicity, carcinogenesis, and other effects of chemicals. However, the fact is that chemicals are potentially hazardous, and any prudent person, whether chemist, engineer, physician, lawyer, or member of the body politic, would be well advised to consider carefully all the evidence without bias.

Toxicity, unlike physical constants, cannot be measured by critical tables or exact mechanisms. It is now recognized that humans differ significantly to a given exposure: age, prior exposures, and even differences in sex are being studied as additional parameters that will assist in more complete understanding of exposure levels and effects.[1–3]

This does not imply that little or nothing is known of the toxic effects of chemicals and other materials; on the contrary, several relevant data bases are now available, both on-line and for access by computer modems, as well as in the more traditional form of the printed page.

Humans and animal systems have several mechanisms for dealing with insults from toxic substances, often called "detoxification." At some point on the dose–effect (or dose–response) curve, either acute or chronic injury can occur, which may or may not affect every other member of the subject group or be immediately obvious. As mentioned in Chapter 5, Dr. Ruth Lilis has noted that the neurotoxicity induced by repeated exposure to organic solvents is real, and may be a deliberate recreational or "sniffing" activity, not related to occupational exposures. It is recognized that some materials potentiate or enhance the toxicity of other materials, so the implications for off-the-job right-to-know are as important as on-the-job information. This is also true of the widely publicized "drug" culture, in which pot, crack, angel dust, PCP, morphine, and other drugs that are not prescribed become part of the society, with devastating and often fatal results.

Symptoms of adverse effects from toxic materials include modified or irregular behavior (intoxication), central-nervous-system disorientation, impairment of body functions, allergic reactions, skin and eye irritation or damage, respiratory distress and cardiac collapse, pulmonary edema, or less obvious delayed reactions that may take years before producing carcinogenic, mutagenic, or teratogenic effects in essential organs. Until the toxic dose actually enters the body through one or more routes of entry, including inhalation, ingestion, or cutaneous (skin) absorption, it is probably harmless. The possible exception is the possibility that a one-hit injury may occur; that is, one molecule of the substance contacts and damages the essential DNA and RNA of a critical organ, and may induce carcinogenic activity. This theory of no threshold exposure for chemical carcinogens is widely debated, and impressive arguments may be cited both for and against the concept. It is possible that our understanding of the process is so incomplete that a threshold value exists but has not yet been recognized and accepted. However, for most chemicals and materials, the consensus is that a threshold value exists, based on protection for the majority of the workers who will be exposed over their working lifetime, but the degree of protection it affords any one individual in a group is not clear at this writing.

Since the original presentation of a list of proposed threshold-limit values (TLVs) by Prof. Warren Cook in 1945, changes have been made annually, as the list is revised by the American Conference of Governmental Industrial Hygienists (ACGIH).[4] The 1969 TLVs published by the ACGIH became the OSHA standards for most substances (see *Federal Register*, **36**, No. 105, May 29, 1971). Since then, the annual revisions have been continued by the ACGIH in an advisory capacity, and have been expanded to cover over 700 substances, as well as physical agents, including light, heat, noise, lasers, microwaves, and ionizing radiation. As noted in the preface to the ACGIH compilation for airborne contaminants in the workplace (to which the reader should refer for the most current values), three categories of TLVs are specified.

1. *Time-Weighted Average (TWA):* This is a time-weighted average concentration for a normal 8-hour workday or 40-hour work week to which nearly all workers may be repeatedly exposed, day after day, without ill effects. Because of the wide variation in individual susceptibility, however, a small percentage of workers may experience discomfort from some substances at concentrations at or below the threshold limit; a smaller percentage may be affected more seriously by aggravation of a preexisting condition or by development of an occupational illness. It must be stressed these values are not absolutes.

Typical values from the 1987–88 listing include those given in Table 8.1.

2. *Short-Term Exposure Limit (STEL):* This is the maximal concentration to which workers can be exposed for a period of up to 15 minutes continuously without suffering from (1) irritation, (2) chronic or irreversible tissue damage, or (3) narcosis of sufficient degree to increase the likelihood of accidental injury, impair self-rescue, or materially reduce work efficiency, provided that the daily TLV-TWA is not exceeded. It is not a separate independent exposure limit but supplements the TWA limit where there are recognized acute effects from a substance whose toxic effffects are primarily of a chronic nature. STELs are recommended only where toxic effects have been reported from high short-term exposures in either humans or animals, and are defined as a 15-minute TWA exposure that should not be exceeded at any time during a workday even if the eight-hour TWA is within the TLV. Exposures at the STEL should not be longer than 15 minutes and should not be repeated more than four times a day. There should be at least 60

TABLE 8.1 Exposure Limits of ACGIH

	TLV-TWA			STEL	
	ppm		mg/m^3	ppm	mg/m^3
Acetone	750	or	1780	1000	2375
Acrolein	0.1	or	0.25	0.3	0.8
Allyl chloride	1	or	3	2	6
Ammonia	25	or	18	35	27
Benzene A2	10	or	30*		
Benzyl chloride	1	or	5		
Beryllium and compounds as Be			0.002 A2*		
Carbon tetrachloride	5 A2	or	30 A 2 (skin)*		
Chlorine	(1)	or	(3)		
Chlorine trifluoride	0.1 C	or	0.4 C (C is ceiling*)		
Pentane	600	or	1800	750	2250
Phosgene	0.1	or	0.4		
Zinc-oxide fume	—		5	—	10

*A2 refers to list of industrial substances suspect of carcinogenic potential for MAN; refer to Appendix A, Carcinogens. C refers to ceiling value. OSHA is reducing exposure of benzene to 1 ppm.

minutes between successive exposures at the STEL. An averaging period other than 15 minutes may be recommended when this is warranted by observing biological effects. Typical TLV-STEL for the listings are included in Table 8.1.

3. *Ceiling (C):* This concentration should not be exceeded during any part of the working exposure. In conventional industrial hygiene practice, if instantaneous monitoring is not feasible, then the TLV-C can be assessed by sampling over a 15-minute period, except for those substances that may cause immediate irritation with exceedingly short exposures. For some substances (e.g., irritant gases), only one category, the TLV-C, may be relevant. For other substances, either two or three categories may be relevant, depending upon their physiological action. It is important to observe that if any one of these three TLVs is exceeded, a potential hazard from that substance is presumed to exist.

Examples of the TLV-C are noted in Table 8.2.

TABLE 8.2. Ceiling Values

	ppm	mg/m^3
Boron trifluoride	C 1	C 3
Cyanogen chloride	C 0.3	C 0.6
o-dichlorobenzene	C 50	C 300
Oxygen difluoride	C 0.05	C 0.1
Sodium azide	C 0.1	C 0.3

For some compounds or elements, such as irritant gases, only one category, the TLV-C, may be relevant; for others, the TLV-TWA and TLV-STEL may be appropriate for control. Substances that are known to be toxic through the intact skin (such as acetonitrile, acrylamide, and carbon tetrachloride) are so designated by the addition of the word "skin" after the chemical name.

From the above, it should be obvious that a careful reading and proper interpretation of the values, and the analytical results that are necessary for their use, should be under the supervision of a person trained or experienced in industrial hygiene or toxicology.

In addition to the exposures mentioned above, the degree of toxicity is influenced by several other factors:

Dose. Generally the larger the dose (or the higher the concentration), the faster is the action or reaction;

Rate of Absorption. The faster this rate, the quicker is the action. With oral administration, the intoxicating and the lethal doses may be considerably influenced by the condition of the gastrointestinal tract, especially by the amount of food and other matter in the stomach and intestine. Vehicles, such as oil, also affect absorption of a skin exposure by buffering the contact or diluting the surface areas exposed to the substance.

Route of Administration. For the most part, toxicity is greatest for the route that carries the toxic substance to the bloodstream most rapidly. In *decreasing* order of speed of action, routes for most drugs and other substances, including chemicals, are:

Intravenous

Inhalation

Intraperitoneal

Intramuscular

Subcutaneous

Oral

Cutaneous (skin contact)

Food in the alimentary canal may delay or decrease toxic action. Digestive enzymes may destroy or alter the compounds with resultant changes in toxicity. Certain compounds are virtually harmless if taken orally, but lethal when introduced parenterally; in many other cases, the converse is true. The toxicity of the material or chemical may also vary considerably with the form in which it is administered, for example, solid or liquid, in suspension or in solution. In solution, the toxicity may be influenced by the solvent and the concentration. Synergism (or combined effect) may be an important factor in the action, and probably occurs far more frequently than recognized. In the area of "mixed exposures," knowledge is very uncertain. As an example, exposure by inhalation of hydrogen sulfide or trichloroethylene, followed by ingestion of alcohol, greatly increases the effects of both. As noted before, the increase in toxicity to certain compounds, such as formaldehyde, in the presence of cigarette smoke, is recognized. Apparently particles carry the gaseous materials into more intimate contact with the lung tissues.

Action of toxic exposures is also influenced by:

Site of Introduction. With subcutaneous injections, toxicity may be affected by the density of the subcutaneous tissue. With intravenous administration, whether the injection is made into the femoral or jugular vein may be of importance, but in any case the rate of injection, or the amount of material injected per unit time, will considerably influence the value of the toxic dose.

Other Influences. Disease, environmental temperature, habits, and tolerance (such as smoking, alcohol intake, and other drugs, including over-the-counter, prescription, and controlled, or illegal, substances), low-level exposure to carbon monoxide and other substances, idiosyncrasy or allergy, diet, stress, and season of the year all may influence the toxicity of a substance. The toxicity of chemical also varies with the species of animals used, and sometimes with different strains of the same species. Within the same strain, significant differences between litter mates have been observed. This variation is not unique to laboratory animals, but can be observed in humans as well. As Owen Kubius has pointed out, there is no "average" person, just as the concept of zero defect in quality assurance ignores the real world.

People have a wide variety of exposures from the moment they are born into the air of this unclean contaminated world—including the portmanteau biota, such as weeds and seeds, shoots and fruits, dusts, volcanic ash and other condensation nuclei from rain and snow, fleas and honeybees, rats, cats, dogs, goats, pigs, sheep, asses, horses, and cattle, along with infectious and parasitic disease including smallpox, measles, influenza, tuberculosis, sexually transmitted diseases, worms, and hosts of others unknown and unnamed (see Crosby, A. W., *The Biological Expansion of Europe, 900–1900*, Cambridge University Press, London, 1986), as well as other natural processes beyond the control of humans, And as the defense processes each person possesses may change from time to time, it is seldom possible to attribute the toxic effects of any substance specifically without considering the other forces or effects from previous exposures that have been operating over the years. In discussing the defense processes, which are often the determining factor in human reactions to a chemical, G. R. C. Atherley, in *Occupational Health and Safety Concerns* (Applied Science Publishers, London, 1978), notes respiratory filtration of aerosols and mists, cellular defense, inflammatory response, immune response (which alters sensitivity), homeostasis (in which the internal milieu of the body is maintained in a stabilized condition), stress resistance (linked to the hormone cortisol), thermoregulation of body temperature, and metabolic transformation whereby a toxic substance is rendered less toxic and can be excreted by the kidneys.

Although not occupational, or strictly chemical, the present concern about the acquired immune deficiency syndrome (AIDS) illustrates the complex systems of humans. A World Health Organization release in January 1987 claims that 48,000 cases of AIDS are known, 75 percent of which are in the United States. A drug for the treatment of AIDS, and a kit for its detection (sold by Cellular Products Co. of Buffalo, and by E. I. du Pont de Nemours & Co., Wilmington, Del.), indicate recent progress in this area. Disturbing is the concern that has been expressed that a rare virus capable of causing cancer, and possibly a mysterious nerve disease, is being spread among Americans. The virus can cause a form of adult leukemia, and is transmitted, like AIDS, by an exchange of blood by hypodermic syringes, sexual practices, or blood transfusions.[5] The virus is known as human T-cell leukemia virus one, or HTLV-1, and to date is the only proven human cancer virus, although many patients infected with the AIDS virus develop a previously rare type of skin cancer. The American Red Cross is conducting a nationwide testing of blood to study how deeply the HTLV-1 virus has infiltrated into the United States from Japan, the Caribbean, and the Mediterranean.

Although no known defense is available against some diseases, the epidemiologists, when studying a large number of persons of a given population, such as those employed on similar occupational tasks for a comparable period of time, often point out that they are usually the population with the highest resistance—due partly to preselection, excellent or at least adequate medical attention, adequate and balanced diet, and other factors, that are in favor of good general health. This "bias" toward generally healthy persons is often noted in epidemiological reports.

Although a direct relationship between an occupation (chimney sweeping) and cancer was established by Potts in 1775, and asbestos was shown at autopsy to be a serious problem in London in 1899, the subject of potential carcinogenicity of common chemicals did not receive widespread attention until fairly recent times. Since 1970, when it became a stated policy of the United States government to develop the information necessary to eliminate cancer from its position as one of the leading causes of adult death (along with heart disease and accidents), various approaches have made considerable progress, but the work is still incomplete as far as real understanding and prevention are concerned. The NCI, which is a part of NIH, has been studying cancer both through epidemiology studies of human populations exposed and through studies in animals, beginning with rats and mice, and going up the scale to nonhuman primates. Although activists' groups have directed much attention in recent times to the use of animals for experimental purposes, and claim that the animals are being treated inhumanely, it is difficult to understand how we would proceed without animal data input.

Several hundred chemicals and related substances have been tested for carcinogenic action, and these data have been made available for public use in massive volumes of Public Health Service 149, *Survey of Compounds Which Have Been Tested for Carcinogenic Activity*. The second volume, published in 1951, covered the literature from 1939 to 1947, including references to the first volume. It contains 1329 compounds, of which 322 were reported to cause malignant tumors in animals and 35 others to induce only benign ones, whereas the first volume contained 633 compounds, of which 169 were said to produce cancer and 23 others to yield only papillomas. Since then, the volumes have been issued every two years; the most recent, 1981–82, in two sections, is titled NIH Publication No. 85-2775, November 1985, National Institutes of Health, National Cancer Institute, Bethesda, Md. (for sale by the Superintendent of Documents, U.S. Government Printing Office, Washington, DC 20402). Designated as 1985 0 487-844, Sections I and II, it contains 2150 pages. This is the 12th volume in the overall series. Others will be released when available. Information on the availability of these volumes and other information on the testing data may be obtained from the Office of Information, National Cancer Institute, Bethesda, MD 20892, attention Information Specialist, or call (301) 496-6095 or 496-5583.

Recognizing that the dissemination of information to workers and the public is a very important factor in educating persons to avoid contact with toxic substances, including carcinogens, mutagens, and teratogens, the OSHA Hazard Communication Regulation, supplemented by several state right-to-know laws that are often more comprehensive than the OSHA (which applies only to manufacturing categories SIC 20-39), may advance the cause of education, and hence, it is hoped, prevention.

As public and social pressures increase, more agressive action will be forthcoming. The Toxic Substances Control Act (TSCA) signed by President Ford in October 1976 and effective as of January 2, 1977, is an example of such concern reduced to law, which one hopes will be administered wisely in the national interest. Interest in the control of cigarette smoking is increasing; the health-care costs from lung cancer associated with smoking have been estimated at $17 billion annually for the United States alone. Public awareness of the high cost of smoking is having real effects as more organizations restrict smoking and bills are introduced into Congress to restrict advertising and other inducements—an effort that has been successful in England. If agricultural researchers could recommend a cash crop that could be grown in soils similar to that used for tobacco (especially in North Carolina, Virginia, and Maryland), and yield more cash for the farmers than tobacco currently does, we would eliminate much of the problem of smoking. Another example of a toxic health problem that is controllable is alcoholism. Estimates of the number of alcoholics in the United States range as high as 15 million. Approximately 67 percent of the adult population in the United States uses alcohol on occasion and 12 percent are considered "heavy drinkers." Hepatic (liver) disorders are a major medical finding in heavy drinkers, since in the body alcohol is oxidized to acetaldehyde and hydrogen equivalents. Little appreciated is the fact that each gram of ethanol provided 7.1 calories; 12 ounces of an 86-proof beverage contains 1200 calories, half of the recommended daily dietary allowance for some persons. (See C. S. Lieber, "Hepatic, Metabolic, and Nutritional Complications of Alcoholism," Res. Staff Phys., August 1983, pages 79–96, 15 references.)

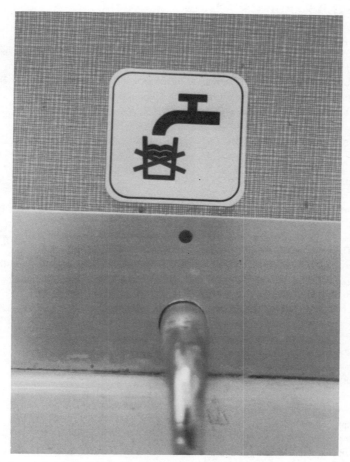

Figure 8.1. International symbol for "Do Not Drink" as used in European railroad cars, April 1987. (Photo by H. Fawcett.)

REFERENCES

1. E. J. Celabrese, *Age and Susceptibility to Toxic Substances,* Wiley-Interscience, New York, 1986.

2. E. J. Celabrese, *Toxic Susceptibility: Male/Female Differences,* Wiley-Interscience, New York, 1985.

3. J. F. Fraumeni, (ed.), *Persons at High Risk to Cancer—An Approach to Cancer Etiology and Control,* Academic Press, New York, 1975.

4. American Conference of Governmental Industrial Hygienists, 6500 Glenway Ave., Bldg. D-7, Cincinnati, OH 45211, annual revision of "TLVs Threshold Limit Values for Chemical Substances and Physical Agents in the Work Environment" adopted by ACGIH.

5. J. E. Bishop, and M. Waldholz, "Concern Grows That Cancer Virus Is Spreading in Same Way as AIDS," *Wall St. J.,* 20 (Jan. 20, 1987).

SUGGESTED READINGS

ADM, "Ad Agencies Join to 'Unsell' Drugs, Alcohol, Drug Abuse and Mental Health News," **XIII,** No. 5, 1, 16 (May 1987), Dept. of Health and Human Services, Room 12-C-15, 5600 Fishers Lane, Rockville, MD 20857.

ADM, "Lab Accreditation Standards Developed for Drug Testing of Urine" (address as above).

J. F. Ahearne, "Nuclear Power After Chernobyl," *Science,* 673–679 (May 8, 1987).

Anon., "Asbestos Control for Industry," booklet, ACTI catalog, P.O. Box 183, Maple Shade, NJ 08052, 1987.

Anon., "Carcinogens," 4th Annual Rep., 1985, U.S. Dept. of Health and Human Services, Washington, D.C.

Anon., *Survey of Compounds Which Have Been Tested for Carcinogenic Activity, 1983–84,* volume in two sections, 2061 pp., National Cancer Institute, National Institutes of Health, Bethesda, Md. (issued annually) (NIH Publication 86-2883), November 1986.

Anon., "Epicure Salt in Spice Sets Is Recalled Nationwide: Seasoning Contains Dangerous Ingredient," *Washington Post,* A11 (Feb. 14, 987).

Anon., "Disclosure Asked on Benzene Study," Occupational Health & Safety, 8 (May 1986); see also "U.S. Tightens Benzene Rule for Workplace," *Wall St. J.,* 24 (Sept. 2, 1987).

Anon., *Fire & Smoke (Understanding the Hazards),* National Academy Press, Washington, D.C., 1986.

Anon, Current Intelligence Bulletin, CIB#47, 4,4'-Methyldiamine (MDA), Revised, 23 p., DHHS (NIOSH) 86–115, 1986

Anon., "EENET Local Receive Site Coordination Guide: Liquefied Compressed Gas: Prescription for a BLEVE—Part II," 12 pp., National Fire Academy, Emmitsburg, Md., Apr. 15, 1987.

Anon., "EPA to Regulate "Inert" Pesticide Ingredients, "*C&EN,* 5 (Apr. 27, 1987).

Anon., *Inconsistent Rules Govern Pesticides in Food, News Report, Regulating Pesticides in Food: The Delaney Paradox,* 288 pp., National Academy Press, Washington, D.C., 1987.

Anon., "Inhalable Insulin," *Wall St. J.,* 33 (July 21, 1987).

Anon., "Jellyfish Research May Soothe the Triggers of Their Sting," *Washington Post,* A3 (July 20, 1987).

Anon., "Reproductive Problems in the Workplace: State of the Art Reviews," *Occupational Medicine,* P.O. Box 1377, Philadelphia, PA 19105-9990, 1986.

Anon., "Skin Disease," *Occupational Medicine,* P.O. Box 1377, Philadelphia, PA 19105-9990, 1986.

ASTM (American Society for Testing and Materials) Philadelphia, Pa., publications: STP 915, "Pesticide Formulations and Application Systems," 156 pp., 1986; STP 440, "Correlation of Subjective-Objective Methods in the Study of Odors and Taste," 112 pp., 1986; STP 834, "Definitions for Asbestos and Other Health Related Silicates," 205 pp., 1987; STP 732, "Health Effects of Synthetic Silica Particulates," 223 pp., 1981; STP 872, "Inhalation Toxicology of Air Pollution: Clinical Research Considerations," 131 pp., 1986.

J. Barron, "6,787 Miles of Gas Line—and It Leaks: Bronx Explosion a Tragic Reminder," *N.Y. Times,* 12 (Apr. 12, 1987).

D. Brahams, "Penicillin Overdose and Deafness," *Lancet,* 1445 (June 20, 1987).

D. J. Burton, "Microbiological Hazards in Laboratories Can Be Controlled (Safe Handling of Biohazards Require Special Equipment, Procedures,) "*Occupational Health & Safety,* 37–38 (May 1986).

T. Burns, "Mass Poisoning Trial Begins in Madrid," *Washington Post,* A23 (March 31, 1987).

G. D. Burrows, T. R. Norman, and G. Rubinstein (eds.), *Handbook of Studies on Schizophrenia,* in two parts: *Part I, Epidemiology; Part II, Management and Research,* 313 pp., Elsevier, Amsterdam, 1987.

E. J. Calabrese. *Age and Susceptibility to Toxic Substances,* 296 pp., Wiley-Interscience, New York, 1986.

E. J. Calabrese, *Toxic Susceptibility: Male/Female Differences,* 336 pp., Wiley-Interscience, New York, 1985.

W. J. Campbell, "Pesticide Endangers Farmers—EPA Regulation of Alachor Flawed—Fatally," *Schenectady (N.Y.) Gazette,* 46 (July 2, 1987).

C. G. Caro, "Effect of Cigarette Smoking on the Pattern of Arterial Blood Flow: Possible Insight into Mechanisms Underlying the Development of Arteriosclerosis," *Lancet,* 11–13 (July 4, 1987).

S. S. Chissick and R. Derricott (eds.), *Asbestos, Properties, Applications and Hazards:* Volume 1, 510 pp., 1979; Volume 2, 652 pp., 1983, Wiley, Chichester, England, and New York.

V. H. Cohn, "Marijuana Disrupts Essential Hormone in Women, Study Shows," *Alcohol, Drug Abuse and Mental Health News,* Dept. of Health and Human Services, **XIII,** No. 3, 7 (March 1987).

H. H. Comly, "Cyanosis in Infants Caused by Nitrates in Well Water," *JAMA,* 2788–2792 (May 22–29, 1987).

J. R. De Paulo, Jr., "Lithium (carbonate)," in Symposium on Clinical Psychopharmacology I, *Pschiatric Clin. N.A.,* **7,** No. 3, 587–599 (Sept. 1984).

F. G. Driscoll, *Groundwater and Wells,* 2nd ed., 1089 pp., Scientific Publications, P.O. Box 23041, Washington, DC 20026-3041, 1987.

C. Durnin, "Carbon Monoxide Poisoning Presenting with Focal Epileptiform Seizures," *Lancet,* 1319 (June 6, 1987).

B. Dvorchak, "Nuclear Plant Dismantled Under Watchful Eyes," *Washington Post,* A7 (July 23, 1987.)

M. G. Ford (ed.), Neuropharmacology and Pesticide Action, Neurotox '85, *Proceedings* of Symposium at University of Bath, England, 1986, VCH Publishers, New York, 1987.

G. P. Forney and L. Y. Cooper, "A Plan for the Development of the Generic Framework and Associated Computer Software for a Consolidated Compartment Fire Model Computer Code," National Bureau of Standards, Washington, D.C., 1987.

J. Francis, et al., "Suspected Solvent Abuse in Cases Referred to the Poison Unit, Guy's Hospital (London), July 1980–June 1981, *Human Toxicology,* **1,** 271–280, 1982 (London).

R. B. Gammage and S. V. Kaye, *Indoor Air and Human Health,* 430 pp., Lewis Publishers, Chelsea, Mich., 1985.

J. Getlin, "Congress Weighs Ban on Home Pesticide Chlordane," *L.A. Times,* 16 (June 25, 1987).

J. E. Greer, "Adolescent Abuse of Typewriter Correction Fluid," *S. Med. J.,* **27,** 297–298, 1984.

B. C. Hacker, *The Dragon's Tail: Radiation Safety in the Manhattan Project 1942–5,* 259 pp., University of California Press, Berkeley, 1987; see also S. W. Bell, "Atomic Bomb's Wastes Find Permanent Home: Burial in Landfill Follows Denial, Years of Fretting, Associated Press report to *Dayton (Ohio) Daily News and Journal Herald,* 16-F (Aug. 9, 1987).

T. J. Haley and W. O. Berndt, *Handbook of Toxicology,* 697 pp., Hemisphere Publishing, New York, 1987.

R. C. Harvey, *Polycyclic Hydrocarbons and Carcinogenesis,* ACS Symposium Series 283, 406 pp., American Chemical Society, Washington, D.C., 1986.

HEEP, "Abstracts on Health Effects of Environmental Pollutants," monthly current awareness newsletter, BIOSIS, 2100 Arch St., Philadelphia, PA 19103-1399.

I. Hertz-Picciotto, "Ethylene Oxide and Leukemia," *JAMA,* 2290 (May 1, 1987).

M. H. Ho and H. K. Dillon, *Biological Monitoring of Exposure to Chemicals, Organic Compounds,* 352 pp., Wiley-Interscience, New York, 1987.

C. Holden, "Industry Toxicologists Keen on Reducing Animal Use," *Science,* 252 (Apr. 17, 1987).

IOM, *Causes and Consequences of Alcohol Problems: An Agenda for Research,* 226 pp., Committee for the Study of Alcohol-Related Problems, Division of Health Sciences Policy, Institute of Medicine, National Academy of Sciences, Washington, D.C.

P. Johnson, "The Border War On Drugs—Congress of the U.S. Office of Technology Assessment, OTA-0-336, Washington, D.C., 1987.

M. R. Kare et al., *Biological and Behavioral Aspects of Salt Intake,* 448 pp., Academic Press, Orlando, Fla., 1980.

M. Karvonen, and M. I. Mikheev, *Epidemiology of Occupational Health,* 392 pp., WHO Regional Publications, European Series No. 20, World Health Organization, Copenhagen and Geneva, 1986.

R. M. Khanbilvardi and J. Fillos, *Groundwater Hydrology, Contamination, and Remediation,* 522 pp., Scientific Publications, P.O. Box 23041, Washington, DC 20026-3041, 1986.

B. C. Levin, "A Summary of the NBS Literature Reviews on the Chemical Nature and Toxicity of the Pyrolysis and Combustion Products from Seven Plastics," 31 pp., National Bureau of Standards, Washington, D.C., 1986.

B. C. Levin et al., "Further Development of a Test Method for the Assessment of the Acute Inhalation Toxicity of Combustion Products," NBSIR 82-2532, 133 pp., National Bureau of Standards, Center for Fire Research, Washington, D.C., 1982.

B. Lewin, *Genes,* 715 pp., Wiley, New York, 1983.

P. Lewis, "Nuclear Europe Is Unswayed by Chernobyl," *Internat'l Herald Tribune,* 5 (Apr. 28, 1987).

A. B. Levy, "Delirium Induced by Inhalation of Typewriter Correction Fluid," *Psychosomatics,* **27,** No. 9, 665–666 (Sept. 1986).

J. W. Lloyd et al., "Background Information on Trichloroethylene," *J. Occup. Med.,* **17,** 603–605 (1975).

H. McDermott, *Handbook of Ventilation for Contaminant Control,* 2nd ed., 424 pp., Butterworth Publishers, Stoneham, Mass., 1985.

E. Marshall, "EPA Indites Formaldehyde 7 Years Later," *Science,* 381 (April 24, 1987).

E. Marshall, "Hanford's Radioactive Tumbleweed," *Science,* 1616–1620 (June 26, 1987).

A. R. Mattocks, *Toxicology of Pyrrolizidine Alkaloids,* 393 pp., Academic Press, Orlando, Fla., 1986.

F. L. Mayer, Jr., and M. R. Ellersieck, *Manual of Acute Toxicity: Interpretations and Data Base for 410 Chemicals and 66 Species of Freshwater Animals,* 506 pp., National Technical Information Service, Springfield, Va., 1987.

B. Meyer, B. A. Kottes Andrews, and R. M. Reinhardt (eds.), *Formaldehyde Release from Wood Products,* ACS Symposium Series 316, 240 pp., American Chemical Society, Washington, D.C., 1986.

R. L. Miller, *Under the Cloud: The Decades of Nuclear Testing,* 547 pp., Free Press (Macmilllan), New York, 1986.

J. M. Montgomery, *Water Treatment Principles and Design,* 696 pp., Wiley-Interscience, New York, 1985.

N. Nelson (Chair), "Report of the Research Briefing Panel on Human Health Effects of Hazardous Chemical Exposures," 10 pp., National Academy Press, Washington, D.C., 1983.

A. Newman, "Expect to See More Cocaine-Induced Psychosis," *Clin. Psychiat. News,* **15,** No. 5, 3 (May 1987).

R. E. Nobel, "Convertible Automobile Touring and Seasonable Allergies from Pollen," *Lancet,* 872 (Apr. 11, 1987).

C. Norman, "Regulating Pesticides: The 'Delaney Paradox,' " *Science,* 1054 (May 29, 1987).

S. Okie, "A Tobacco Warning to Congress," *Washington Post,* A17 (Jan. 27, 1987).

R. W. Old and S. B. Primrose, *Principles of Gene Manipulation,* 3rd ed., 409 pp., Blackwell Scientific Publications, Oxford, England, 1985.

C. Peterson, "EPA's Nuclear Disposal Rules Voided (for High-Level Waste)," *Washington Post,* A19 (July 21, 1987).

J. J. Pignatello et al., "EDB: Persistence in Soil," *Science,* 898 (May 22, 1987).

J. Pointer, "Typewriter Correction Fluid: Inhalation: A New Substance of Abuse," *J. Toxicol. Clin. Toxicol.,* **19,** 483–489, 1982.

P. L. Polakeff, "Notification Process Raises Dilemmas," *Occupational Health & Safety,* 36–37 (Apr. 1986).

J. Powers, "Plant Operator Training Simplified with Use of Digital Simulator," *Chem. Proc.,* 77–78 (Mid-March 1987).

D. P. Rall, "Carcinogenicity of p-Dichlorobenzene," *Science,* 897–898 (May 28, 1987).

N. M. Ram, E. J. Calabrese, and R. F. Christman, *Organic Carcinogens in Drinking Water: Detection, Treatment and Risk Assessment,* 542 pp., Wiley-Interscience, New York, 1986.

C. Ramel et al., *Genetic Toxicity of Environmental Chemicals,* in two parts, 637 and 569 pp., Liss, New York, 1985.

B. Rensberger, "Fraud and Laxity in Research Are Detailed: Controversial Report Questions Effectiveness of Scientists' Self-Regulation, *Washington Post,* A4 (Jan. 27, 1987).

R. Rhodes, *The Making of the Atomic Bomb,* 886 pp., Simon & Schuster, New York, 1987.

A.H.T. Robb-Smith, "Thallium and a Pale Horse," *Lancet,* 872 (Apr. 11, 1987).

C. G. Rousseaux, "The Use of Animal Models for Predicting the Potential Chronic Effects of Highly Toxic Chemicals," *J. Hazardous Mat.,* **14,** 283–292 (March 1987).

M. Rutter and R. R. Jones, *Lead Versus Health, Sources and Effects of Low Level Lead Exposure,* 379 pp., Wiley, Chichester, England, and New York, 1983.

L. Sage, "Damage from Drink: A Chemical Link," *Outlook,* Washington University School of Medicine, **XXIV,** No. 1, 26–7 (Spring 1987).

M. T. Sampson, "Every Day About 1 Young Person Between 15 and 24 Commits Suicide Using Carbon Monoxide," *Clin. Psychiat. News,* **15,** No. 5, 1, 15

J. L. Sever and R. L. Brent, *Teratogen Update: Environmentally Induced Birth Defects Risks,* 248 pp., Liss, New York, 1986.

I. Shigematsu and A. Kagan, "Cancer in Atomic Bomb Survivors," 196 pp., GANN Monograph on Cancer Research No. 32, Plenum Press, New York, 1987.

P. Shrivastava, *Bhopal: Anatomy of a Crisis,* 185 pp., Ballinger, Cambridge, Mass., 1987.

D. Shuse and S. Burrell, "A Review of Solvent Abuses and Their Management by a Child Psychiatrist Outpatient Service," *Human Toxico.,* **I,** 321–329, 1982.

D. Streitfeld, "Pet Spray Controversy: EPA Studying Effects of Hartz 'Blockade,' " *Washington Post,* B5 (Sept. 11, 1987).

I. H. Suffet and M. Malaiyandi, "Organic Pollutants in Water: Sampling, Analysis, and Toxicity Testing," ACS Advances in Chemistry Series 214, 797 pp., American Chemical Society, Washington, D.C., 1987.

L. Tato, "Unexpected Less from Chernobyl (Importance of Iodized Salt in Preventing Congenital Hypothyroidism)," *Lancet,* 803 (Apr. 4, 1987).

P. Taylor, *Practical Teratology,* Academic Press, Orlando, Fla., 1986.

C. C. Travis et al., "Potential Health Risk of Hazardous Waste Incineration," *J. Hazardous Mat.,* **14,** 309–20 (March 1987).

J. S. Von Aspern, "Special Monitoring Precautions Needed for Workers Exposed to Hydrogen Sulfide," *Occupational Health & Safety,* 62–66 (May 1986).

J. M. Von Bergen, "Ironworkers Sue Over Lead Level in Blood," *Philadelphia Inquirer,* 8-B (Sept. 17, 1987).

R. D. Weiss, "Crack—A New Drug?," *Psychiat. Times,* 2–4 (July 1987).

M. Weisskoph, "Persistent Pervasive Pollutant Found in Soil, Water and Food, Lead Increasingly Seen as Health Peril," *Washington Post,* 1, 6 (June 15, 1987).

M. Weisskoff, "EPA to Strengthen Water Rules—Proposal Would Require Suppliers to Report Lead Content," *Washington Post,* A7 (March 31, 1987).

M. Weisskoff, "Smokers a Dwindling Minority in U.S.: Only 26.5 percent Puff Cigarettes Admit Health Concerns, Social Pressure," *Washington Post,* A9 (Sept. 11, 1987).

P. Wexler, *Guide to Toxicology Information Resources,* 2nd ed., Elsevier, New York, 1988.

C. P. Wickersham, "Decommissioned Transport Drums Decontaminated, Eliminating Concern over Disposal Procedures," *Chem. Proc.,* 74 (Mid-March 1987).

R. G. Zika and W. J. Cooper, "Photochemistry of Environmental Aquatic Systems," ACS Symposium Series 327, 288 pp., American Chemical Society, Washington, D.C., 1987.

9

Long-Term Toxicity

Elizabeth K. Weisburger

In the past decade there have been several legal actions that have attempted to increase the information about occupational hazards and to regulate possible carcinogens. These include the Toxic Substances Control Act of 1976, the adoption by OSHA of a list of regulated carcinogens, and the passage of the right-to-know laws that aim to inform workers of the hazardous materials to which they may be exposed. There is the possibility, however, that trade names may disguise the actual substances in commercial mixtures or formulations. Therefore, it is wise for those involved in such situations to be informed as to the nature of various compounds, especially with respect to the extent of their carcinogenicity and other long-term effects.

CARCINOGENICITY

Carcinogens are compounds that eventually cause some type of cancer in exposed animals or humans. Testing compounds for possible carcinogenic activity is generally done in groups of laboratory rats, mice, or sometimes hamsters. Exposure may be by inhalation, feeding, applying to the skin, or sometimes by injection. Usually the route that most closely resembles that by which people may be exposed is selected. Such tests are generally conducted over a period of about two years, which is the greater part of the life span of these animals.

The situation is more complicated when attempting to study carcinogenic effects in humans. The life span of humans is longer and often a period of 20–30 years may elapse before any differences in tumor incidence are noted between exposed people and the general population. Animals can be exposed to higher levels of test compounds than workers are likely to receive. Over a period of years, exposure levels in occupational settings may change, generally to lower levels. Industrial hygiene surveys of actual exposure levels may be incomplete so that reconstruction of actual exposure is difficult.

Despite all these uncertainties, surveys of exposed people, called epidemiologic studies as opposed to the experimental studies in animals, do indicate that certain industrial processes or discrete chemical compounds are likely to increase cancer in humans. These are listed in Table 9.1, with the organs or tissues generally affected. Various groups, such as the International Agency for Research on Cancer (IARC)[1] and the National Toxicology Program (NTP),[2] publish lists of such compounds on a periodic basis.

The industrial use of many of the substances that are definitely associated with an increase in human cancer has been banned or severely restricted in many countries. In addition, there are other compounds concerning which the evidence from

TABLE 9.1 Recognized Human Carcinogens

Compound	Site Affected or Tumor Type
4-Aminobiphenyl	Urinary bladder
Analgesic mixtures containing phenacetin	Kidney, urinary bladder
Arsenic and certain arsenic compounds	Skin, lung, liver
Asbestos	Lung, peritoneum or pleura (mesothelioma)
Azathioprine	Lymphoma; skin
Benzene	Leukemia
Benzidine	Urinary bladder
N,N-Bis(2-chloroethyl)-2-naphthylamine (chlornaphazine)	Urinary bladder
Bis(chloromethyl)ether and technical grade chloromethyl methyl ether	Lung
1,4-Butanediol dimethylsulfonate (Myleran)	Breast; Leukemia
Certain combined chemotherapy for lymphomas	Leukemia
Chlorambucil	Leukemia
Chromium and certain chromium compounds	Lung
Coke oven emissions	Lung, urinary tract
Conjugated estrogens	Liver, endometrium, ovary, breast
Cyclophosphamide	Leukemia; urinary bladder
Diethylstilbestrol	Vagina (in utero)
Melphalan	Leukemia
Methoxsalen with ultraviolet A therapy (PUVA)	Skin
Mustard gas	Respiratory tract
2-Naphthylamine	Urinary bladder
Nickel refining	Nasal cavity, lung
Thorium dioxide	Liver
Vinyl chloride monomer	Liver, brain, lung

epidemiologic studies is not so firm but for which animal studies do indicate a possible hazard. In the absence of information to the contrary, it is prudent to assume that an animal carcinogen may also be a human carcinogen. Substances in this category are listed in Table 9.2.

There also are several hundred compounds that have shown some carcinogenic effects in animals, but whose likelihood of appreciable exposure in the general population is low. In a few cases, epidemiologic surveys of exposed populations have been negative, but for most of these compounds there are no data. Nevertheless, it is wise to limit exposure to these compounds by means of good industrial hygiene measures and to treat them as if they might present a hazard (Table 9.3).

Recognition that natural and life-style factors may determine or influence the incidence of cancer in various populations is also needed. With regard to life-style, smoking is the one personal habit that has the most influence with respect to cancers. Smoking alone is considered responsible for up to 30 percent of male cancer deaths each year, comprising mostly lung, but also esophageal, bladder, and other cancer. Furthermore, a high proportion of heart disease also results from the use of smoking materials, as well as emphysema and other ailments. Passive smoking—that is, exposure to smoke from another's cigarette—also increases the risk of various types of cancers, especially lung and breast. Use of smokeless tobacco, as in snuff, is a dangerous habit as snuff contains fairly potent carcinogens, and epidemiologic studies have shown that snuff users may have up to a 50-fold higher incidence of cancer of the mouth than nonusers.

Smoking also enhances manyfold the action of some carcinogens, especially that of asbestos and the natural radioactivity of uranium mines. The combined action of smoking and using ethyl alcohol, which appears to be a very weak carcinogen itself, leads to an increased risk of cancer of the esophagus.

Another factor that has an appreciable influence on cancer rates is exposure to sunlight. Some sunlight is required to convert sterols to vitamin D in the skin. Nevertheless, an excess is harmful and increases the risk of skin cancers and melanoma.

There are other life-style factors that are less definitive than those mentioned but may likewise increase somewhat the possibility of developing cancer. These include diet, congenital and genetic diseases, drug use, acquired disease, familial susceptibility, behavioral patterns established by socioeconomic class and cultural conditions, and the presence of a precancerous state of some organ or tissue. There

TABLE 9.2 Probable Human Carcinogens

Acrylonitrile	Nickel and certain nickel compounds
Aflatoxins	Nitrogen mustard
Benzo(a)pyrene	Oxymetholone
Beryllium and beryllium compounds	Phenacetin
Combined oral contraceptives	Procarbazine
Diethyl sulfate	*o*-Toluidine
Dimethyl sulfate	

TABLE 9.3 Substances that Are Carcinogenic in Animals

2-Acetylaminofluorene	Estrogens (not conjugated): 3. Ethinyles-tradiol
Adriamycin	
2-Aminoanthraquinone	Estrogens (not conjugated): 4. Mestranol
1-Amino-2-methylanthraquinone	Ethylene oxide
Amitrole	Ethylene thiourea
o-Anisidine and o-anisidine hydorchloride	Formaldehyde (gas)
Aramite	Hexachlorobenzene
Benz(a)anthracene	Hexamethylphosphoramide
Benzo(b)fluoranthene	Hydrazine and hydrazine sulfate
Benzotrichloride	Hydrazobenzene
Bischloroethyl nitrosourea	Indeno(1,2,3-cd)pyrene
Cadmium and certain cadmium compounds	Iron dextran complex
Carbon tetrachloride	Kepone® (Chlorodecone)
1-(2-Chloroethyl)-3-cyclohexyl-1-nitrosourea (CCNU)	Lead acetate and lead phosphate
	Lindane and other hexachlorocyclohexane isomers
Chloroform	
4-Chloro-o-phenylenediamine	2-Methylaziridine (propyleneimine)
p-Cresidine	4,4'-Methylenebis(2-chloroaniline) (MBOCA)
Cupferon	
Cycasin	4,4'-Methylenebis(N,N-dimethyl) benzen-amine
Dacarbazine	
DDT	4,4'-Methylenedianiline and its dihydro-chloride
2,4-Diaminoanisole sulfate	
2,4-Diaminotoluene	Methyl iodide
Dibenz(a,h)acridine	Metronidazole
Dibenz(a,j)acridine	Michler's ketone
Dibenz(a,h)anthracene	Mirex
7H-Dibenzo(c,g)carbazole	Nitrilotriacetic acid
Dibenzo(a,h)pyrene	5-Nitro-o-anisidine
Dibenzo(a,i)pyrene	Nitrofen
1,2-Dibromo-3-chloropropane	2-Nitropropane
1,2-Dibromoethane (EDB)	N-Nitrosodi-n-butylamine
3,3'-Dichlorobenzidine	N-Nitrosodiethanolamine
1,2-Dichloroethane	N-Nitrosodiethylamine
Diepoxybutane	N-Nitrosodimethylamine
Di(2-ethylhexyl)phthalate	p-Nitrosodiphenylamine
3,3'-Dimethoxybenzidine	N-Nitrosodi-n-propylamine
4-Dimethylaminoazobenzene	N-Nitroso-N-ethylurea
3,3'-Dimethylbenzidine	N-Nitroso-N-methylurea
Dimethylcarbamoyl chloride	N-Nitrosomethylvinylamine
1,1-Dimethylhydrazine	N-Nitrosomorpholine
1,4-Dioxane	N-Nitrosonornicotine
Direct Black 38	N-Nitrosopiperidine
Direct Blue 6	N-Nitrosopyrrolidine
Epichlorohydrin	N-Nitrososarcosine
Estrogens (not conjugated): 1. Estradiol 17β	Norethisterone
	Phenazopyridine and phenazopyridine hy-drochloride
Estrogens (not conjugated): 2. Estrone	

TABLE 9.3 (*Continued*)

Phenytoin and sodium salt of phenytoin	Sulfallate
Polybrominated biphenyls	2,3,7,8-Tetrachlorodibenzo-p-dioxin
Polychlorinated biphenyls	(TCDD)
Progesterone	Thioacetamide
1,3-Propane sultone	Thiourea
β-Propiolactone	Toluene diisocyanate
Propylthiouracil	Toxaphene
Reserpine	2,4,6-Trichlorophenol
Saccharin	Tris(1-aziridinyl)phosphine sulfide
Safrole	Tris(2,3-dibromopropyl)phosphate
Selenium sulfide	Urethane
Streptozotocin	

is much controversy over many of these factors, but epidemiologic studies clearly indicate that the effects cannot be discounted.

Studies of migrant populations have shown the differing effects of these factors, specifically diet. Japanese diets, for example, have led to a high rate of stomach cancer but low colon cancer rates. Typical American diets have tended to decrease stomach cancer and increase colon cancer. Migrants from Japan to the United States have intermediate rates; migrant populations eventually acquire the typical rates of the new country.[3]

Congenital and genetic diseases seem to predispose individuals to developing cancer, often leukemia. Drugs, especially those employed in the treatment of neoplastic diseases, may increase the risk of cancer. In this situation, the risk versus the benefit to the patient must be considered. Other drugs, such as immunosuppressives, androgenic-anabolic steroids, overuse of phenacetin, and one treatment for psoriasis, have been associated with somewhat higher cancer rates in the patients. An illicit drug, specifically heroin, is thought to be linked to Hodgkin's disease in addicts.[4]

Acquired diseases, including infectious diseases, inflammatory states, endocrine and nutritional disorders, and trauma, have been implicated in the predisposition to later development of cancer. An example is schistosomiasis, which often leads to bladder cancer in affected individuals. Familial susceptibility leads to the clustering of certain types of cancer in families, a phenomenon that has been well documented for several hundred years. For example, close female relatives of breast cancer patients usually have a twofold risk of developing the same type of cancer. For relatives of those with melanoma, the risk may be up to eight times greater than in the general population.

Behavioral patterns may play a role in tumors of endocrine-related organs. Women of higher socioeconomic class and nuns have a higher risk of developing breast cancer. In contrast, women of lower socioeconomic status, those who have frequent sexual partners, or who initiate sexual activity at an early age have a lower risk of breast cancer but an increased risk of cancer of the uterine cervix. Increased risk of prostate cancer among men has also been associated with multiple sexual

TABLE 9.4 Proportions of Cancer Cases Attributed to Different Factors

Factor	Percent of Cancer Cases	
	Males	Females
Tobacco	28–30	7–8
Tobacco/alcohol	4–5	1–3
Diet	40	57
Life-style	30	63
Occupation	4–6	2
Sunlight	10	10
Ionizing radiation	1	1
Iatrogenic	1	1
Exogenous hormones	-	4
Congenital	2	2
Unknown	15	11

partners. The age at first pregnancy and the number of pregnancies have a bearing on risks for cancer of the breast and ovary.

Estimates have been made by several groups of epidemiologists on the percent of cancer cases that can be attributed to various factors and have been summarized by Doll and Peto (Table 9.4). Although there are slight variations, all indicate that tobacco is responsible for the greatest percentage of cancer cases among males. In contrast, the estimates for cancer due to occupational exposure range from 2 to 8 percent.

Nevertheless, there should be no slackening of industrial hygiene standards or a decrease in the use of protective devices when handling chemicals in the workplace or elsewhere in the environment. However, there is a need for each of us personally to assume a greater responsibility for preventing cancer and to adjust our life style accordingly.

OTHER TYPES OF TOXICITY

Although the main concern regarding exposure to chemical compounds seems to be carcinogenicity, other toxic effects should not be disregarded. The acute toxicity of the intermediates methyl isocyanate, phosgene, hydrogen cyanide, phosphorus, hydrogen fluoride, chlorine, hydrogen sulfide, and arsenic oxide, to name a few, is recognized (cf., Chapter 8). Other compounds or their metabolites are neurotoxins, and in some cases may lead to irreversible effects; for others, the neuropathy may be reversible. Neurological effects result from exposure to hexane, acrylamide, lead, or mercury, among others (Table 9.5).

In addition to acute toxicity and neurotoxicity, the possible mutagenicity of industrial materials, as well as their teratogenic and reproductive effects, should be considered. The workforce is now more likely to be composed of both men and

TABLE 9.5 Neurotoxic Agents

A. Defined Agents

Acrylamide	Hexachlorophene
Aluminum	Lead
Arsenic	Leptophos
Barium	Manganese
Cadmium	Methanol
Carbon disulfide	Methyl-n-butyl ketone
Chlorodecone	Methyl mercury
Clioquinol	Tellurium
Dimethylaminopropionitrile	Thallium
Doxorubicin	Triethyl tin
Hexane (metabolites)	Zinc pyridinethione

B. Natural or Not Well-Defined Products

Animal toxins
    Amphibians (toads, frogs, salamanders)
    Mammalian (anteater, shrew)
    Piscine (puffer fish, sting ray, toad fish, weever fish)
    Reptilian (cobra, rattlesnake, coral snake)
Plant toxins
    Buckthorn, jimson weed, peyote

women. Although teratogenic actions are of concern to women, reproductive toxicity should be a subject of concern for both men and women.

MUTAGENICITY

Mutagens are compounds that can cause abrupt and heritable genetic changes. Although some mutations are beneficial, the concern is that most may lead to deleterious effects that may be either immediate or expressed over many generations. Since it may require many generations to determine the effect of some mutagens in mammals, most such tests are performed with bacteria as the test organisms. One of the most widely used is the Ames test, in which specially developed sensitive strains of the bacterium *Salmonella typhimurium*, grown in a defined culture medium, are exposed to the test compound. The specific strains of *S. typhimurium* generally employed are histidine dependent; when the bacteria mutate, they no longer require histidine and form growing colonies. The count of these colonies on the culture dish constitutes a measure of the mutagenic activity of the test compound. The effect of metabolic activation by mammalian enzymes is determined by adding an aliquot of a liver homogenate from rats, mice, or hamsters pretreated with an enzyme inducer. Such tests are run in parallel with those where not liver homogenate is added. Details on the procedures to be followed are given by Brusick.[4]

REPRODUCTIVE EFFECTS

The subject of reproductive toxicity is complicated by the diverse systems involved: the male reproductive system, the female reproductive system, and the germ cells. Various types of chemicals have been shown to affect these systems. For the purposes of this chapter, industrial and environmental agents that are associated with human reproductive toxicity will be mentioned.

Lead is a confirmed reproductive toxicant; occupationally exposed men have shown disturbances in spermatogenesis while there has been a higher incidence of spontaneous abortions and stillbirths in exposed women. Inorganic mercury has been linked to reproductive disorders. Workers exposed during manufacture or formulation of the pesticides 1,2-dibromo-3-chloropropane and chlordecone (Kepone) had decreased spermatogenesis in one exposed population, but another study on workers who had a very low exposure showed no reproductive effects. Ethylene oxide has been associated with infertility in exposed women but not in men. Other compounds implicated as reproductive toxicants are aniline, benzene, chloroprene, formaldehyde, probably polychlorinated biphenyls, styrene, toluene, and vinyl chloride. Many other compounds have shown effects on reproductive capability in laboratory animals but human data are inconclusive or lacking. In this category are arsenic, boron, cadmium, manganese, chromium compounds, selenium, thallium, DDT, 1,2-dibromoethane, hexane, ethylene glycol monomethyl and monoethyl ethers, phthalic acid esters, and tris(2,3-dibromopropyl)phosphate. In addition, there are many drugs that have some action on reproductive systems, especially alkylating agents used as chemotherapeutic agents. Such habits as smoking, use of ethanol, and illicit drugs may also have reproductive effects.[5]

TERATOGENICITY

Teratogenicity relates to the capability to induce a congenital malformation in a developing system. The deviation may be of either a structural or a functional nature. There are both physical and chemical teratogens, as well as other less well-defined factors, such as maternal disease or malnutrition, that can have a teratogenic effect (Table 9.6).

Experimentally, teratogenesis is usually studied in rats and rabbits but no common laboratory species is a perfect model for humans. The period of gestation when there is exposure has a great influence, depending on which organ system is developing (organogenesis)—the time when this system is most sensitive. Exposure before the cells of the developing organism have differentiated into specific organ systems usually does not lead to a teratogenic effect, whereas after these systems have developed, there is an increased resistance to teratogenesis. Physical teratogens include X-rays, heat, and pressure. Among maternal factors are infection, excess or deficiency of certain nutrients, rubella or other viral diseases, long-term malnutrition, and age. The known chemical agents that have shown a teratogenic effect in humans are listed in Table 9.7. A great number of viral, chemical, and

TABLE 9.6 Causes of Developmental Defects in Humans

Genetic transmission
Chromosomal aberration
Environmental causes
    Radiation
        Therapeutic, diagnostic
Infections
    Rubella virus
    Cytomegalovirus
    Herpes virus
    Toxoplasma
    Syphilis
Maternal imbalance
    Endemic cretinism
    Diabetes
    Phenylketonuria
    Virilizing tumors
Drugs and environmental chemicals

TABLE 9.7 Human Teratogens

Compound	System Affected
A. Recognized	
Aminopterin	Skeletal
Androgenic hormones	Pseudohermaphroditism
Antithyroid compounds	Hypothyroidism
6-Azauridine	—
Busulfan	Renal and central nervous system
Chlorambucil	Urogenital
Coumarin anticoagulants	Nose and skeletal
Cyclophosphamide	Digits
Cytarabine	Limb and ear
Diethylstilbestrol	Uterine lesions
Fluorouracil	Multiple
Mechlorethamine/procarbazine	Renal, limbs, ear
Methotrexate	Skeletal
Methyl mercury	Brain and nervous system
Streptomycin/dihydrostreptomycin	Inner ear
Thalidomide	Limbs
Trimethadone/paramethadione	Face, mental retardation
B. Suspected	
Barbiturates	Metronidazole
Diazepam	Quinine
Hydantoins	Tetracycline
Quinine	Valproic acid
Lithium carbonate	Vitamin A and analogs (excess)

Source: Data from Schardein.[5]

other agents have been tested for teratogenicity in laboratory animals and cataloged in appropriate fashion for easy reference by Shepard.[6]

To decrease the possibility of a teratogenic effect, pregnant women should not receive X-rays, should have an adequate diet, and should be given the lowest effective dose of any necessary drugs. Exposure to unknown factors, chemical or physical, should be eliminated to the greatest possible extent.

REFERENCES

1. International Agency for Research on Cancer, IARC Monographs on the "Evaluation of the Carcinogenic Risk of Chemicals to Humans. Chemicals, Industrial Processes and Industries Associated with Cancer in Humans." IARC Monographs Supplement 4, IARC, Lyon, France, 1982.

2. U.S. Department of Health and Human Services, Public Health Service, National Toxicology Program, Fourth Annual Report on Carcinogens, 1985.

3. R. Doll and R. Peto, "The Causes of Cancer: Quantitative Estimates of Avoidable Risks of Cancer in the United States Today, *J. Natl. Cancer Inst.*, **66,** 1191–1308 (1981).

4. D. Brusick, *Principles of Genetic Toxicology,* Plenum Press, New York, 1980.

5. J. L. Schardein, *Chemically Induced Birth Defects,* M. Dekker, New York, 1985.

6. T. H. Shepard, *Catalog of Teratogenic Agents,* 4th ed., John Hopkins University Press, Baltimore, Md., 1983.

SUGGESTED READINGS

R. L. Dixon (ed.), *Reproductive Toxicology,* Raven Press, New York, 1985.

J. F. Fraumeni, Jr. (ed.) *Persons at High Risk of Cancer. An Approach to Cancer Etiology and Control.* Academic Press, New York, 1975.

Identifying and Estimating the Genetic Impact of Chemical Mutagens. National Academy Press, Washington, DC, 1983.

H. Kalter (ed.), *Issues and Reviews of Teratology,* Vol. 1, Plenum Press, New York, 1983.

P. S. Spencer and H. H. Schaumburg, (eds.), *Experimental and Clinical Neurotoxicity,* Williams & Wilkins, Baltimore, Md., 1980.

R. W. Tennant et al., Prediction of Chemical Carcinogenicity in Rodents from in Vitro Genetic Toxicity Assays, *Science,* 933–941 (May 22, 1987).

U.S. Department of Health and Human Services, Public Health Service, Office on Smoking and Health. "The Health Consequences of Smoking; A Report of the Surgeon General," 1982.

U.S. Department of Health and Human Services, Public Health Service. "The Health Consequences of Using Smokeless Tobacco. A Report of the Advisory Committee to the Surgeon General," 1986.

J. G. Wilson, *Environment and Birth Defects,* Academic Press, New York, 1973.

J. G. Wilson and F. C. Fraser (eds.), *Handbook of Teratology,* Vol. 1, Plenum Press, New York, 1977.

10

Dioxin and Related Substances

Howard H. Fawcett

Dioxin, an imprecise term for one or more of the 75 isomers that constitute variations on the basic molecule, has been the subject of many "horror" stories, in both the print and the electronic media. Often overlooked is the fact that dioxins (TCDDs) are not deliberately synthesized molecules but are formed as the unwanted (and often unsuspected) by-products of trichlorophenols, polychlorinated biphenyls (PCBs), and certain herbicides that contain the specific atomic configuration that responds to unusual conditions of temperature, pressure, concentrations, and time, to form, often in only small concentrations, TCDDs and related molecules.

Dibenzo-p-dioxin

2,3,7,8-Tetrachloro-
dibenzo-p-dioxin (TCDD)

Other molecules closely associated with the dioxins are the dibenzofurans, formed by the condensation reaction involving tetrachlorobenzene and sodium trichlorophenate, 2,3,7,8-tetrachlorodibenzofuran (TCDF). Various degress of chlorination and substitution make a variety of isomers possible.

The most elementary source of these and related compounds is in the manufacture of 2,4,5-trichlorophenol, essential to the production of 2,4,5-T, both a useful herbicide and an established component of the widely discussed Agent Orange, about which there is little agreement even two decades after its use as a defoliant in Vietnam.

Pentachlorophenol manufacture also produces both dioxins and PCDFs as by-products.

PCBs are excellent heat-transfer agents and were widely used in a variety of electrical equipment, including transformers and fluorescent lighting and other capicators, until banned in the United States in 1977. Thousands of such pieces of equipment and accesories are still in service, but PCB-containing transformers must be removed from buildings by 1990 by law. PCBs were considered relatively innocuous materials in the United States and Europe until 1968, when severe illness was reported in Japan's Fukuoka prefect that was said to result from the ingestion of cooking oils contaminated during manufacture with PCBs and PCDFs. First noted was the peculiar skin rash the contaminated oils produced, which was called *Yusho* (oil) disease. The contamination apparently occurred when PCBs (Kanechlor 400) were used to heat oil under reduced pressure, they leaked into the oil, which, at the elevated temperatures, produced by-products and small amounts of the dioxins, furans, and other impurities. As a result, the handling and disposal of PCBs became a major concern of environmentalists, and many laws and regulations were instituted to prevent improper transfer of these products to humans via the environment (see Suggested Readings).

Depending on the reaction rate, concentrations, and temperature control, various combinations of the dioxins and the dibenzofurans are formed. Should the temperature rise in the initial reaction stages, a condensation reaction involving tetrachlorobenzene and 2,4,5-sodium trichlorophenate would take place, and 2,3,7,8-TCDF would be formed. Professor C. Rappe, University of Umea, Sweden, the recognized authority on such reactions, feels that an accident during this reaction at an early stage favors PCDF formation, and at the end of the reaction favors TCDD production. At Seveso, Italy, in what is widely cited as a classic case of inadequate control, the accident occurred six and a half hours after the completion of the production run. Analysis of the soil around the factor that was affected by the "fallout" confirmed that 2,3,7,8-TCDD was the major contamination.[1]

TOXICITY AND HUMAN EXPOSURES

Not all animal species or all humans react in the same way to a given dose or exposure of a chemical or drug.

The statement that dioxin is "one of the deadliest substances known" or that it is "one of the deadliest man-made substances" is very misleading, and is based on its extreme and unusual toxicity to guinea pigs. As little as 0.6 μg/kg (microgram) per kilogram of body weight given orally will kill half the male guinea pigs receiving the dose (or oral LD 50). Illness occurs immediately and death within a week or 10 days after the dose is administered.

Dioxin is much less toxic to mice than to guinea pigs. The guinea pig is 500–10,000 times more sensitive to TCDD than is the hamster (which is the least sensitive animal tested). Rabbits, mice, and monkeys are roughly 200 times less sensitive than guinea pigs and 50 times more sensitive than hamsters. All such comparisons must be made with great care, since other, as yet unrecognized factors may have an influence on these numbers.

The single does LD50 for monkeys for TCDD is 50 μg/kg body weight. Human LD50 is estimated to be in the same range of 50–100 μg/kg body weight. Using the figure 50 μg/kg, TCDD is about 10 times as toxic as hydrogen cyanide (HCN). As noted above, all such comparisons must be used with caution, since the ability of HCN to enter the body is many times greater than that of TCDD.

The single doses LD50 for several substances may be compared as in Table 10.1.

Dioxin is stable to heat, acids, and alkali. Its solubility in water is very low (2 $\times$ 10^{-4} ppm) (parts per million). It is slightly soluble in fats (44 ppm in lard oil); and is 570 ppm in benzene and 1400 ppm in 0-dichlorobenzene. In soil, where the soil microbes slowly degrade or decompose the substance, the half-lives of TCDD in Utah and Florida are 320 and 230 days respectively. The dioxin half-life at Seveso, Italy, where soil and bacteria are different, as estimated as two to three years, or possibly longer.

At temperatures of 700°C (1292°F), only 50 percent TCDD is decomposed in 21 seconds, while at 800°C (1472°F), the decomposition is reported to be complete. A residence time of at least two seconds in an incinerator has been required in such operations. Considerable uncertainty exists in the literature as to the TCDD formation (if any) from the burning of vegetation sprayed with 2,4,5-T. In forest fires, where a temperature of 1200°C (2192°F) is possible, the dioxins probably are completely, or nearly, destroyed. Pyrolysis of technical-grade PCB mixtures will yield some 30 major and 30 minor polychlorinated dibenzofurans.

The most widely publicized incident to date in which PCBs were directly involved was a February 1981 fire in the basement of the 17-story State Office Building in Binghamton, N.Y. As will be noted later in this chapter, completion of cleanup and reoccupancy of the building are not anticipated until January 1988 due to the widespread contamination of the building and its contents by the smoke, which deposited decomposition products on all parts of the building.

It is known that when PCBs are directly involved in fire, furans, including 2,3,7,8-tetrachlorodibenzofuran or TCDF (the most toxic furans), as well as the dioxins, are formed. Uncontrolled burning of the PCBs can be an environmental hazard. Dr. Otto Hutzinger of the University of Amsterdam has found that, upon burning, lignin and PVC produce dioxins. At least one state, New York, has

TABLE 10.1

Substance	Dose, μg/kg
Dioxin (TCDD)	50 μg/kg
HCN	500 μg/kg
Cyanide salts	2000 μg/kg
Cantharidin	300 μg/kg
Nicotine	600 μg/kg
Colchicine	300 μg/kg
Digitoxin (or digitalis)	35 μg/kg

seriously considered writing combustion toxicity standards as part of the state building code, to encourage the use of material that, in a fire, will not produce especially toxic products.

Much study has been devoted to the potential and actual health hazards of commercial-grade PCB as used in the electrical industry, including studies of persons exposed for many years in the handling and filling of capacitors and transformers, at such locations as Hudson Falls and Fort Edward, N.Y. Severe PCB contamination in the Hudson River—reportedly more than 100 times greater than in any other major river system—has been identified. Edible portions of fish collected from this area often exceed the FDA tolerance level of 5.0 ppm fresh weight. Carcich and Tracy Tofflemire, Senior Santary Engineers for New York State, estimated that more than 272,000 kg (perhaps as much as 603,000 kg) of PCBs was discharged into the river, and that most of this still resides in sediments north of Troy, N.Y. In the Hudson River, levels of higher chlorinated PCB components typical of Aroclor 1254 have stabilized during 1977–1981, suggesting that a dynamic equilibrium has been reached, and that these compounds may continue to exist at concentrations close to prsesent levels. Removal of PCB-contaminated sediments by dredging from the Hudson River is now being studied, with greatest effort confined to the most highly contaminated 8 percent of the river bed. Disposal, by total containment and isolation of contaminated materials within a land-burial facility, is one of the preferred options.

Dr. Seymour Friess has reviewed the data, and has summarized many of these findings: "At human exposure levels as high as those previously encountered in occupational settings, PCBs can cause chloracne and increases in one or more liver enzymes. Neither represents a serious or life-threatening problem. From present evidence, no firm associations can be made between PCB exposures and any other human health effects." Dioxins have also been noted in fires that do not contain PCBs.

Dioxin can be decomposed by ultraviolet (UV) light if dissolved in a suitable solvent such as methanol. Twenty-four hours were required for complete photolysis using artifical UV light; 36 hours were needed when using natural sunlight. Dioxin-containing substances, such as Agent Orange [a 1:1 mixture of butyl esters of 2,4-dichlorophenoxyacetic acid (2,4-D) and 2,4,5-T], can be chlorinated at high temperatures and pressures, producing carbon tetrachloride. Oxidation by ruthenium tetraoxide ($RuO4$) will also degrade TCDD.

HUMAN ASPECTS OF CLINICAL FINDINGS

Known or suspected effects of exposure to TCDD have been studied by records and observation of 1000 persons who had been exposed since 1949 in industrial accidents during the production of chlorinated phenols or 2,4,5-T. Three of these 17 incidents occurred in the United States, and may have involved a total of 317 persons. The data reveal:

1. *Chloroacne:* This eruption of the skin causes blackheads, usually associated with small pale-yellow cysts. In severe cases, papulas or pustules may be observed. The major area involved is usually the face, under the eyes and behind the ears. It may persist for several years, perhaps as many as 15 years after the last exposure. It should be noted that chloracne in humans can be produced by exposure to chlornaphthylenes (CNs), polychlorinated biphenyls (PBCs), polybrominated biphenyls (PBB), polychlorinated dibenzo-p-dioxins (PCDDs), polychlorinated dibenzofurans (PCDFs), 3,4,3,4-tetrachloroazobenzene (TCAB), 3,4,3,4-tetrachloroazoxybenzene (TCAOB).

The Dow Chemical Company toxicology laboratory has performed extensive research on the chloracne problem.

2. *Enlarged Liver and Impairment of Liver Functions:* Increased transaminase values in serum over the normal may be found after exposure to TCDD, but this is not considered a reliable diagnostic tool. Clinical signs of liver dysfunction have been noted in up to 50 percent of persons with known TCDD exposures.

3. *Neurology:* Severe muscle pains aggravated by exertion, especially in the calves, thighs, and chest area, and impairment of sight, hearing, smell, and taste have also been noted. In the central nervous system, lassitude, weakness, impotence, and loss of libido have been reported.

LONG-TERM EFFECTS OF TCDD-RELATED EXPOSURES

Long-term effects have been observed as follows:

1. *Immunocapability:* Persons exposed in the Coalite TCP explosion (1969 in England) and studied 10 years later, who still had chloracne, showed some changes on immunological tests, but were in a health state comparable to those of other workers exposed but without chloracne and of an unexposed control group. Forty-five children exposed during the Seveso, Italy, incident with maximum exposures of 235 $\mu g/m^2$ of soil (20 of whom had chloracne) had comparable levels of effective pathology compared with 44 controls, three years later.

2. *Teratogenic Effects:* Studies of several thousand women of childbearing age exposed to a known level of TCDD in Seveso have shown that the frequency of spontaneous abortions per number of calculated pregnancies and per number of women of childbearing age did not change either immediately after the accident or in the following three years as compared with previous years.

3. *Carcinogenic Aspects:* TCDD causes cancer in rats and mice; however, cancer-mortality studies of five groups of exposed persons (410 workers) indicate no excess in mortality over the matching population 14–30 years after exposure. Increased stomach-cancer mortality was reported from the 71 workers exposed during the BASF accident in 1953, but peer review has questioned the significance of this study.

In Sweden, frequency of soft-tissue sarcoma seems to be higher for railway workers spraying 2,4,5-T and other herbicides, but not in a similar group in Finland, or in agricultural workers in New Zealand. The issue is unresolved.

On July 29, 1983, a UPI press report quoted Philip Landrigan of NIOSH as saying that an association has been found between dioxin and soft-tissue sarcoma, but no absolute proof is yet available. Soft-tissue sarcoma attacks muscles, fat, nerves, and/or connective fibers. On March 26, 1987, Dr. M. Fingerhut of NIOSH informed the writer that, in spite of much research, the subject has not yet resolved.[2]

4. *Chromosome Aberrations:* No abnormal chromosome aberrations have been reported in the cytogenic studies in four exposed populations.

ACCEPTABLE DAILY INTAKE (ADI)

The acceptable daily intake (ADI) is the amount that can be regularly absorbed through all possible routes for the small concentrations absorbed for the entire life span via diet or other means of environmental contamination. In 1980, the Scientific Advisory Panel of the EPA stated that a dose of 0.001 μg/kg body weight per day of TCDD is, for all practical purposes, a no-observable-effect level, including carcinogenic, tetraogenic, and reproductive risk. The FDA recommended in 1981 that fish containing TCDD at a level of more than 50 parts per trillion should not be consumed.

In this context, it is worthy of note that biomagnification of PCBs through marine food chains in an Australian estuary became increasing important with upper-level carnivores, such as gulls and pelicans, but was relatively unimportant at lower trophic levels. A similar situation was observed in Central Puget Sound in Washington State in 1979. PCB body burdens in marine organisms, especially benthic organisms, were directly related to the log of PCB concentration in sediments. Furthermore, PCBs were found in every tissue analyzed from fish and invertebrates in Puget Sound in 1979. High PCB levels, especially in sediments, have been recorded from highly industrial areas worldwide.[3]

The CDC recommends one part per billion (1 ppb) as an acceptable level of TCDD in soil. This is not intended as an all-purpose standard, but primarily for residential properties and other areas where children may ingest soil on a daily basis. Each contaminated site should be reviewed on a case-by-case basis. (The highest level of dioxin to date was found in Missouri, which forced evacuation of three families near St. James. The EPA found levels up to 1800 ppb, six times higher than those initially found in Times Beach, Mo.)

PCB burdens in waters, sediments, soils, disposal sites, and deployed transformers and other containers of PCB is estimated at 82 million kilograms. At this time, total PCB residues in organisms appear to be a more reliable measure of environmental PCB levels than measurements of any commercial mixtures. In light of the demonstrated differential toxicities within the array of PCB congeners, existing standards and criteria may need to be modified in order to reflect the more toxic PCBs.

PCB tolerance levels have been recommended for protection of various environmental resources and human health.[3,4] The recommended freshwater aquatic life protection criterion of 0.014 μg/l (micrograms per liter) (24-hour average) is lower than 0.1 μg/l, a concentration known adversely to affect the growth of freshwater algae and fish. This criterion would probably afford a satisfactory degree of protection to freshwater life if it were changed from 0.014 μg/l (24-hour average) to 0.014 μg/l (maximum). Criteria based on average daily concentrations usually indicate that high doses of toxicants may be absorbed within a short period. Unfortunately, data bases existing for PCBs are inadequate to predict long-term effects on growth, uptake, and other variables when repeated high doses take place in short intervals.

The criterion of 0.03 μg/l (24-hour average) recommended for saltwater aquatic life protection is unsatisfactory. Concentrations of 0.1 μg/l of Arochlor 1254 are fatal to sheepshead minnows in 21 days, and concentrations as low as 0.006 μg/l result in significant uptake by oysters over a period of 65 days. Until additional data become available, the saltwater aquatic life protection criterion should not differ from the freshwater criterion (0.014 μg/l, maximum).

Sound management of fishery and wildlife resources—including those resources that are artificially propagated and released—requires noninterference with desired uses such as those for the health and well-being of humans and other organisms at various trophic levels. Before the legislative restrictions on PCB use, substantial losses to the atmosphere resulted from evaporation of plasticizers and from improper incineration, directly affecting occupational workers, as well as aquatic ecosystems. In recent years, PCB levels have significantly declined in all human food items, with the possible exception of fish; most samples of fish containing more than 5.0 μg PCBs per kilogram fresh weight originated from the Great Lakes area. In Michigan, all of a sample of 1057 mothers had measurable PCBs in their breast milk at an average level of 2.3 μg/kg. Nursing infants from Michigan mothers might consume 10–25 times the maximum daily dose rate of 1.0 μg/kg currently recommended by the FDA for human adult intake. The Michigan Department of Public Health has since established a Public Health Advisory related to fish consumption. It recommends that children, pregnant women, nursing mothers, and women who expect to bear children should not consume fish from the Great Lakes area.

Canadian PCB tolerance levels in food items for human health protection are markedly lower than those of the United States. In one case, the current U.S. health tolerance level of 5.0 μg/kg fresh weight in fish and shellfish presents a distinct hazard to piscivorous teleosts and fish-eating birds and mammals. A lowering from 5.0 to 2.0 μg PCB per kilogram fresh weight in fish and shellfish has been proposed by the FDA, but the tolerance level has not yet been changed; the delay appears to be based on economic reasons. In the Great Lakes, for example, 55 percent of the domestic fish samples collected in 1979–80 exceeded 2.0 μg PCBs fresh weight; in 1980–81, this figure was 17 percent; and in 1981–82, 10 percent of the samples exceeded 2 μg/kg, including chinook salmon and their eggs and lake trout. In every collection year, measurable PCB residues were recorded in at least 28 percent of the Great Lakes fish samples collected. At present, three courses of action appear warranted: continuation of the nationwide monitoring program of fish and wildlife for PCBs and other environmental pollutants; additional investigations on the fate of PCBs under conditions prevailing in the natural environment; and controlled studies on the toxicological significance of chlorinated dibenzofurans and other trace impurities found in commercial PCB mixtures and PCB-containing fluids.

EPA has established criteria for 2,3,7,8-TCDD in surface water of 1.3×10^{-8} μg/l.[4] For 2,4,5-T, a joint committee of the Food and Agriculture Organization and the World Health Organization stated in 1980 that the "no-effect level" is 3 μg/kg/day, and the ADI for humans is 0.003 μg/kg/day when the TCDD content of the 2,4,5-T is 0.05.

Personnel should not be exposed to air containing more than 1 μg of PCBs per cubic meter released by electrical equipment fires. This is the lowest level at which PCBs can be accurately detected. PCBs can cause abnormal reproduction of animals, and cancer in laboratory mice and rats; some isomers may be human carcinogens, and also may cause liver injuries. After an electrical fire, air and wipe samples should be taken and analyzed by an approved laboratory. Personnel doing cleanup need protective clothing and respiratory protection, in addition to' strict personal hygiene and other appropriate controls on exiting from the facility in question.

The Seveso incident prompted the European Economic Community to initiate studies on a directive aimed at preventing "the risk of incidents." The purpose of the directive (known as the Seveso directive) is the establishment of general criteria for the regulation of hazardous industrial activities in the 10 member countries. Note this was five years *before* the Bhopal, Chernobyl, Challenger, and Miamisburg (Ohio) incidents that led to the Title III section of PL 99-499 in the United States on emergency planning and response.

REMEDIAL ACTION

Once it has been determined that excessive levels of dioxins and/or other comparable hazardous materials are present in soil or ground areas, several approaches may be considered.

1. *Stabilization in Place:* This involves sealing or otherwise covering the soil with a cover inside an impermeable barrier around the perimeter. A clay cap at least 4 feet thick must be placed over the whole area to ensure that no groundwater will move through or into the area. As an alternative, cement or fly ash or organic polymers may be considered as soil-stabilization agents.

2. *On-Site Storage:* A landfill may be created directly on site, using a concrete building or structure, or an above-ground cell with an impermeable clay or synthetic liner. A leachate collection system and monitoring wells are also required.

3. *Transport to Secure Landfill:* This refers to excavation of the contaminated

soil and removal by truck or rail to an acceptable secure landfill where the soil would be covered and monitored to ensure that there will be no leakage of leachate to the environment. The transport mode introduces additional risk and significantly increases the overall cost and the exposure of people.

4. *Dredging from a Stream and Burying on Land in a Secure Landfill:* This method has both advantages and disadvantages. The removal from the contaminated stream, such as the Hudson River above Troy, N.Y., for example, would be highly desirable, but has met with considerable citizens' resistance out of fear that the dredging will contaminate local water supplies. A landfill would be established, in this case, at Fort Edward near lock 7 and Rogers Island. The slurry would be brought by scow to a pumping facility, before the PCBs are repumped to the "containment site," and the water returned to the Hudson River. A sum of $20 million has been set aside for this project under the Clean Water Act of EPA if the state realizes a May 10, 1989, construction start date. The state plans to dredge about 24,000 pounds of PCBs from a five-mile stretch of the Hudson just south of Fort Edward. The work would remove about half of the PCBs located in a five-mile stretch known as the Thompson Island Pool. The plan would require seven years to complete.

BINGHAMTON STATE OFFICE BUILDING

Early on the morning of Thursday, February 5, 1981, a fire occurred in the electrical equipment in the basement area of the 17-story building when it was unoccupied except for a security guard and a stationary engineer. The fire services responded quickly and extinguished the fire.

Each of two transformers contained 1060 gallons of cooling oil containing PCBs, of which 180 gallons had leaked out from cracked insulators. A complete inspection of the building by the Department of Environmental Control revealed that a fine soot had been distributed throughout all areas of the upper floors via the air-conditioning system. At that time, the estimated cleanup time was several days to several weeks. Air samples taken by the N.Y. State Department of Health contained 6–62 μg of PCB per cubic meter, and the soot registered PCB levels of from 10 to 20 percent. A few days later, the State Health Department informed the Office of General Services that analyses firmly indicated that, in addition to the PCBs, the soot also contained lesser amounts of dioxin and dibenzofuran. Since this was a unique problem, a panel of experts (chemists and physicians) assembled to focus on such questions as:

What level of human exposure to the various chemicals identified is acceptable?

Which chemical compounds should be the main target of the cleanup?

Should guidelines be established separately for different routes of exposure, such as dermal, ingestion, and inhalation?

Should all areas of the building be subject to the same guidelines regardless of differences in potential human exposure?

What safeguards are necessary to prevent exposure in noncontaminated areas?

Establishment of proper controls for entry and exit of cleanup personnel and others followed the standard recommendations that might be employed when working with biochemicals or radiological materials.

To repeat the details of the cleanup, which has been much slower and more costly than originally predicted, is hardly necessary.[5,6] According to David Rings of the New York General Services, Albany, as of March 15, 1987, it was estimated that the building would be ready for occupancy in January 1988, at a total cost of $37 million for the cleanup and related services.

Several companies are offering their services to remove and replace the PCB fluid with other electrical insulating fluids that now are available to the industry. However, it should be noted that this changeover (or retrofit) introduces an increased risk of fire, since the newer substitutes are less fire resistant than PCB-containing fluids.[4]

REFERENCES

1. C. Rappe, Analysis of Polychlorinated dibenzofurans and Dioxins in Ecological Systems, 304, and Compositions of PCD's Formed in PCB Fires, 252, *Abstracts of 186 National Meeting, American Chemical Society, Division of Environmental Chemistry,* Vol. 23, No. 2, August 28–Sept. 2, 1983, Washington, D.C.

2. anon, PCB health effects challenged, *Pollution Engineering,* Vol. XIX, No. 10, 48, October 1987

3. D. G. Barnes, "Regulatory Actions on Dioxins and Related Compounds," pp. 23–31, in *Human and Environmental Risks of Chlorinated Dioxins and Related Compounds,* edited by R. E. Tucker, A. L. Young, and A. P. Gray, Plenum Press, New York and London, 1983.

4. *Federal Register,* **49,** No. 32, 5831 (Feb. 15, 1984).

5. H. H. Fawcett, *Hazardous and Toxic Materials,* 1st ed., pp. 229–242, Wiley-Interscience, New York, 1984. (Includes numerous citations to literature before 1984.)

6. NFC, National Fire Codes, 1987, Article 450, "Transformers and Transformer Vaults; 450-23 (Less Flammable Liquid Insulated Transformers, Fire Point Above 300 Degrees C); 450-24 (Non-flammable Fluid Insulated Transformers); 450-25 (Askarel Insulated Transformers).

SUGGESTED READINGS

R. Albrecht, "Food Contamination by PCBs: Toxicological Aspects, *Med. Nutr.,* **22** No. 2, 115–119.

A. L. Alford-Stevens, "Analyzing PCBs," *Environ. Sci. Tech.,* **20,** No. 12, 1194–1199 (1986).

J. F. Anderson and M. A. Wojtas, "Honey Bees Contaminated with Pesticides and PCBs." *J. Econ. Entomology,* **79,** No. 5, 1200–1205, (1986).

M. R. Anderson, and J. F. Pankow, "A Case Study of a Chemical Spill: PCBs, PCB Sorption and Retardation in Soil Underlying the Site, *Water Resour. Res.,* **22,** No. 7, 1051–1057, (1986).

Anon., "Bugs Eat Their Way Through PCBs," *Chem. Eng.,* **92,** No. 3, 21–22 (1985).

Anon., "A Kit for Removing PCBs," Environ. Sci. Tech., **19,** No. 4, 297 (1985).

Anon., "PCB Contamination of Ceiling Tiles in Public Buildings in New Jersey," *JAMA,* 1297–1301 (March 13, 1987).

T. Awogi, et al., "Comparisons of Inhibiting Activity on Cell-Cell Communication Between Some Tumor Promoters in Chinese Hamster V79 Cells," *Mutat. Res.,* **130,** 361 (1984).

J. F. Brown, Jr., "Polychlorinated Biphenyl Dechlorinated in Aquatic Sediments," reprint, General Electric R&D Center, K-1, Room 3B35, Schenectady, NY 12309.

H. Bucholz et al., "Capillary Gas Chromatography of "Significant" Chlorobiphenyls," *Landwirtsch. Forsch.*, **39** (1–2). 104–108 (1986) (German).

D. Brunelle et al., "Reaction Removal of PCBs from Transformer Oil: Treatment of Contaminated Oil with Polyethylene Glycol/Potassium Hydroxide," *Environ. Sci. Tech.*, **19** No. 8, 740–746 (1986).

L. Burkhard, A. Andren, and D. Armstrong, "Estimation of Vapor Pressures for Polychlorinated Biphenyls: A Comparison of Eleven Predictive Methods," *Envir. Sci. Tech*, **19**, No. 6, 500–507 (1985).

E. R. Christensen and C. L. Lo, "PCBs in Dated Sediments of Milwaukee Harbor, Wisconsin, USA," *Environ. Pollut. Ser. B*, **12**, No. 3, 217–232 (1986).

L. Coleman, "Foe of Dumping PCBs at Fort Edward Calls His Stand 'Justifiable,' " *Schenectady (N.Y.) Gazette*, 5 (Feb. 10, 1987).

L. Coleman, "No Increase in Cancer Incidence from PCB Exposure, Study Shows," *Schenectady (N.Y.) Gazette*, 16 (June 20, 1987).

P. A. DesRosiers and A. Lee, "PCBs Fires: Correlation of Chlorobenzene Isomer and PCB Homolog Contents of PCB Fluids with PCDD and PCDF Contents of Soot, *Chemosphere*, **15** (9–12), 1313–1323 (1986).

EPA, "PCBs: Toxics Information Series, OPA 59/0, Office of Pesticides and Toxic Substances, TS-793,; see also PCB Regulations under TSCA: Over 100 Questions and Answers to Help You Meet These Requirements, TSCA Assistance Office and Exposure Evaluation Division, Office of Toxic Substances, Revised Edition No. 3, U.S. Environmental Protection Agency, Washington, D.C.

R. Eisler, "Polychlorinated Biphenyl Hazards to Fish, Wildlife and Invertebrates," Contamination Hazard Reviews Report No. 7, Biological Report 85 (1.7) April 1986. Fish and Wildlife Service, U.S. Dept. of the Interior, Patuxent Wildlife Research Center, Laurel, MD 20708, 72 pp., 1987.

Federal Register, March 31, 1979, Part VI, EPA: Polychlorinated Biphenyls: Criteria Modifications; Hearings, 31514–31588; Aug. 25, 1982, 37342–37360; July 17, 1985, 29170–29201; Oct. 21, 1982, 46980–46996; March 23, 1984, 11070–11083; July 10, 1984, 28154–28209; Dec. 31, 1986, 47241–47309.

R. A. Femia et al., "Fluorescence Characteristics of PCB Isomers in Cyclodextrin Media," *Environ. Sci. Tech.*, **19**, No. 2, 155–158 (1985).

A. Fischbein, and J. N. Rizzo, "Health Effects of PCBs—A Brief Review," *NE Environ. Sci.*, **5** (1–2), 64–69 (1986).

G. W. Gibson, "Apparatus and Method for Solar Destruction of Toxic and Hazardous Materials," U.S. Patent 4549528 A, Oct. 1985

M. Gough, *Dioxin, Agent Orange: The Facts,* 289 pp., Plenum Press, New York, 1986 (reviewed in *Wall St. J.,* Nov. 11, 1986).

P. Gustavsson et al., "Short-Term Mortality and Cancer Incidence in Capacitor Manufacturing Workers Exposed to PCBs, *Am. Jr. Indust. Med.*, **10**, No. 4, 341–344 (1986).

K. Haraguchi, F. H. Kuroki, and Y. Masuda, "Capillary Gas Chromatographic Analysis of Methyl Sulfone Metabolites of PCBs Retained in Human Tissues," *Jr. Chromatogr.*, **361**, 239–252 (1986).

D. L. Hazelwood, F. J. Smith, and E. M. Gartner, "Assessment of Waste Fuel Used in Cement Kilns," project summary, 3 pp., U.S. EPA Industrial Environmental Laboratory, Cincinnati, Ohio (EPA-600/S2-82-013), Oct. 1982.

G. G. Hess et al., "Selective Preconcentration of Polynuclear Aromatic Hydrocarbons and Polychlorinated Biphenyls by In Situ Metal Hydroxide Precipitation," *J. Chromatogr.*, **366**, 197–203 (1986).

E. Huschenbeth, "The Contamination of Fishes from the North and Baltic Seas and the Lower Elbe with Organochlorine Pesticides and PCBs," *Arch. Fischereiwiss.*, **36**, No. 3, 269–286 (1986).

M. Kedlecek, "Cleanup Offers a Second Chance," *Conservationist*, **39**, No. 5, 32–35 (1985).

L. Kokoszka and J. Flood, "A Guide to EPA-Approved PCB Disposal Methods," *Chem. Eng.*, **92**, No. 14, 41–43 (1985).

F. Kredl and K. Kren, "Residues of Chlorinated Pesticides and PCBs in the Eggs and Fatty Tissues of Wild Birds," *Vet. Med. (Prague)*, **31**, No. 7, 423–432 (1986) (Czech).

P. Larsson, "Change in PCB (Clophen A50) Composition When Transported From Sediment to Air in Aquatic Model Systems," *Environmental Pollution (Series B)*, **9**, No. 2, 81–94 (1985).

P. Larsson, "Sedimentation of PCBs in Limnic and Marine Environments," *Water Res.*, **18**, No. 11, 1389–1394 (1984).

G. Laule, R. Hawk, and D. Miller, "Oxidation of 4,4'-Dichlorobiphenyl at a Ruthenium Dioxide Anode," *J. Electroanal. Chem. Interfacial Electrochem.*, **213**, No. 2, 329–332 (1987).

R. E. Lawn and S. A. Toffel, "Determination of PCBs in Waste Oil by Gas-Liquid Chromatography," *Analyst (London)*, **112**, No. 1, 53–56 (1987).

M. C. Lee and T. G. Erler, "PCB-Contaminated Site Cleanup," *Proceedings of 1984 Specialty Conference*, June 25–27, Environmental Engineering, University of Southern California., Los Angeles, ASCE, 711–713 (1984).

R. G. Lewis et al., "Measurement of Fugitive Atmospheric Emissions of Polychlorinated Biphenyls from Hazardous Waste Landfills," U.S. EPA, Research Triangle Park, N.C.

J. D. McKinney, "Biological Activity of PCBs Related to Conformational Structure," *Biochem. J.*, **240**, No. 2, 621–642.

L. Matter, "PCBs in Fuel Oils," *Form Staedte-Hyg.*, **37**, No. 4, 260–261 (1986) (German).

Y. Mesuda et al., "PCDFs and Related Compounds in Humans from Yusho and Yu-Cheng Incidents," *Chemosphere*, **15** (9–12), 1621–1628 (1987).

A. Mikulik and M. Vavrova, "PCBs in the Production Environment from the Point of View of Animal Production," *Cesk Hyg.*, **31** (7–8), 383–387 (1986) (Czech).

M. M. Nemac, "Sunohio Offers Onsite Solution for PCBs," *Hazardous Mat. Waste Mgt.*, **3**, No. 1, 24–26 (1985).

L. Oatman, and R. Roy, "Surface and Indoor Air Levels of PCBs in Public Buildings," *Bull. Environ. Contam. Toxicol.*, **37**, No. 3, 461–466 (1986).

P. Orris et al., "Exposure to PCBs from an Overheated Transformer," *Chemosphere*, **15** (9–12), 1305–1311 (1986).

I. Pavan, L. Operti, and R. Orazietti, "Hazards Involved in the Use of Mineral Oils for Heat Treatment of Metals," *Chem. Abs.*, **104**, No. 20, 173604u

J. K. Post, "Hudson PCB Dredging Plan to Get Final Review," *Schenectady (N.Y.) Gazette*, 5 (Feb. 10, 1987).

J. K. Post, "Waterford Water Panel Plots Strategy in PCBs Dredging, Seeks Guarantees from State," *Schenectady (N.Y.) Gazette*, 5 (Feb. 10, 1987).

L. A. Rich, A. Hope, et al., "Burning of Toxics Faces Rising Protests Worldwide," *Chem. Week*, **136**, No. 21, 18–20 (1985).

S. Sassa et al., "Chloro-Substituent Sites and Probability of Coplanarity in PCBs in Determining Uroporphyrin Formation in Cultured Liver Cells," *Biochem. J.*, **240**, No. 2, 622–623 (1986).

M. Schreiner et al., "Determination of PCBs and Other Chlorinated Hydrocarbons in Context with Examinations of Dioxins in Waste Incinerators," *Chemosphere*, **15**, (9–12), 2093–2097 (1986).

P. H. Schuck, *Agent Orange on Trial*, 347 pp., Belnap (Harvard University Press), Cambridge, Mass., 1986.

A. M. Sepp et al., "Reversible Nerve Lesions After Accidental Polychlorinated Biphenyl Exposure," *Scand. J. Work, Environ. Health*, **11**, No. 2, 91–95 (Apr. 1985).

J. Sevcik et al., "PCB Load in Children," *Cesk. Hyg.*, **31** (7–8), 378–383 (1986) (Czech).

W. Shain et al., "A Congener Analysis of PCBs Accumulating in Rat Pups After Perinatal Exposure," *Arch. Environ. Contam. Toxicol.*, **15**, No. 6, 687–707 (1986).

C. G. Shultz, "Destruction of PCBs and Other Hazardous Halogenated Hydrocarbonas, *Chem. Abst.,* **105** No. 6, 48445n.

A. D. Stark et al., "Health Effeacts of Low-Level Exposure to PCBs," *Environ. Res.,* **41,** No. 1, 174–183 (1986).

P. A. Stehr and D. L. Forney, "Amateur Radio Operators and Exposure to PCBs," *Arch. Environ. Health,* **40,** No. 1, 18–19 (1985).

P. A. Stehr-Green et al., "A Pilot Study of Serum PCB Levels in Persons at High Risk of Exposure in Residential and Occupational Environments, *Arch. Environ. Health,* **41,** No. 4, 240–244 (1987).

F. C. Whitmore and J. D. Barden, "A Study of PCB Destruction Efficiency and Performance for a Coal-Fired Utility Boiler," U.S. EPA 1 p., (EPA-600/S2-83-101a/b), Industrial Environmental Research Laboratory, Research Triangle Park, N.C., Nov. 1983.

L. B. Willet, T. Y. Liu, et al., "Quantification and Distribution of PCBs in Farm Silos," *Bull. Environ. Contami. Toxicol.,* **35,** No. 1, 51–60 (1985).

T. K. Wong, T. Sloop, and G. W. Lucier, "Nondetectable Concentrations of Human Placental Ah Receptors Are Associated with Potent Induction of Microsomal Benzo[a]pyrene Hydroxylase in Individuals Exposed to PCBs, Quaterphenyls, and Dibenzofurans, *Toxicol. Appl. Pharmacol.* **85,** No. 1, 60–68 (1986).

11

Personal Protective Equipment

Howard H. Fawcett

Supplementing good engineering and prudent work practices, personal protective equipment has an important role as "secondary" or backup protection where chemicals and other hazardous materials or substances are encountered. It is generally understood that proper engineering, adequate attention to good safety and health practices, and education of both personnel and management so that control is reduced to standard operating procedures, even if carefully followed, cannot completely protect personnel or property, since unusual incidents, spills, and failures not anticipated with the most complete analyses do occur in the real world. Personal protective equipment is then called upon to provide that extra measure of operational health and safety to personnel who must cope with the problem.

The injurious effects on skin, body, eyes, and respiratory system of contact with chemicals and other materials have been well documented elsewhere, but should be emphasized again as ranging from acute injury, such as skin irritation, inflammation, or lung involvement (which could even result in pulmonary edema or cardiac impairment) to chronic injuries, which may become manifest many years later.

Exposures or contacts may range from one-time splashes or inhalation to continuous wetting by liquids or chronic inhalation of background "odors," as well as direct contact with solids. Clothing should be an effective barrier for more than a few minutes, to permit the contaminated person to retreat, remove the protective gear and/or clothing, and then wash and decontaminate. This washing should be very thorough. The Chemical Manufacturers Association for years has recommended at least 15 minutes of irrigation with running water. In areas where safety showers are available, this may create a local flood unless an adequate drain is nearby—a frequently overlooked design and construction deficiency. Nevertheless, cleanup by water is preferable to the serious medical treatment that becomes necessary if the washing is inadequate. For outside use, portable decontamination showers are now available, and these would be most suitable where facilities are remote, as are most loading docks and chemical hazardous-waste sites. The initial decontamination must be planned depending on the clothing, the contaminant, and the degree of contamination. An industrial hygienist or health professional, such as an occupational health nurse or an industrial physician, should be consulted in situations or plans involving chemicals.

Where a formal decontamination facility is not available, as when the fire services respond to a leaking tank car or tank truck at a remote location, human ingenuity must be invoked.

Captain John Maleta of the Los Angeles Fire Department has developed a relatively simple but effective approach to the decontamination of personnel working to control a leak in a railway car. The department is very conscious of the necessity to protect its personnel, and Captain Maleta's remarks are most timely:

"The on-site personnel subject to contamination when spills/releases go down and the emergency responders, such as fire department and emergency response personnel, are the ones who must put pressure on manufacturers of personal protective equipment to upgrade that cocoon, better known as the encapsulating suit. We have all watched NASA send people to the moon but it requires years for that same technology to become available to the emergency service. We have upgraded these ensembles [protective suits] from butyl rubber to Viton to Teflon, and in the near future you may see a suit made of Mylar. The materials mentioned are not impervious to many chemicals found in the workplace or in transit . . . The manufacturer does not put a label inside the collar instructing us how to wash away chemicals. In other words, these suits are not 'wash and wear.'

"I have developed a decon system that will clean the suits but will not purify, sterilize, or disinfect. The procedure calls for a series of plastic blow-up [childrens'] wading pools set on a laid-out plastic sheeting strip (10 feet × 30 feet). The base material, water, is from a reel line (pumper) and you walk your people through the series of pools. (The water may be hot.) The person rinsing uses a 4-foot metal gardening sprinkler wand [long-handled shower head] and moves with the suited person as he is washed and scrubbed at each pool site. Various chemicals can be used to clean, but some that should be available are TSP [trisodium phosphate], soap, and, most important, water.

"The pools are not used to sit in and wash down; they are only used to catch/hold the rinse water. Since the pools are relatively inexpensive, more pools are easily added as needed . . . Innovative and resourceful responders have fabricated, out of plastic pipe, portable showers in which the runoff water is captured by using a catch basin made out of ladders and salvage covers. Others prefer to use a portable tank (fold-a-tank). There is also the commercially made decon unit which is set up like a mobile trailer with shower, dressing area, and a holding tank for the wash water. However, these mobile units cost up to $20,000. You must remember, if you have civilians or employees contaminated, you will have to strip them down and wash and rinse them off before you put them in an ambulance or admit them into a medical facility . . .

"The personnel protective equipment does degradate. It is also susceptible to permeation and, because these suits can have an accumulative problem, the chemicals can in some cases cause the individual wearing the suit great harm. In summary, because we are removing chemicals from the suit's pores, seams, and zippers, we are performing *chemical reduction,* not decontamination."[1]

While Captain Maleta's approach may be unusual, it does touch on important factors in the real world, and deserves serious consideration. The question of how to dispose of the contaminated water resulting from the captain's approach is another issue, but obviously can be discussed with more leisure than when personnel are trying to get out of contaminated suits.

Protective clothing, including coveralls of protective suits, gloves, boots or other appropriate safety shoes, and head and face protection all deserve critical attention. While the makers and vendors may assure buyers that their products are adequate for the exposures anticipated, and often can supply, on specific request, test data that show the ability of their products to withstand certain exposures, the buyer should carefully and critically review such data, and be certain it is appropriate to his or her specific requirements. We must recognize that we cannot know what potential exposures may be encountered at chemical hazardous-waste disposal sites, or during transportation accidents, until incidents such as the Miamisburg, Ohio, derailment bring the unknown reality without advance warning.

One often-overlooked aspect of protection is just how hazardous a material might be if, for some reason, it were to contact the skin. Five skin-permeation predictive models have been evaluated for 10 drugs with a wide range of physical properties. Dr. David W. Osborne of the Upjohn Company, Kalamazoo, Mich., has reported his efforts to date. He notes that all five models evaluated predict the flux of a drug from a saturated aqueous solution. The first model considered was B. Berner's two-parallel—pathway model for skin permeation. This model separates permeation through the skin barrier function into two paths, a polar (aqueous) and a nonpolar (lipophilic) path. The second model was the three-parallel-pathway model of Berner and E. R. Cooper, which combines not only the polar and lipophilic, but also an oil–water multiaminate pathway. Reports on these two modules are in preparation. The next model considered was the structural model of A. S. Michaels, S. K. Chandrasekaran, and J. E. Shaw (*AIChE J.,* **21,** 985–996, 1975). This model requires knowledge of the drug's mineral-oil/water partition coefficient and water solubility. The last two models were taken from a theoretical description of percutaneous absorption by W. J. Albery and J. Hadgraft (*J. Pharm. Pharmacol.,* **31,** 129–139, 1979). This treatment is very detailed and is applicable to both continuous and pulse applications, where pulse implies that the drug is applied for a time and then removed. All of these models assume that the stratum corneum is the barrier function for the skin, and all are for drugs delivered from a saturated aqueous solution.

It was concluded that theoretical models that use water solubility, molecular weight, and partition coefficient data can usually predict the flux of a drug through the barrier function of the skin. All of the models examined occasionally predicted fluxes that were unacceptably high or low compared with the experimentally determined flux, and for this reason it is necessary to use more than one of the predictive models. For some of the models, an increase in the partition coefficient caused an increase in the predicted flux as compared with the experimental flux. Such trends were not seen for molecular weight or water solubility. For substances that become aligned with the bilayers at the interface, such as steroids, the predicted fluxes may be orders of magnitude larger than experimentally determined fluxes. Albery's combined model can be used to predict the permeation of concentrated systems such as solvents provided that the thermodynamic activity is used rather than the water solubility. With appropriate care regarding these limitations, the use of this type of modeling can be beneficial to researchers concerned with "ballpark" skin permeability predictions.[2]

Protective clothing and gloves are fabricated from a variety of materials—ranging from disposable paper suits designed to be used once to more expensive, better-made suits and gloves that usually can be reused many times. Each material, fabrication, and combination has limitations. Normally, for routine occupational exposures, it would be recommended that any materials used in gloves, suits, or footwear to protect the wearer from contaminants should be tested for permeation before use. However, often the nature of the contaminants and mixtures, and the degree of exposure to be encountered, are unknown. The prudent wearer must rely on test data for general classes of substances as analogous as possible to the combinations or expected exposures. For some substances, such as benzene or the aliphatic hydrocarbons such as hexane, good data on the permeability will be found in the literature. For many others, and for combinations of chemicals that may be encountered in the field, corresponding data should be sought, but often will be unavailable. In that case, the opinions of an industrial hygienist or health professional competent in this area should be sought and followed.

The ASTM Committee F-23 on Protective Clothing has been considering an appropriate approach to testing materials for penetration by liquids, gases, and molten substances. The following ASTM standards should be consulted for details of these tests.

F-739-85: Standard Test Method for Resistance of Protective Clothing Materials to Permeation by Liquids or Gases

F-903-84: Standard Test Method for Resistance of Protective Clothing Materials to Penetration by Liquids

F-955-85: Standard Test Method for Evaluating Heat Transfer Through Materials for Protective Clothing Upon Contact with Molten Substances

F 1001-86: New Standard Guide for the Selection of Chemicals to Evaluate Protective Clothing Materials

F 1002: New Standard Performance Specification for Protective Clothing for Use by Workers Exposed to Specific Molten Substrates and Related Thermal Hazards.

Copies of these standards may be obtained from the American Society for Testing and Materials, 1916 Race Street, Philadelphia, PA 19103.

The MSDSs required by the OSHA Hazard Communication regulation and by some state laws often contain specific recommendations on protective materials that should be carefully noted, but should be cross-checked to be certain the data are both complete and up to date.

The routine maintenance of such equipment should not be overlooked. When not in use, suits should be hung or stored in a clean, well-ventilated area, and after every wearing, or weekly, should be carefully inspected for tears, leaks, or other defects, which should be promptly repaired before the next use. Carefully written logs should be kept of such inspections, and all defects or problems noted, as well as when corrected and by whom.

Impervious clothing and respiratory devices are expensive, and also uncomfortable when worn for long periods of time at work. Hence heat stress, as well as normal work stress, should be considered. The ACGIH has recognized the problem of heat stress and has established threshold limit values (TLVs) for conditions to which, it is believed, nearly all workers may be repeatedly exposed without adverse health effects. The TLVs shown in Table 11.1, taken from the 1987–88 ACGIH publication, are based on the assumption that nearly all acclimatized, fully clothed workers with adequate water and salt intake should be able to function effectively under the given working conditions without exceeding a deep body temperature of 38°C. To determine these factors in the "real world", wet-bulb globe temperatures are taken in the environment, and then calculated by the following formula for indoors or outdoors with no solar load:

$$WBGT = 0.7\ NWB + 0.3\ GT$$

where WBGT is wet-bulb globe temperature index, NWB is natural wet-bulb temperature, DB is dry-bulb temperature, and GT is globe temperature.

The opposite condition, cold stress, has also been recognized as a serious health and safety problem, from either exposure to the air or in water.[3] Hypothermia can develop without warning, and the ACGIH recommends adequate insulating clothing to maintain core temperatures above 36°C. Protection must be provided to workers if work is performed in air temperatures below 4°C (40° F). Wind-chill factor or the cooling power of the air is a critical factor; the higher the wind speed and the lower the temperature in the work area, the greater the insulation value of the protective clothing that will be required. Table 11.2 notes these data in detail. Table 11.3 presents the progressive development of hypothermia.

TABLE 11.1. Permissible Heat Exposure Threshold Limit Values (Values Given in degrees Celsius WBGT)

Work–Rest Regimen, per Hour	Light	Moderate	Heavy
Continuous work	30.0	26.7	25.0
75% work/25% rest	30.6	28.0	25.9
50% work/50% rest each hour	31.4	29.4	27.9
25% work/75% rest each hour	32.2	31.1	30.0

Source: ACGIH TVLs 1987–88, p. 69.

TABLE 11.2. Wind-Chill Table
(Indicates the WIND-CHILL INDEX [equivalent in cooling power on exposed flesh])

WIND SPEED (MILES/HOUR)	AIR TEMPERATURE °F																
	35	30	25	20	15	10	5	0	-5	-10	-15	-20	-25	-30	-35	-40	-45
4	35	30	25	20	15	10	5	0	-5	-10	-15	-20	-25	-30	-35	-40	-45
5	32	27	22	16	11	6	0	-5	-10	-15	-21	-26	-31	-36	-42	-47	-52
10	22	16	10	3	-3	-9	-15	-22	-27	-34	-40	-46	-52	-58	-64	-71	-77
15	16	9	2	-5	-11	-18	-25	-31	-38	-45	-51	-58	-65	-72	-78	-85	-92
20	12	4	-3	-10	-17	-24	-31	-39	-46	-53	-60	-67	-74	-81	-88	-95	-103
25	8	1	-7	-15	-22	-29	-36	-44	-51	-59	-66	-74	-81	-88	-96	-103	-110
30	6	-2	-10	-18	-25	-33	-41	-49	-56	-64	-71	-79	-86	-93	-101	-109	-116
35	4	-4	-12	-20	-27	-35	-43	-52	-58	-67	-74	-82	-89	-97	-105	-113	-120
40	3	-5	-13	-21	-29	-37	-45	-53	-60	-69	-76	-84	-92	-100	-107	-115	-123
45*	2	-6	-14	-22	-30	-38	-46	-54	-62	-70	-78	-85	-93	-102	-109	-117	-125

Category bands (left to right, increasing severity): COLD, VERY COLD, BITTER COLD, EXTREME COLD.

*Wind speeds greater than 4 MPH have little additional cooling effect.
EXAMPLE- A 30 MPH wind, combined with a temperature of 30 degrees F, (-1 degree Celsius), can have the same chilling effect as a temperature of -2 degrees F, (-19 degrees Clesius), when it is calm.

126

TABLE 11.3. Progressive Clinical Presentations of Hypothermia

Core Temperature		Clinical Signs
°C	°F	
37.6	99.6	"Normal" rectal temperature
37	98.6	"Normal" oral temperature
36	96.8	Metabolic rate increases in an attempt to compensate for heat loss
35	95.0	Maximum shivering
34	93.2	Victim conscious and responsive, with normal blood pressure
33	91.4	Severe hypothermia below this temperature
31–32	89.6–87.8	Consciousness clouded; blood pressure becomes difficult to obtain; pupils dilated but react to light; shivering ceases
30–29	86.0–84.2	Preogressive loss of consciousness; musuclar rigidity increases; pulse and blood pressure difficult to obtain; respiratory rate decreased
28	82.4	Ventricular fibrillation possible with myocardial irritability
27	80.6	Voluntary motion ceases; pupils nonreactive to light; deep tendon and superficial reflexes absent
26	78.8	Victim seldom conscious
25	77.0	Ventricular fibrillation may occur spontaneously
24	75.2	Pulmonary edema
21–22	71.6–69.8	Maximum risk of ventricular fibrilation
20	68.0	Cardiac standstill
18	64.4	Lowest accidental hypothermia victim to recover
17	62.6	Isoelectric electroencephalogram
9	48.2	Lowest artificially cooled hypothermia patient to recover

Source: ACGIH TLVs 1987–88, p. 76.

Additional details on evaluation and control measures for low-temperature activities will be found in the Table 11.2 citation.

The discomfort involved with wearing various types of protective clothing resulting from excessive heat and lack of ventilation may be minimized by using air-supplied circulation to the suits to permit more nearly normal body heat and perspiration to be dissipated. A vortex air injector has been used successfully to provide both internal air and cooling. The location of the air intake must always be monitored for possible intake of air that is not of breathing quantity.

If an air supply is considered for breathing or cooling of an impervious suit, the problems associated with air purity should be carefully analyzed. Diaphragm compressors or other devices that cannot generate carbon monoxide or excessive oil (from oil lubrication) should be used. Cross-connections to a plant air supply where the air is used for plant purposes must be avoided, since gases other than air have been introduced into breathing air supplies in this way, with tragic results. This is especially true of gases that are recognized asphyxiants and have little or no odor, including acetylene, argon, ethane, ethylene, helium, hydrogen, methane (natural gas), neon, propane, propylene, and nitrogen. In the fatalities in the past, plant engineers had modified the system without informing the personnel who might be using the air for breathing purposes. Odor alone cannot be depended upon to serve as a warning. Even with substances of significant odor, such as hydrogen sulfide, olfactory fatigue can prevent any evaluation of the change, either an increase or a decrease, in the concentration being detected with the nose. Olfactory receptors are specialized bipolar neurons located in the pigmented part of the upper nasal cavity. Like taste cells, the receptor portion is continually renewed, but with a turnover time that averages 30 days. according to Dr. S. S. Shiffman, professor of medical psychology, Department of Psychiatry, Duke University Medical Center, the turnover occurs as bundles of axons of bipolar neurons course through small holes in the cribriform plate, making connections in the olfactory bulb in bushy masses called "glomeruli." Glomeruli atrophy with age and take on a "moth-eaten" appearance as fibers degenerate and disappear.

Olfactory thresholds are more vulnerable to aging than taste thresholds. Thresholds for food flavors were found to be 11 times higher in the elderly than in the young. Suprathreshold odors are perceived as less intense by older persons. The elderly are also less able to identify foods correctly on the basis of smell in blindfolded testing conditions. In addition, the ability to discriminate among odors of different qualities is greatly reduced. These perceptual changes result not only from normal aging but also from disease states and drugs.

HEAD PROTECTION

For chemical and related operations, especially in facilities with extensive overhead piping, wiring, tanks, columns, and related equipment that may occasionally fail, head protection is clearly indicated. In addition, head protection offers protection against impact, flying particles, and electrical shock. Properly designed and engineered head protection can protect the scalp, the face, and the neck, as well as the head, and can be compatible with other protective devices, such as ear muffs, noise protectors, goggles, and face pieces of masks.

NIOSH has noted that safety helmets are rigid headgear made of various materials, such as polycarbonate plastic and even aluminum. Two basic types are recognized: full brimmed and brimless with peak. Both types are further divided into four classes:

CLASS A: Limited voltage resistance for general service;

CLASS B: High-voltage resistance;

CLASS C: No electrical voltage protection (i.e., metallic)

CLASS D: Limited protection for fire-fighting use.

Class A helmets are made without holes in the shell, except for those used for mounting suspensions or accessories, and have no metallic parts in contact with the head. They must pass voltage tests of 2200 volts ac (rms) at 60 Hz for one minute, with no more than 9-mA leakage. In addition, they should not burn at a rate greater than 3 inches/minute. After 24-hour immersion in water, the shell should absorb no more than 5 percent by weight. These helmets are designed to transmit a maximum average force of not more than 850 pounds. Class A helmets do not weigh more than 15 ounces, including suspension, but excluding winter liner and chin strap.

Class B helmets are designed specifically for use around electrical hazards, with the same impact resistance as Class A helmets. They pass voltage tests of 20,000 volts ac (rms) at 60 Hz for 3 minutes, with no more than 9-mA leakage. In addition, no holes are allowed in the shell for any reason, and no metallic parts can be used in the helmet. The burning rate of the thinnest part is not greater than 3 inches/minute. After 24 hours in water, absorption of the shell will be no more than 0.5 percent by weight. The maximum weight of Class B helmets is 15.5 ounces.

Class C metallic helmets do not offer the same degree of protection, but are preferred by many because of their lighter weight. They should not be used in the vicinity of electrical equipment, or near acids, alkali, and other substances that are corrosive to aluminum and alloys.

Brims are an optional feature of helmets. A brim completely around the helmet affords the most complete head, face, and back-of-neck protection. The brimless-with-peak helmet may be used where a brim may be objectionable and the brimless may be equipped with lugs to support a face mask or face shield to provide face and eye protection.

The key to protection from impact is proper helmet suspension, since the suspension distributes and absorbs the impact force. Examples of suspensions include a compressible liner or a cradle formed by the crown straps and headband, or a combination of the two. To function properly, the adjustment of straps must keep the helmet a minimum distance of 1.25 inches above the head.

To restrain the helmet from dislodging during normal use, various leather, fabric, and elastic chin straps are used. Helmet liners are optional equipment, often used with ear protectors in colder weather.

In recent times, the "bumb" cap has been introduced to be worn by persons working in cramped quarters. In general, it is thin shelled and made of plastic. No specifications exist for these caps, and they are not a safe substitute for the helmets discussed above.

Another aspect of head protection that must be considered is the length of head hair in both males and females. This becomes especially critical where moving parts and machinery are involved or flammable materials and ignition sources may be present. Hair nets or "snoods" are often specified, but worn only with reluctance by most workers. When combined with a cap, they are more appealing, and hence have increased acceptance. In areas where sparks or hot metals are encountered, such as in welding or cutting operations, the nets or caps or other head covering should be flame resistant and have a visor sufficiently long to afford protection from the exposures coming from above or on an angle.

A wide variety of plastics, fiberglass, and other materials is available for helmet construction, and many are available in various colors. The use of colors can help identify various groups or crafts, such as millwrights, electricians, pipefitters, and machinery repairmen, and also is a type of security clearance for the worker, especially in a large facility. The addition of the employee's name on the hat is also a useful incentive for each person to keep his or her hat in a proper condition of readiness and cleanliness. Ear muffs or ear protectors are often integrated into hats, and when properly adjusted, can be worn for long periods.

It is important that the headgear be comparable to other personal protective equipment, and be properly maintained and cleaned.

HEARING PROTECTION AND LOSS

Hearing is an important human personal function that often is overlooked as possibly involving safety issues. The ability to hear, adequately and completely, conversations, shouted warnings, or audible signals (such as backing-up signals, horns, sirens, or other warning devices) constitutes a protective factor not to be overlooked if accidents are to be avoided.

We live in a very noisy world, especially in cities and other congested areas, where heavy vehicular traffic, subways, radios, television, sterios, public address systems, outboard motors, powered lawn-care equipment (including mowers and blowers), airplanes, helicopters, rocket engines, and supersonic booms contribute to our "background," to say nothing of the rock-and-roll music played at high levels of sound that is currently popular with the younger generation. Within the chemical and related industries, one can occasionally find noisy agitators, grinders, mixers, pulverizers, compressors, fans, blowers, crushers, and other equipment. At what point the noise becomes a problem can only be determined by measurements that analyze both the frequency and the length of exposure. An industrial hygiene engineer or an acoustical engineer may be helpful in carrying out this task.

Engineering improvements can often solve noise problems. To reduce the noise of the air-cooling fans of electric motors, a "multiple-disk" fan that satisfies the motor's double-rotation direction requirement has been tested in the Department of Mechanical Engineering of the University of Santa Catarina, Brazil. Professor S. N. Y. Gerges described the fan and test results at Inter-Noise '86 held in Cambridge, Mass., July 21–23, 1986.

The multiple-disk fan consists of a stack of closely spaced disks. Air enters the spacing from the central hole, acquires acceleration by friction on the disks, and is collected radially or axially. The absence of blades provides a quiet operation. Flow characteristics of this fan mounted on a 15-horsepower TEFC, 3560-rpm motor were studied. The motor was placed on a 60 by 60-cm tube and the pressure measured at the inlet where a standard calibrated nozzle is used. The multiple-disk fan has the same external diameter and rotation speed as that of the motor. An internal diameter of 120–130 mm with an 0.8-mm spacing between the disks gives the maximum flow rate.

The sound power radiated was determined in the 405-meter reverberation room at the acoustics and vibration laboratory. Six microphones were used, and the captured signals were processed by the HP4541C Fourier analyze using a one-third-octave band digital filter. The sound power spectrum, together with a variation of plus or minus 1.0 standard deviation, was determined for the following cases: (1) the motor with the original fan; (2) the motor with no fan; and (3) the motor with the proposed multiple-disk fan. The results showed that the major noise source was the cooling fan. The overall sound power level was reduced from 97 dBa to 78 dBa.

In another paper delivered at Inter-Noise '86, H. S. Sagoo, J. E. T. Penny, and R. T. Booth described the testing of a low-cost alternative to commercially available signature-analysis systems for identifying noise sources in rotating machinery. Applying their technique to a vacuum cleaner, they found the following to be prominent: first order—motor out of balance; second order—imbalance second harmonic; seventh order—number of blades on centrifugal fan; 12th order—number of slots on rotor; 19th order—number of blades on cooling air fan; and 24th order—commutator elements. Apart from two resonances at 2800 Hz and 7600 Hz, most of the activity was below 2 kHz. From the response for 0–2 kHz, it could be deduced that (1) response in the range 600–2200 Hz was due to airflow turbulence; (2) structural resonances occurred at 345 Hz, 460 Hz, 520 Hz, and 1540 Hz; and (3) the first order (the worst) diminished slightly for motor speeds above 290 Hz (17,400 rpm). In addition, this analysis illustrated the machine's critical speeds. The vacuum cleaner speed varied due to the fluctuations in the domestic electrical supply and the condition of the dust bag, carpet, and bearings; however, speed control is possible via a rheostat. Thus this technique can be quite useful as a quick-look tool when only simple equipment is available.[5]

The ACGIH has considered noise, and has set TLVs for sound-pressure levels and durations of exposure that represent conditions under which it is believed that nearly all workers may be repeatedly exposed without adverse effect on their ability to hear and understand normal speech. Prior to 1979, the medical profession had defined hearing impairment as an average hearing threshold level in excess of 25 dB (ANSI-S3.6-1969) at 500, 1000, and 2000 Hz; the limits in Table 11.4 have been established to prevent a hearing loss in excess of this level. These values should be used as guides, and due to individual susceptibility, should not be regarded as fine lines between safe and dangerous levels. The application of the TLV for noise will not protect all workers, but a hearing-conservation program with audiometric testing is highly desirable when workers are exposed to noise at or above the TLV levels. Table 11.4 presents the data.

The medical departments of larger organizations may elect to institute a regular program of audiometric testing, during which an employee is tested at regular intervals, such as annually or semiannually, for his or her response to various frequency tones corresponding to normal speech. The records of such testing can then constitute an important part of the employee's overall medical records, and can be referred to in the future to determine if a tendency toward hearing loss is occurring, and whether it may be from occupational or nonoccupational causes, such as disco music in the range of 100–120 dBa. Once a program is agreed upon, the medical department may recommend the proper fitting of protective devices, such as ear plugs, ear muffs, helmets, or combinations of these, so the person is

TABLE 11.4 Threshold Limit Values for Noise

Duration per Day, Hours	Sound Level dBa*
16	80
8	85
4	90
2	95
1	100
½	105
¼	110
⅛	115†

*Sound levels in decibels are measured on a sound level meter, conforming as a minimum to the requirements of the ANSI Specification for Sound Level Meters, S1.4 (1971) Type S2A, and set to use the A-weighted network with slow meter response.

†No exposure to continuous or intermittent noise in excess of 115 dBa.

Source: ACGIH TLVs, 1987–88, pp. 100–101.

matched to specific job requirements. It is vital that the employee understand the importance of this program to him or her personally, and actually cooperate. Ear plugs, which are the simplest and least expensive control, have only a limited ability to attenuate sound, and, if used, should be carefully fitted. For higher sound levels, ear plugs must be supplemented by muffs or helmets with built-in muffs, and built-in earphones may be added to attached microphones to permit the use of telephones or two-way radio equipment. This is especially important, during a fire or other emergency, in areas where personnel may be separated but must maintain contact with a central control area.[6]

As with odor, noted previously, hearing perception changes with age. Age-related structural and physiological changes lead to perceptual hearing losses, according to Dr. Schiffman. The loss of sensitivity to pure tones occurs early (at approximately 20 years of age). Most of the losses are at 1000 Hz and above; frequencies above 4000 Hz are especially vulnerable. As a group, males experience greater losses than females. The ability to discriminate among frequencies also declines with age, and the losses are greatest in the higher frequency ranges. The elderly have greater difficulty localizing sounds, especially those with higher frequencies. The ability to distinguish a pure tone or other signal from a masking background noise diminishes with age. A person who reports normal loudness for sounds of low intensity but elevated, or even painful, loudness for sounds of moderate to high intensities is said to suffer from loudness recruitment. This condition occurs in about 50 percent of the elderly population and makes the use of hearing aids problematic in situations where high-intensity background noise occurs along with wanted signals of low intensity.

The most serious problem for the elderly is comprehending speech. This is partially due to the loss of high-frequency sounds that are crucial in identifying consonants. Extensive experimental work suggests that losses are not only peripheral; decrements in the central nervous system are also responsible for this loss in understanding speech.

Data on noise, heat stress, cold, and nonionizing radiation for personnel and area measurements can be recorded, stored, and retrieved in report form through the physical hazards module of the Westinghouse Information System for Health, Environment and Safety (WISHES).

The physical hazards module system is completely menu driven. One can input data, edit data, produce hard copy of the input form, generate reports, and inactivate records. The system has specific reports for each physical hazard—noise, heat stress, and nonionizing radiation. It can indicate threshold levels for noise dosimeter samples. Sound level meter and octave band analyzer samples do not have a threshold entry. The time frame in which the sample was collected is noted. This parameter remains blank for sound level meter and actave band analyzer samples. It indicates partial day or time-weighted averages for noise dosimeter samples. Status indicates whether or not an overexposure has occurred. The heat-stress report calculates a one-hour time-weighted average wet-bulb globe temperature and references it to the appropriate ACGIH TLV. Here status indicates whether the TLV has been exceeded. An unusual feature of the nonionizing radiation report is that it indicates the body part where the measurement was collected.

The employee report, which is designed to be given to the employee, indicates the results of all physical hazards monitoring—noise, heat stress, and nonionizing radiation—for the specific employee. It lists department and job title for each monitoring result. The sampling summary report indicates all sampling results between any two dates. It is designed for posting results and lists the departments where monitoring took place. The noise statistical report generates log normal data with separate categories for sound level meter data, noise dosimeter data by threshold, and octave band analyzer data. It can also generate data by department and job title. The heat-stress statistical report tells what percent of samples exceeded the appropriate TLV.[7]

SAFETY FOOTWEAR

Safety shoes and boots have wide acceptance in the chemical and allied industries, since the intrinsic value of the steel safety cap, which weighs just over an ounce, has been demonstrated many times in prevention of serious toe and foot injuries. In addition, safety shoes and boots, in styles for both women and men, are attractive and well made, and represent an excellent value. Many companies encourage the use of safety shoes by granting partial or total credit for safety shoe purchases, and several shoe vendors have trucks or vans that make on-the-job fitting convenient.

NIOSH has classified protective footwear into five categories:

1. Safety-toe shoes (the most commonly accepted)
2. Conductive shoes (to leak off static charges)
3. Foundry or molders' shoes

4. Explosive-operations shoes (nonsparking)
5. Electrical hazard shoes

One other type of shoe is the acid shoe. These shoes are made completely of such materials as neoprene or other elastomers, and resist attack by acids, alkali, and other corrosive materials. They are especially important in acid- or caustic-handling operations, including tank car, truck, or barge loading and discharging.

OSHA requires the use of safety-toe shoes for persons who work with heavy materials, since the shoes afford protection against impact and rolling objects, and against the hazard of inadvertently striking sharp sheet metal or glass. Safety-toe shoes have been divided into three groups, namely, 75, 50, and 30, which represent the minimum requirements for both compression and impact. The usual material for the safety toe is carbon tool steel iron, but brass or other metals of comparable strength may be substituted in nonsparking shoes if desired. For additional protection against extremely heavy impacts, metatarsal (or over-feet) guards may be used in conjunction with safety-toe shoes. These guards are made of heavy-gauge metal, flanged, and corrugated to protect the feet to the ankles. They are also referred to as protective leggings.

In locations where a potential exists for fire or explosion, as in the liquefaction or use of hydrogen or methane (LNG) or in the handling of highly volatile substances such as diethyl ether or acetone, conductive shoes are recommended. These shoes are engineered to dissipate static charges, reducing the possibility of static spark, when used in connection with a conductive flooring, and the shoes and floors are properly maintained to ensure real conductance. Although there has been much controversy as to whether a static discharge from a human would institute or cause ignition, the evidence is sufficiently strong that every precaution should be taken, including wearing of clothing that generates less static (dry cotton versus synthetic fibers, for example). Periodic tests should be performed, using proper equipment, to ensure that the maximum allowable resistance of 450,000 ohms is not exceeded. To guard against slippage, all shoe soles should have a tread pattern to minimize the instability possibility.

Foundry shoes protect against molten-metal splashes, and are made so they can be removed easily and rapidly if a spill occurs. The tops of the shoes should be closed by the pants leg, spats, or leggings to preclude splashes entering from the top.

Electrical hazards, such as those presented by the potential with an electrical current from point of contact to ground, may be minimized by wearing electrical shoes. These shoes contain no metal, except for the toe box, which is insulated from the remainder of the shoe. Dampness or significant wear will definitely decrease the protection provided by these shoes.[8]

EYE AND FACE PROTECTION AND CARE

Although it would seem self-evident that eye and face protection, with related care, would be high on the list of concerns, both to the employee and to the employer, such is not always the case. We tend to take our face and eyes for granted until some incident arises that makes them of concern.

A well-engineered and planned eye-and-face protection program has at least four elements—all of which must be operable if the program is to prevent or reduce injuries:

1. Prevention of injuries in general by hazard communications and inspiring a respect for chemicals and related eye and face hazards.

2. Protection of the eye and face, using barriers that are engineered (in place) or worn by the person.

3. Minimization of any injury by immediate action, including thorough irrigation with water and prompt referral to an medical specialist who is thoroughly grounded in chemical injuries.

4. Regular eye examinations, to recognize the changes that all persons experience with age, and to correct vision problems before they become serious.

Five basic types of eye and face protectors are available, and should be carefully considered in the context of the materials and possible exposure routes:

1. Spectacles or "safety glasses," either with or without side shields.

2. Eye cups (goggles).

3. Helmet-type protectors (usually associated with welding, cutting, and other operations where full-face protection is required as well as protection from radiant energy.

4. Hand-shield type (usually used for very short exposures at a local hazard site).

5. Transparent (plastic) face shields.

Each of the above types has its advantages and drawbacks. Certainly the basic "safety glasses" can be worn by most persons without difficulty, if they are properly fitted and adjusted, and, if corrective lenses are needed, are up to date insofar as the individual's vision requirements are concerned. Both the frame and the lenses (which may be either plastic or tempered glass) must conform to the ANSI Z87 code on eye protection, or ISO 4849 (International Organization for Standardization, Geneva, 1981 personal eye protectors, specifications). The importance of proper fitting by a competent optical specialist cannot be overemphasized, if wearers are to use eye protection on a regular basis. In some instances, occupational health nurses and safety specialists have been trained for this function, but the services of a real professional are often justified by the increased acceptance of the eye protectors. Industrial safety spectacles with glass lenses were found by NIOSH to be in general compliance with the primary requirements of the ANSI Z87.1-1968, U.S.A. Standard Practice for Occupational and Educational Eye and Face protection, ANSI in a series of tests involving 12 specimens of each of 22 models.[9]

Cup-type (or acidproof) goggles are preferable for liquid chemical exposures, since they fit snugly and will prevent any splash, either directly into the eye or by liquid running from the head or forehead. These are not overly appealing from a comfort viewpoint and are sometimes uncomfortable unless carefully adjusted, but have proved their worth many times when actually used. The washing, sterilization, and drying of these goggles become extremely important to ensure that any remaining splashed material does not find its way into the eye of the next user. Many companies find it desirable to issue, clean, and store the goggles properly for each shift, and to make sure that the personnel actually have a clean device ready for use on the job at shift time. Goggles provide only limited face protection.

Helmets, which are comprehensive coverage for the front and sides of the face and neck, are usually associated with operations where filter lenses are required, as with the radiation from welding, gas cutting, or plasma arc cutting, or from lasers. The filter lenses are rated in efficiency on a scale of 1 through 16, and care should be taken to use the correctly rated lens for the intensity and wavelength of light to be encountered.[10]

Face shields of the transparent, plastic type are very useful when properly used and maintained. Unfortunately, often they are not used correctly because of indifference, or the poor visibility they permit. Often the latter is attributable to inadequate cleaning before and after each use, as well as to scratches. One excellent face shield is the Nitrometer Shield, which has been used successfully for years when operating a nitrometer, where exposures to mercury, sulfuric acid, and even flying glass are real possibilities. This shild, with a replaceable plastic face piece, has an adjustible headband attached to the aluminum frame, but is still very light and strong. Without a frame, many plastic face shields become warped and unusable.

Dr. Schiffman has reminded us of the salient losses in sight due to age, and the importance of frequent eye examinations to detect eye changes so that corrective measures can be taken in time. In evaluating vision, several aspects may be considered by the optician or ophthamologist:

1. *Visual Threshold*: Also called detection threshold, this is the minimal amount of energy that can be detected in a darkened room or at night. Detection sensitivity decreases 4 percent per year, especially for the shorter wavelengths. Greater differences in brightness are required by older persons in order to detect a change.

2. *Glare:* Aging increases susceptibility to glare due to increased dispersion of light that occurs in all the ocular media. Glare makes vision less distinct and decreases the ability to perceive detail. This loss can be compensated for by increasing either the contrast or the size of an object relative to its background.

3. *Image Persistence:* Images persist longer for the elderly than for the young as measured by critical flicker frequency (CFF), which is the frequency at which a rapidly flashing beam of light is perceived to reach constant steady state. There is a linear decline in CFF with increasing age, indicating a reduced capacity for regeneration. This is probably due to slower retinal metabolism and slower information processing in the central nervous system.

4. *Acuity:* After 60 years of age, there is a decline in visual acuity as determined by the snellen decimal, a measure of the smallest letter that can be read on the Snellen chart. This decrement in acuity results from reduced light input due to

narrowing of the pupil and proliferation of the lens; light scattering and as neutral losses also play a role. Raising the luminance level and increasing contrast between the object and its surroundings can overcome some of the decrements.

5. *Accommodation:* Accomodation is the process by which the ciliary muscle adjusts the focal length of the lens such that the lens becomes thicker for viewing near orjects and thinner for distant objects. The loss in the ability to accommodate as a function of age is called "presbyopia." The decrement in the ability to focus on near objects begins at 40 years of age and is predominantly due to changes in lens structure rather than weakness of the ciliary muscle.

6. *Visual Field Size:* The size of the field of vision decreases with age. Subjects, while fixating at one point, report when they first detect that a target has moved into their field of vision. Loss of peripheral vision tends to begin after 55 years of age and can have a deleterious effect on such tasks as driving an automobile.

7. *Depth Perception:* The ability to perceive depth is based both on monocular cues, such as texture and overlap of objects, and binocular cues, including retinal disparity and ocular convergence. Defects with age have been reported for both types of depth perception.

8. *Color Perception:* Deficiencies in color vision can begin as early as 40 years of age and tend to be limited to shorter wavelengths. After 60, however, losses are found in the longer wavelengths as well. It should be noted that about 8 percent of American males and 2 percent of American females are color deficient to some degree, especially in red–green perception, and this may be acquired from previous generations through the male genes.

In summary, eye and face protection require a detailed study and analysis both of the exposures and of the personnel who may be exposed, and a strong conviction, backed by daily actions, that eye and face injuries, like other injuries, can be prevented and controlled. With computerized record-keeping of the type described, information will be more useful than before, and the overall result should be better protection for the employee.[11]

HAND AND ARM PROTECTION (GLOVES)

The importance of hand and arm protection may be noted in that approximately 25 percent of all industrial injuries involve the hand or arm. Chemicals are only one of the several major causes of hand and arm injuries; others are fire and heat, cold, electromagnetic and ionizing radiations, electricity, impacts, cuts, abrasions, and infections.

Gloves and mittens are available in a wide variety of styles, types, and materials. For this reason, proper concern must be given to selecting the proper type and style for the task at hand.

Two basic methods are used in manufacturing liquidproof gloves, namely, the latex-dipped process and the cement-dipped process. In the former, particles of rubber, suspended in water, are coagulated onto a glove form. Since numerous tiny air pockets may develop that have resulted from the incomplete contact of rubber particles with the form, the latex-tipped gloves have a higher penetration or permeation rate than do the cement-dipped gloves. In the latter process, the rubber is dissolved in an organic solvent before it is deposited on the form. This permits a more complete joining of rubber particles, resulting in fewer air pockets and greater resistance to permeation.

NIOSH has noted other factors that affect the rates of permeation, namely, glove thickness and solvent concentration. To this should be added the type of solvent, since some materials may be highly resistant to a solvent while others are not. Permeation rates are indirectly proportional to glove thickness and directly proportional to solvent concentration, as well as to time of contact and area involved.

When selecting apparel for chemical resistance, information on the following factors should be established:

1. Ability of the apparel to resist penetration of the chemical.
2. Chemical composition of the solution to be handled.
3. Degree of concentration of the solution at various processing stages.
4. Abrasive effects of the apparel material on the skin.
5. Temperature conditions.
6. Time cycle of usage.

Once a glove or mitten has been selected and is in use, monitoring for any undesired effects should be instituted. Compared with protective clothing, gloves are much easier to test for the ability to resist penetration by a solvent or material of choice.

First, the gloves are tested for leaks by filling them with air and immersing them in water. They are then washed, dried, turned inside out, weighed, and measured (polyvinyl alcohol gloves are wiped with dry paper towels and stored in a dessicator to await testing). The reusable gloves are filled with a measured amount of a given solvent and after 24 hours are measured for length and their gross weights are determined. They are then emptied, wiped as dry as possible, reweighed, washed, and examined for physical condition. With this procedure, information is obtained concerning the permeability of the glove, solubility of the glove material, resistance to change of shape, hardening characteristics, and resistance to stretching and tearing.[12]

As noted previously, manufacturers and suppliers should provide the requested information, as well as a copy of the test data on which the recommendations were made. ASTM (1916 Race Street, Philadelphia, PA 19103) has several recommended test methods for glove permeability.

An important factor often overlooked is the thickness of the glove—obviously, the thicker the glove, the more restrictive it will be to the fingers. In general, the thickest glove practical should be specified, if it is not excessively stiff and will not introduce an additional hazard into the work. The length of the glove is also important, especially in operations in which the worker must handle parts or items in a liquid, such as in electroplating baths. Long gloves permit the wearer to turn down the tops of the gloves to form cuffs, thereby preventing the liquid from passing down the arms when the hands are raised.

SAFETY BELTS, LIFELINES, LANYARDS, AND SAFETY NETS: PERSONAL PROTECTION AGAINST FALLS FROM HEIGHTS

The tendency to "build in height," or to seek higher buildings and structures, including stacks, process towers and communications equipment towers, has increased interest in working at heights, with its attendant hazards. If obvious protection such as handrails and other physical restraints cannot be applied, personal protection for personnel should be considered.

Safety belts, harnesses, lifelines, and related restraint systems all have certain features in common:

1. A device or belt/harness firmly attached to the wearer's body, with the other end secured to a building element or pole (anchoring point), which will restrain the wearer if the wearer should fall.
2. The anchoring point must be rigid structure near the raised workplace where accessible and reliable anchoring points can be established.
3. The device and attachments must work automatically, so that the wearer becomes protected immediately upon losing normal grips or footings.

For climbing poles or trees, a self-restrained system is used, in which the vertical element is considered prima facie to be sufficiently stable for an anchoring point.

During normal operations, such as hoisting or lowering the wearer, or providing steady support while at work, the belt or lifeline may be considered part of the routine equipment and procedure for the job. This includes the lowering and lifting of personnel into and out of utility holes, tanks, large drainage or sewer pipes that must be inspected or sampled, and other places where the worker is unable to use a ladder or steps. Under these normal operations, comparatively mild stresses are applied to the belt, and are usually less than the total static weight of the wearer. In emergencies, however, such as preventing the wearer from falling further than the slack in the line, or if the wearer becomes unconscious for any reason, the belt or line is subjected to impact loading, which can amount to many times the weight of the user. The amount of impact force developed in stoppng a fall depends on:

1. Weight of the wearer
2. Distance of the fall
3. Speed of deceleration or stopping

To limit the distance of the fall, the wearer should never tie off below waist level. Some shock absorber or decelerating device (such as a spring or an elastic rope) should be incorporated into the systsem to bring the fall to a gradual stop. The impact load on the equipment and the wearer will thus be reduced.

Four classes of safety belts have been recognized:

CLASS I: Body belts for limited movement and positioning to restrict the worker to a safer area in order to prevent a fall.

CLASS II: Chest harnesses used where freedom of movement is paramount, and only limited fall is possible. These are not recommended for vertical free-fall hazard situations.

CLASS III: Body harnesses used when the worker must move about at dangerous heights. In the event of a fall, the harness distributes the impact force over a wide body area, reducing the injury potential.

CLASS IV: Suspension belts used when working from a fixed surface. The user is completely supported by the suspension belt. These are used in shipboard and bridge painting and maintenance, stack maintenance, and tree trimming.

Of the four classes, the body harnesses are preferred for many operations, since they more completely absorb impact and will keep the wearer upright during a fall. When choosing belts and harnesses for protection and selecting personnel for the job, all aspects of the hazards should be recognized—the possible distance to fall, the limitations against restricted mobility, and the health and stability (physically and emotionally) of the wearer.

To judge the safety of a belt, NIOSH recommends several criteria. The belt should be of sufficient strength to withstand the maximum possible free fall of the wearer. The lanyard of the safety belt should be a minimum of 0.5 inch nylon or equivalent with a maximum length that limits a fall to 6 feet or less. The rope should have a nominal breaking strength of 5400 pounds. Also, the belt should be equipped with some form of shock absorber to limit the impact loading. The stopping distance of the belt should be such that it will prevent the user from striking some dangerous obstruction before the fall is arrested. There must also be a sufficient safety margin on all of the above criteria to cover all unknowns, including the weight and physical condition of the wearer, the distance of the fall, the distance to dangerous obstructions, variations in the strength or elasticity of materials, and deterioration of the materials due to wear or other causes.

Lifelines, which attach the user of a safety belt to an anchorage, such as when below the surface or in window washing and similar maintenance, should be secured above the point of operation. This positioning will limit the fall of the wearer, thus reducing the impact loading. All lifelines should be capable of supporting a minimum dead weight of 5400 pounds. The most important criteria for lifelines are their shock-loading strength and energy-absorption ability. Shock absorbers should be used to assist the lifeline in these critical areas. Lifelines should be secured so that the wearer is subjected to as little shock as possible. This will limit the free-fall distance.

Numerous materials are available for lifelines, including nylon, Dacron, and manila. Each has specific characteristics, and lifelines should be selected based on the specific situation in which they will be used.

Safety nets represent another approach to minimization of the effects of falls. Safety nets should be used wherever the use of safety belts and lifelines is impractical or infeasible, but where the danger of a serious fall is nevertheless significant.

Safety nets are usually designed for specific purposes and are therefore custom-made from various natural or synthetic materials. These materials are used in the form of rope or webbing, and in numerous combinations of rope or webbing in various mesh sizes. Each net and section of net should have broader ropes of the same material, but of larger diameter. The Associated General Contractors of America, 1957 E Street, N.W., Washington, DC 20006, and the U.S. Corps of Engineers, Department of the Army, Washington, DC 20315, have established minimum sizes for safety net materials, as well as specific performance standards for nets of various sizes and dimensions.

Where the use of safety nets is considered, extra care should be exercised to arrange the nets so that sufficient clearance exists to prevent them from coming into contact with surfaces or structures below or to each side when the anticipated impact load is applied. When using safety nets near electrical power lines, this factor becomes especially critical.

When more than one net is employed and they are joined to form a larger net, they should be laced or otherwise secured so that they will perform properly. For all nets, perimeter suspension systems should be designed and installed in such a manner that the suspension points either are level or slope toward the building so that a rebounding load will be directed into a protected area. Perimeter nets should always follow the work upward as it progresses, and should never be more than 25 feet below the working level, and closer if possible.

To ensure that nets perform as anticipated, daily inspections are essential. Inspections should be made prior to and after installation, after any alterations, and after impact loading occurs. Recommended test procedures are available. All defects should be repaired promptly and properly.[13]

SUMMARY REGARDING PERSONAL PROTECTIVE EQUIPMENT

Selection, regular use, care, cleaning, maintenance, and proper storage of personal equipment of all kinds must be based on a comprehensive understanding of the hazards to which the worker is exposed. For example, a worker exposed to electrical hazards, as well as foot and head injuries, should be equipped and actually wear a Class B, electrical-hazard-resistant safety helmet, and with special electrical-hazard shoes that do not have soles of flexible metal. In addition, the worker must be adequately and periodically instructed in proper use of the equipment, the importance of the equipment to his or her health and safety on the job, and the proper methods and materials recommended for proper and adequate maintenance. The worker must understand that a protective device for one job is not always adequate or safe for another, and hence should not lend or borrow equipment. A paint-spray respirator, for example, is not efficient or safe against acid gases. Gloves that may be completely adequate for paint dipping may not be the proper protection for wearing around a trichloroethylene degreaser.

No protection equipment is without some disadvantages, but should be made as comfortable as possible by proper sizing and frequent fitting, and be maintained to encourage use. The equipment should not increase or introduce additional hazards to the job—gloves that are excessively thick or become slippery in use may cause more problems than they eliminate. Visibility, weight, and appearance are often factors that determine "real-world" use. A full-brimmed hard hat used in close quarters (as in underground work, for example) may limit visibility to the point the wearer is prone to additional hazards.

Unless the protective devices are accepted for their intrinsic value, and actually used, a false sense of security may arise, which can produce even more serious problems. Careful and intelligent selection of equipment, cooperation with the wearers, frequent checks to be sure that the devices are actually being used and are comfortable, as well as adequate and thorough cleaning, maintenance, storage, and availability are all important. Most of all, however, the wearer must be told WHY he or she is being asked to wear the device, in simple truthful terms.

REFERENCES

1. J. Maleta, *Industrial Fire World*, **1**, No. 2, 39–41 (July–Aug. 1986).

2. D. W. Osborne, *Industrial Hygiene News Report*, **29**, No. 9, 3 (Sept. 1986).

3. Anon., "People Lie in Fridges, Stand in Ice Water to Help Study Cold," *Wall St. J.*, 1, 14 (Feb. 9, 1987).

4. S. Schiffman, M. Orlandi, and R. P. Erickson, "Changes in Taste and Smell with Age: Biological Aspects," pp. 247–268, in *Sensory Systems and Communication in the Elderly*, vol. 10, *Aging*, J. M. Ordy and K. R. Brizzee (eds.), Raven Press, New York, 1979.

5. H. S. Sagoo, J.E.T. Penny, and R. T. Booth, *Industrial Hygiene News Report*, **29**, No. 9, 1 (Sept. 1986).

6. L. N. Skarinov, "Hearing Protection," *Encyclopaedia of Occupational Health and Safety*, 3rd rev. ed., pp. 1013–1015, Geneva, 1983.

7. K. M. Goellner, L. J. Fleming, and M. A. Perriello, "WISHES," presented to American Industrial Hygiene Association Annual Meeting, Dallas, Texas, May 18–23, 1986. Authors are with Westinghouse Information System for Health, Environment and Safety (WISHES), 1310 Beulah Road, Pittsburgh, PA 15235.

8. T. Miura, "Foot and Leg Protection, *Encyclopaedia of Occupational Health and Safety*, 3rd rev. ed., pp. 904–905, International Labour Organization, Geneva, 1983.

9. Anon., "NIOSH Technical Information, Tests of Glass Plano Safety Spectacles, DHEW (NIOSH) Publication No. 77-136, National Institute for Occupational Safety and Health, 944 Chestnut Ridge Road, Morgantown, WV 26505, Feb. 1977.

10. Anon., ISO/DIS 4850, Personal Eye Protectors for Welding and Related Techniques—Filters— Utilisation and Transmittance Requirements, International Organization for Standardization, Geneva 1987. See also publications of the American Welding Society, 2501 Northwest Seventh St., Miami, FL 33125, 1988.

11. D. L. Smith, "Eye Protection," pp. 819–822, and T. Miura, "Eye and Face Protection," pp. 822–825, *Encyclopaedia of Occupational Health and Safety*, 3rd rev. ed., International Labour Organization, Geneva, 1983.

12. W. A. Prowse and D. Williams, "Hand and Arm Protection," pp. 992–994, *Encyclopaedia of Occupational Health and Safety*, 3rd rev. ed., International Labour Organization, Geneva, 1983.

13. J. F. Ulysse, "Falls from Heights, Personal Protection Against," pp. 832–836, *Encyclopaedia of Occupational Health and Safety,* 3rd rev. ed., International Labour Organization, Geneva, 1983.

SUGGESTED READING

R. Reid, How Three Companies Confront Eye, Head, and Face Hazards, *Occupational Hazards,* 35–39 (Oct. 1987).

12

Respiration: System and Protection

Howard H. Fawcett

The most essential input to the human system is air, which is supplied by the respiratory system and eventually to the cells by the circulatory system, which removes the carbon dioxide from cell metabolism. Without food, one can exist for weeks, and without water, for many days, but without air, for only a very few minutes.

Air is a mixture of gases, predominately nitrogen (about 78 percent), oxygen (about 20.9 percent), and approximately a percent of several other gases, including argon, carbon dioxide, krypton, radon, and sulfur dioxide. The essential element for life is the oxygen. Even air that is completely safe for human breathing contains some "impurities"; "pure air" is far scarcer than "pure gold."

The gas-exchange function of the human lung is essential to a healthy, well-functioning respiratory system; any interference with the exchange mechanism can trigger serious illness or death. The gas exchange occurs in the microscopic air sacs deep within the lungs. Here the inhaled gas is separated from the bloodstream by a very thin, delicate membrane. In normal lungs, both oxygen and carbon dioxide pass the membranes without difficulty. The bloodstream carries oxygen from the lungs to the other organs of the body, where it picks up carbon dioxide to be returned to the lungs, and ultimately exhaled. Lungs, bloodstream, and the heart are all closely interrelated elements of the entire oxygen-supply system. Disease or blockage in any part can result in serious illness or death.

CHANGES IN ATMOSPHERIC "AIR"

In the real world, air is constantly being modified or changed by numerous agents, processes, and activities. Included are the natural forces: (1) precipitation, which contributes moisture; (2) winds, which are carriers of dusts, pollen, seeds, spores, salt, and other particulates; (3) changes or stagnation (lapses) in atmospheric pressures, which contribute to air movements or stillness; (4) volcanic activity such as that of Mount St. Helens in Washington State, and the recent volcanic activity in Hawaii and Central America; (5) decay of naturally occurring radioactive nuclides of long half-life, which evolve radon-222 and other disintegration products (see below); (6) fire (started by humans and also by nature, such as lightning), which adds carbon dioxide, carbon monoxide, and particulates (smoke); (7) biological processes, including fermentation and decay, which contribute carbon dioxide, and sometimes carbon monoxide, hydrogen sulfide, and methane by action of bacteria, enzymes, and other agents; and (8) the sun, which contributes ultraviolet, visible, and infrared radiation. Solar radiation is an important ingredient of this complex mixture by providing light and heat and the energy for plant photosynthesis (essential to the oxygen–carbon dioxide balance), as well as catalyzing the action of oxidizers, such as ozone and oxides of nitrogen, on hydrocarbon gases and vapors with particulates to synthesize "smog" (smoke and organic matter).

Since 1950, atomic testing by the United States and several other nations has contributed to the radiation background, as did the Chernobyl fallout after the nuclear power plant disaster. While most of the nuclides are of relatively short half-life, some are sufficiently long-lived to increase the overall background level. Another substance that may be present in significant concentrations in certain areas is radon-222.

RADON-222

Radon (Rn-222) is an inert radioactive gas, without color or odor, evolving from naturally occurring uranium, thorium, and radium soils and rocks such as granite, shale, phosphate, and pitchblende. Radon may also be found in soils contaminated with certain types of industrial wastes, such as the by-products from uranium or phosphate mining.

The main concern about this gas is that it has been shown to be a contributing factor to lung cancer, since the radon attaches itself to particulates and, when inhaled, exposes the lungs, and to a limited extent the bones, to alpha 5.489-MeV radiation. Although the half-life of Rn-222 is only 3.8235 days, continuous inhalation of the gas (and other progeny radionuclides from the emissions and their decay) may be a serious health problem, depending, of course, on the concentration of the gas and the length of exposure. The exposure limit recommended by the EPA is 4.0 pCi/l (picocuries per liter) for a 70-year exposure. No master or comprehensive survey has been made to date, but EPA estimates that one to five million private residences may be affected by exposures to radon over this level. The wide variance in estimates arises from the fact that the danger cannot simply be calculated by looking for uranium or radium-bearing rocks, and assuming that everyone living above that rock is at risk. One house in a given neighborhood may be heavily contaminated while another a few doors away may be within acceptable limits. It should be noted that the EPA believes that radon levels in most houses can be reduced to about 0.02 WL (working level) or 4 pCi/l, which would bring the estimated number of lung cancer deaths due to radon exposure to between 13 and 50 per 1000. Such recommendations are based on an occupancy of the house for 70 years. While pollution-related deaths in the United States caused by tobacco are much higher (350,000 deaths per year compared with an estimated 5000 to 20,000 for radon), the magnitude of these numbers suggests that much more attention should be directed to smoking, and that the areas where radon is shown by properly supervised testing to be significantly above the EPA recommended level deserve serious concern. Only by testing an area with one or more of the devices recognized for this purpose can one have assurance that the radon concentration is within the assigned recommended level.[1]

Another substances not normally associated with the air is bromine. A repeatable springtime burst occurs in solid (aerosol) and gas-phase bromine in Arctic air troposphere. At Point Barrow, Alaska, it was found that the aerosol fraction of tropospheric samples averaged about 5 ppt (parts per trillion). During the springtime, particulate bromine levels exceeded 82 ppt. Gas-phase bromine averaged 7 ppt over the spring bloom, and total bromine in Arctic air jumped to 133 ppt. Bromides are also found in air due to the association between vehicle-emitted lead and bromide concentrations of atmospheric particulates. Lead is added to gasoline as organic tetraethyl (or methyl) lead, an antiknock agent, which during combustion reacts with ethylene dihalide "scavengers" in the gasoline to emit the lead in an inorganic particulate form, predominantly $PbBrCl$. While "unleaded" gasoline seems to be the fuel of the future, undoubtledly it will be years before the phase-out from the antiknock agent is complete. Bromine also is introduced into the atmosphere by the burning of coal and emissions from plants producing organohalogen compounds. Methyl bromide (used as a fumigant) and marine aerosols also contribute to the low natural background of bromine.[2]

AIR-POLLUTION CHEMISTRY

An excellent discussion of air pollution chemistry can be found in R. M. Harrison, and R. Perry's *Handbook of Air Pollution Analysis* (2nd ed., Chapman & Hall, Methuen, New York, 1986, pages 133–154). Both inorganic and organic reactions are noted. A variety of chemical processes in the atmosphere transform the relatively small number of inorganic primary pollutants, and the much larger number of organic compounds emitted from anthropogenic sources, into a diverse spectrum of secondary air pollutants. 'Trace components' in the atmospheric system may have significant, but as-yet-undefined, roles in visibility, vegetation, and human health.

INDOOR AIR

It has been estimated that humans spend 75 percent of their time indoors. If that time is spent in an environment of poor air circulation, with possible localized concentrations of such substances as formaldehyde, oxides of nitrogen, carbon dioxide and carbon monoxide, sulfur compounds, particulates from fuel and tobacco smoke, radon and progeny radionuclides, cooking fumes, greases, oils, spices, toilet odors, and related by-products of human activities, as well as the smoke from indoor wood-burning or coal-burning fireplaces or stoves, indoor air quality assumes an important factor in our personal lives. Adequate ventilation and air movement, together with heat and cooling, should be considered if the air we breathe is to be considered safe to breathe.

The proper and efficient burning of fuels for home or office warming in colder seasons requires some attention to the combustion products that are produced, and assurance that they are properly vented. 3M Engineering Analysts, Ltd., of St. Charles, Ill., has suggested that flue gas readings be made for various fuels to serve as an indicator, not only of efficiency of combustion, but also of the need for adequate ventilation. Under date of September 1986, 3M Engineering noted the following.

The only way to discover how to burn fuel efficiently is to conduct a combustion gas analysis on the flue gases passing out of the combustion chamber. Portable instrumentation can be temporarily connected to the heating appliance, which will indicate the products of combustion for the type of fuel being burned. (See Table 12.1.)

The Bacharach Portable Test Kit (Orsat method of volumetric analysis) is useful for measuring carbon dioxide and oxygen in flue gases or in the atmosphere of the habitable zone where a heating appliance is installed. The Bacharach equipment includes a universal gas sampler for testing carbon monoxide and other gases in the flue gas stream or at remote locations in the local environment. A Scott model S100 portable oxygen-measuring instrument is available for measuring oxygen concentration in aircraft cabin spaces, ship holds, boiler and fire rooms, offices, and residences. A Monitox portable hydrogen cyanide gas detector and warning system is available for indicating in parts per million the quantity of HCN gas present in burned or confined compartments afloat or ashore that contain plastic materials that produce HCN on combustion.

A Hioki model M-1008 General Appliance Tester is available for measuring flue gas temperatures from 75 to 1100°F or refrigeration temperatures from −100 to 75°F, and is also capable of measuring pilot generator performance in the range of

TABLE 12.1. General Values for Flue Gas Readings

	Gas	Oil	Coal or Wood
Carbon dioxide, %	16	16	8.5
Carbon monoxide, %	0	0	0
Oxygen, %	10–20	10–20	10.5
Smoke (indicator), %	0	Trace	No limit
Fuel gas temperature, °F	500–600	600–750	750–950

750 cs mV scale, dc voltage in the range of 5 mV to 300 volts, ac voltage in the range of 5–1200 volts, dc amperage in the range of 30 μA to 600 mA, and resistance in the range of 0–30,000 ohms.

A portable Drager MultiGas Detector will detect, identify, and determine the quantity of various vapors present in the local atmosphere. Drager tubes are available for testing the 130 most often encountered industrial vapors. A probe is also available for measuring the emissions from internal combustion engines.

Used properly, these instruments provide information that is useful in adjusting burning conditions to a satisfactory life-support environment.

Too much oxygen (an oxygen-enriched atmosphere) tends to accelerate burning, which increases the rate of heat release from the fuel, but wastes the heat. Insufficient air (an oxygen-deficient atmosphere) reduces the rate of heat release from the fuel and results in incomplete combustion, which produces unburned carbon (soot), carbon monoxide, and other toxic fire gases. A fuel cannot be burned in either the liquid or solid staate. For the proper combustion reaction (burning) to occur, the fuel (carbon commpound) and the oxidizer (oxygen) must be brought into contact in the gaseous state at the molecular level.

With the onset of the heating season, the competition for oxygen between the human body and the combustion reaction of burning fuel, all within a confined habitable atmosphere such as found inside most houses, becomes critical. Homes and businesses are winterized with the intention of "keeping the cold air out." This is accomplished by adding storm windows, insulating glass, plastic film envelopes, and additional insulation, and by closing off ventilation. "Keeping the cold air out" reduces the amount of air available for human respiration and the combustion reaction in the confined atmosphere inside the home or business. The addition of mechanical or automatic devices to the flue in order to retard the flow of warm air up the flue and transfer additional heat from the flue gases reduces air movement in the local environment and reduces the amount of oxygen available for life support and for the combustion reaction in the heating appliance. Heat conservation projects are often accomplished without regard for the provision of adequate combustion air for the central and other heating appliances.

Portable, unvented fuel-burning appliances added to a confined environment to supplement the central heating plant consume oxygen when operating and produce toxic fire gases that are expelled into the confined local atmosphere. If the fuel being burned is wood or coal, visible smoke will appear and the occupants will be driven out of the space by the smoke. If the combustion process produces an invisible flue gas, the occupants will not notice or become alarmed. These invisible, odorless but toxic gases cause asphyxiation in an atmosphere the average person considers safe because the senses of sight, smell, touch, taste, and hearing are not affected.

When buildings are winterized or weather-proofed it is mandatory to provide a safe, habitable atmosphere for the occupants and for the effective burning of the heating fuel. Infiltration and exfiltration of the air into the confined space must be provided to maintain a habitable atmosphere.

IMPORTANCE OF VENTILATION

Occasionally, in large office buildings, employees will complain of irritation or illness due to inadequate ventilation. Often this can be traced to dirty air filters, poor control of solvents (such as typewriter and computer cleaning fluids), and the unresolved question of possible ill effects from cathode-ray display tubes on computers and electronic equipment. Fluorescent lighting has also been suspected as a possible cause of irritation, although research has suggested that this is unlikely. However, eyestrain of persons working without proper illumination, and without corrective lenses when needed, has been known to contribute to disruption of employee morale. Frequent inspections of these areas by health professional teams (including industrial physicians, occupational health nurses, safety engineers, and industrial hygienists) often can resolve problems before they become critical.

The air "impurities" suggested above, in either atmospheric or indoor air, must be viewed with the knowledge that most humans can tolerate a significant deviation from "pure air," regardless of the source of the contamination, since most healthy humans have the ability to adjust to or tolerate respiratory "insults." It is only when the summation of the various pollutants in the breathing zone reaches an intolerable level that human life is threatened by respiratory hazards, whether of artificial or natural origin. Serious effects may be observed in seconds from a few breaths of certain gases, such as arsine, phosgene, chlorine, hydrogen sulfide, or the oxides of nitrogen, while the effects of chronic exposures to other materials, such as an aerosol-containing bis-dichlorodiethyl ether, asbestos, beryllium compounds, or benzene, may not be apparent until years later.

It is recognized that the human system in generally good health has remarkable tolerance or ability to cope with assaults from inhalation insults; hence the term "threshold" is applied to limits above which airborne contaminants may be expected to produce injury or ill effects of some type. However, this threshold is not a "go/no-go" concept. For a small but very real percentage of persons who constitute a high-risk population, including the very young, the aging, and persons with severe respiratory diseases, such as bronchial asthma, chronic bronchitis, pulmonary emphysema, or pneumonia, exposures that may be acceptable and tolerated by most healthy persons may have serious effects.

ASBESTOS

Recent action on reducting the limits of exposure to asbestos illustrates that "threshold limits" are not "cast in concrete" but are adjusted as new data become available. OSHA has ordered a 10-fold reduction in worker exposure to asbestos, a material whose effects on the lungs have been known since 1899 at autopsy in London, but whose dangers were largely ignored or deliberately overlooked until the shipbuilding program of World War II brought hundreds of serious, and often fatal, exposures. OSHA has now set an "action level," which demands protective and training measures, at concentrations of 100,000 microscopic asbestos fibers per cubic meter of air. This means that under the new regulations, the permissible occupational-exposure ceilings fall from two million particles for each 1000 cubic meters to 200,000 particles. Construction companies, garages, and other businesses where workers are exposed to asbestos, as well as manufacturing organizations, now are required to alert employees to the dangers of assbestos and to explain how to work with it. The added annual cost to business in meeting the new standard is $352 million for construction firms and $108 million for general industry. The new limit is expected to decrease from 6.4 percent to less than 1 percent excess cancer dangers among about 1.3 million workers exposed to the "action level."

SYNERGISTIC EFFECTS

Respiratory hazards have been studied for over a century, especially in Germany and England, but even today much is not known.[3,4] We are limited in our understanding of the synergistic or combined effects of air contaminants. We do know that several substances have enhanced toxicity when inhaled with a "carrier." However, studies of real-world air, including the concentrations of the various gases, vapors, and particulates encountered in daily exposures, especially when aggravated by smoking, alcohol, bacteria, and physiologically active aerosol drugs (often administered through the nose by a nebulizer, in a saline solution), are seldom directly applicable ot an individual because our data base is usually too incomplete as applied to a specific person.

AEROSOLS

Aerosols consist of solids or liquids suspended in air as pointed out, it is recognized that the human system in generally good health has remarkable tolerance or ability to cope with assaults from inhalation insults; hence "threshold" limits are established for the average person's exposures. Again, however, for the high-risk population, including the very young, the aging, and persons with severe respiratory diseases, including bronchial asthma, chronoc bronchitis, pulmonary emphysema, or pneumonia, exposures that may be acceptable and tolerated by most healthy persons may be unacceptable.

Aerosols may be defined as a mixture of gases and particulates that exhibit some stability in a gravitational field. In atmospheric aerosols, this gravitational stability excludes particules with a diameter greater than several hundred micrometers. Table 12.2 gives the names and characteristics of aerosol particles.

A particle is any minute piece of solid or liquid. Many particles important in studies of air pollution are unstable, and can change or even disappear upon contact with a surface. Precipitation, whether rain, sleet, hail, or snow, begins with condensation nuclei, and "cloud seeding" or "rain making" is based on the introduction of particles, such as silver iodide, to the selected cloud or other saturated air mass. Other examples of air-borne particles are raindrops striking a surface and

TABLE 12.2 Names and Characteristics of Aerosol Particles

Name	Unique Physical Characteristics	Effects	Origin	Predominant Size Range (μm)
Coarse particle			Mechanical process Condensation	>2
Fine particle			Condensation	<2
Dust	Solid	Nuisance and ice nuclei	Mechanical dispersion	>1
Smoke	Solid or liquid	Health and visibility	Condensation	<1
Fume	Solid	Health and visibility	Condensation	<1
Fog	Water droplets	Visibility reduction	Condensation	2–30
Mist	Water droplets	Visibility reduction and cleansing air	Condensation or atomization	5–1000
Haze	Exists at lower RH than fog— hygroscopic	Visibility reduction		<1
Aitken or condensation nuclei (CN)		Nuclei for condensation at supersaturation <300%	Combustion and atmospheric chemistry	<0.1
Ice nuclei (IN)	Has very special crystal structure	Causes freezing of supercooling water droplets	Natural dusts	>1
Small ions	Stable particle with an electric charge	Carries atmospheric electricity	All sources	>0.0015
Large particles	Special name			0.1–1
Giant particles	Special name			>1

coalescing, a loose aggregate of carbon black disintegrating upon contact with a surface, and an ion losing its charge after contact with a surface or an oppositely charged particle.

EFFECTS OF AEROSOLS

Eye irritation is one of the more conspicuous and obvious effects of the aerosols that constitute smog. Olefins are especially reactive when oxides of nitrogen react photochemically with the hydrocarbons to produce smog. Solvents play a major role in such formation, and have been rated for their tendency to produce a smog capable of eye irritation at 20 ppm and 5 ppm exposures. At the 20-ppm level, the following ranking of substances has been reported in decreasing order of irritation:

Methyl isobutyl ketone

Trichloroethylene

Xylene

Methyl ethyl ketone

Hydrocarbon fractions (six representative samples with boiling ranges from 264°F to 488°F constituted the hydrocarbon fractions in this study)

Methanol

Toluene

Hexane

Ethanol

Isopropanol

The composition of gases and aerosols in the air may be measured and monitored by well-established analytical methods, and hence a cause/effect relationship of relative safety or potential hazards, such as oxygen deficiency or carbon monoxide concentrations, can be performed relatively easily. On the other hand, most particulate or aerosol matter is measured by its total suspended particulate context, which includes all filterable particles. Molecular and ionic species are often lumped together, including cause/effect studies where chemical composition is important. For this reason alone, one must examine carefully any analytical data on air for implications as "breathing air."

TRAVEL OF AEROSOLS

Often overlooked is the fact that aerosols, as well as gases, can and do travel long distances. Long before the tragic Chernobyl nuclear accident in 1986—whose fallout produced significant measurable contamination in parts of the northern hemisphere, including milk supplies in Germany, other foods in Japan, raindeer in Finland, and livestock in nothern England, as well as being detected in the United States at least as far as the Washington, D.C., area (in rainwater)—nuclear testing from the Nevada Test Site had contributed increased radioactivity in the northeastern United States, including the tricity area of Albany, Schenectady, and Troy, N.Y. Strontium-90 and iodine-131 were definitely identified in such fallouts. The World Climate Conference in Geneva in 1983 heard reports suggesting that the smog and dust from industrial Europe and China may account for the haze that persists over Alaska, Greenland, and the Arctic Ocean every spring. "Acid rain," or acidic deposition of emissions from coal-burning power plants in the U.S. Midwest, has been linked to the continuing "fish kills" and pollution of lakes in New York State, New England, southern Canada, and even further south into Virginia and the Carolinas. The role of aluminum in this polllution process as affecting fish and other wildlife, as well as trees, and other vegitation, is still under study.

On August 5, 1980, Canada and the United States signed a Memorandum of Intent (MOI) concerning transboundary air pollution. President Reagan affirmed his commitment to the MOI during a visit to Canada in March 1981, after which both countries concluded an agreement on transboundary air pollution and work groups were established to develp documents of such an agreement. Reports of these work groups were available in an executive summary form in February 1983. On March 18, 1987, President Reagan announced he had approved $2.5 billion for further activities in this area.[5]

THE HUMAN RESPIRATORY SYSTEM

To appreciate the problems of evaluating the actions and effects of respiratory hazards, consider the complexity of the human respiratory system. Air normally enters the body through the nostrils. Larger particles or aerosols may be retained on the unciliated anterior portion of the nose, while other particles or aerosols, as well as the gases, pass through a web of nasal hairs and then flow through the narrow passages around the turbinates. The "inspired air" is warmed, moistened, and depleted of particles with aerodynamic diameters greater than 1 μm by sedimentation and impaction on nasal hairs and passages. The beating action of the cilia propels the inspired air toward the pharynx. Deposited insoluble particles are transported by the mucus and soluble particles may dissolve.[6]

Particles inhaled through the nose and deposited in the nasopharynx or inhaled through the mouth and deposited in the mouth and oropharynx are swallowed within minutes and go into the gastrointestinal tract.

The inspired air now proceeds down the trachea, or windpipe, which divides into two branches, or primary bronchi, leading in turn to upper and lower lobar bronchi for the right and left. The airway diameter decreases, but the number of tubes increases. The total cross section for flow increases and the air velocity decreases.

At the smaller velocities in the smaller airways, particles deposit by sedimentation and diffusion. Inert nonsoluble particles deposited on normal ciliated airways are cleaned within one day be transport on the moving mucus to the larynx. Soluble particles are cleaned much faster, presumably by bronchial blood flow.

Gas exchange occurs in the acini of the lung parenchyma, or the partions of the lungs from the first order of respiratory bronchioles down to the alveoli. These respiratory bronchioles originate from the terminal bronchioles, which are the smallest airways not concerned with gas exchange. The system of airways leading to the acini does not participate in the gas exchange and is called the "dead space." Inhaled particles may be deposited either in the lung parenchyma (the bronchioles, atrial sacs, and alveoli) or in the dead space. Smaller inhaled partices may be breathed in and out of the respiratory tract without deposition.

DETECTION OF ATMOSPHERIC CONTAMINANTS

Odor is the simplest sense for detecting certain contaminants in the air, since *pure air* should be odorless, or, as after a thunderstorm with lightning, perhaps contain a slight odor of ozone. Odor, however, is not a dependable or reproducible criterion of air quality, since it is often misleading and unreliable. Certain substances, such as acrolein, ammonia, bromine, chlorine, formaldehyde, acetic acid, acetic anhydride, sulfur dioxide and sulfur trioxide, hydrogen chloride, and the mercaptans, for example, have distinctive odors at relatively low concentrations. Some gases and vapors, such as fluorine and hydrogen fluoride, are so immediately corrosive to the upper respiratory tract that odor is not a safe warning. Other gases, including arsine, phosphine, stibine, hydrogen cyanide, nitric oxide, and hydrogen sulfide, may be encountered at concentrations far beyond their "permissible safe inhalation limits" before a "fresh nose" can respond. The ability of several of these gases, especially hydrogen sulfide, to cause olfactory fatigue, is now recognized. The olfactory nerves are rapidly overcome, and they no longer can sense changes in concentrations. A concentration of 1000 ppm hydrogen sulfide causes loss of consciousness in seconds from a few breaths. The ability of hydrogen sulfide rapidly to overcome detection by odor is undoubtedly a factor in the continuing fatalities that have been seen over the years in many locations as a result of exposure to this gas.[7]

At the other end of the odor scale, carbon monoxide is, for all practical purposes when reasonably pure, odorless and colorless. Inhalation can often result in significant, and even fatal, consequences. The action of CO is attributable to its ability to compete with oxygen for hemoglobin-binding sites in the blood, and subsequent transfer to the body tissues. The degree of competition of oxygen versus carbon monoxide is reflected in the fact that CO has an affinity for the hemoglobin complex that is over 200 times greater than is the oxygen-hemoglobin affinity. Once carboxyhemoglobin is formed, a considerable amount of time is required for the complex to dissociate. Until this happens, oxygen binding or transport is not possible. Thus the main effect of increased blood–CO levels is tissue hypoxia, or oxygen deficiency.

As the tissue demand for oxygen increases, increased stress on the heart is experienced because of an increased cardiac output. Therefore, the heart is the first target organ during CO inhalation. This is especially significant for those individuals who may already be experiencing cardiovascular difficulty. The other organ system most rapidly affected by hypoxia is the central nervous system (CNS).

As the carboxyhemoglobin level increases, a progression of symptoms is noted. Nausea and headache symptoms start at blood–carboxyhemoglobin levels of 15 percent. At levels of 25 percent, changes in the electrocardiogram occur. At 40 percent, unconsciousness will usually ensue. Blood–carboxyhemoglobin levels of 66 percent or higher are usually considered fatal, although death has resulted from extended exposures at levels in the 30 percent range, such as when attempting to escape from fire gases that may contain high percentages of CO.

After intense, high-level exposure to CO has ceased, several pathologic events can take place. The most serious is the development of cerebral edema, which can be life threatening if left untreated. This excessive accumulation of fluid in the brain is a result of increased permeability of the capillaries due to the change in oxygen tension. Within several days, confusion and other signs of mental deterioration can ensue. Serious mental deficits that are often irreversible may result from prolonged intense exposure. In addition, transient cardiac arrhythmias and enzyme elevations may also develop. The danger of asphyxiation in the unconscious person is increased by such serious complications as aspiration pneumonia and laryngeal edema.[18a-c]

Carbon monoxide is not the only gas that can bind the blood hemoglobin with serious results. Sulfhemoglobin is a green-pigmented molecule with a sulfur atom incorporated into the porphyrin ring and a markedly reduced oxygen affinity that makes it ineffective for oxygen transport. It has been associated with drug abuse, occupational exposure to sulfur compounds (such as zinc ethylene bis-dithiocarbamate), and environmental exposure to polluted air. Since the altered blood hemes in sulfhemoglobin and methemoglobin do not transport oxygen, affected persons may suffer the physiologic effects of anemia in extreme cases of methemoglobinemia and sulfhemoglobinema or when an additional cause for a low hemoglobin level exists. However, the clinical effects of nonfunctional hemes are not limited to their inability to transport oxygen. Small amounts of nonfunctional hemes can have additional clinical importance if their presence produces a physiologically dysfunctional change in the oxygen affinity of neighboring unmodified subunits. This is the case with methemoglobinemia, in which relatively mild degrees can cause a left-shifted oxygenation curve, impaired oxygen delivery to the periphery, and respiratory distress. In the case of sulfhemoglobin, the isoelectric-focusing experiments reported demonstrate the separation of partially sulfurated from unmodified hemoglobin on the basis of the fact that the sulfurated subunits are held in an unliganded conformation.

Drs. Park and Nagel[8] note that although their patient's hemolysate contains only 12 percent modified hemes, the distribution of these hemes among partly sulfurated tetramers results in a larger percentage of the tetramers being abnormal. Since the green half-sulfurated hemoglobin species is a symmetric tetramer, the clinical sample contains only two dimer types, unmodified and singly modified. In solution, these associate to form unmodified tetramers, singly modified tetramers, and doubly modified tetramers. Thus between 24 and 48 percent of the hemoglobin tetramers in the patient's blood were partially modified, having no more than one or two sulfurated subunits.

Sulfhemoglobinemia and methemoglobinemia have been reported together in a number of cases of drug-induced hemoglobinopathy, and the lists of causative agents overlap. In the case cited, the sulfhemoglobinemia presumably resulted from taking phenacetin (in the Darvon compound), since neither barbiturates (amobarbital) nor amphethamines (dextroamphethamine) have been associated with this disorder. Acetanilid (formerly in a commonly used over-the-counter drug for gastric discomfort) and phenacetin were the main offenders in 62 cases of sulfhemoglo-binemia seen at the Mayo Clinic. Metabolites of these drugs serve as reducing agents in a cyclic process that generates both sulfhemoglobin and methemoglobin. The origin of the sulfur atom in the former remains unclear, but both hydrogen sulfide released by intestinal organisms and glutathione have been suggested. Although the acetanilid and phenacetin have both been acted upon by the FDA, sulfonamides, dapsone, and ointments containing sulfur are reported offenders and are still widely used. Further, accidents involving occupational exposure to hydro-gen sulfide still occur. Park and Nagel note that laboratory documentation of sulfhemoglobinemia is often inadequate and that it is probably underdiagnosed, and so a proper diagnostic approach is needed to determine the true frequency of this disorder.[8]

While hydrogen sulfide and carbon monoxide present extremely acute problems in the real world,[9] other gases must be given full respect as well.

Sulfur dioxide[10] (Table 12.3), oxides of nitrogen, and ammonia (Table 12.3) have serious potential as far as respiration is concerned. The first two are acidic and the third is basic. If a person is occupationally exposed to these gases, the entire respiratory tree is affected, with reactions ranging from sneezing and coughing to severe bronchoconstriction and cessation of respiration. Because of this induced change in normal respiratory physiology, cardiovascular responses include in-creased blood pressure and pulse rate.

Acute, intense (high-level) exposure to these gases may also produce pulmonary edema, manifested as an increase in intercellular and intestitial fluid. This edematous condition may result in a variety of physiologic malfunctions, including decreased lung compliance, hypoxemia, ventilation/perfusion mismatch, and res-piratory alkalosis followed by metabolic acidosis.

As continuous exposure to these irritant gases increases, definite clinical disease patterns may be seen, such as bronchiolitis, bronchitis, and pneumonia, as well as adverse changes in the teeth, eyes, and skin. A person who has respiratory disease and who continues to be exposed to these irritant gases may ultimately experience irreversible respiratory pathology (see Table 12.3).

The effect of exposure to gases is enhanced by such factors as heavy labor, high environmental temperature, and increased altitude (over 2000 feet or 610 meters). Susceptibility to the effects of gases is greatest in the very young, the elderly, persons with cardiac or chronic respiratory disease, and pregnant women. Cold air can also make breathing more difficult, and this is especially true if a person has chronic heart disease or respiratory difficulty. Wearing a mask or scarf over the mouth and nose is helpful in such situations. This will lessen irritation to the body's airways as well as warm the air and make breathing easier. Wind also complicates the ability to survive cold; wind-chill factor is a very real danger (see the wind-chill conversion chart of the National Weather Service, Table 11.2). Another complicat-ing condition for breathing, especially in contaminated atmospheres, is asthma.[11]

The odor intensity and physiological response produced by paraffin hydrocar-bons have been studied in terms of the potential warning of possible concentration

TABLE 12.3 Symptoms of Exposures to Selected Gases

Effect	Concentration (ppm)
a. Carbon Monoxide	
TLV-TWA/STEL	50/400
Slight headache in some cases	0–200
After 5–6 hours, mild headache, nausea, vertigo, and mental symptoms	200–400
After 4–5 hours, severe headache, muscular incoordination weakness, vomiting, and collapse	400–700
After 3–5 hours, severe headache, weakness, vomiting, and collapse	700–1000
After 1.5–3 hours, coma, and breathing still fairly good unless poisoning has been prolonged	1100–1600
After 1–1.5 hours, possibly death	1600–2000
After 2–15 minutes, death	5000–10,000
b. Ammonia	
TLV-TWA/STL	25/35
Least detectable odor	53
Least amount causing immediate irritation to the eyes	698
Least amount causing immediate irritation to the throat	408
Least amount causing coughing	1720
Maximum concentration allowable for prolonged exposure	100
Maximum concentration allowable for short exposure (½–1 hour)	300–500
Dangerous for even short exposure (½ hour)	2500–4500
c. Sulfur Dioxide	
TLV-TWA/STEL	2/5
Least amount causing detectable odor	3–5
Least amount causing immediate eye irritation	20
Least amount causing immediate throat irritation	8–12
Least amount causing coughing	20
Maximum concentration allowable for prolonged exposure	10
Maximum concentration allowable for short (30-minute) exposure	50–100
Amount dangerous for even short exposure	400–500
d. Hydrogen Sulfide	
TLV/TWA/STEL	10/15
Eye and respiratory tract irritation after exposure of 1 hour	50–100
Marked eye and respiratory tract irritation after exposure of 1 hour	200–300
Dizziness, headache, nausea, etc., within 15 minute and loss of consciousness and possible death after 30–60 minute exposure	500–700
Rapidly produces unconsciousness and death occurs a few minutes later	700–900
Death is apparently instantaneous	1000–2000

(Apparent death from H_2S is not irreversible as prompt and efficient artificial respiration may restore life.)

buildup leading to an explosive mixture with air. The odors of heptane and hexane are easily noticed in concentrations below their lower flammable context of the atmosphere in which they will be used. (See Figure 6.1.)

CLASSIFICATION AND DESCRIPTION OF RESPIRATORS (FIGURE 12.1)

Self-Contained Breathing Apparatus (SCBA)

The self-contained breathing apparatus (Figure 12.2), which, as the name implies, is completely independent of an outside source of breathing air during the time the air supply is in proper service, furnishes the maximum protection against respiratory hazards. It is designed to supply complete respiratory protection, except for those gases or vapors that may penetrate the skin (see personal protective clothing, pages 121–143). When used in atmospheres where gases or vapors with significant action of toxicity through the skin penetration are encountered, such as hydrogen cyanide, the respiratory protective device must be supplemented by complete clothing of the type impervious to the substance or materials involved. Until there is general agreement as to what constitutes impervious material to chemicals, suspicion of the effectiveness of protection should always be raised, especially when details of what is involved and the concentration are unknown (as encountered in the fire services and in hazardous waste-site remedial operations).

Since the SCBA has no external connection to an outside air supply, it is obviously the device of choice for emergency operations and for entry into or escape from oxygen-deficient areas. Heptane and hexane vapors produce distinct symptoms. The odor of pentane is indistinct, and that of ethane and propane practically absent in mixtures at lower flammable limits. Recently the widespread interest in self-service gasoline service stations has been accompanied by several studies pertaining to the concentration of hydrocarbons and additives the average consumer inhales when refueling a motor vehicle at a self-service pump.

Historically, animals such as canaries and Japanese waltzing mice have been used as warning indicators for "bad air" in mines and other confined spaces. The Davy mine safety lamp, which is an indicator of oxygen deficiency and of methane-containing atmospheres, has been largely displaced by portable as well as fixed-station instrumentation to detect and record low or changing concentrations of gases, vapors, dusts, and aerosols. The availability of gas-detector tubes for use with personal samplers worn by exposed personnel has been a major advance, as has the personal gaseous "film badges" now in use for monitoring many gases and vapors.

The "Odor Threshold Manual" of ASTM contains an excellent compilation of published data on odors. However, it must always be kept in mind that some persons have very limited ability to detect an odor, while others have a high sensitivity; this difference in the ability to recognize odors may contribute to serious physiological as well as emotional effects, as has been noted where mass hysteria

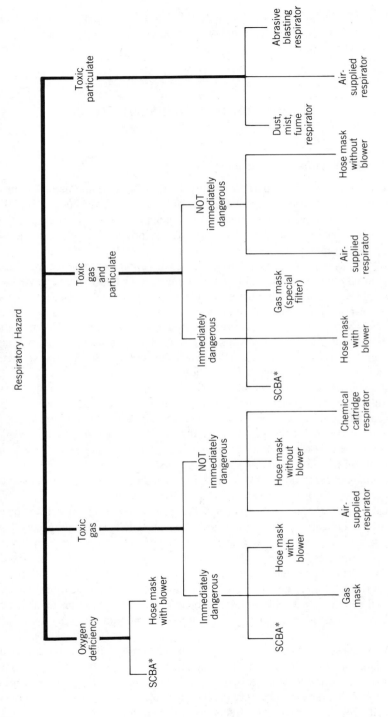

Figure 12.1. Major respiratory hazards and the classes of protective devices available.

*SCBA = Self-contained breathing apparatus

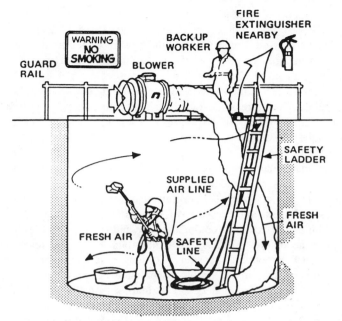

Figure 12.2. Entry of personnel into confined spaces (such as lakes, sewers, and other areas of restricted air movement) should include an SCBA and a backup person also wearing an SCBA for possible rescue. Instant communicators should be established while person is in the confined space, and emergency response must move immediately. (Courtesy of *Plant Engineering*.)

has developed with only marginal cause. (See *Ventilation '85,* Proceedings of the first International Symposium on Ventilation for Contaminant Control, October 1–3, 1985, Toronto, Canada, edited by H. D. Goodfellow. *Chemical Engineering Monographs,* **24,** Elsevier Science Publishers, Amsterdam, The Netherlands, 1986, 870 pages; and *Advanced Design of Ventilation Systems for Contaminant Control* by H. D. Goodfellow, *Chemical Engineering Monographs,* **23,** Elsevier Science Publishers, Amsterdam, The Netherlands, 1985, 746 pages.)

Increased sophistication and accuracy in instrumentation for measurement of very low concentrations of gases and vapors may prove the long-range solution to many of these problems. For example, absolute measurements of ambient nitric acid and ammonia by kilometer path-length Fourier transform infrared (FT-IR) spectroscopy have been conducted by Dr. Ernesto C. Tuazon of the California Statewide Air Pollution Research Center. An FT-IR spectrometer interfaced to an open-path multiple-reflection optical system compared the current analytical methods for determining nitrogenous species concentrations in the atmosphere. Signals averaging about five minutes at a path length of 1150 meters and spectral resolution of 0.125 cm^{-1} afforded detection sensitivities of approximately 4 ppb for nitric acid and 1.5 ppb for ammonia. The nitric acid levels were above the FT-IR detection limit most of the daytime hours during a smoke episode on September 14, when ozone peaked at greater than 0.2 ppm and the highest nitric acid concentration of 26 ppb was recorded at approximately 3:45 P.M. Background ammonia levels were generally 2–4 ppb, but concentration "spikes" as high as 84 ppb were measured when the wind direction was from nearby agricultural sources. (Anon. "Measurements of ambient nitric Acid and Ammonia," *Industrial Hygiene News Report,* **29,** No. 11, 3, 4, Nov. 1986.

The growing interest in indoor air quality, including the prohibition of smoking in the workplace, has already evinced several interesting related aspects. Dr. Kenneth M. Wallingford of NIOSH Hazard Evaluations and Technical Assistance Branch presented some of his data at a meeting of the Indoor Air Quality Symposium in Atlanta, September 23–25, 1986. In more than 300 indoor air-quality investigations, inadequate ventilation was found in 50 percent of the sites. Some of the ventilation problems commonly encountered were (1) insufficient fresh outdoor air supplied to the office space; (2) poor air distribution and mixing, which causes stratification, draftiness, and pressure differences between office spaces; (3) temperature and humidity extremes or fluctuations; and (4) filtration problems caused by improper or no maintenance. Another important factor was inside contamination, found in 19 percent of the sites. Copying machines were found to be a significant source. Other inside problems included (1) pesticides, such as chlordane, that were improperly applied; (2) dermatitis from boiler additives such as diethyl ethanolamine; (3) improperly diluted cleaning agents such as rug shampoo; (4) tobacco smoke (cigarettes, cigars, pipes); (5) combustion gases from sources common to cafeterias and laboratories; and (6) cross-contamination from poorly ventilated sources that leak into other air-handling zones.

Outside contamination was the major problem at 11 percent of the sites. Problems due to motor vehicle exhaust, boiler gases, and previously exhausted air were essentially caused by reentrainment. Other outside contamination problems included contaminants from construction or renovation, such as asphalt, solvents, and dusts.

As an example that even health experts react strongly to inadequate ventilation and lack of cooperation with contractors, the *Rockville, Md. Gazette* of April 1, 1987, pages 1, 14, noted that employees at the Department of Health and Human Services, entrusted with guarding the nation's health, had claimed that a roofing project at the Rockville, Md., building was making them sick. Pots of hot tar on the roof were contaminating the air that feeds into the building's ventilation system, causing workers to suffer from headaches, dizziness, skin rashes, and even nose bleeds.

"The smell has been really bad, I've been feeling really tired and yawning all the time. Other people are saying that they are having trouble breathing and are getting rashes," testified one secretary who worked on the 11th floor. As a result, some division supervisors sent employees home, sometimes as early as 10:30. Workers attended the infirmary more frequently.

The building, built in 1968, has no windows to open. Employees depend entirely on the circulation system for fresh air. "Either they cut off the airflow and we suffocate, or they keep the vents open and we have to breathe the tar fumes," said a 12th-floor worker.

Complaints about water leaks from the roof instituted the roof repair, which was completed in three weeks. Safety officials said the problem was caused by the placement of a tar pot next to an intake duct. It has been suggested that future reroofing could be done on weekends or at night.

Also, gasoline fumes infiltrating the basement and/or sewer system (where drain traps can evaporate or drain without replacing the water for the trap) sometimes caused problems. Biological contamination was involved at 5 percent of the sites. Though not a common cause of office problems, biological contamination can result in a potentially severe medical condition known as hypersensitivity pneumonitis. This can be caused by organisms such as bacteria, fungi, protozoa, and microbial products. Building fibric contamination was the major problem at 4 percent of the sites. Formaldehyde can off-gas from urea-formaldehyde foam insulation, particle board, plywood, and some glues and adhesives commonly used during construction. Other fibric contamination problems included (1) dermatitis resulting from fibrous glass erosion in lined ventilating ducts; (2) various organic solvents from glues and adhesives; and (3) acetic acid as a curing agent in silicone caulking.[12]

Protection

The classic approaches to reducing or eliminating personnel exposure to hazardous airborne materials (gases, vapors, fumes, or other aerosols) are (1) to confine the contamination to closed systems and/or (2) to remove it by properly designed, maintained and intelligently operated vents or fume hoods. In fact, these approaches are not simple in their application.

The movement of the hazardous substances, fumes, or other materials outside the building away from air intakes and from inhabited areas is often not considered carefully in terms of the possible involvement of both on-site and off-site personnel. If Bhopal has taught anything, it is that space and distance must be adequately considered, as well as wind roses, to understand more completely how even a relatively small release can travel significant distances before dilution to a relatively "safe" concentration. With the appearance and acceptance of computerized systems on site to be immediately available in case of an accidental release, such as the TRACE system (Toxic Release Analysis of Chemical Emissions) in many plants, the frequent hesitation and confusion that arise when an emergency occurs may be minimized or better controlled. Depending on the materials involved, dilution, filtration, scrubbing, or flaring to reduce levels of discharge may be considered. The filters and other pollution-control devices should be carefully engineered.[21] To illustrate, discharge to the roof level may be satisfactory most of the time, but if the wind-directional rose indicates that, even for a small percentage of time, the effluent gas may be recycled or reach a populated area, serious concern should be given to the air movements. In one specific operational problem, ethylene dibromide (EDB) was being exhausted from an animal inhalation bioassay laboratory at a concentration of 20 ppm. Since the roof-level discharge was near a populated office-building complex, it was desired to reduce the stack concentration to 1 ppm. Activated charcoal bed filters were installed in the vent system at a cost of $10,000, part of which was for the changes in the vent to accommodate the filters. The filters performed successfully, as planned, and frequent monitoring was instituted to ensure that saturation or breakthrough did not occur between the scheduled monthly filter replacements. The importance of periodic monitoring, coupled with a maintenance schedule that ensures replacement and other necessary repairs as required, cannot be overemphasized.

Engineering controls should always have the first consideration in planning protection for personnel both on- and off-site. Properly designed and maintained engineered strategies are far more dependable than dependence on the on-the-spot decisions of what to do in a plant emergency, especially if a respiratory threat is involved. A competent industrial hygienist or ventilation, heating, and cooling engineer should design or, in older facilities, retrofit systems for control of hazards.

If engineering controls, such as mentioned above, cannot be trusted to control adequately or to confine the material (and it must be admitted that no system is perfect), personal protective equipment must be considered, at least on a temporary basis. We stress the word "temporary" since respiratory protection cannot be relied on for long periods of time for hazardous exposures, unless highly unusual control procedures are established and rigorously enforced. As will be noted later in this discussion, all protection has limitations, expense, and discomfort.

Time is also an important factor, especially in work with hazardous and toxic wastes, where the practical limits of time may seriously limit productivity. The special package of recirculating oxygen-breathing apparatus with protective clothing, which has been developed by the EPA for workers at waste sites and in other situations, may ultimately be approved by NIOSH for a working limit of 2½ hours, and should greatly expand the horizon of self-contained equipment/clothing. Where the risks are known to be high, as in the possibility of breathing dioxin, plutonium, or aerosols containing carcinogens, programs of respiratory protection have been successfully instituted. In areas where occasional (often infrequent) emergencies involve less obvious or inadequately characterized materials, respiratory protection is successful only if well-planned and implemented programs of education, maintenance, and enforcement are in actual use. Now that MSDS, supposedly are available for each material on the site, it is hoped the information from these sheets, together with the education of the workers and the community, will improve the acceptance of prevention, or at least place greater emphasis on backup, including respiratory protection and other personnel protection, and the community understanding of the risks involved within the plant and outside (Figures 12.3 and 12.4). However, we must suggest that unless the MSDSs are complete and scientifically accurate, this gain may not be as extensive as it should be. In a recent study of 476 MSDSs for the Seattle Area Hospital Council, only 46.6 percent of the sheets reviewed had all the blanks filled in only 70 percent were internally consistent. Only 3.2 percent had all required elements present, and finally, only 2.9 percent of the reviewed sheets were found to be acceptable for employee use. The author of the study feels there is a real danger that the workers may think they are protected, only to find they are not when they must rely solely on what may be incomplete MSDS information. An additional data-base check or a phone call to the supplier should be made to clean up any ambiguities or to fill in incomplete data.[13]

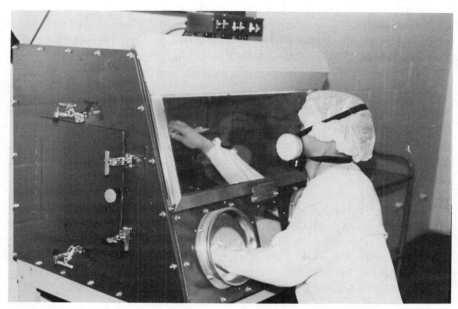

Figure 12.3. Even when working with toxic carcinogenic substances in enclosed hoods, respirators may be indicated as additional protection. (Photo by H. Fawcett.)

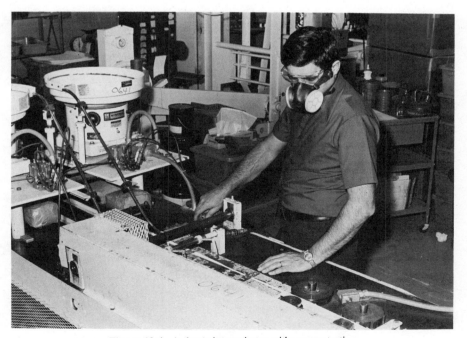

Figure 12.4. A dust/mist respirator with eye protection.

The idea that stock off-the-shelf answers will adequately cover certain aspects of all MSDSs is highly questionable. For example, a major compilation of 867 MSDS forms, available commercially, used the same wording for the "First Aid" section of each form. A prudent occupational health physician or nurse would have suggested a separate review of each material for medical aspects, since the compounds covered differ widely in their properties.

Air Supply

Where air-supplied respiratory protection is used, the important problem of the purity of the breathing air must be considered. In the past, fatal accidents have occurred when an air-supplied respirator was connected to a plant air supply, which, without notice or warning, had been changed to a nitrogen supply to ensure instrument "air" while work was being done on a compressor. In other cases, cylinders of breathing air were, in fact, charged with nitrogen, carbon dioxide, and butane. In some instances, air has been produced by mixing compressed oxygen with compressed nitrogen; such mixtures are useful but must always be suspect until it can be shown by analysis that they do contain a mixture that is within the recognized limits for breathing air.

While oxygen deficiency is the more obvious potential error in such synthetic air mixtures, the fire hazard created when oxygen is above 25 percent must be considered as well. For short-duration tasks, air-supplied hoods are often used successfully, but must not be used with oxygen. See Figure 12.5.

Legal standards exist for air supply from a compressor. OSHA specification 1910.94(6) notes that the air for abrasive-blasting respirators shall be free of harmful quantities of dusts, mists, or noxious gases, and shall meet the requirements for air purity in ANSI Z9.2-1960 or a more recent edition. The air from the regular compressed-air line of the plant may be used for the abrasive-blasting respirator if (1) a trap and carbon filter are installed and regularly maintained to remove oil, water, scale, and odor; (2) a pressure-reducing diaphragm or valve is installed to reduce the pressure to the requirements of the particular type of abrasive-blasting respirator; and (3) an automatic control is provided to either sound an alarm or shut down the compressor in case of overheating.

In OSHA specification 1910.134, the quality of the air is specified. Oxygen shall meet the requirements of the *U.S. Pharmacopoaedia* for medical or breathing oxygen. The breathing air shall meet at least the requirements of the specifications for the Grade D breathing air as described in Compressed Gas Association (CGA) Commodity Specification G-7, 1973, or the most recent revision. Compressed oxygen shall never be used with air-line hoods or respirators. If a compressor is used, it shall be of the diaphragm or other breathing-air type, constructed and situated so as to avoid entry of contaminated air into the system, and suitable in-line air-purifying absorbent beds and filters shall be installed to further assure the breathing-air quality. If an oil-lubricated compressor is used, it shall have a high-temperature or carbon monoxide alarm, or both. If only a high-temperature alarm is used, the air from the compressor should be frequently tested for carbon

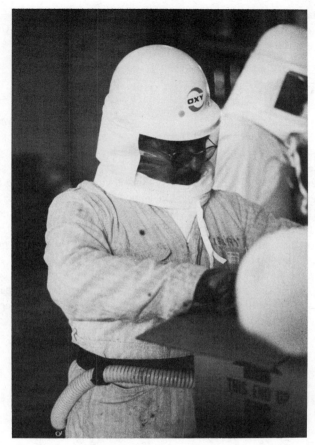

Figure 12.5. Air-supplied hood used near grinding/polishing operation. Note text for standards on the air supply.

monoxide to ensure that it meets the specifications. Where air is used for diving, the specifications of the U.S. Navy Diving Manual, NAV-SHIPS 250-538, should be followed. CGA and Navy Standards for breathing air are summarized in Table 12.4.

TABLE 12.4 Standards in Breathing Air

	Maximum Allowable Level	
Contaminant	CGA Grade D	U.S. Navy
Carbon monoxide (ppm)	20	20
Carbon dioxide (ppm)	1000	500
Oil vapor (mg/m^3)	5	5

Several states, including California, New Hampshire, New Jersey, New York, and Washington, have even lower limits, and specify that the air for SCBAs be free from odors and other contaminants.

RESPIRATORY PROTECTIVE DEVICES

Based on the mode of operation, several types of respiratory protective devices are available and should be considered in such atmopheres as sewers, tanks (vented or not), and other spaces where situations that can be immediately dangerous to life may be present. As noted in Figure 12.2, the entry into a confined space should never be attempted alone, since a "buddy" or backup colleague, also fitted with a SCBA and ready to rescue the first person, must be on hand at all times and give his or her undivided attention to the operation; see also Figures 12.6 and 12.7.

In recent times, there has been a movement away from the so-called "demand" SCBA, in which the air was made available to the wearer in the face piece only on inhalation, to the so-called closed-circuit SCBA, in which air is continuously supplied into the face piece. This is especially important in highly contaminated atmospheres, as in fire-fighting smoke conditions or serious chemical gas leaks, since, under some conditions, the gas or smoke could enter the face piece during the exhalation cycle, when no air was being supplied to maintain a positive pressure in the face piece. Positive-pressure devices are safe.

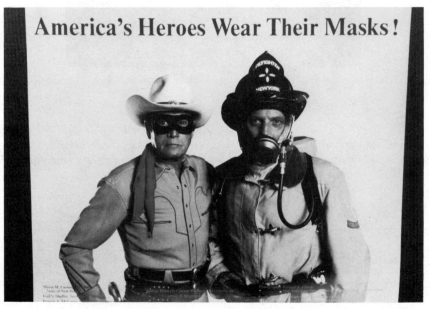

Figure 12.6. Heroes wear their masks. (Courtesy New York State Office of Fire Prevention and Control.)

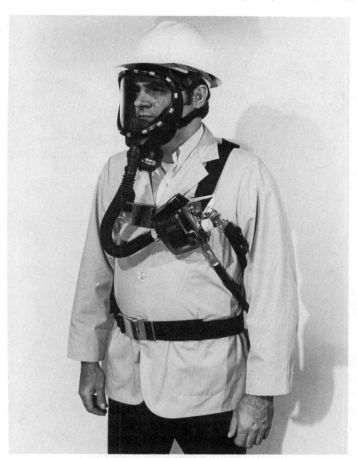

Figure 12.7. Typical SCBA (self-contained breathing apparatus) employing the positive-pressure mode to ensure no leakage of outside gases into face piece. Air cylinder is carried on back. (Courtesy Scott Aviation Co.)

Another concern in recent years is that the so-called 4500-psi aluminum fiber-glass-wrapped air tanks, especially the DOT 7235 series, have been known to leak, and in two recorded cases, to rupture at the neck. These tanks should all have been retrofitted with steel bands around the neck to minimize this problem. Users of such tanks should be very vigilant as to leaks or other malfunctions, and should immediately report any such incidents to NIOSH and the Department of Transportation, as well as to fire and emergency services.

If the atmosphere does not require SCBA equipment, gas masks of various types are available. For gases that have poor warning-odor properties, gas masks are clearly not indicated, and are not certified for such use. In choosing a gas mask, one must be very certain that the canister is the proper one for the intended use, considering the materials to be encountered as well as the length of time and concentrations involved. All gas masks assume that sufficient oxygen is present at all times.

Going up the scale, we find respirators of various kinds, from relatively simple one-use devices (which, in the writer's view, are more cosmetic than protective) to high-efficiency masks for use against small particles, including radioactive dusts, Figure 12.8. In choosing a respirator, consult the latest certification and approval certificate issued for the device by NIOSH to be certain that it is the proper one for the intended service. In addition, a very careful record should be made of its use to ensure that the cartridges or filters are "fresh" and not contaminated. The practice of issuing respirators demands careful control. Each respirator should have its own number, and should be returned to a central cleaning station after every shift. The

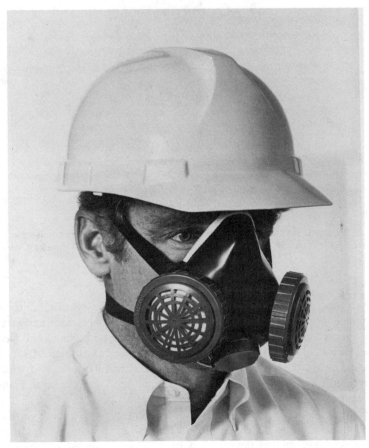

Figure 12.8. Typical "dust mask" for dusts for which standards have been established by NIOSH. Masks must be compatible with other protective equipment.

cleaning and disinfecting, as well as inspection to ensure that all parts are in proper condition or replaced, must be thorough—a respiratory device is not a screwdriver or other tool, but a vital adjunct to human health.

For additional details on respiratory protection, which is a rapidly changing and complex area, contact NIOSH at the address given under "Suggested Reading." Independent verification of the sales representative's claims may well be entirely justified.

Note the cartridge or canister capability and the length of time it may be used before contaminant breakthrough can occur. (If test data are not available, the manufacturer of the device should be required to furnish such data or an air-supplied device used instead.)

For communications between workers, the use of in-mask microphones or throat mikes external to the mask should be considered. Either amplifiers or two-way radio equipment may be used where necessary [see H. H. Fawcett, "Speech Transmission Through Respiratory Protective Devices," *Am. Ind. Hyg. Assoc. J.,* **22,** No. 3, pp 170–174 (June 1961)].

REFERENCES

1. M. Eisenbud, *Environmental Radioactivity, From Natural, Industrial, and Military Sources,* Academic Press, Orlando, Fla., 1986; see also G. Weisburg, "Front Range Residents Face Radon Gas Danger," *The Colorado Statesman,* **88,** No. 14 1, 10 (Apr. 3, 1987). (10 percent of the houses in the Colorado Front Range area have high levels of radon gas.)

2. B. Saltzman, R. Benzi and A. C. Wiin-Nielsen, *Anomalous Atmospheric Flows and Blocking,* Vol. 29 of *Advances in Geophysics,* Academic Press, Orlando, Fla., 1986, and R. A. Pielke, *Mesoscale Meterorolgical Modelling,* Academic Press, Orlando, Fla., 1984.

3. A. C. Stern, *Air Pollution,* Vol. VI, *Supplement to Air Pollutants, Their Transformation, Transport and Effects,* 496 pp. *Supplement to Measurements, Monitoring, Surveillance and Engineering Control,* Vol. VII, 544 pp., 1986; *Supplement to Management of Air Quality,* Vol. VIII, 240 pp., Academic Press, Orlando, Fla., 1986.

4. T. E. Graedel and L. D. Claxton, *Atmospheric Chemical Compounds: Sources, Occurrence, and Bioassay,* 816 pp., 1986.

5. L. Ember, "Acid Rain Focus of International Cooperation," *C&EN,* 15–17 (Dec. 3, 1979); see also "U.S. Raising Acid Rain Spending," *Washington Post,* A25 (March 19, 1987).

6. N. Muica, "Respiratory System," pp. 1926–1930; G. Morse and W. B. Miller, "Respiratory Protective Equipment," pp. 1919–1926; P. Brochard and J. Bignon, "Respiratory Cancer—Occupational," pp. 1916–1919, *Encyclopaedia of Occupational Health and Safety,* 3rd ed., International Labour Office, Geneva, Switzerland, 1983.

7. W. W. Burnett, E. G. King, M. Grace, and W. F. Hall, "Hydrogen Sulfide Poisoning: Review of Five Years' Experience," *Canad. Med. Assoc. J.,* **117,** 1277–1280 (1977.); see also H. H. Fawcett, "Hydrogen Sulfide—Killer That May Not Stink," *J. Chem. Ed.,* **25,** 511 (Sept. 1948).

8. C. M. Park and R. L. Nagel, "Sulfhemoglobinema: Clinical and Molecular Aspects, *N. E. Med.,* **310,** No. 24, 1579–1584 (June 14, 1984) (32 references).

9. M.H.G. Medeiros et al., "Oxygen Toxicity and Hemoglobinemia in Subjects from a Highly Polluted Town," *Arch. Environ. Health,* **38,** 11–16 (1983).

10. J. E. McFadden and M. D. Koontz, "Sulfur Dioxide and Sulfates Materials Damage Study," *Geomet,* ES-812 (Feb. 1980), U.S. Environmental Protection Agency, Research Triangle Park, N.C.

11. A. W. Weinstein, *Asthma*, McGraw-Hill, New York, 1987.

12. Anon., "Indoor Air Quality Investigations in Office Buildings," *Indus. Hyg. News Rep.*, **29**, No. 11, 1 (Nov. 1986).

13. Anon., "Material Safety Data Sheets Rated in Hazard Communication Program," *Indus. Hyg. News Rep.*, **29**, No. 11, 1, 2 (Nov. 1986).

SUGGESTED READINGS

AIChE, *Guidelines for Use of Vapor Cloud Dispersion Models*, 176 pp., American Institute of Chemical Engineers, New York, 1987.

E. V. Anderson, "EPA Is Set to Propose Tough Fuel Volatility Regulations," *Chem. Eng. News*, 7–13 (July 6, 1987).

Anon., "Colorado to Restrict Gasoline Use in Winter," *Chem. Eng. News*, 8 (June 29, 1987).

Anon., "Aerosols: *Antropogenic and Natural Sources and Transport*," *Ann. N.Y. Acad. of Sci.*, **338**, 1980.

P. Brimblecombe, *The Big Smoke, A History of Air Pollution in London since Medieval Times*, Methuen & Co., New York, 1987, reviewed in *Sci. Am.*, 112 (Aug. 1987).

G. Brooks, "The 70 Million Sheep roving New Zealand Create Quite a Stink," *Wall St. J.*, 1, 19 (June 30, 1987).

M. Ghassemi and A. Panahloo, "Physical and Chemical Characteristics of Some Widely Used Petroleum Fuels: A Reference Data Base for Assessing Similarities and Differences Between Synfuel and Petrofuel Products, *Energy Sources*, **7**, No. 4, 377–401 (1984).

R. J. Cicerone, "Changes in Stratospheric Ozone," *Science*, 35–42 (July 3, 1987).

R. E. Forster II, *The Lung: Physiologic Basis of Pulmonary Function Tests*, 3rd ed., 329 pp., Year Book Publishing Co., Chicago, Ill., 1987.

S. K. Friedlander, *Smoke, Dust and Haze*, Wiley, New York, 1977.

M. H. Ho and H. K. Dillon, *Biological Monitoring of Exposure to Chemicals, Organic Compounds*, 532 pp. Wiley-Interscience, New York, 1987.

P. Hochstein et al., "Mechanisms of Copper Toxicity in Red Cells," pp. 669–681 in G. J. Brewer, *The Red Cell*, Liss, New York, 1978.

ILO, *Occupational Exposure Limits for Airborne Toxic Substances*, No. 37, 3rd rev. ed., International Labour Organization, Geneva, Switzerland, 1987.

C. L. Keller, "Future Requirementes for Unrestricted Entry into Confined Spaces," *Plant/Operations Prog.*, **6**, No. 3, 142–145 (July 1987).

G. W. Kling et al., The 1986 Lake Nyos Gas Disaster in Cameroon, West Africa," *Science*, 169–175 (Apr. 10, 1987).

W. Meyer and N. Heister, *Topics in Respiratory and Comparative Physiology*, 157 pp. VCH Publishers, New York, 1987.

E. Marshall, "Tobacco Science Wars," *Science*, 250–251 (Apr. 17, 1987).

R. W. Shaw, "Air Pollution by Particles, *Sci. Am.*, 96–103 (Aug. 1987).

J. H. Seinfeld, *Atmospheric Chemistry and Physics of Air Pollution*, 738 pp., Wiley-Interscience, New York, 1986.

R. K. Stevens et al "Characterization of the Aerosol in the Great Smoky Mountains," *Environ. Sci. Technol.*, **14**, No. 12, 1491–1498 (Dec. 1980).

A. C. Stern, *Air Pollution*, 3rd., Vol. VI, 496 pp,; Vol. VII. 544 pp.; Volume VIII, 206 pp., Academic Press.

R. E. Taylor, EPA Deals Blow to Auto, Truck Makers in Ruling on Handling Gasoline Fumes," *Wall St. J.*, 18 (July 23, 1987).

L. Wahlin, *Atmospheric Electrostatics*, 134 pp., Wiley-Interscience, New York, 1986.

L. Slote, *Handbook of Occupational Safety and Health,* 744 pp., Wiley-Interscience, New York, 1987.

V. M. Steiner, Meeting Clean Air Standards with Regenerative Fume Incinerator, *Plant Engr.,* Oct. 22, 87, 32 Orlando, Fla., 1986.

R. E. Taylor, "Nominee Bork Helps Reverse His EPA Ruling (on vinyl chloride), *Wall St. J.,* 1 (July 29, 1987) (Federal Appeals Court partly reversed a ruling on regulation of vinyl chloride by EPA; court requires EPA to consider what level of a chemical's emissions presents unacceptable health risks).

M. Weisskoff, "EPA Proposes New Auto Pollution Device: Industry Opposes Trap for Gasoline Fumes, Limits on Fuel Volatility," *Washington Post,* A1 (July 23, 1987).

Testings Approval of Respirators

Bulletins and Letters issued by the Certification Branch, Centers for Disease Control, National Institute for Occupational Safety and Health, 944 Chestnut Ridge Rd., Morgantown, WV 26505 (issued as indicated). Among recent issues:

Ethylene Oxide Canister Bench Tests, Aug. 15, 1984. Special Report to Respirator Users on NIOSH Respirator

Problem Investigation, Oct. 15, 1984. Notice to All Respirator Manufacturers with MSHA/NIOSH Approved Respirators, Nov. 6, 1984.

Respirator Users' Notice: Use of Unapproved Subassemblies, Nov. 6, 1984.

Letter to All Respirator Manufacturers (Supplied-air respirators and escape air purifying respirators), July 21 1986.

Use of Bureau of Mines Approved Gas Mask Canisters (approved under Schedule 14F for protection against highly toxic substances such as hydrogen sulfide, hydrogen cyanide, and phosphine, Nov. 15, 1985.

Letter to All Respirator Manufacturer's (regarding combination of pressure-demand supplied air (SAR) and escape high efficiency particulate respirator), March 10, 1986.

NIOSH Certified Equipment List—Respirators, Coal Mine Personal Sampler Units, Oct. 1, 1985, or most recent issue, National Institute for Occupational Safety and Health, 944 Chestnut Ridge Road, Morgantown, WV 26505-2888

G. Rajhans and D. S. Blackwell, *Practical Guide to Respirator Usage in Industry,* 176 pp. Butterworth Publishers, 80 Montvale Ave., Stoneham, MA 02180, 1984.

Training Aids

The following are available from ITS Industrial Training Systems Corporation, 20 West Stow Road, Marlton, NJ 08053-9990:

"The Breath You Save," 680-01, slide tape or video, 16 minutes.

"Air Purifying Respirators," 680-2, slide tape or video, 19 minutes.

"Atmosphere Supplying Respirators," 680-3, slide tape or video, 19 minutes.

Asbestos: Breathe Easy," slide tape or video, 14 minutes.

"Don't Let It Get You Down," slide tape or video with handout, 17 minutes.

"Matter of Minutes," 601-05, slide tape or video, 21 minutes, (hazards of H_2S in pulp and paper industry).

"Matter of Minutes," 601-06, slide tape or video, 21 minutes (Hazards of H_2S in the waste-water treatment industry.)

"Occupational Medical Surveillance," 600-22, 13 minutes.

13

Laboratories—Source of Knowledge and Information

Howard H. Fawcett

Laboratories, like the people who inhabit and manage them, vary greatly in size, shape, function, philosophy, and dedication to safety and health. A variability in purpose accounts for the first four of these aspects, while health and safety (or their lack) may be traced to ancient times., Then people were motivated only by the goals of eternal life or extreme wealth (gold)—objectives that, even today, escape the grasp of most chemists. History records that many alchemists succumbed to their cavalier handling of mercury, lead, tin, antimony, and other elements and natural products that are now recognized as demanding control measures far in excess of what was then considered necessary. Like alchemists, even today some laboratory personnel (including chemists, engineers, physicists, technicians, and mathematical modelers) see little reason for health and safety measures, and openly resent, almost to the point of sincere disbelief and contempt, attempts by others to preserve and protect their lives. It is human nature to resist change, but the open-mindedness that scientific personnel are expected to exhibit to scientific affairs is often not present when safer and healthier approaches or changes in procedures are recommended.

Each of us, including scientific personnel, is mortal. Our time on this earth is limited, but can be even shorter than intended if poor work practices, indifference to hazards, and a closed mind so preoccupied with the immediate task and dedication to work that the human interface is forgotten or underemphasized.

Laboratory work, including routine analyses, experimentation, research and development, and innovative processes and procedures, all have hazards that must be recognized if serious difficulty is to be avoided. Hazards are not confined to "chemical" laboratories; a 1980 survey suggested that in research and development laboratories, hazardous conditions are the rule rather than the exception. Flammable chemicals and toxic materials present the hazards most frequently encountered. One out of 11 laboratories surveyed had no safety program at all; three out of 10 no effective safety program; one out of five had experienced a serious work-related injury in the past year. All this even though "safety" is supposed to be a *sine qua non* of laboratory investigations.[1]

It is hoped that the OSHA Hazard Communication Regulation[2] plus the numerous local and state right-to-know regulations for communities as well as the public under the Superfund Reauthorization and Amendment Act of 1986[3]—together with the sobering effects of the Bhopal release, the Chernobyl nuclear disaster (with its very broad contamination and long-range potential for biological effects not yet fully appreciated), and the train derailment in Miamisburg, Ohio[4]—will convince even the most cynical and independent person that prevention is better than widespread chronic illness or fear of chemicals and nuclear materials, to say nothing of economic loss.

The writer fully appreciates that the quantities of chemicals, reagents, and related substances found in an average laboratory are small compared with large industrial operations or the bulk movement of chemicals by sea, barge, rail, or highway. However, even a small amount of some materials can cause much confusion and wasted nonproductive time, even if the potential hazard is relatively low.

In the first edition of this book, we noted how 2 grams of thallium acetylide caused major a disruption of a large research center.[5] On February 11, 1987, at a research facility connected to a hospital in Washington, D.C., near hysteria was generated when an employee, recently appointed to the local safety committee, discovered that the scientists around her were using picric acid in their research. It is certainly true that picric acid is an explosive when dry and crystalized, but the 250-gram bottle in this laboratory was properly hydrated, and did not warrant the evacuation of 90 persons (12 in hospital beds) outdoors into freezing weather for over two hours while the fire department and the bomb squad removed, and eventually destroyed, the bottle, using a detonator to initiate the explosion. Picric acid is a valuable reagent, but must be treated with respect, and should be kept moist with not less than half its own weight of water; it is commonly used in alcohol solutions. The incomplete analysis of a potential hazard and undue concern for a problem do not advance the cause of safety, but raise anxiety. On February 27, 1987, the safety task force, which had become critical of the laboratory's handling and disposal of chemicals, instituted another inspection. In this case, three bottles of picric acid were found; again the fire department and the bomb squad were called, 30 mentally ill patients under treatment were bussed to another location, and the staff was evacuated for one and a half hours. The three bottles were duly detonated in a safe location. With a little more experience and understanding, both incidents could have been handled without unnecessarily alarming the personnel, and respect for, not fear of, the substances could have been generated. [An excellent reference on picric acid is the National Safety Council (NSC) Data Sheet I-351-79 "Picric Acid," available from the National Safety Council, 444 N. Michigan Ave., Chicago, IL 60611.]

Letters to the editor of *Chemical and Engineering News* continue to contribute to our knowledge of hazardous chemical reactions. The most complete reference to date in this field is the third edition of the *Handbook of Reactive Chemical Hazards*, which describes nearly 30,000 reactions reported over the past 50 years.[6] Obviously, these constitute but a small percentage of the little publicized reactions or decompositions that have been encountered with the seven million compounds known. If a more open reporting of experiments that went astray, or did not produce the expected results, could reach such publications as the *Chemical and Engineering News,* the American Chemical Society Division of Chemical Health and Safety files, as a contribution to the NFPA 491-M Committee on Hazardous Chemical Reactions, the Center for Chemical Process Safety of AIChE, the files of the AIC, the National Science Teachers Association, and the NSC's Chemical and R&D Sections, the cause of chemical health and safety would be greatly advanced. Such reports can be made anonymously, as long as they can be independently verified for accuracy. A formal system of reporting hazardous reactions is needed to ensure that information actually reaches all the various data bases in a timely fashion. The *International Journal of Hazardous Materials* (published by Elsevier in Amsterdam, The Netherlands), and the quarterly *Hazardous Waste and Hazardous Materials* (published by Mary Ann Liebert, 1651 Third Ave., New York, NY 10128), as well as the chemical safety publications of both the Chemical Abstracts Service (United States) and the Royal Society of Chemistry (England) are valuable in disseminating health and safety information worldwide, including to the developing countries that are seeking to built a better world.

Experimental efforts in the laboratory or elsewhere can never be completely "safe," since by the very nature of the operation, unknown factors can be expected to arise. Many of the misunderstandings that have developed when a health and safety professional suggests even obvious deficiences to a dedicated researcher were attributable to a lack of appreciation on both sides—the reseacher not wanting to be bothered or to admit the risk involved, and the health and safety professional not wanting to overlook what, to him or her, is an obvious hazard.

If one or two subgram or gram-scale reactions have shown promise, and extensive investigations are planned that involve a system of chemicals, certain fundamental health and safety information should be assembled, if at all available. It is fully recognized that only limited data exist for many chemicals, and these data may be difficult to locate even with the many "computer data bases" now available. However, with the ultimate goal of large-scale manufacture and marketing, the potential liabilities this will impose upon the company, and the laboratory base being the foundation on which future activities must be built, the prudent investigator or laboratory management should consider the assembly of such parameters as the following.

1. If the material is a gas or liquid at STP, what is its flammability with air, oxygen, and other gases and over what range? For liquids, what are the flash- and fire-point data, and by what method were they obtained? What are the boiling point and the freezing point? Examples of flammable limits for common gases and liquids are shown in Figure 6.4.

2. If flammable, what is the auto- or self-ignition temperature? What are the products of combustion?

3. If not defined as flammable, does the material undergo decomposition or pyrolysis into flammable or toxic products on exposure to fire or heat?

4. What is the vapor density compared with air (useful in determining vapor movements from releases and in ventilation calculations)?

5. What are the hazards and/or effects of inhaling the gas or vapor (acute and chronic exposures)? Does the material have an odor threshold below or above what is considered a permissive concentration?

6. What bioelimination mechanism is known? Does this suggest monitoring of blood, urine, feces, or other body fluids or tissues, such as hair?

7. What respiratory protection is required, if any?

8. Is skin contact harmful (irritation, absorption)?

9. Should the experiment be conducted only under a hood with a known monitored air flow, or can it be set up on an open bench?

10. What first-aid treatment is known, both for on-the-scene use and for use by paramedics, the occupational health nurse, and the industrial physician who will respond to any serious emergency? (As an example, penicillin injections are *not* the proper treatment for hydrofluoric acid burns.) It must never be assumed that even a registered medical doctor has extensive knowledge and experience in the treatment of exposures to chemicals in general, and to specific research chemicals in particular. This matter should be discussed in detail with the physician and nurse *before* their services are needed in an emergency.

11. What analytical instrumentation is available for determining injurious concentrations of the gas or vapor in air, assuming it has been determined what is a harmful concentration (permissive or threshold limit) for short-term exposures?

12. What type of fire-extinguishing agent is effective on the material, and what methods are acceptable for cleanup for spills, and for disposal of the residue?

13. Will the waste from the cleanup be considered a hazardous waste? Is so, how will it be disposed of?

Only in recent times has sufficient interest been generated to justify the time and expense for compilation of such and related information. It will be recognized that the material safety data sheets (MSDSs), which ultimately must be prepared if the material is to be sold, as well as the requirements of the emergency services and community right-to-know provisions under the Superfund Amendments and Reauthorization Act of 1986 (PL 99-499), suggest the information will be invaluable, especially in an emergency situation or on off-shift, holidays, and weekends when technical personnel are usually not available for consultation. An active and sincere attempt should be made to develop as much of these data as possible and practical, *and to make the data accessible.*

A selection can now be made, based on even the limited data accumulated to date, as to some basic aspects of the laboratory operations and experiments.

If the liquid is relatively free of serious fire and health hazards, such as the higher alcohols, ethers, and ketones, the normal care that an experienced, prudent, and cautious chemist normally exercises should suffice. However, even chemists and other scientists will differ in their understanding of what these terms mean and of their implications.

If serious health or fire hazards are present, as with the lower alcohols, ethers, and aldehydes; nitro and amino compounds; and many aromatics, including benzene, toluene, xylenes, and common monomers, handling and reaction procedures should be carefully reviewed and developed to include protection of personnel from excessive exposures to either vapor, gas, or liquid, or to eliminate exposure completely by proper facilities and procedures. Note Figure 6.4, which illustrates the wide range of flammability for common chemicals. Closed systems should be utilized as much as possible, and personal protective equipment—including face shield, gloves, apron, and, if needed, respiratory protection equipment—should be available. To cite a specific example, the reaction of acetylene with OF_2 was to be investigated. The research chemist obtained from the safety office a heavy-duty reinforced "nitrometer" face mask as a precaution. After a few preliminary attempts, the reaction was achieved, in the form of a violent explosion. The researcher was cut on the arms and hands, but escaped face injuries completely due to his foresight in anticipating that the reaction might not be controllable. This was in 1948; the chemist, now happily retired, is without visible scars from his experiments and enjoys full vision.

As experience is gained with a reaction or process, procedures should be reviewed further to refine or change measures related to health and safety as necessity dictates. For example, adequate protection may have been provided against the gross concentrations associated with fires and explosions, but experience may show that sufficient vapor or gas is being released to the laboratory air to cause headaches, occasional dizziness, and upset stomachs. Obviously, additional attention must be given to reducing releases or improving the ventilation system, including the efficiency and proper use of hoods. *Reliance on a hood to remove or to disperse flammable vapors for disposal purposes may also be a serious error.* A college student was instructed by a graduate instructor to boil off excess toluene using an open beaker and a Bunsen burner in the fume hood. After the student attempted this, he was instructed to pour the contents of the beaker into a smaller beaker so it would boil faster. During the transfer of the hot solvent from one beaker to the other, with the flame nearby, an explosion occurred in which the student was burned. A distillation apparatus or a rotary evaporator is obviously the preferred method of solvent removal. Disposal of solvents "up the hood" by evaporation is also dangerous since the possibility of travel of the vapors to other locations, as well as the potential for fire of many materials, is too great to ignore. Other flammable solvents, including ethanol, methanol, ethyl acetate, and acetone, have been improperly handled in this regard. The Alpha Chi Sigma fraternity safety program was established in 1942 as a direct result of the death of a fully qualified and experienced brother alchemist working in the laboratory of a major industry, who was transferring ethanol during a distillation, in the presence of an open flame. Several of the original safety posters widely sold and circulated by the fraternity since 1948 stressed the danger of accidental fire, which even today remains a major occupational potential hazard in many laboratories that is frequently ignored or overlooked.

The vapors from a flammable solvent can travel surprisingly long distances and flash back from an ignition source. As noted above, the *evaporation of spent or waste solvent as a disposal method should not be attempted*. In addition to the pollution aspect, the potential for ignition by static electricity during the pouring where nonconductive materials, such as glassware and plastics, are involved, must be considered. Collection of spent or waste solvents is the desired alternative, in spite of the expense such disposal engenders. Recycling or reclamation by filtration or distillation under controlled conditions should also be encouraged, for both safety and economic reasons. A major research center recently noted that it had spent over $100,000 in one year for chemical-waste disposal, in addition to other charges for disposal of low-level radioactive wastes.

Once it has been determined that a material has properties that classify it as having unusual or questionable effects on life or the environment, or produces unusual reactions, it is essential that these properties be given full consideration by the experimenter and pilot-plant management before large-scale manufacture is attempted. To illustrate the importance of the need for serious attention in this context, a new insecticide was developed about 1950. The process itself was not without hazard, and was documented in a 1952 U.S. Patent that mentioned the use of liquid sulfur trioxide, sodium hydroxide solution, and sulfuric acid neutralization as reactants with hexachlorocyclopentadiene to produce the product. In 1961, a study was reported in a major journal on the acute and subacute toxicity of 22 insecticides proposed to be added to chicken feed as potentially effective against house fly larvae in poultry manure, including the insecticide in question. The LD_{50} for female chicks was determined as 480 mg/kg for the material; 440 mg/kg in the feed produced a mortality of 11/11. In discussing the results, the report noted that "affected chicks exhibited a typical syndrome characterized by a violent shaking of the entire body. The onset of the syndrome was rapid, the intensity varying with dosage level. At the highest levels, the chicks were unable to walk; they sat and trembled. At lower dosage levels, the animals walked in an ataxic gait, yet appeared to feed and drink at the normal rate. The intensity of the syndrome gradually diminished with time." In the general discussion, the report continued: "This is the only insecticide of the 22 tested that caused a distinctive syndrome in all chicks, regardless of the concentration level. The continuous ingestion of feed containing smaller concentrations resulted in delayed symptoms which increased in intensity with time. This demonstrates the cumulative effect. The gradual diminution of the syndrome after withdrawal indicates that although the effects of this material were reversible, the chick metabolized and eliminated it slowly."[7]

The product was manufactured for several years. By 1975, questions began to be raised when the city into whose effluent the plant waste drained found its sewage-treatment plant to be inoperative, and the city was eventually fined by the state. In 1976, a report by the bioassay group of the National Cancer Institute produced even more discussion. National attention was directed to the substance and its manufacture when the lower James River was closed to fishing for many months, and a Senate panel investigated. Although the ban on fishing was lifted in 1985, several former employees are claiming disability resulting from exposure to the material.

We cite this unfortunate case history to note that the 1961 report existed, and had it been fully appreciated and the material recognized as requiring unusual care in handling and disposal, this tragic sequence of events would have been prevented. The laboratory, experimental chemist, and supervision should have followed the herbicide's production and its consequences more closely, including the exposure of employees and the disposal of waste products from the operation.

The product and the eventual fate of the reaction of the experimental program, which began in a laboratory, may also be questioned in terms of:

1. Impact sensitivity.
2. Stability in storage and transport, especially under excessive moisture or heat, as in a fire or other emergency situation.
3. Bioaccumulation or biodegradability, useful in suggesting disposal methods that do not create long-term problems.
4. Melting and freezing point (including flash point).
5. Acute and chronic dosages as required by both OSHA and the Toxic Substances Control Act of EPA.
6. Fire hazard, including the ease of ignition and the nature of the combustion or pyrolysis products.
7. Whether there are data or reasons to suspect the material to be carcinogenic (either in animals or in humans), mutagenic, or teratogenic, or that it interferes with reproduction.
8. Whether in handling the substance, anyone has experienced any abnormal effects on skin, eyes, or general health.
9. Whether first-aid and clinical treatment for possible exposures have been developed and communicated, in case of misuse or spills that may affect personnel.
10. The fire-extinguishing agent of choice and other emergency control aspects that should be considered, such as the effect of water or moisture on the substance.
11. Whether the essential medical and emergency control information developed above has been communicated to the emergency services (fire and rescue) as well as to the local government units as required under PL 99-499.[8]

Usually a review of these and related items will be made during the transition of the process from the laboratory to the pilot plant, and much of this, and the data suggested on the reactants and the reaction, will be passed on with the process *before* pilot-plant or operating personnel attempt to conduct the process operations. From these data should evolve both an MSDS and a warning label that should clearly define, in simple language understood by the employees (using foreign-language translations, if necessary), the main hazards of the material; this should be displayed prominently on every container, regardless of size. The failure to transmit all the known information about a process or product can result in serious problems. For example, during the transfer, under Army contract, from one company to another of a pilot plant for the preparation of diborane (B_2H_6) as a possible rocket fuel, inadequate attention was given right-to-know by not warning the second company that a serious potential hazard was known to exist in the use of carbon tetrachloride (at that time a commonly used fire extinguisher,) and the diborane under fire conditions. A fire broke out shortly after the new personnel began operations, carbon tetrachloride was applied by the uninformed chemical engineers, and the resulting explosion was fatal to both. Although carbon tetrachloride (Pyrene) fire extinguishers are no longer approved, the possibility exists of a reaction between water and carbon dioxide or the several variations of dry chemical powders with the process materials, intermediates, and waste products, and should be investigated in the interest of protecting not only laboratory and plant personnel and local fire fighters but also emergency personnel from outside the laboratory or plant who may be called upon in an emergency. The classic example of the fire services not heeding the recommendations of reputable sources during an emergency was seen at Somerville, Mass. on April 3, 1980, when, while controlling a rupture in a phosphorous trichloride rail tank car, water clearly was not indicated but was used, forcing the evacuation of 23,000 persons because of the acidic fumes and fog. At Miamisburg, Ohio, on July 8, 1986, railroad personnel waited 30 minutes before informing the fire department that one of the ruptured tank cars contained white phosphorus, which self-ignited on contact with air. This contributed to a five-day emergency situation that involved 30,000 persons, who were evacuated for various periods, and a billion-dollar lawsuit against the railroad by residents of the area; Figure 13.1. These two incidents illustrate that even in modern times, with the communication equipment and data sources available, relatively common chemicals can and do create serious problems. The *Hazardous Materials Emergency Guidebook,"* DOT P5800.2, 1986 edition, U.S. Department of Transportation, Washington, D.C. 20590, is of limited assistance since it covers relatively few of the seven million chemicals extant. The new HIT system available from the Chemical Manufacturers Association, 2501 M St., N.W., Washington, DC 20037, which provides, on short notice, a printout via a modem linked to a computer over a telephone linkup should improve the communication gaps. Meanwhile, CHEMTREC emergency information is available on a 24-hour basis by calling 800-424-9300 or (202) 483-7616.

Over 2000 emergency response guidance reports are available on the HIT data base for transmission. In addition to this, CHEMTREC has over 170,000 MSDSs from which the communicators can provide verbal information on commercial products. A personal computer is not required to use this service; a simple modem/ printer arrangement provides an inexpensive link with the data. Details of HIT registration, which is a prerequisite for the service, are given in the booklet "HITS," available from the Chemical Manufacturers Association, at the above address.

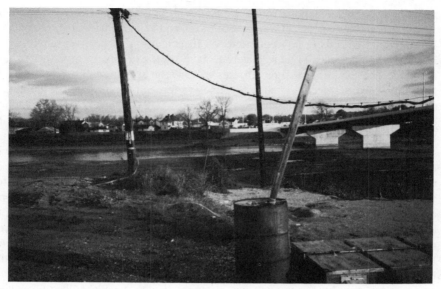

Figure 13.1. Now peaceful scene in Miamisburg, Ohio, where derailment and ignition of white phosphorous tank car resulted in major evacuation (see text). (Photo by M. M. Fawcett.)

It is difficult to predict exactly when exhaustive and expensive tests should be undertaken as the experiment is scaled up. In the toxicological area, data must be developed and submitted to establish that the new material does not pose an unreasonable risk. The current regulations of the EPA and OSHA in the United States and the Health and Safety Executive in England should be consulted to ensure that the rapidly changing legal requirements are in compliance, to say nothing of the responsibility to employees and the shareholders involving costly "tort" liability.[18]

When a new product is first isolated, the usual elementary and structure analyses, GC, AA, NMR, and other analytical techniques will at least suggest possible structures. Particular attention should be directed to those groups that create explosive tendencies, known as "plosophores." These include ONO_2 nitrate; $R - NO_3$, aliphatic nitro; $NH - NO$ primary nitramine; $Ar - NO_2$, aromatic nitro; and $N—NO$, secondary nitramine; in addition to organic salts of the following: chlorates, perchlorates, picrates, nitrates, and iodates.

Less powerful but quite sensitive compounds may contain: N_3, azide; NO, nitroso; $N = N$, diazo; $N = N - S - N = N$, diazosulfide; $O - O$, peroxide; $N - X$, halamines; $C \equiv C$, acetylides. In considering the explosive potential, in general the more plosophore groups represented in the molecule, the more powerful will be the explosive.

Explosives are not always recognized as such if they are formed in solutions intended for another purpose. A case in point is the widespread use of electrolyte solutions containing perchloric acid in electropolishing metallic samples for metallographic examination. Perchloric acid with organic liquids deserves special attention. Perchloric acid is a widely recognized and valuable laboratory chemical.[9] However, its hazards at concentrations of 70 percent or higher, especially when heated in contact with organic material, have been extensively investigated and reported. The explosion in Los Angeles in 1947, in which perchloric acid/acetic anhydride mixtures decomposed with explosive force in the presence of aluminum and a plastic used as a tank lining, clearly demonstrated the power of the perchlorate decomposition.[10] Previously, the hazards of mixing perchlorates and chlorates with reducing materials had been described.[11]

No reference had been made in the literature to relatively dilute perchloric acid in ethyl alcohol other than a statement that electrolytes of the DeSy and Haemer type, used in a commercial electropolisher, were *completely harmless*. The writer investigated the mixture of 62 ml perchloric acid, 70 percent, sp. gr. 1.67, 137 ml distilled water, 700 ml ethanol, with 100 ml butylcellosolve, prepared according to the instructions: "The perchloric acid should be added to the previously prepared mixture of ethanol and water. This mixture must be delivered in a separate one-liter flask and the butylcellosolve in another flask, and not be added to the rest of the mixture until immediately before use."

The flash point of the mixture was determined with the Fisher-Tag Cleveland open-cup tester (ASTM D-92) and found to be 81°F or 27.2°C. The fire point coincided with the flash point, producing a faint blue flame typical of ethanol fires. In view of this, the mixture should be treated as a flammable liquid. However, the corrosive nature of the mixture prevents the use of metal safety cans and makes glass or plastic bottles and beakers mandatory. Adequate protection to protect the glass or plastic from breakage, fracture, or other damage to release the mixture is obviously desirable. Wheaton "Second Skin" safety containers, which are glass bottles and jars treated with an impact-resistant high-tear thermoplastic, are designed for such service where glass must be used for purity reasons. (For details, contact Wheaton Safety Container Co., Mays Landing, NJ 08330.)

Depending on the temperature and rate of evaporation, 10-ml portions of the solution in an open evaporating dish were observed either to ignite spontaneously with a bright flash and to continue burning, or else actually to decompose with explosive force. Evaporations up to seven minutes on a moderate hot plate usually ignited spontaneously and continued to burn. If the evaporations were allowed to proceed on a low heat for more than eight minutes, explosions were observed. These explosions ranged from "mild" to "violent," but in no case were the evaporating dishes broken. The explanation for the above is that small amounts of ethyl perchlorate were formed, which is recognized as a violent explosive, coupled with the very rapid action of the strong oxidating effect of the acid at concentrations over 70 percent as the evaporation of the mixture proceeded.

Both as a method of disposal and as a means of studying the burning characteristics, several outdoor fires were instituted and observed, each involving 1 liter of used mixture (following the recommendations that mixtures should be discarded one week after the butylcellosolve was added). The liquid was poured in a metal waste can lid and ignited by throwing a burning paper towel into the liquid. The blue alcohol flame was almost invisible in the early stages of the burning, but as the burning progressed, the areas where organic matter from the paper had entered the liquid became small eruptions resembling pyrotechnics in color, noise, and smoke. The fire could be extinguished using a carbon dioxide extinguisher, but tended to reignite. Smothering with another lid was only partly effective since reignition occurred. Dry chemical from a dry-powder bicarbonate-based fire extinguisher provided the best extinguishing with no reignitions.

Paper towels of the type widely used in laboratories were used in the experiments, and were found to burn approximately twice as fast as uncontaminated towels, suggesting the importance of keeping the mixture from splashing on paper or clothing.

Animal tests using rabbits were conducted to evaluate the degree of hazard the mixture produced for the eye. One drop of the mixture was instilled into the rabbit eye without any washing out. Twelve hours later, ulcerative keratitis of the entire cornea, with necrosis of the conjunctiva, was observed. Four days later, scar tissue was present in the preplay area and the eye was not completely healed. Based on the above, the strict use of approved eye protection, such as side-shield safety glasses or a face shield, was recommended. No obvious effects were observed when the mixture was applied to denuded rabbit skin, other than reddening and irritation. No obvious effects from skin absorption were observed in the animals.[12] The overall conclusion drawn clearly suggests that the mixture is *not* "completely harmless."

Another molecule that over the years has caused serious injury to chemists and other process workers is peroxide. Organic peroxides, which vary widely in their sensitivity and fire potential, have been evaluated for hazards, but are occasionally mishandled with resulting tragedy.

Less obvious even today is the peroxide formation in various chemicals, including some ethers and alcohols. Although diisopropyl ether is perhaps the most hazardous from a standpoint of peroxide formation, several other compounds have been shown to form peroxide, especially when the can or bottle is opened and air contacts the substance for long periods. For that reason, it is important that all substances known or suspected of peroxide formation be recorded on arrival, carefully labeled and dated, and within a year (or less) disposed of safely regardless of how much or how little of the material remains in the container. Numerous references are available on peroxide formation, (which should be read and their message as to any potential hazard observed.[13]

Certain fundamentals as recommended by the NFPA, especially in NFPA 45, "Fire Protection in Laboratories," may be of interest. If a laboratory or unit has an explosion hazard (such as high-pressure equipment or experiments with rocket motors), protection should be provided for both the laboratory personnel and occupants of the surrounding areas. Protection designs should be based upon the hazard as defined in terms of (1) blast effects (including considerations of impulse, rate of pressure rise, peak pressure developed, duration of pressure, velocity of the pressure-wave propagation, and residual overpressures), and (2) missiles, classed according to mass, size, shape, and velocity.

Protection should consist of one of the following: (1) using special preventive or protective measures for the reactions, equipment, or materials themselves, such as explosion suppression, high-speed fire detection with deluge sparklers, or explosion-resistant enclosures; (2) providing blast- and missile-resisting shields or blast hoods between small-scale explosion hazards and laboratory personnel; (3) using remote control to minimize personnel exposure; (4) carrying out experiments in a detached or isolated building, or, even better, outdoors; (5) providing explosion-resistant walls or barricades for the hazardous laboratory; (6) limiting amounts of flammable or reactive chemicals exposed by experiments; (7) providing explosion venting in outside walls sufficient to maintain the integrity of the walls separating the hazardous laboratory unit from adjoining areas; and/or (8) disallowing the use of hazardous laboratories for other operations or storage of any type.

Laboratory personnel may be protected by explosion-resisting shields or by hoods with an equivalent resistance to a few grams of TNT. Specially designed explosion-vented hoods may afford protection for slightly larger explosion hazards. Explosion-resistant construction, isolated location, and other protective means should be considered for larger-scale explosion hazards.

When explosion-resistant construction is used, adequately designed explosion resistance should be achieved by one of the following methods:

1. Reinforced concrete walls of a thickness proportional to the energy level of the "worst case" explosion.
2. Rodded and filled concrete block walls.
3. Steel walls.
4. Steel plate walls with energy-absorbing lining.
5. Barricades, as used for work with explosives, constructed of reinforced concrete, sand-filled wood sandwich, wood-lined steel plate, earth, or rock berm.

Explosion-resistant construction should be based upon the anticipated explosion impulse defined in terms of the peak pressure impulse and duration, and the worst-case shrapnel mass, shape, and velocity. It is possible to achieve velocities of 10,000 ft/s with missiles of a mass equal to the TNT equivalence of a detonated explosive. Although these velocities may not be achieved during accidental explosions, velocities of 1000–4000 ft/s would be expected.

The NFPA recommends that a laboratory be classified as to explosion hazard on the basis of the substances present that have been rated in the NFPA 704-M system. Using this criterion, a laboratory shall be considered to contain an explosion hazard if the violent accidental release of energy in the following items could cause serious or fatal injuries to personnel within the laboratory in an explosion:

1. The storage of materials with a reactivity of 4 on the NFPA 704 scale.
2. The use or formation of materials with a reactivity of 3 or 4.
3. Highly exothermic reactions, for example, polymerizations, oxidations, nitrations, peroxidations, hydrogenations, or organo-metallic reactions.
4. The use or formation of materials whose structure indicates a potential hazard but whose properties have not been established.

5. High-pressure reactions, usually considered to be over 200 lb/in.

6. High-pressure experimental and test vessels.

7. High rotational velocity equipment, such as a centrifuge.

Three types of chemical reaction explosions are recognized: thermal explosions, deflagrations, and detonations.

Thermal explosions are exothermic self-heating accelerating reactions (often decompositions) that take place throughout the substance (no separate distinct reaction zone is obvious in the material). Substances that can cause a thermal explosion are organic peroxides, nitro compounds, and nitrates, as well as mixtures of oxidizing and reducing agents.

When the exothermic rate exceeds the cooling rate, the temperature of the material rises exponentially with time and a thermal explosion results with a sudden evolution of very hot vapors and decomposition gases (without combustion).

A test that measures the minimum unsafe storage temperature at which a self-accelerating temperature will occur in the material is the SADT (self-accelerating decomposition temperature) test.

The pressure-vessel test determines the rate of evolution of decomposition gases and vapors. The rate is given by the maximum venting-orifice diameter, which is just insufficient to prevent rupture of a 100-psi burst disk when the sample is heated.

The homogeneous explosion test measures the peak pressure and rate of rise of presssure when a sample is heated and expands into a large expansion (1000:1) vessel. These values are a measure of the energy and power of the thermal explosion and are scaled to MJ/kg and MW/kg respectively.

The peak pressure and rate of rise of pressure for thermal explosions are *directly proportional to the amount of material per unit volume of container*.

This is quite unlike gas or vapor explosions where the loading density is normally fixed by the combustion mixture at one atmosphere. Combustion of 5 percent propane–air mixture, for example, has a peak pressure of 96 psi with a rate of rise of 1700 psi/s. These values may be compared with the totally confined thermal explosion of tert-butyl peroxy isopropyl carbonate:

Loading	kg/cubic meter	7.5	0.75	75
Peak pressure	psi	125	12.5	1251
Rate of rise of pressure	psi/s	1631	163.1	16,313

Adequate venting, however, can reduce the values of both of these explosions.

Additional tests useful in characterizing thermal explosions are DTA-TGA studies and the determination of kinetic parameters of the reactions.

The Frank-Kamenetskii theory is useful for evaluating the critical mass in the thermal explosion of solids.

Deflagrations are characterized by a progressing reaction zone (flame front) with a velocity of 10^{-5}–100 ms/s (subsonic velocity). Energy is transferred ahead of the flame front by conduction, convection, and radiation.

The rate of burning R is significantly increased by an increase in pressure as

$$R = a + bp^r$$

This fact makes possible the very high burning rate of propellant in the cartridges of firearms without producing a detonation. The transition of a deflagration into a detonation is influenced by compression of combustion products under confinement by the advancing flame front and the accelerating influence of pressure on the combustion rate. Experimental measurements of deflagrations are of two types, the Crawford bomb test and the deflagration tube test.

Detonations are characterized by a constant supersonic rate of propagation of the reaction zone through the substance ($1\frac{1}{2} - 9$ km/s. A shock wave leads the reaction front, which produces gaseous reaction products of very high temperature and pressure (3000–5500°C, 1–4 psi $\times 10^6$) and sets up a shock wave in the surrounding media.

The rate of pressure rise of the shock wave in air is of the order of microseconds close to the charge, with a duration of a few milliseconds. The air-shock velocity is also supersonic. This is to be compared with deflagration and thermal explosion subsonic rates of propagation, with rates of pressure rise of 10 to hundreds of milliseconds.

Safety tests basic to the evaluation of a detonation are measurements of the supersonic shock velocity propagating in the reacting substance such, as the steel-tube test. Since a detonable substance has a critical diameter below which a detonation cannot propagate, there is a possibility that the tube diameter chosen is not large enough for a suitable test. Detonation sensitivity tests are the impact (drop-weight), friction, and shock (card-gap) tests.

Explosion venting may be utilized to lower the peak pressure of a thermal explosion or deflagration. This does not apply to detonations because of their more rapid rise of pressure rise and supersonic shock wave. Excellent reviews of testing for chemical stability are given by R. D. Coffee ("Chemical Stability," Chapter 17, pp. 305–321, in H. H. Fawcett and W. S. Wood (eds.), *Safety and Accident Prevention in Chemical Operations,* 2nd ed., Wiley/Interscience, New York, 1982) and J. J. Cudahy and W. L. Troxier, ["Autoignition Temperature as an Indicator of Thermal Ignition Stability," *J. Hazard. Mat.,* **8,** No. 1, 59–68 (June 1983).]

High-pressure experimental reactions should be conducted behind fix barriers able to withstand the calculated lateral forces. The barricades should be firmly supported at the top and bottom to take these loads. At least one wall should be explosion vented.[14]

Experimental reactions that are known to involve materials inherently unstable, such as reactions of acetylene with thallium, copper, bromine, chlorine, potassium, nitric acid, and mercury (II) salts, and certain oxidations, such as halogenations and nitrations should be barricaded. The attempted experiment with acetylene and OF_2 was noted previously.

Routine reactions where pressures and temperatures are expected between predetermined limits based on long experience or routine work need not be conducted behind barricades if the vessels comply with the following: (1) they are built of suitable construction materials with an adequate safety factor; and (2) they are provided with pressure relief in the form of a dependable tested safety relief valve or a rupture disk.

The explosive energy in a vessel containing fluid (gas or liquid) under pressure is the sum of the energy of pressurization in the fluid and the strain energy in the cylinder due to pressure-induced expansion.

In pressurized gas systems, the energy in the compressed gas represents a large proportion of the total energy released in the vent of a pressure vessel rupture. As noted previously, an aluminum cylinder being charged to 2000 pounds pressure with breathing air ruptured; parts of the cylinder were found six blocks away and the main cylinder traveled two blocks. This was an older cylinder. It is hoped that application of a steel ring on the neck of the cylinders (which are rated for 4500 psi) will prevent such failures. Many thousands of these and other cylinders are in use by fire departments and others on self-contained breathing apparatus for emergency control. Aluminum fiberglass-wound cylinders with the Department of Transportation (DOT) designation DOT 7235-4500 should be removed from 4500-psi breathing air service until checked with the manufacturer, Luxfer, Ltd., 1995 Third St., Riverside, CA 92507, unless they have been modified by a steel ring around the cylinder neck.

Liquid systems with pressures over 5000 psi, large volumes at lower pressures, or vessels made of materials exhibiting high elasticity should be evaluated. This should not imply that nonelastic vessels are preferred. Liquid systems in which air or any other gas is entrapped will store more energy and are more hazardous than the liquid alone.

The blast criteria applicable to detonations of small charges (0.1–100 gram weights) are shown in Table 13.1.

Not all explosions are from obvious causes. While acetylene is a known flammable gas that can be expected to explode under certain conditions (note its flammable range of 2.5–80 percent by volume in air), the role of acetone, which is always present in acetylene cylinders, is not always appreciated. Dr. Robert J. Everson, Animal Disease Diagnostic Laboratory, Purdue University, recently reported to *Chemical and Engineering News* an explosion of the atomic absorption spectrophotometer (AA) in his laboratory. A full unused acetylene tank had been connected to the instrument. During operation of the AA, a sudden surge of liquid acetone came from the acetylene tank all the way to the flame. The fuel was quickly shut off and the manufacturer's service representative contacted. He said that the acetone may have, and eventually would, cause damage to the diaphragms and tubing within the instrument and that these needed to be replaced.

The gas-control module was serviced at the manufacturer's facility and returned to the laboratory for installation in the AA. After testing with a soap solution to check for leaking connections, and during a brief 15-minute operating period when the burner alignment was being optimized, the instrument exploded. Subsequent investigation determined the cause to be a pinhole-size leak in one of the plastic fuel lines that allowed acetylene to accumulate slowly within the instrument to an explosive concentration (above 2.5 percent by volume in air). When and how the hole developed is not clear.

TABLE 13.1 Blast Criteria Applicable to Detonations of Small Charges

Blast Effect	Range Indicated Explosive Yield (ft)				Criteria*
	0.1 g	1.0 g	10 g	100 g	
1% eardrum rupture	1.1	2.4	5.2	11	$P_i = 3.4$ psi
50% eardrum rupture	0.47	1.0	2.2	4.7	$P_i = 16$ psi
No blow-down	0.31	1.3	6.9	~30	$I_i + I_q = 1.25$ psi · ms $V_{max} = 0.3$ ft/s
50% blow-down	<0.1	0.29	1.1	4.1	$I_i + I_q = 8.3$ psi · ms $V_{max} = 2.0$ ft/s
1% serious displacement injury	<0.1	<0.2	<0.5	~1.1	$I_i + I_q = 54$ psi · ms $V_{max} = 13$ ft/s
Threshold lung hemorrhage	<0.1	<0.2	<0.5	~1.8	$I_i + I_q = 26$ psi · ms
Severe lung hemorrhage	<0.1	<0.2	~0.5	1.1	$I_i + I_q = 52$ psi · ms
1% mortality	<0.1	<0.2	<0.5	~1	$I_i + I_q + 85$ psi · ms
50% mortality	<0.1	<0.2	<0.5	<1	$I_i + I_q = 130$ psi · ms
50% big (16–25 ft²) windows broken	0.26	1.1	5.7	~30	$I_r = 3$ psi · ms
50% small (1.3–6 ft²) windows broken	0.17	0.49	1.9	9.9	$I_r = 8$ psi · ms

*P_i—peak incident overpressure (psi); V_{max}—maximum translational velocity for an initially standing man (ft/s); I_i—impulse in the incident wave (psi · m); I_q—dynamic pressure impulse in the incident wave (psi · ms); $I_r =$ the impulse in the incident wave upon reflection against a surface perpendicular to its path of travel (psi · ms).

Dr. Everson notes that this is the seventh laboratory in Indiana and Illinois to experience acetone damage to an AA that had been repaired. A second AA in Illinois also exploded after being repaired. He suggests a more refined procedure for testing new acetylene tanks in the laboratory for acetone discharge (briefly venting to a hood or the AA exhaust with a hose connected to the pressure regulator) before connecting to the AA; a filter device to follow gaseous acetylene or acetone to pass but not liquid acetone; an indicating filter to indicate when acetone vapors are coming through the acetylene hose; and a sensor for acetylene gas within the AA instrument that will turn off the acetylene when it detects the presence of acetylene within the AA instrument.

In view of the intensity of the sound, Dr. Everson recommends that all laboratory personnel be given hearing tests upon employment so that any permanent damage from such explosions can be determined. At the writer's suggestion, Dr. Everson has circulated the essential details to several organizations, including the ACS (*Chemical and Engineering News* and Division of Chemical Health and Safety), the NFPA, the Chemical and R&D Sections of the NSC and to the Compressed Gas Association; Figure 13.2.

Explosions can also occur from many other combinations, not always widely known. Dr. K. L. Stuart, chair of the Department of Chemistry Safety Committee, Simon Fraser University, Burnaby, B. C., Canada recently reported an explosion

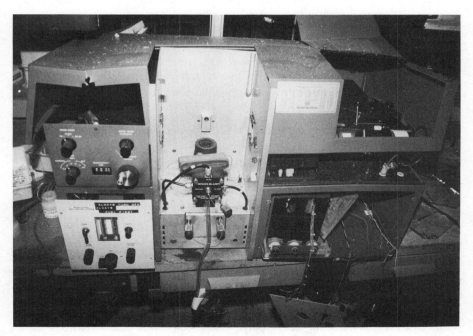

Figure 13.2. Exploded AA spectrophotometric instrument at Purdue University. See text for details. (Photo courtesy Dr. Everson, Purdue.)

that took place when trans-2-pentanoic acid was reacted with performic acid using the reaction conditions outlined in *Organic Reactions,* vol. VII. The explosion happened after about 30 mL of water and formic acid was removed by vacuum distillation at 45°C. It destroyed a hot plate, along with the glass equipment and some adjacent fluorescent lamps outside the reaction fume hood. The accident was believed to be due to the presence of unreacted excess performic acid, or formation of the peracid. Fortunately no one was injured.

Even attempted synthesis from elementary materials may result in explosions. Dr. Carolus M. Cobb, American Science and Engineering, Cambridge, Mass., has commented on a letter of G. Denes in *Chemical and Engineering News,* February 16, 1987, by noting a similar explosion during an attempted synthesis of TiI_2 in the 1950s. The synthesis used titanium metal and elementary iodine and followed a procedure described by J. D. Fast [*Rec. Trav. Chim.,* **58,** 174 (1939)]. A sealed glass system was used that was pumped down under high vaccum before seal-off. The synthesis proceeded according to plan for two days, when a violent explosion occurred. At the time, he believed an unstable iodide of titanium was involved. *No literature references to violent decompositions of titanium iodides could be found.* The probable cause, then, was considered to ba a crack in the apparatus, or possibly the synthesis of a small amount of nitrogen tri-iodide formed from contaminant nitrogen in the titanium. A graduate student narrowly missed losing her sight since she had removed her safety glasses moments before the explosion, which sprayed the reaction mixture over her face and eyes. Again, the importance of precautionary information in the literature is noted.

Even moderately dilute concentrations of some materials can cause serious problems. Dr. Paul A. Haas, senior research engineer with Oak Ridge National Laboratory, has reported to *Chemical and Engineering News* that aqueous nitric acid and organic solutions of moderate concentrations at room temperature can show sudden bursts of reactions. The principal lessons to be learned from his experience are:

1. Dozens of repetitions without an incident do not mean that the reactions will never occur.

2. Long periods of waste accumulation are an invitation for trouble.

Waste materials from a series of process development tests were acidified with nitric acid to dissolve hydrous metal oxides. Urea and hexamethylenetetramine were also in solution. The hexamethylenetetramine will hydrolyze at low pH values to form NH_4NO_3 and formaldehyde.

The estimated concentrations of the stored wastes were about 2M HNO_3, 2M HCHO, 1M NH_4NO_3, and 0.5M metal nitrate. Because of a change in waste-disposal procedures, a polyethylene bottle of waste was held for two months with the bottle cap barely closed. One night when the laboratory was unoccupied, there was a very high rate of reaction, with a discharge of contents through the loose cap followed by a rupture of the heavy polyethylene bottle wall and a vigorous jet or spray of the solution through the rupture. The polyethylene bottle was contained in a hood, and no significant damage resulted. Similar acidifications of wastes by nitric acid had been used for about six years. *One similar incident had occurred on a small scale, but had not been recorded or reported.*

This incident does not reveal any new chemical information as the potential chemical reactivity of the solutes would be commonly recognized. Instead, it illustrates a common problem: *long acquaintance with a potential hazard results in a relaxation of precautions, or "familiarity breeds contempt."*

CHEMICALS IN THE CLASSROOM OR SCHOOL LABORATORY

In view of the wider awareness in what a hazardous chemical is and who should be exposed to it, the National Science Teachers' Association recently announced a film on school safety.[15] In Delaware, the DuPont Company has cooperated with schools to improve safety and encourage the removal of hazardous or potentially dangerous reagents.

The publication in 1986 of the fourth edition of an authoritative book by the Royal Society of Chemistry (London) should also be of significant assistance in laboratory safety.[16]

The ACS, through the Council Committee on Chemical Safety and the Division of Chemical Health and Safety, has continued its strong leadership in this area.[17] The ACS Safety Referral Service continues to serve callers on (202) 872-4511, as does Dr. Maurine Matkovich, ACS Safety Coordinator, on (202) 872-4515 or (202) 872-6000.

Examples of current practices at a large university are shown in Figures 13.3 to 13.7.

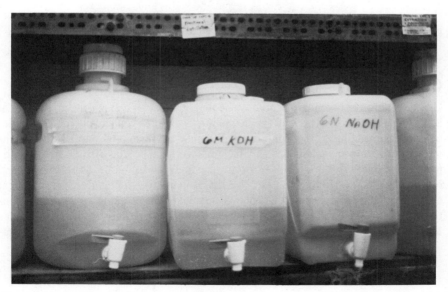

Figure 13.3. Identification of chemicals in plastic containers present problems that permit no error.

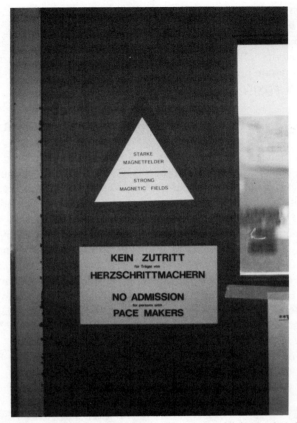

Figure 13.4. Interference with pacemakers by certain frequencies plainly noted on laboratory door.

Experiments in School and College Labs

Classic courses in chemistry at some schools use a teaching experiments that are at least questionable from a safety viewpoint, and often give students an inadequate understanding of the importance of safety and health as part of their training—information they will need in the real world. The classification of experiments was published originally in *Education in Science*, 16–18 (Apr. 1980), and reprinted in *Chem 13* (Oct. 1980) by the University of Waterloo, is a critical evaluation of experiments and contains an interesting grading of hazard potentials by which chemists can evaluate the safety of their experiments (Tables 13.2 and 13.3). As noted, the categories of restrictions, while directed to the academic situation, can easily be adapted to other environments.

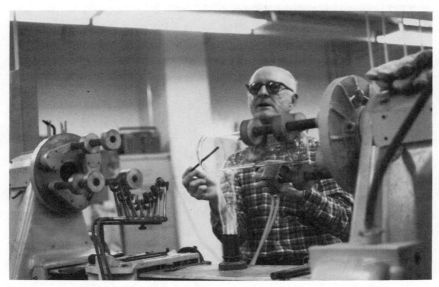

Figure 13.5. Shielding of eyes from radiation such as glass-blowing and lasers is an important part of hazard control.

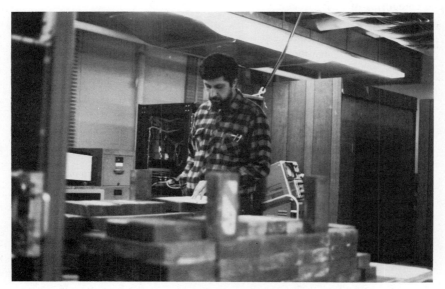

Figure 13.6. Shielding of gamma radiation from experimental facilities is essential to protection of personnel.

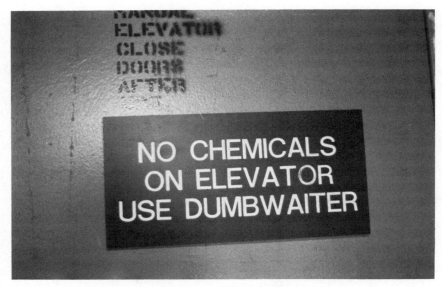

Figure 13.7. Chemicals must be excluded from passenger elevators.

The categories of restrictions are:

N Unsuitable. The experiment is considered unsafe for use in schools.

T For teacher demonstration only. Teachers should be thoroughly familiar with the technique to be used. It is assumed that these experiments will have been rehearsed before being done in front of a class for the first time.

S Considered suitable for supervised senior pupils. Some of these could perhaps be entrusted to responsible pupils in the final year of a 0-level, 0-grade, CSE, or similar course.

O Considered safe as a class experiment in the last two or three years of 0-level, 0-grade, or CSE and similar courses. It is essential here for the teacher to exercise his or her discretion as to the responsibility of a particular class. Any experiment listed here may present dangers to irresponsible pupils. The use of a fume cupboard is recommended. Teachers may have to use their discretion and allow experiments classified in this way to be carried out in a very well-ventilated room with small quantities of materials.

Hazards of Laboratory Chemicals

Although intended primarily for guidance of academe, the study by the *Education in Science*, 19–26 (April 1980) and reprinted in *Chem 13* (November 1980) gives a gradation of hazards, in terms of schools. As listed, the categories of restriction are:

X Chemicals to be excluded from schools.

N Chemicals not recommended to be normally held or stored.

E Chemicals restricted to small quantity for observation or exhibition only.

R Chemicals restricted to small quantities—in storage.

T Teachers use only.

S Senior pupils, that is, post '0' Grade and post '0' level use.

O '0' grade, '0' level, or CSE and above (meaning the last two/three years of these and similar courses).

t Years 1 and 2 of secondary school (11/12 years upward) with close teacher supervision.

F To be used in fume cupboard (hood).

(F) To be used in fume cupboard (hood) if in open vessels on a scale other than small.

L Short safe shelf-life.

TABLE 13.2 Hazardous Experiments in Laboratories

Experiment	Restriction
Ammonia, oxidation using oxygen in an enclosed apparatus	N Use air (T). Oxygen may be used in an open vessel (T).
Ammonium dichromate(VI), heat ("Volcano experiment")	T, F A fume cupboard is needed to avoid possible inhalation of chromate(VI) dust
Ammonium dichromate(VI), heat with aluminum or magnesium powder	N
Ammonium nitrate, heat	T Heating a mixture of ammonium chloride and sodium nitrate is considered safer. Use safety screens
Ammonium nitrite, prepare and heat	T In solution only, concentration less than molar
Aryl and acyl halides, reactions	S, F
Cadmium iodide, electrolysis of molten	N Lead bromide preferable
Carbon monoxide, reductions with	T, F Use safety screens
Carbonyl chloride, preparation	N
Chlorine, reaction with ammonia	N
Chlorine, reaction of a mixture with hydrogen	N This refers to the gas syringe and similar experiments. It is possible to demonstrate the reaction in, for instance, a plastic bag. Burning hydrogen at a jet in chlorine is safe for teacher demonstration.
Chlorine, reaction with ethyne	N The reaction where the gases are generated simultaneously by adding dilute hydrochloric acid to a mixture of bleaching powder and calcium dicarbide is acceptable as a teacher demonstration (T, F Use safety screens).
Chlorine, preparation	S, F See Potassium manganate(VII), reaction with concentrated hydrochloric acid.
Chlorine, reaction with metals	S, F

(continued)

TABLE 13.2 *(Continued)*

Experiment	Restriction	
Chlorine oxides, preparation	N	
Crude oil, distillation	O, F	
Cyanogen, preparation	N	
Ethene or ethyne, explosion of a mixture with oxygen	N	
Ethene or ethyne, igniting in a gas jar or test-tube	T	
Explosives (*e.g.*, mixtures of chlorates, manganates(VII) or nitrates with combustible substances)	N	
Hydrogen, large scale generation and collection	T	
Hydrogen, generation and testing for, on a test-tube scale	O	
Hydrogen, burning in air	T	
Hydrogen, burning in chlorine	T	Use safety screens.
Hydrogen, explosion with air	T	
Hydrogen, explosion with oxygen	T	
Hydrogen, reductions using	T	Use safety screens for the normal scale experiment. Reduction of metal oxides may be performed on a test-tube scale using, for example, a mixture of zinc powder and calcium hydroxide in the same tube as the oxide to generate the gas. Such experiments may be classified 0.
Hydrogen cyanide, preparation	N	
Hdrogen sulphide, preparation	T, F	
Hydrogen sulphide, use of gas	S, F	
Hydrogen sulphide, use of aqueous solution	O	
Iodine, heating in air	T or S, F	
Lead bromide, electrolysis	T or O, F	in which case the fume cupboard is essential.
Lead(II) carbonate, heating	O	
Lead(II) nitrate, heating	O, F	
Lead oxides, heating	O	
Lithium, heating	T	Use safety screens
Mercury, heating	T, F	The fume cupboard is essential and must be left on for the duration of the experiment (*i.e.* while the mercury is above room temperature).
Mercury(II) oxide, heating	T, F	The fume cupboard is essential.

TABLE 13.2 *(Continued)*

Experiment		Restriction
Natural gas, enrichment for reductions	T	If ethanal tetramer (metaldehyde or "meta fuel") is used as the enriching agent, in a test-tube scale experiment, it may be classified 0.
		The large-scale experiment has proved dangerous, probably because of the extra dead volume introduced into the apparatus.
Nitrations, organic	S, F	In some cases when only a mild nitrating agent, such as dilute nitric acid, is necessary, a fume cupboard is not needed (*e.g.,* nitration of phenols)
N-nitrosamines, preparation from amines	N	See previous article on carcinogens (*Education in Science,* September 1979)
Oxygen mixture, use of	T	See 'Potassium chlorate(V) and manganese(IV) oxide, heating mixture'
Phosphine, preparation	T, F	
Phosphorus halides, reaction with water	S, F	
Phosphorus, red, burning	O, F	
Phosphorus, white, burning	T, F	
Plastics: heating polyurethanes and polystyrene	O, F	
Plastics: heating PVC	T, F	The fume cupboard is essential
Plastics: polymerization and depolymerization of acrylics	S, F	
Plastics: polymerization of phenylethene	S, F	
Plastics: preparation of nylon "rope"	O	Note that if a solution of dioyl chloride in tetrachloromethane is used this must be classified T, F. 1,1,1-trichloroethane may be used as solvent if the solution is freshly prepared.
Potassium, reaction with water	T	Use safety screens
Potassium chlorate(V) and manganese(IV) oxide, heating mixture	T	Many safer alternatives for oxygen preparation. Use demonstration as illustration of catalysis only. Use safety screens.
Potassium manganate(VII), heating	O	Eye protection essential. Heat in small test-tubes fitted with a loose ceramic wool plug to prevent splitting
Potassium manganate(VII), reaction with concentrated hydrochloric acid	S, F	Cover the manganate(VII) with water first. This experiment is highly dangerous if sulphuric acid is used by mistake instead of hydrochloric. It is safer to use bleaching powder or sodium chlorate(I) and dilute hydrochloric or sulphuric acid.

(continued)

TABLE 13.2 *(Continued)*

Experiment	Restriction
Rocket fuels, preparation	N
Silicon(IV) oxide, reduction with magnesium or aluminum	S The reactants must be dry. Use safety screens
Sodium, reaction with water	S Use safety screens
Sodium hydroxide (molten), electrolysis	T, F
Sodium peroxide, preparation of oxygen from	T Use safety screens
Sulphur and zinc, reaction	T Do not confine the mixture in any way, *i.e.* heat the mixture on a ceramic centered gauze or mineral fibre paper. Use safety screens.
Sulphuric acid, concentrated, reactions	O With close supervision, otherwise S. Use a fume cupboard if corrosive or toxic gases are likely to be evolved
Thermite reaction	T Use safety screens (or perform outdoors). Fe_2O_3, Mn_3O_4, Cr_2O_3 are safe oxides to use. Do not use CuO, MnO_2 or CrO_3.
Zinc, burning	O, F

TABLE 13.3 Hazardous Chemicals in Laboratories

Name	Restriction
Acetonitrile (methyl cyanide)	R, S, F
Aerosol sprays	R, Ot, F
Alcohols other than ethanol	R, O, (F)
Aldehydes other than methanal	R, O, (F)
Alkyl halides	R, Ot, (F)
All unlabeled bottles which contain substances of unknown composition	X
Aluminum powder	Rt
Aluminum bromide, anhydrous	R, S, L
Aluminum carbide	R, T, L
Aluminum chloride, anhydrous	R, S, L
4-aminobiphenyl	X
Ammonia '880'	Ot, (F)
Ammonical silver nitrate (Tollens reagent)	X Prepare as required and immediately dispose of excess

TABLE 13.2 *(Continued)*

Experiment	Restriction
Ammonium chlorate(VII) (perchlorate)	X
Ammonium dichromate(VI)	S
Ammonium nitrate	R, St
Ammonium peroxodisulphate(VI) (persulphate)	St avoid raising dust
Ammonium sulphide	Ot, (F)
Anhydrone	N, L alternative are calcium sulphate, calcium chloride (both anydrous) and molecular sieves
Anthracene	E
Antimony	E
Antimony compounds	S
Aromatic amines (except aminobiphenyls or naphthalenamines)	R, St, F
Arsenic	E
Arsenic compounds	N if Marsh's Test needs to be shown use impure zinc
Asbestos, soft forms (paper, fibre, mats, platinised, centred gauzes)	X ceramic wool forms of paper, wool and platinized wool available. Calcium silicate matrix heat resistant mats and ceramic centred or stainless steel gauzes available.
gloves	use heat resistant leather
Azo dyes	R, Ot See article on Carcinogens in *Education in Science,* September 1979, p. 17
Barium metal	T
Barium compounds, solid	S
Barium compounds, dilute solution	t
Barium chromate(VI)	N should not be isolated from any preparation
Barium peroxide	R, T, L
Barium sulphate	O
Benedict's solution	O
Benzamide	S
Benzene, use as a solvent	X use methylbenzene as alternative solvent. Use cyclohexane for change of state experiment.
Benzene, use as reagent	R, St, F (small scale preparative work) (in hood)
Benzenecarbaldehyde (benzaldehyde)	R, S, (F)
Benzenecarbonyl chloride (benzoyl chloride)	R, S, F
Benzene-1,3-diamine (m-phenylenediamine)	R, S, F

(continued)

TABLE 13.3 *(Continued)*

Name	Restriction
Benzene-1,4-diamine (p-phenylenediamine)	R, S, F
Benzene-1,2-diol (catechol)	S
Benzene-1,3-diol (resorcinol)	Ot, F
Benzene-1,4-diol (quinol or hydroquinone)	S
Benzenesulphonic acid	St
Benzene,1,2,3-triol (pyrogallol)	S
Benzonitrile	R, S, F
Beryllium	E
Beryllium compounds	X
Biphenyl-4,4'-diamine (benzidine)	X
Bis (4-isocyanatophenyl) methane (Caradate 30)	R, St, F
Bismuth	S
Bismuth compounds	O
Bleaching powder	R, O, L
Bromates	R, S
Bromine, element	R, St, F
dilute solutions	O
Bromobenzene (phenyl bromide)	S
1-bromobutane (n-butyl bromide)	R, S, (F)
2-bromobutane (sec-butyl bromide)	S, (F)
Bromoethane (ethyl bromide)	R, S, (F)
2-bromo-2-methylpropane (t-butyl bromide)	R, S, (F)
Bromomethane (methyl bromide)	R, T, F
Bromopropane (propyl bromides)	R, S, (F)
3-bromoprop-1-ene (allyl bromide)	R, S, F
Butanal	R, O, (F)
Butane cylinder	N not recommended in lab.
Butanoic acid	R, S
Butan-1-ol (n-butanol)	O, (F)
Butan-2-ol (sec-butanol)	O, (F)
Butanone (methyl ethyl ketone)	O, (F)
Cadmium	R, St
Cadmium compounds	R, St
Calcium, metal turnings	R, Ot
Calcium dicarbide	R, St, L
Calcium hydride	R, St, L
Calcium oxide	R, Ot, L
Calcium phosphide	N

TABLE 13.3 *(Continued)*

Name	Restriction
Calcium sulphide	R, S, F
Calcium dioxide, solid	Ot
Carbon monoxide	X small scale preparation St, F
Carbon disulphide	N use dimethyl-benzene as solvent for preparing rhombic sulphur and ethyl cinnamate for prism experiment.
Camphor	S
Chlorate(I) (hypochlorites)	R, Ot, L purchase sodium salt as solution; ensure cap is vented
Chlorates(III) (chlorites)	N
Chlorates(V) (chlorates)	R, St
Chlorates(VII) (perchlorates)	N small quantities may be isolated as in fractional crystallisation of disproportionation products of potassium chlorate(V)-not to be stored
Chloric(VII) acid (perchloric acid)	X
Chlorine cylinder	N
Chlorobenzene	S
Chlorobutanes (butyl chlorides)	R, S, (F)
Chloroethane (ethyl chloride)	R, S, (F)
Chloroethane (vinyl chloride monomer)	X
(Chloromethyl) benzene (Benzyl chloride)	R, S, F
Chloropropanes (propyl chlorides)	R, S, (F)
Chlorosulphonic acid	R, St, F
Chromates(VI) and dichromates(VI)	
solutions	O
solids	S
Chromium(VI) oxide (chromium trioxide)	R, S
Chromium(III) compounds (chromic compounds)	O
Cleaning mixture (dichromate(VI)/conc. sulphuric acid)	T Do not store. Decon 90 good alternative
Crude Oil	Ot, F
Cyanates	R, T
Cyanides	N
Cyclohexane	O, (F)
Cyclohexanol	S, (F)
Cyclohexanone	S, (F)
Cyclohexene	O, (F)

(continued)

TABLE 13.3 *(Continued)*

Name	Restriction
DDT	N
Decanedioyl dichloride (sebacoyl chloride)	Ot, F
Devarda's alloy	O
N,N'-dialkylphenylamines (N,N'-dialkylanilines)	R, S, F
Di(benzenecarbonyl)peroxide (benzoyl peroxide)	N di(dodecanoyl)peroxide is alternative polymerisation catalyst
1,2-dibromoethane (ethylene dibromide)	N may be formed as in test for unsaturation, but should not be isolated
1,2-dibromopropane (propylene dibromide)	R, S, F
Dichlorobenzenes	R, S, F 1,2-isomer most toxic of the three isomers
Dichlorobiphenyl-4,4'-diamines (chlorobenzidines)	X
Dichlorodimethylsilane	R, T, F
1,2-dichloroethane (ethylene dichloride)	R, T, F
Dichloroethanoic acid	R, S
2,4-dichlorophenols	R, S
Di(dodecanoyl)peroxide (lauroyl peroxide)	R, Ot
Diethylamine	R, Ot, F
Diethylamine, dilute solution	O
Diethyl sulphate	X
Diiodine hexachloride (iodine trichloride)	R, St, F
3,3'dimethoxybiphenyl-4,4'-diamines	X
Dimethylamine	R, Ot, F
Dimethylamine, dilute solutions	O
3,3'-dimethylbiphenyl-4,4'-diamine (o-tolidine)	X
Dimethyl formamide	R, S, F
Dimethyl sulphate	X
Dinitrobenzenes	R, St
3,5-dinitrobenzoic acid	R, S
4,4'-dinitrobiphenyl	X
2,4'-dinitrobromobenzene	R, T
2,4-dinitrochlorobenzene	N
2,4-dinitrofluorobenzene	N
Dinitrophenols	R, St
2,4-dinitrophenylhydrazine	R, S
Dioxan	R, St, L
Dipentene	R, O

TABLE 13.3 *(Continued)*

Name	Restriction
Diphenylamine solution for redox indicator	R, St otherwise N
Esters (general)	R, O, (F)
Ethanal (acetaldehyde)	R, O, (F)
Ethanal tetramer (metaldehyde)	Ot
Ethanal trimer (paraldehyde)	R, S, F
Ethane cylinder	N
Ethane-1,2-diamine (ethylene diamine)	R, S, F
Ethanedioic acid and salts (oxalic acid and salts)	
solid	R, S
dilute solution	R, Ot
Ethanoic acid, glacial (acetic acid, glacial)	Ot, (F)
Ethanoic anhydride (acetic anhydride)	R, S, (F)
Ethanol	O, (F)
Ethanoyl chloride (acetyl chloride)	S, F
Ethene cylinder (ethylene)	N
Ethers (general)	R, S, F
Ethoxyethane (diethyl ether)	R, S, F, L
Ethoxyethanol (cellosolve)	S, F
Ethylamine	R, Ot, F
Ethylamine, dilute solution	O
Ethylbenzene	O, (F)
Ethyl benzoate	O, (F)
Ethyl carbamate	N
Ethyl ethanoate (ethyl acetate)	O, (F)
Ethyl methanoate (ethyl formate)	O, (F)
Ethyne cylinder (acetylene)	X
Fehlings solution No. 2	Ot Use water bath. Alternative is Benedict's or Barfoed's solution
Fluorine	N
Fluorene	N
Fluorenone	N
Fluorides, solid	R, T
Fluorides, solutions	Ot
Germanium tetrachloride	R, S, F
Heptane	R, O, (F)
Hexacyanoferrates(II) (ferrocyanides)	S
Hexacyanoferrates(III) (ferricyanides)	S
Solutions of hexacyanoferrates	Ot no heating, no addition of strong acids

(continued)

TABLE 13.3 *(Continued)*

Name	Restriction
Hexamethylcosane (squalene)	O
Hexamine	R, S, F
Hexane	R, O, (F)
Hexane-1, 6-diamine (hexamethylene-diamine)	Ot
Hexanedioic acid (adipic acid)	O
Hexanedioyl dichloride (adipoyl chloride)	Ot, F
Hexenes	O, (F)
Hydrazine	X
Hydrazine chloride	R, St
Hydrazine hydrate	R, T
Hydrazine sulphate	R, St
Hydrides, metal	R, St
Hydriodic acid	R, S
Hydrobromic acid	R, S
Hydrocarbons, aliphatic	O small scale, (F)
Hydrocarbons, aryl	S, (F)
Hydrochloric acid, conc	Ot
Hydrofluoric acid	X
Hydrogenation catalysts	R, St
Hydrogen cyanide	X
Hydrogen cylinder	T
Hydrogen peroxide 20 volume	t, L
Hydrogen peroxide 100 volume	R, T, L
Hydrogen sulphide gas	S, F aqueous solutions may be used outside fume cupboard
2-hydroxybenzoic acid (salicylic acid)	O
Indicator powders	T
Indium compounds	S
Iodates(V)	S
Iodic(V) acid	R, T
Iodine, solid	O, lower levels t, if heated t, (F)
Iodine(V) oxide (iodine pentoxide)	N
Iodoethane (ethyl iodide)	R, T, F
Iron(III) chloride, solid	O
Iron(II) sulphide	O
Isocyanates	R, T, F
Lead alkyls	N
Lead(II) bromide	Ot, if fused for electrolysis F

TABLE 13.3 *(Continued)*

Name	Restriction
Lead(II) chloride	Ot
Lead(II) chromate(VI)	N
Lead(II) ethanoate (lead acetate)	Ot
Lead(II) methanoate (lead formate)	Ot
Lead oxides	all levels t
Lithium	R, Ot if heated T
Lithium compounds	R, S lithium borohydride or sodium borohydride are more stable and are suitable for some applications
Lithium aluminium hydride	R, St, F, L
Lithium hydride	R, T, F, L
Lithium hydroxide	R, S
Magnesium powder	Ot
Magnesium ribbon	t
Mercury	R, St in well ventilated room on spillage tray
Mercury alkyls	X
Mercury salts, solid	St
Mercury salts, solution	Ot
Methanal (formaldehyde, formalin)	R, Ot in F unless very dilute. Do not use in presence of hydrogen chloride
Methanoic acid (formic acid)	Ot, (F)
Methanol	Ot, (F)
2-methoxyphenylamine (o-anisidine)	R, S, F
4-methoxyphenylamine (p-anisidine)	R, S, F
Methylamine	S, F
Methylamine, dilute solution	O
Methylbenzene (toluene)	Ot, (F)
3-methylbutanol (iso-amyl alcohol)	O
3-methylbutyl ethanoate (isoamyl acetate)	S, (F)
Methyl ethanoate (methyl acetate)	O, (F)
Methyl ethyl ketone peroxide	Ot
Methyl methanoate (methyl formate)	O, (F)
Methyl 2-methylpropenoate (methyl methacrylate)	R, S, F, L
Methylphenols (cresols)	R, S
N-methylphenylamine (N-methylaniline)	R, St, F
Millon's reagent	R, S alternatives are Albustix, Cole's Modification of Millon's reagent or Sakaguchi Test

(continued)

TABLE 13.3 *(Continued)*

Name	Restriction
Molybdenum	R, S
Naphtha	R,T, F liquid paraffin is preferred for storing alkali metals
Naphthalen-1-amine (1-naphthylamine)	X
Naphthalen-2-amine (2-naphthylamine)	X
Naphthalene	O For cooling curves use hexadecan-1-ol, octadecan-1-ol, hexadecanoic or octadecanoic acid
N-naphthylethane-1, 2-diamine as solution (N.E.D. or N-naphthylethylenediamine)	R, St
Naphthylthiourea (ANTU)	R, T
Nessler's reagent	R, S
Nickel, dust	R, St
Nickel salts, solid	S avoid raising dust
Nickel salts, solution	O
Ninhydrin, solid	R, T
Ninhydrin, aerosol spray	R, Ot, F
Nitric acid, conc	Ot
Nitric acid, fuming	R, St, F
Nitrobenzene	R, S, F
4-nitrobiphenyl	X
Nitrocellulose	X
Nitrogen dioxide	O, F
Nitrogen triiodide	X
Nitromethylbenzenes (nitrotoluenes)	N
Nitronaphthalenes	X
Nitrophenols	R, St
4[(4-nitrophenyl)azo] benzene-1,3-diol solution (Magneson 1)	O
4[(4-nitrophenyl)azo] napthalen-1-ol solution (Magneson II)	O
Nitrosamines	X
Nitrosophenols, 2- and 3-isomers	X
4-nitrosophenol	R, St
Octane	R, O, (F)
Oct-1-ene	R, S, (F)
Oleum	N
Orthophosphoric acid	S
Orthophosphoric acid, dilute	O
Osmic acid	N alternative stains for microscope work are the Sudan dyes

TABLE 13.3 *(Continued)*

Name	Restriction
Oxygen mixture (potassium chlorate(V)/ manganese(IV) oxide)	N alternative preparation is decomposition of 20 vol hydrogen peroxide catalyzed by manganese(IV) oxide
Paraffin oil	O
Paraquat	R, T
Pentane	O, (F)
Pentan-1-ol and 2-ol (n- and sec-amyl alcohol)	O, (F)
Pentan-3-one (diethyl ketone)	O, (F)
Pentyl ethanoate (amyl acetate)	R, O, (F)
Peroxides, inorganic (excluding H_2O_2)	S
Peroxodisulphates(VI) (persulphates)	St
Petroleum ether, BP below 80°C	S, (F)
Petroleum ether, BP above 80°C	Ot, (F)
Phenols	St
Phenols, dilute solutions (e.g., indicators)	O
Phenylamine (aniline)	R, St, F
Phenylammonium salts	R, S (F)
Phenylethene (styrene)	R, S, F
Phenylhydrazine and salts	R, S
Phenylthiourea (P.T.U.) also phenylthio-carbamide (P.T.C)	Ot see *Education in Science,* September 1979, page 17.
Phosphides, metal	N
Phosphorus, red	R, Ot, F
Phosphorus, white	R, T, F, L
Phosphorus(V) oxide	R, St, F, L
Phosphorus pentabromide	R, St, F, L
Phosphorus pentachloride	R, St, F, L
Phosphorus tribromide	R, St, F, L
Phosphorus trichloride	R, St, F, L
Phosphorus trichloride oxide	R, St, F, L
Photographic developer	t
Potassium	R, T, L
Potassium amide (potassamide)	N, L
Potassium hydrogen-sulphate (potassium bisulphate)	O
Potassium hydroxide, solution <2 molar	Ot
Potassium hydroxide, solid, melt or concentrated solution	St

(continued)

TABLE 13.3 *(Continued)*

Name	Restriction
Potassium manganate(VII) (potassium permanganate)	t
Potassium nitrate	t
Potassium nitrite	R, S
Potassium sulphide	R, Ot
Propanal (propionaldehyde)	O, (F)
Propanoic acid (propionic acid)	O, (F)
propan-1-ol and -2-ol (n-propyl and isopropyl alcohols)	O, (F)
Propanone (acetone)	O, below O if t, (F)
Propylamine	S, F
Propylamine, dilute solution	O
Propyl ethanoate (propyl acetate)	O, (F)
Pyridine	R, St, F
Quinine	R,T cold tea is alternative for taste buds experiment
Selenium and compounds	R, S, F
Silicon tetrachloride	R, St, F, L
Silver nitrate	R, S
Silver nitrate solution	Ot
Sodamide (sodium amide)	N, L
Sodium	R, St
Sodium amalgam	R, S
Sodium azide	R, S
Sodium chlorate(I) solution (hypochlorite)	Ot Ensure container is vented
Sodium hydroxide, solution <2 molar	Ot
Sodium hydroxide, solid, melt or concentrated solution	St
Sodium hydrogen sulphate (bisulphate)	O
Sodium nitrate	t
Sodium nitrite	R, S
Sodium pentacyanonitrosylferrate(II) (sodium nitroprusside)	S
Sodium peroxide	R, St, L
Sodium sulphide	R, Ot
Strontium	R, T
Sulphides, heavy metal	Ot
Sulphur chlorides	R, St, F
Sulphur dioxide canister	St, F
Sulphuric acid, conc.	Ot

TABLE 13.3 *(Continued)*

Name	Restriction
Sulphuric acid, dilute	t
Tellurium metal and compounds	E
Tellurium compounds	X
Tetrachloromethane (carbon tetrachloride)	R, St, F 1,1,1-trichloroethane is less harmful substitute for solvent applications
Thallium and compounds	X
Thermite mixture	T Do not store
Thiocyanates, solid	S Do not heat to decomposition or add strong acids
Thiourea (also thiocarbamide)	R, S *See Education in Science,* September 1976, p. 17
Tin(II) chloride (stannous chloride)	O
Tin(IV) chloride (stannic chloride)	R, S, F, L
Titanium(IV) chloride (titanium tetrachloride)	R, T, F
1,1,1-trichloroethane as solvent	t, (F)
Trichloroethanoic acid (trichloroacetic acid)	S
Trichloroethane (trichloroethylene)	N 1,1,1-trichloroethane is a less harmful substitute for solvent applications
2,2,2-trichloroethanediol (chloral hydrate)	R, S, F
Trichloromethane (chloroform)	R, St, F 1,1,1-trichloroethane is a less harmful substitute for solvent applications
3,4,5-trinitrobenzoic acid (gallic acid)	R, S
2,4,6-trinitrophenol (picric acid)	R, S
Turpentine	R, t, F
Uranium compounds, solid	R, T
Uranium compounds; solution	S
Vanadium(V) oxide (vanadium pentoxide)	T
Vanadates(V)	S
Xylene cyanol solid	R, S
Zinc powder	R, t
Zince chloride	S
Zinc chromate(VI)	X

Note: t indicates close supervision by teacher.

EXTREMELY HAZARDOUS SUBSTANCES

When planning laboratory or plant chemistry, the Emergency Planning and Community Right-to-Know Programs, 40 CFR Part 300, under the EPA, should be noted. Section 302 of the Superfund Amendments and Reauthorization Act of 1986

(SARA), signed into law on October 17, 1986, required the Administrator of EPA to publish a list of extremely hazardous substances. In the *Federal Register* (**52,** No. 77, April 22, 1987), this list constitutes 402 chemicals, and it would be well to consult the full text of this regulation before undertaking laboratory or plant operation (see Appendix A)

Title III of SARA (PL 99-499) mandates the type of program advocated by the EPA's CEPP. It requires state and local governments to establish the infrastructure needed to facilitate emergency planning and provides technical support to these programs. It also requires certain facilities to supply the information on chemicals present at the facility that is necessary for contingency planning.

The "extremely hazardous substances" list and its threshold planning quantities are intended to help the local community focus on the chemicals and facilities of the most immediate concern from a community emergency planning and response perspective. EPA strongly emphasizes, however, that while the list published April 22, 1987 includes 402 of the chemicals that may pose an immediate hazard to a community upon release, it is not to be considered a list of all chemicals that are hazardous enough to require community emergency response planning. There are tens of thousands of compounds and mixtures in commerce in the United States and elsewhere, and in specific circumstances, many of these could be considered toxic or otherwise dangerous.

A revised and corrected version of the original November 17, 1986 list was published in the *Federal Register,* **52,** No. 77, Wednesday, April 22, 1987, pages 13397–13410, and is included in this book as Appendix A. Until robots have come into wide use, this list should be considered required reading (Figure 13.8). Meanwhile, animals must be used (Figure 13.9).

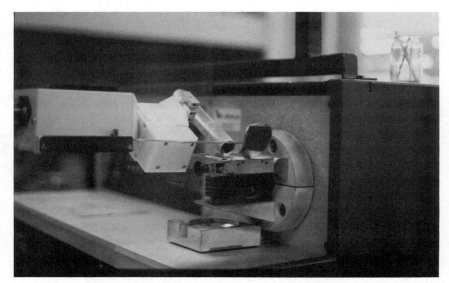

Figure 13.8. Robot in analytical laboratory of Laborlux S.A. Esch-sur-Alzette, Grand Duchy of Luxembourg. Robot was performing complete cycle of sampling, putting sample in flask, heat treating it in furnace, withdrawing, and labeling at 15 times/hour. (Photo by H. Fawcett.)

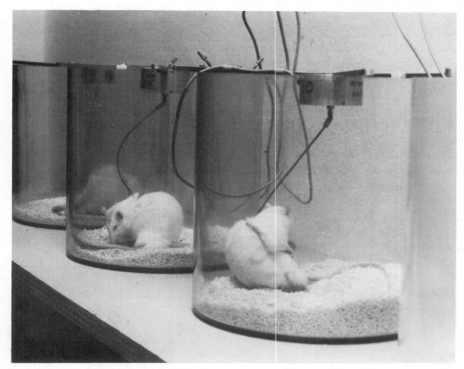

Figure 13.9. Animals contine to supply basic data needed to evaluate chemicals. These mice are being monitored for motion frequency. (Courtesy of National Institute for Mental Health Research.)

Subtitle A of PL 99-499 established under section 302 that each facility where any extremely hazardous substance is present at any time in a quantity equal to or above the threshold planning quantity established for that substance must notify the state emergency response commission, and this notification must be provided within seven months after the enactment of SARA (now May 17, 1987) or within 60 days from the time that the facility first becomes subject to the notification requirements in section 302, whichever is later. Section 303(d) requires these facilities to designate a representative who will participate in the local emergency planning effort as a facility emergency response coordinator. This designation must have been made by September 17, 1987, or 30 days after establishment of the local emergency response committee, whichever is earlier. The facilities are required to provide the committee with information relevant to the development or implementation of the local emergency response plan.

Section 304 requires notification by a facility at which a hazardous chemical is produced, used, or stored to the local planning committee and the state emergency response commission upon release of a reportable quantity (RQ), in pounds, of a any extremely hazardous substance identified under CERCLA section 101.[15] This notification is required even if a threshold planning quantity of a substance is not present at the facility. These extremely hazardous substances for which an RQ has not been established under CERCLA are given an RQ of 1 pound. These will be adjusted in later regulation by EPA. Section 304 requires both an immediate release notification to the local committee and state commission and a follow-up report providing additional information on the release, and any actions taken in response. (See Appendix C for states.)

The above is not just legal or academic; under section 325, failure to comply may result in the imposition of civil or criminal penalties. States, local governments, and citizens may also bring suit to enforce many section of the act. Any person who fails to comply with the requirements of section 300-94 shall be subject to civil penalties of up to $25,000 for each violation in accordance with section 325(b)(1) of the Act; continuing violations will be subject to civil penalties of up to $25,000 for each day during which the violation continues, and in the case of a second or subsequent violation, any such person may be subject to civil penalties of up to $75,000 for each day. Any person who knowingly and willfully fails to provide notice in accordance with section 300.94 shall, upon conviction, be fined not more than $25,000 or imprisoned for not more than two years, or both (or, in the case of a second or subsequent conviction, shall be fined not more than $50,000 or imprisoned for not more than five years, or both, according to 325(b)(4). If actually enforced, this Act will be an interesting example of "pro bono publico" in action.

REFERENCES

1. R. R. Jones, "Readers Reveal the Dangerous Lives of R&D Scientists," *Ind. Res. Devel.* 127–130 (July 1980).

2. "Occupational Safety and Health Hazard Communication: Final Rule," *Federal Register,* **48,** No. 228, 53280–53348 (Nov. 25, 1983) (29 CFR Part 1910.1200). [Specifically directed toward SIC 20-39 (manufacturing) but obviously with significant effect even on laboratories]; see also H. H. Fawcett, "The OSHA Hazard Communication Standard or 'Right to Know,' " *J. Chem. Ed.,* **63,** No. 3, A70–A73 (March 1986), and H. H. Fawcett, "Secrecy of Alchemists Threatened," *Hexagon of Alpha Chi Sigma,* Spring 1986 issue, 8 (1986).

3. Superfund Amendments and Reauthorization Act of 1986, P.L. 99-499, signed into law Oct. 17, 1986, Title III—Emergency Planning and Community Right-to-Know; see also E. L. Quarantelli, "Chemical Disaster Prepardness at the Local Community Level," *J. Hazard. Mater.,* **8,** No. 3, 239–250 (Jan. 1984); Symposium on Right-to-Know, L. Meck, presiding, seven papers presented at the 193 ACS National Meeting, Denver, Col., April 5–10, 1987, abstracts of which are in the meeting abstract book.

4. Derailment of a train on the Chessie System in Miamisburg, Ohio, resulted in release of fumes from burning white phosphorous, during a five-day period, affecting, at various times, 30,000 persons. For detailed video presentation of this event, see *American Heat,* Vol. 1, Program II, Aug. 1986, 8001 Clayton Road, St. Louis, MO 63117. The National Transportation Safety Board report on this accident is being prepared.

5. H. H. Fawcett, *Hazardous and Toxic Materials,* 1st ed., pp. 1–3, Wiley/Interscience, New York, 1984.

6. L. Bretherick, *Handbook of Reactive Chemical Reactions,* 3rd ed., Butterworths, London, 1985; see also Manual 491-M, National Fire Protection Association, Quincy, Mass.

7. U.S. Patents 2,616,825 and 2,616,928, Nov. 1952. One mole hexachlorocyclopentadiene in 1.5

moles of liquid SO_3 forms a dark red viscous intermediate, which, on hydrolysis in an excess of 6 percent NaOH followed by neutralization with H_2SO_4, gives the product. See also M. Sherman and E. Ross, "Acute and Subacute Toxicity of Insecticides to Chicks," *Toxicol. Appl. Pharm.*, **3**, 521–533 (1961), "Report on Bioassay of Technical Grade Chlordecone," National Cancer Institute, Bethesda, Md., 1976; "Senate Panel Probes Kepone Disaster," *Chem. & Eng. News*, **54**, No. 5, 17–18 (Feb. 2, 1976); S. B. Cannon, "Epidemic Kepone Poisoning in Chemical Workers," *Am. J. Epidemiol.*, **14**, No. 7, 534 et seq. (1978); R. J. Huggett and M. E. Bender, "Kepone in the James River," *Environ. Sci. Technol.*, **14**, No. 8, 918–921 (1980).

8. *Federal Register,* Nov. 17, 1986, Part III, Environmental Protection Agency, 40 CFR Part 300, Emergency Planning and Community Right-to-Know Program; Interim Final Rule and Proposed Rule Cross-Reference, pages 41570–41594 (see also reference 17).

9. A. A. Schilt, *Perchloric Acid and Perchlorates,* 189 pp., G. Frederick Smith Chemical Co., Columbus, Ohio 1979.

10. O'Connor Electro-Plating Corp., Los Angeles, Calif., Feb. 20, 1947. Seventeen fatalities and serious building damage resulted. See also F. A. Herr, "Los Angeles Plating Plant Explosion," *Metal Finish.*, **45**, No. 3, 72–73, 107, (1947).

11. I. Kabik, "Hazards from Chlorates and Perchlorates in Mixtures with Reducing Materials," Report I.C. 7340, U.S. Bureau of Mines, Washington, D.C., 1945.

12. H. H. Fawcett, "Perchloric Acid–Ethyl Alcohol Electropolishing Mixtures," Report RL-1185, Class 1, unclassified, General Electric Research Laboratory (now R&D Center), Schenectady, N.Y., 1954.

13. D. Swern, *Organic Peroxides* (3 vol.), Wiley-Interscience, New York, 1970–1980; also Noyes Data Corp., Organic Peroxide Technology, Park Ridge, N.J., 1983.

14. NFPA-68-1987, "Guide for Explosion Testing," National Fire Protection Association, Quincy, Mass. 02269, 1987.

15. "School Lab Safety," 16-mm color sound film, 20 minutes, prepared under the supervision of Franklin D. Kizer and Deloy Stromme, Handel Film Corp., 8730 Sunset Boulevard, West Hollywood, CA 90069, 1987 (grade level: J, H)

16. L. Bretherick, *Hazards in the Chemical Laboratory,* 4th ed., 604 pp., Royal Society of Chemistry, London, 1986. (In addition to a major section for fast reference to several hundreds of compounds and reactions, the volume contains chapters on England's health and safety act of 1974, safety planning and management, fire protection, reactive chemical hazards, chemical hazards and toxicology, health care and first aid, hazardous chemicals, precautions against radiations, and an American view.)

17. *Safety in the Academic Chemical Laboratory,* 4th ed., American Chemical Society, Washington, D.C. 20036 (prepared by the ACS Council Committee on Chemical Safety). The Division of Chemical Health and Safety of ACS presents frequent sessions on laboratory safety and health problems, such as the Symposium on Fume Hoods and Laboratory Safety, S. H. Pine, presiding, at the 193rd ACS National Meeting, Denver, Colo., April 5–10, 1987.

SUGGESTED READINGS

EPA, *"Lab Compliance with RCRA"*, ½-inch video tape prepared for EPA by Booz-Allen, Job 2359, 22:45 min., March 18, 1987

EPA, "Hexamethylphosphoramide and Urethane: Significant New Uses of Chemical Substances," 40 CFR Part 721, *Federal Register* **51**,(53), 9450–9453 (March 19, 1986).

K. E. Fischer, Contracts to Dispose of Laboratory Waste, *Jour. of Chem. Ed.*, **62**, A118–A122 (April 1985).

K. E. Fischer, Managing Hazardous Laboratory Wastes, *Haz. Mats. & Waste Manag.*, 44–47 (Sept.–Oct. 1986).

C. P. Fundacentro, Data sheets published by CEP 05499, Sao Paulo, Brazil.

L. Grover, A written eye safety policy reduces risks and prevents injuries, *Occu. Health Safety,* **55**(5), 31–48 (May 1986).

D. Hanson, "Academic Labs Face Compliance with Emergency Planning Rules," *Chem. Eng. News,* **65**, No. 20, 19–20 (May 18, 1987).

Health Safety Bulletin., "Accident Reporting: The Good and Bad News," (ACTU-VTHC) **47**, 11–16 (Apr. 1986), (Australia).

M. H. Ho and H. K. Dillon, *Biological Monitoring of Exposure to Chemicals—Organic Compounds,* 352 pp., Wiley/Interscience, New York, 1987.

W. C. Hollinsed and S. T. Ketchen, Waste Reduction Through Minimization of Reagent Usage, *Hazardous Waste and Hazardous Materials,* **4**(4), 357–361 (Fall 1987).

C. P. Priesing, "Environmental Impairment Liability Insurance: Is It an Endangered Species?" *Toxic Subst. J.,* **6**(2–3), 127–140 (Autumn–Winter 1985).

S. Pure, "What's in a Name? More Than You Might Think," *Lab. News,* (351), 10 (May 23, 1986).

F. Schmidt-Bleek, "Government Attitudes Towards Risk Assessment of Chemicals," *Toxic Subst. J.,* **6**(2–3), 115–118 (Autumn–Winter 1985).

M. Scott, *Prof. Saf.,* **31**(4), 25–27 (April 1986).

B. Z. Shakhashiri, *Chemical Demonstrations: A Handbook for Teachers of Chemistry,* vol. 2, University of Wisconsin Press, Madison, Wis., 1985; *Educ. Chem.,* **23**(6), 187 (Nov. 1986).

J. Tripodes, *"Low-Level Nuclear Waste Disposal,"* *Environ. Sci. Technol.,* **20**(11), 1071 (Nov. 1986).

E. L. Walls, "The Dos and Don'ts of Fume Hood Safety," *Scientist,* 18 (Aug. 10, 1987).

R. J. Wood, "A Proper Computer Program Can Enhance Health, Safety Practices, *Occu. Health Safety,* **55**(5), 20–24 (May 1986).

W. Worthy, "Shock Sensitivity of Explosives Clarified, *Chem. Eng. News,* 25 (Aug. 10, 1987).

Appendix: Real-World Accidents

Dr. James Kaufman, of the Chemistry Department of Curry College, Milton, Mass., conducted a national survey during 1984–1985 of college and university chemistry departments as part of his activities in connection with the Laboratory Safety Workshop, which is a national center for training and information. With his permission, the following incidents can be recorded with the hope that they will inspire increased chemical health and safety.

CHEMICAL INCIDENTS

1. A fire in a volatile storage area resulted from a defective container of white phosphorus that apparently lost the water because of a leak, cracked container, or evaporation. The phosphorus ignited, causing damage to containers and chemicals on metal shelves above it. The sprinkler system cooled and restricted the damage, which was less than $1000.

2. A student was evaporating ethyl alcohol, which ignited. He pulled the beaker toward himself and burned his hand.

3. An explosion occurred when propionic acid, pyrrolidine, and benzaldehyde were heated to form porphrins.

4. A student was heating a flask of nitric acid when she reached around the stand to adjust the gas, tipping the acid over her arm. She received second- and third-degree burns. No litigation resulted.

5. A student attempted to put a test tube containing concentrated nitric acid into a centrifuge located at eye level. The centrifuge was running, and shattered the tube, causing burns to face, hands, and other body parts. Safety glasses prevented permanent damage.

6. A student worker opened a new 5-gallon can of pentane. He was not wearing eye protection. When the pentane warned to room temperature, it exploded. Eye injury resulted, and his eyes were bandaged for a few days.

7. A 4-liter glass bottle of cyclohexanone fell from a lab cart and shattered. The area was evacuated because of the high-level odor. No injuries resulted.

8. A student, in a hurry to complete a recrystallization, increased the heat on a hot plate. He than put an ethanol solution on the hot plate. The ethanol boiled over and burned. No injuries resulted.

9. A student inhaled trace amounts of bromine vapor.

10. A chemistry instructor was moving a plastic bottle of concentrated nitric acid to the sink for disposal when it collapsed in her hands, splashing nitric acid over her hands, legs, arms, and face. She was wearing goggles. No shower was available so she could not promptly dilute or wash off the acid. Severe burns resulted.

11. A major spill of 2 ml mercury resulted from a broken thermometer. The spill covered the tile floor and bench top. The spill area was treated with a hand-water aspirator for large quantities of mercury and was wiped with a mercury pillow sponge. Pillow and aspirator are still in storage with past mercury-spill material in stockroom. The entire stock of dirty mercury is around 10 ml.

12. A student sniffed a small amount of chlorine. It was not a significant amount, but when he inquired what chlorine does, he was told, "It kills you." The student went to the hospital and was checked there. No litigation resulted.

13. An organic "unknown" was spilled on the hand of a student. Irritation developed but was gone in two days.

14. A student set aside safety glasses and proceeded to drop a beaker of dilute hydrochloric acid. Some hit her eye. She flushed it for 15 minutes; there was no apparent damage.

15. A faculty member was exposed to nitrogen dioxide gas through a leaky seal on a furnace. He spent a day in the hospital but suffered no complications.

16. Two glassblowers spent several days in the hospital after inhaling nitrogen dioxide generated while dissolving copper packing from a glass column with nitric acid. No permanent damage resulted.

17. An acid-soaking bucket cracked and a student spilled 3 liters of 1:1 nitric acid in a hood. One slight burn occurred. A case of sodium bicarbonate was required to neutralize the acid.

18. A student spilled acid on his leg. He ran to the nurse, and the burn became significant in the transit time. There would have been no injury if the student had asked the instructor for assistance.

19. A graduate student added what was thought to be hexane to a hexane still. An exothermic reaction immediately occurred. The top of the still was blown off and hit the ceiling. The student jumped back and was uninjured.

20. A student spilled concentrated sulfuric acid down the front of his trousers. His trousers were ruined but he escaped any skin burns.

21. A student poured concentrated sulfuric acid directly onto his face. He did not have any permanent damage, but did wear a patch and take medication for two weeks.

22. A student plunged a test tube containing ethanol in boiling water. (The procedure called for placing the tube in tap water and then to "heat gently and then record the B.P.") The hot ethanol vapor caused second-degree burns to the student's face and affected one eye. No permanent damage occurred. The student was not wearing safety glasses.

23. Three students were burned (one receiving second-degree burns on hands and arms) by chlorosulfonylic acid. The students did not check to see if water was still in the reaction vessel. The fluid blew up out of the containers, splattering acid around the lab.

24. A student was carrying out a polymer synthesis in a glass apparatus that was heated in a salt bath containing 3 pounds of sodium nitrite and 1 pound of sodium thiocyanate. The bath was heated above 270°C using a hot plate. The bath exploded with a force estimated to be equal to that which would result from a pound of dynamite, causing over $200,000 damage to the laboratory. The student escaped probable death only because he was bending over a vacuum pump at the time of the explosion. He did receive serious cuts and burns, but has since recovered.

25. A visiting scientist prepared an adduct of neodymium perchlorate and acetonitrile, and was removing the last portion from a glass flask when the material exploded. The scientist lost two fingers and was blinded by the explosion. The scientist had removed his safety glasses just before the accident because the lenses had fogged.

26. A technician added sulfuric acid to water in a large, graduated cylinder. Insufficient initial mixing caused heat buildup and bumping of the mixture. Minor burns resulted on the upper part of his body. There was no permanent damage.

27. A dehydration experiment in organic chemistry caused noxious gases to form in a flask. This suggests that the person added the wrong reagent. He suffered breathing problems, but returned to school the following day.

28. A student removed a 100-ml round-bottom flask from a heating mantle. The flask was dropped, hit the hood table top, and bounced. The boiling liquid hit the student in the face and neck area and down the front of her blouse. Her face, neck, and breast were burned. After continuous rinsing and washing with soda solution and water, the deep redness began to dissipate. No harm resulted to the student and no litigation followed.

29. Students were generating hydrogen with mossy zinc and 6M sulfuric acid. They added concentrated sulfuric acid in excess. An explosion occurred. Since the glassware was wrapped with toweling, no shattering occurred.

30. Two burns resulted when students did not follow instructions. They boiled concentrated nitric acid in crucibles and were spattered on their hands, requiring treatment by a doctor.

31. An undergraduate student splashed some 6M hydrochloric acid into her eye. The professor had her use the eye-wash fountain for several minutes after the accident. No permanent damage resulted.

32. In 1984, a pint bottle half-full of chromic acid cleaning solution exploded within two to three minutes after the solution had been poured back into the bottle with the cap tightened. No injuries resulted.

33. Three students were "cleaning up" a research lab and were collecting organic chemical waste in a large glass bottle. One of them placed a diluted solution of nitric acid into the same bottle. It was then capped. Shortly after, it exploded, showering glass throughout the lab and on the students. Injuries included tendon cuts on fingers, head abrasions, a severe abdominal laceration, and minor cuts.

34. In a procedure walnut shells were ground in a small amount of pet ether in a regular blender, when the rubber gasket either failed or loosened becaused it had not been tightened properly. A spectacular, but easily contained, fire resulted. No injuries occurred."

35. Chemicals splashed in the face causing burns; an abrupt pressure change spilled chemicals on the hand of a student.

36. In 1980, a student was doing an experiment on the chemical properties of the elements. In noting the properties of chlorine gas, she made two mistakes. She combined 10 times the proper amount of potassium permanganate with concentrated hydrochloric acid, and then she inhaled the fumes (rather than wafting them to her nose). She was hospitalized for three days with a severe lung problem. No permanent damage resulted.

37. A student was using ether in the course work. Earlier in the day he had been using a hot plate, but had turned it off. Not realizing that it might still be hot, the student placed the container with the ether on the hot plate. The ether boiled over and ignited. Minor burns resulted.

38. A student was titrating unsaturated lipids with 5 percent bromine in a cyclohexane solution when the stopcock component separated from the buret barrel. The bromine solution ran out on her hand and arm. The separation was attributed to an aged "O" ring, which did not hold the components securely. A professor was nearby and immediately placed her hand under water, and then treated it with glycerol. No permanent damage resulted.

39. An organic diazide compound was prepared without incident up to the final stop, following all safety rules and advisories. Goggles, shields, etc., were not in place when the final dried product was being transferred from the funnel to a permanent container. An explosion then occurred, shattering glassware nearby and propelling the funnel into the wall. The researcher was injured by flying glass.

40. On a Sunday afternoon, faculty members discovered that the stockroom was full of smoke. Its source was a can of white phosphorous sticks, previously unopened. The unused can, purchased some time prior to 1976, had corroded, which apparently punctured the can, causing the phosphorus to contact air and burn. No injuries occurred. Damage was confined to the shelf.

OTHER LABORATORY INCIDENTS

41. An impacted toenail was the result of a crushing blow from a laboratory table top that was being moved.

42. An organic chemistry student attempted to insert a thermometer into a rubber stopper without lubrication. The thermometer broke and cut the students finger. No litigation resulted.

43. A student attempted to push glass tubing through a rubber stopper, sustaining a major cut when the tubing shattered and cut his palm. Surgery was required. No litigation resulted.

44. A student was placing a thistle tube through a rubber stopper and failed to lubricate the tube. He applied pressure on the end of the tube, and it broke, cutting his finger. Stitches were required. No litigation resulted.

45. A postdoctoral student was filling two lecture bottles of ammonia from lecture bottles of liquid nitrogen. He filled the cylinders completely; when they warmed to room temperature, they exploded.

46. A student, operating a Bunsen burner, pulled the burner loose from the rubber tubing. Gas escaping from the tubing ignited and melted the end of the tubing. The student suffered minor blistering. There was no litigation.

47. A laboratory assistant released a built-in overhead screen and it escaped from the support hook. The screen swung down and struck her on the cheek at the gum line. Damage to her salivary glands required corrective surgery.

48. A fire was intentionally set to trash in a large plastic trash can in the chemical storage area. It was discovered in time to avoid what could have been a disaster. Increased security was instituted.

49. Graduate students were aligning optics at low power and did not believe they needed to wear protective goggles. The reflected laser light caused corneal abrasion and some retinal damage. No permanent damage to the eyes resulted.

50. A bottle of toxic material cracked during a weekend, possibly because of heat-control problems in the stockroom. A stockroom supervisor inhaled the material before noticing the spillage. He was admitted to the hospital for observation, but did not develop any symptoms.

51. Despite a departmental ban on pipetting by mouth, a faculty member ordered students to do so. One student, following orders, suffered a chipped front tooth.

52. Students mishandled glassware, which broke in their hands and injured their fingers. Microsurgery was needed to correct the thumb tendons that were severed.

53. A professor fell off his chair while seeking the source of an odor believed to be due to burning.

54. A Tyrell-type burner flame blew out enough gas that collected and mixed with proper amount of air to cause an explosion, ignited from the red-hot wire gauze and/or ring. A beaker shattered, resulting in minor cuts to the students conducting the experiment. One student required minor surgery to remove glass particles from neck and arms.

55. A fire occurred in a trash can after someone had placed sodium paper waste in the trash and the safety officers on campus, in inspecting the eyewash and showers in the laboratory, used the trash can as a reservoir, thus igniting the papers. No injuries resulted.

56. An explosion took place as the result of a chemical being placed in a supposedly explosionproof oven, which apparently malfunctioned. When the oven kicked on to heat, a sparking occurred and caused the explosion, which ruined the oven.

57. In glassware operation by a lab worker, momentary exposure to the high-heat flame resulted in a third-degree burn to the back of his right hand when the burner was dropped from his left hand.

58. A student, with no formal training, was using a muffle furnace. The controls were set so high that the interior of the furnace melted.

59. A student broke a piece of tubing and rammed it into his palm, breaking off a section in his hand. No litigation resulted.

60. A student removed his goggles to inspect a precipitate, and spilled alkaline sample in his eyes. His eyes were rinsed thoroughly and vision was normal. There would have been a serious problem (student was wearing contact lenses against regulations), but another student was skilled in removing contact lenses.

61. A lab assistant evaporated waste solvent on a hot plate in the hood. Some was spilled on his hand and also caught fire. He received a first-degree chemical burn. No further damage resulted.

14

The Shad Return to the Delaware

Phillip J. Wingate

From the Atlantic Ocean to Philadelphia via the Delaware River and Delaware Bay is only 100 miles. This body of water has perhaps better natural cleansing facilities than any other major estuary in the United States.

The Chesapeake Bay is more than twice as long from Baltimore to the Atlantic and the tides that twice daily dump billions of gallons of clean ocean water into the Chesapeake could not as easily purge the Chesapeake of pollutants pouring into it, as similar tides flowing into and out of the Delaware might be expected to do for this shorter body of water. Nevertheless, during the past three-quarters of a century, the Delaware Bay and Delaware River became substantially more contaminated than the Chesapeake, and both shellfish and finfish, as well as other types of marine life, suffered more in the Delaware than in the Chesapeake.

Why? The full answer to this question is very complex but can be summarized in a single word: people. Three times as many people live along the shores of the Delaware from Trenton, N.J., to the ocean as live along the Chesapeake from Baltimore to the ocean, and these additional millions of people along the Delaware more than offset the better natural cleansing operation that nature has provided there.

During the past 50 years, the city of Washington and its suburbs have grown enormously, and the pollutants from the two million people in and around Washington flow down the Potomac River and then into the Chesapeake, but the point of entry is so far down the Chesapeake and so much nearer the Atlantic that the Chesapeake has suffered far less than it would have if the Potomac had entered the Chesapeake at a point 100 miles north of where it actually does. While Washington and suburbs cannot be ignored as a source of pollution for the Chesapeake, the effect is lessened greatly by its entry point.

Most people living in Philadelphia, Trenton, Camden, Wilmington, and smaller communities along both sides of the Delaware River would express surprise if they were accused of having contributed to fouling the Delaware and making it a less healthy body of water than the Chesapeake. Some would probably say that they have never come within a mile of either the river or the bay. Nevertheless, they have all been guilty to some degree, even those living in apartment houses 10 miles from the river.

The municipalities along the Delaware, and on the smaller streams feeding it, have never fully cleaned up the waste waters that all cities and towns generate, and some of the smaller towns and villages have done no cleanup at all. In addition, all metropolitian areas create thousands of small businesses, such as garages, service stations, paint shops, printing plants, beauty parlors, dry-cleaning facilities, and restaurants, all of which have, in the past, found it convenient to dump small amounts of unwanted materials into the sewers. Detergents and other chemicals from the millions of washing machines and dishwashers, as well as pesticides from farms and gardens, have added a heavy burden of pollution to the Delaware.

More conspicuous than the above contributions is pollution from six major oil refineries located along the Delaware to supply fuel oil and gasoline to the millions of homes and automobiles owned by residents of the area. And the most highly publicized pollution of all has come from the dozens of chemical plants—small, large, and huge—which grew up along the Delaware during the first half of this century. The Du Pont Company's Chambers Works at Deepwater, N.J., for many years was the largest chemical plant in the world.

For a period of nearly 40 years, the Chambers Works was a significant contributor to pollution of both to the Delaware River and Delaware Bay, even though it probably never provided as much as 1 percent of the total. However, it did afford a greater variety of chemical pollutants than any other single source simply because it manufactured more different chemicals than any other plant in the nation, and for years washed the impurities and unwanted by-products into its ditches that flowed into the river.

It is probable that the Delaware River had a greater variety of chemicals feeding into it during the 1950s than any other river in the world except one—the Rhine River in Germany. This was so because the Chambers Works was then producing slightly more than half of all the dyes being manufactured in the world, and dyes require more chemical intermediates than any other branch of organic chemistry. A full list of the individual chemicals being used at Chambers Works would exceed 2000, but some idea of the diversity can be given by naming just a few of the derivatives of benzene alone: chlorobenzene, bromobenzene, fluorobenzene, dichlorobenzene, trichlorobenzene, nitrobenzene, dinitrobenzene, trinitrohydroxy-benzene (picric acid), orthochloronitrobenzene, parachloronitrobenzene, hydroxy-benzene (phenol), benzoic acid, hydroxybenzoic acid (salicyclic acid), aminobenzene (aniline), methyl aniline, dimethyl aniline, paranitroaniline, orthonitroaniline, orthochloroaniline, parachloroaniline, etc, etc. Then there was naphthalene and a long list of its derivatives, including at least 20 naphthalene sulfonic acids, such as peri acid, J acid, H acid, and S acid. Next came anthraquinone and its derivatives; climaxing the whole array were the 700 or so azo dyes.

All of these chemicals found their way into the Delaware in varying amounts, ranging from a few ounces per year to a few tons per month, with the naphthalane sulfonic acids in the second category.

The Rhine River had an even greater diversity of chemicals going into it but it took half a dozen plants in Germany and two in Switzerland to match Chambers Works alone.

The English poet Samuel Taylor Coleridge took note of the fact that the Rhine was badly polluted long before the Germans began to manufacture chemicals. He visited Cologne about 1800 and wrote a brief poem on the subject. While in Cologne he said that he counted "twenty stenches, all well defined, and several stinks." He closed his poem as follows:

> The Rhine, it is well known
> Doth wash your city of Cologne
> But tell me, nymphs, what power divine
> Shall henceforth wash the River Rhine?

Unfortunately, most of the Rhine is not washed by anything except its own waters flowing down from the Alps. Some saltwater from the North Sea does wash a few miles of the Rhine in the Netherlands, but this amount is tiny compared with the vast quantities that flow into the Delaware twice daily.

The Delaware also has benefited from the fact that the Chambers Works no longer manufacturers dyes and has installed what is probably the most efficient water—treatment facility in the world. It was developed for approximately $5 million, cost $40 million to install in 1974, and has a replacement value of about $120 million.

The key element in the process is a patented procedure called "PACT" (powder-activated carbon technology), which uses carbon as a base for the growth of a complex strain of bacteria that will consume just about any organic chemical, except a few bacteriocides. The first step neutralizes the water to be treated, since most water treated at the Chambers Works is acidic. This step also precipitates most of the metals that might interfere with the next two steps, which are biological in nature. In these next two steps, the unwanted chemicals are consumed in a manner very similar to what formerly occurred in the Delaware River itself. The final stream has always bettered the standards set by the national pollution division of the government, has always passed the live-fish test, which goes on constantly, and has always been cleaner then the effluents coming from the many municipal waste-water-treatment plants along the Delaware River.

In 1920, less than half as many people lived along the Delaware from Trenton to the ocean as today. They used less than a 1/10 as much household detergent *per capita,* the chemical plants and oil refineries were less than a 1/10 as numerous, the garages and service stations were less than a 1/50 as numerous, dry cleaning was just getting started in America, and farms along the Delaware used much smaller amounts of fertilizers and insecticides, some of which, naturally, ran off into the streams and smaller rivers that fed the Delaware.

The Delaware River and Delaware Bay were then much more hospitable places for nearly all forms of marine life—from diatoms to oysters and shad fish (alosa sapidissima).

Shad were then so plentiful in the Delaware every spring that they were an important source of food for hundreds of thousands of people living in Philadelphia, Camden, Wilmington, and dozens of small towns in southern New Jersey.

Shad fishing for this large market became such a profitable business that when Du Pont started up its plant at Deepwater in 1917 to manufacture dyes, and hired many of the fishermen to work at the plant, some of the new workers would quit abruptly or take "sick leave" every spring when the shad began their run up the Delaware to their spawning grounds. To retain its work force, Du Pont found it necessary to pay a "shad bonus" amounting to 20 percent of base pay. Even this bonus did not hold all the former fishermen, but it held enough of them to ensure the operation of the plant during shad season.

Oysters (crassostrea virginica) were also a plentiful crop in the bay during the first quarter of this century, particularly on the New Jersey side, near the mouth of the Maurice River. Even blue crabs (calinectes sapidus) grew there in considerable numbers, although for reasons not fully understood, the blue crabs obviously liked the Chesapeake Bay better, since they were 10 to 20 times more plentiful in the Chesapeake.

Shad fish liked the Delaware as much as any estuary on the East Coast, and the people living along the Delaware liked to catch and eat the shad. This was particularly true of the inhabitants of Salem County in New Jersey, where they developed a procedure for cooking shad that inspired a Philadelphia food critic to remark that "planked shad is one of the noblest dishes known to man."

"Planked shad" referred to the fact that the cleaned fish was split and nailed to a plank and then baked by holding the plank before a hot fire until the fish was fully cooked. At the Wild Oaks Country Club and the Salem Country Club in New Jersey, the cooks always used an oak board for the plank and the positioned the plank before a roaring hot fire of oak wood. Whether gases from the hot oak plank or the burning hot oak coals gave a special flavor to the shad, or simply holding the fish in a vertical position while it cooked allowed some of the oils to drain from it to give a dry mealy texture, or some other factor was responsible for the taste, has never been scientifically determined, but there is no doubt about the fact that Salem County planked shad is indeed a noble dish. Visiting diners from as far away as New York City and Charleston, S.C., have all testified to its unique taste.

Unfortunately, regardless of how tasty planked shad may be, people and industries began to proliferate along the Delaware during the 1930s amd 1940s and pollution factors to increase, and the Delaware became a less hospitable body of water for all forms of marine life. The shad did not disappear entirely but became increasingly scarce, and shad feasts and festivals along the Delaware became fewer all the time. Du Pont's Chambers Works, employing more than 10,000, no longer found it necessary to pay a "shad bonus" to hold its work force during the early spring. The operators were earning several times as much money per hour as they were during the 1920s, and the shad were too scarce to represent an opportunity to make big money.

Later, during the 1960s, pollution became still more severe, and even the oysters far down the Delaware Bay became scarce. They did not disappear entirely, but were concentrated chiefly near Lewes, Del., close to the ocean, and in the section of the bay near the mouth of the Maurice River on the New Jersey side. In this area, near the Maurice River cove, the oysters were somewhat protected from the pollution flowing down the Delaware since the main flow stayed near the Delaware shore of the bay. It is true that runoff from the farms along the Maurice River and other pollution from the increasing number of people along the Maurice probably hurt the oysters, but they were not entirely wiped out as was the case on the Delaware side of the bay down to Lewes, which was cleansed twice daily by ocean tides.

The time had finally arrived when action had to be taken to keep both the Delaware River and Delaware Bay from becoming dead bodies of water, and slowly most people became aware of the problem.

During the 1950s, the Du Pont Company, for many years a leader in matters of chemical health and safety, had contracted for studies to determine how Chambers Works' effluents were affecting the diatoms—microscopic forms of life that constitute the first rung in the food ladder or the protein chain. These studies revealed that the diatoms were still alive and well in the Delaware as it flows past Deepwater Point, and even indicated that the Chambers Works' effluents had a negligible effect, or none at all, on their health and variety. Dr. Ruth Patrick, celebrated limnologist of the Philadelphia Academy of Science, pointed out it was the sum total of all pollution in the Delaware that must be considered. It would always be difficult, she said, for any one source of pollution to be singled out as a dominant factor in the health of the Delaware.

The Du Pont Company, acting on this theory, then began a series of actions designed to clean up its effluents from the Chambers Works, and in the late 1970s completed a waste-water-treatment plant at Deepwater that has become a model for chemical plants all over the world. Effluents from this water-treating system not only add nothing to the average level of pollution but actually decrease it, since these effluents are cleaner than those coming from all the municipal water-treating plants from Trenton to Lewes. Du Pont even found a way to realize a profit on its water-treatment plant, and other chemical companies now pay Du Pont for cleaning up some of their polluted wastes that are shipped to the Chambers Works'; Figure 14.1.

Under pressure from a multitude of public forces, municipalities and hundreds, or perhaps thousands, of industrial concerns, large and small, along with millions of private homes, have made conscious efforts to reduce their flow of pollutants into the Delaware. Some still have a considerable way to go before they match the Chambers Works treating system, but nearly all have made some improvement.

The Delaware River and Delaware Bay have both responded well. Both are now considerably cleaner bodies of water than they were in 1970, and both are consider-

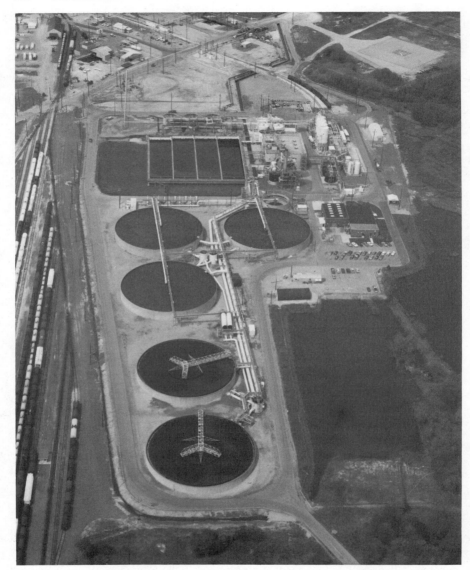

Figure 14.1. Aerial view of waste-processing facility at DuPont Chambers Works, Deepwater, N.J. (Courtesy, E. I. du Pont deNemours & Co., Inc.)

ably more hospitable to all forms of marine life than 10 years ago, according to Dr. Carolyn Thoroughgood, dean of the College of Marine Studies of the University of Delaware, which has a large campus at Lewes.

Oysters have shown a small improvement in numbers and in prospects for the future, but, as Dr. Thoroughgood points out, they have a long way to go before they return to their numbers in the 1920s. Such complete recovery may never occur, or may take several decades, because, Dr. Thoroughgood says, the support chain, going all the way back to the diatoms, may have been seriously damaged by having certain species killed off completely. The ecology of oysters, which cannot move or even duck when pollution approaches, is one of the most complex of all marine studies.

Shad are doing much better in their recovery than the oysters and shad feasts in Salem County are again popular as compared with the 1960s.

Today some people look upon any efforts to use the oceans to clean up pollution—even such natural procedures as tides flowing in and out of the Delaware and the Chesapeake—as unwise, or even immoral. They argue that such movements will only foul the oceans and kill all marine life, but these same people forget that the difference in size between the Atlantic Ocean and the Delaware Bay is so great that it is a difference in kind, not just a difference in magnitude.

The oceans of the world contain about 1500 million billion tons of water, and have dissolved in them enough lead, arsenic, and mercury to poison all life on earth if these elements could be collected and fed in concentrated doses to all forms of animal life. However, in the concentrations in which they are found in the oceans they pose no hazards at all. Ocean water contains about 0.01 mg of arsenic per kilogram of water, for example, for a total of about 15 billion tons of arsenic—easily enough to poison everyone if pulled together in one place. That is no reason why anyone should be afraid to take a swim in the ocean or eat a lobster from the sea. The arsenic in seawater apparently does not bother the shad either; they probably would miss it if it were all removed from the oceans.

As to the future of Delaware Bay, it will continue to be a struggle, because the population density along the bay is expected to continue to grow. By the year 2050 there may be twice as many people living along the Delaware as there were in 1950, and all people and industries will then have to cut their amount of pollution per capita in half just to keep even with the way things were in 1950. Further improvement in the health of the Delaware will require more than a 50 percent cut in pollution by everyone, people and industry alike. It will not be easy—but, with a reasonable chance and a little encouragement by all, the shad will continue to swim up the Delaware. Industry is well aware of its responsibilities (see Appendix E).

SUGGESTED READINGS

E. I. du Pont de Nemours & Company, Chambers Works, pp. 279–309, in *Cutting Chemical Wastes: What 29 Organic Chemical Plants Are Doing to Reduce Hazardous Wastes,* by D. J. Sarokin, W. R. Muir, C. G. Miller, and S. R. Sperber, edited by P. Stryker and P. Lone, an INFORM Report, 535 pp., paperbound, Inform, Inc., New York.

"Du Pont's Waste Business Is Cleaning Up," *Wilmington (Dela.) Sunday News J.,* C5 (Dec. 28, 1986).

P. L. Layman, "Rhine Spills Force Rethinking of Potential for Chemical Polution," *Chem. Eng. News,* 7–11 (Feb. 23, 1987).

S. O. Rohmann and N. Lilienthal, Tracing a River's Toxic Pollution—A Case Study of the Hudson, Phase II, 209 pages, Inform, 381 Park Ave. South, New York, NY 10016, 1987

T. Shelton and B. Hamilton, "Landscaping for Water Conservation," 24 pp., Rutgers Cooperative Extension, New Jersey Agricultural Experimental Station, Rutgers, The State University of New Jersey, New Brunswick, N.J. 1987.

M. Weisskopf, A Fourth of U.S. Waterways too Polluted for Recreation, *Washington Post,* Nov. 11, 1987, A-14

15
Hazards of Home Chemistry

Howard H. Fawcett

"Home chemistry" implies the use of chemicals and chemical-containing substances or mixtures for domestic, personal, or recreational purposes, under conditions where formal control measures or supervision may be limited or nonexistent.

The past few decades, especially since World War II, have witnessed a remarkable increase in the use of chemicals formulated and packaged for home use. They are intended to make life pleasant, to minimize work, or to increase efficiency. The additional attention that has been focused recently upon science and technology (such as amateur rocketry and powered toy cars, boats, and airplanes) has encouraged experimentation, especially by young people with infinite enthusiasm but limited knowledge of·the hazards. With the benefits have come undesirable by-products, where incomplete information or wanton disregard of labels, instructions, and fundamental precautions has resulted in injuries. This discussion presents the case for more sophistication in the use of chemicals, especially in domestic and recreational situations. As applied here, a chemical is defined as any element, compound, mixture, or formulation, of known or unknown composition, possessing properties that make it potentially beneficial to society *if properly utilized and disposed* of.

AMATEUR PYROTECHNICS, ROCKETS, AND EXPLOSIVES

The fascination of a beautiful pyrotechnics display is undeniable, as provided for centuries by firecrackers, rockets, Roman candles, and related pieces. Although there is no federal fireworks law as such, there are innumerable local, state, and city codes, ordinances, and other regulations at various governmental levels with regard to the manufacture and use of "explosives." In spite of these various laws, designed

231

to remove dangerous materials from the hands of amateurs, pyrotechnics are still part of the scene, and can be justified if made and displayed safely. Unfortunately, young children, as well as overzealous adults, become so enamored with pyrotechnics and explosives that they have little or no regard for their own safety or for the safety of on-lookers.

Even educators have fallen prey to the lure of "popular" science; in a special student course in a Washington, D.C., school, a professor (not trained in chemistry) assigned a group of eight- and 9-year-old students the task of mixing metal powders with oxidizers to produce a paste, which, when placed on a wire, would become "sparklers," with little or no supervision or instructions. Three of the students were burned, one seriously, when the bowlful of mixture ignited. The question of academic responsibility was again raised, and a lawsuit was instituted.

Complex chemistry and hard-to-obtain ingredients are not necessary to pursue this potentially dangerous hobby. Substances as familiar and available as dry ice or match heads, if confined, as in a stoppered bottle, pipe, tube, or closed can, will expand and the container will burst, with possibly tragic effects. One common explosive combination consists of weed-killer mixed with powdered sugar. Powdered zinc mixed with sulfur is another hazardous system. Even sodium bicarbonate with vinegar can develop considerable pressure if allowed to build up in a confined space. Such mixtures became very popular after the launching of the first man-made satellites in 1957, and are still employed, in spite of the opposition of the American Rocket Society (now the American Institute of Aeronautics and Astronautics). Explosives research is *not* a field for amateurs, and rocket propellants and pyrotechnics, by whatever names, are truly *explosives*.[1a]

Explosives may even fascinate more mature students well grounded in the sciences, as demonstrated by two unrelated incidents, each involving three 20-year-old college students. The unusual nature of these two incidents suggest that human ingenuity is boundless when coupled with youthful enthusiasm.

1. In one case, an engineering college freshman brought two classmates home for a weekend, and, to demonstrate his technical knowledge and ability, prepared to launch signal rockets from a high bluff along the Mohawk River. Ignition was to be by remote control, using a short-wave radio signal transmitted from a moving automobile and received by the preset ignition system. The flare mixture, which was powdered metals with oxidizing agents, ignited prematurely, resulting in serious injuries to all three; the young engineer was permanently blinded.

2. In another real-world incident, five college students were riding in a compact automobile, two in front and three in the rear. From available information it appears that the three occupants of the rear seat were filling plastic bags with a commercially available disinfectant (calcium hypochlorite base) to which they added model airplane fuel (which contained 10–15 percent nitromethane). The delayed reaction permitted the closed bags to be tossed from the moving automobile, with "spontaneous ignition" occurring several minutes after the automobile had passed. This was especially interesting when the bag landed in a dense shrub. However, one reaction mixture ignited prematurely inside the automobile, resulting in a vigorous

fire; ignited other combustibles, including the seat and floor mat; and caused the driver to lose control of the vehicle. The two occupants of the front seat escaped with minor injuries but the three students in the rear seat were fatally burned. The vigorous oxidation from the chemical disinfectant with organic matter is well documented.[1-3]

These incidents, selected from many on record, emphasize again that, unless respect for chemicals can be implanted at an early age, such tragedies will continue. This education must start in the home, and *must* be extended through schools and colleges. The Institute of Makers of Explosives[4] has long been engaged in a vigorous campaign to teach children and adults to recognize misplaced or stolen dynamite and blasting caps, and to surrender any suspicious object to the police or other authorities. The military has the same attitude about war souvenirs; a bullet, bomb, or grenade may explode after many years on a mantle or game-room shelf. Radioactive materials (such as the luminous cords used as directional indicators during black-out conditions) contain radium and should not be treated as toys. Neither should any other material or object containing radiation be treated casually. Objects of the type described greatly increase the hazard for emergency personnel, especially during a fire, where explosive, radioactive, or toxic substances may be released without warning.

"TOY" CHEMISTRY SETS

If it is agreed that young people should be encouraged to experiment in the sciences (and it should be noted that some authorities feel this should be a natural selection process, and that a wide distribution of our best talent on *all* fronts, *both scientific and sociologic,* is more important in the national long-term interest than excessive pressure to produce more scientists and engineers), organized and well-documented experiments with supplied reagents and detailed instructions may be considered. Thanks to the Consumer Products Safety Commission, the National Science Teachers Association, and other concerned groups, much progress has been made in "foolproofing" chemistry sets sold in stores for home use. Chemistry sets, reflecting our expanding technology and improved merchandising techniques, are now available in a glittering array of sizes and types, including instructional manuals that closely parallel a high school chemistry course. Of the sets examined recently, dangerous and potentially explosive ingredients have been excluded, and the labels reflect the newer laws on precautions for hazardous and toxic substances. It is strongly emphasized in the manuals that directions should be followed to the letter, and that reagents or other substances not supplied and specified should never be added to experiments.

Over 20 years ago, the Chemical Section and Toy Safety Committee of the NSC Home Conference developed and distributed a Fact Sheet that reviewed the fundamentals of safe use and was widely accepted by toy-set makers and parents. It pointed out that competent supervision is necessary, even with relatively simple sets. This precaution is especially important for sets that include open flames, such as an alcohol lamp, for glass-blowing and heating. In addition, it urged that eye protectors be provided with the sets and specified that they were *to be worn* when performing any experimental work—excellent preparation for industry and OSHA, state, and local school regulations, where the value of no nonsense eye protection has been demonstrated many times. It would further create a respect for *all* chemicals, and establish patterns of conduct that would be useful in later scientific careers as well as in the home use of chemicals.[5] The National Society for the Prevention of Blindness has documented the eye effects of 1600 chemicals, including the more severe eye hazards such as acids and caustics. The wearing of contact lenses while working with chemicals or dusts, even while wearing eye protectors, should be discouraged to have to remove contact lenses first can waste valuable time when irrigating an eye injury.[6] (The "youthful chemist" pictured in the NSC fact sheet elected to become a professional actor and writer, and is currently host of a popular television program viewed nationally.)

Another recommendation of the fact sheet to increase safety is to classify chemistry sets and other scientific toys by age brackets, and to state in large, clear print the range of suggested ages for each specific set. Clearly, a parent buying a large complicated set for a child too young to comprehend it is not doing the child a favor, but is encouraging waste and arousing frustrations. If the ages for which the set is intended could be clearly and conspicuously displayed on the box or carton, the prospective buyer would have some basis for a more intelligent selection, and the young student would be more likely to learn from, as well as enjoy, the experiments. Scientific "sets" should be the beginning of a long-range educational experience, and not treated as "toys" to be used frivolously and then promptly discarded.

HOME CHEMICALS

In one sense, there are no "home chemicals," as chemicals have identical properties and hazards whether used in the home or in industry. However, two differences may be noted between domestic and industrial use: (1) The containers used in the home are usually smaller, more attractive, made of paper, plastic, or glass, and less substantial. Also, the precautionary labeling and ingredients information is much less conspicuously displayed, usually in small print so that the legal, but hardly the user, requirements are met by the maker. (2) Recommended precautions, are less likely to be observed in the home because they are less well understood, and the motivation for observing them is less than clear. Such instructions as "Use with adequate ventilation" or "If spilled on skin, wash thoroughly with water" are too vague to be more than suggestions. The ingredients, when given, are often described in technical rather than common generic terms, to aid in proprietary security. Advice to call a physician implies that the physician will know what to do immediately when, in fact, very few physicians have the needed information at hand, and moreover will only make house calls in the most unusual circumstances.

The local poison control centers (of which more than 700 exist in the United States and Canada) are better geared to provide prompt information and suggest actions. Where possible, the maker's hot-line should be called immediately. With the wide interest in OSHA and state right-to-know laws, and the stipulation that medical personnel (including physicians and nurses) must have immediate access to technical aspects of the chemicals involved at the site so that they can institute adequate and complete care and treatment at once, it is to be hoped that much of the time wasted in previous cases while legal counsel was brought into the picture will be obviated.

One cardinal rule regarding all "home chemicals" is that they must be kept out of the reach or grasp of children, just as with medicines and drugs. Children have no understanding of the nature or effects of a substance and may just as well sprinkle cleaning solvents about (some of which are quite flammable and all of which are toxic to some degree) as sugar or flour. Until the age of five or six, when other interests begin to overtake the *"let's spill, drink, or eat it"* syndrome, children *must be protected from self-descruction*.

Solvents and Cleaners

Chemically, such materials range from aliphatic and aromatic hydrocarbons to halogenated hydrocarbons, with a variety of mixtures and blends included. Many now appear as "aerosols" in pressurized containers, either alone or in combination with propellants. The latter range from highly flammable (such as propane and butane) to the chlorofluorocarbons, about which much concern has been expressed, especially as related to the long-term effects on the ozone layer even in the relatively uncontaminated Antarctic. The range of hazards is wide, and each "package" should be considered on its own merits. To illustrate that the problem of home chemicals are not new, under date of October 11, 1963, the FDA warned against home use of a water repellent containing silicones mixed with gasoline. Flash fires had occurred following the application of the mixture to a masonry wall in a home basement to eliminate water seepage. The revised label, which was recommended by the FDA, contained the statement:

> The potential hazard from the use of this product is so great that it is recommended the user, before applying the material, consult with a professional expert in handling such highly hazardous materials to minimize the chance of personal injury or property damage.

At the time, the FDA pointed out it had no authortiy to remove such items from sale but only to insist on adequate labeling. Today, the Consumer Products Safety Commission would have the authority to order the product from the market.

Even with adequate warning on a container, however, the human element must be considered. On January 6, 1987, in an apartment in Aspen Hill, Md., a man was not satisfied with the rate of discharge of a pesticide from an aerosol container. He used a screwdriver to puncture the container, resulting in the release of large volumes of the propellant (propane), which ignited at a stove pilot light, and resulted in a $300,000 fire loss to several apartments. The man was lucky and escaped with no injuries. *"Read the label carefully"* is still a wise prelude to the use of any product.

Bleaches

When liquid bleach contacts acids, acid-containing, or strongly alkaline substances, gases, including chlorine, are evolved. It is difficult to understand how one commercial compound on the market (1987) used for cleaning tile in bathrooms meets all the requirements for a "safe" product, since both the sodium hydroxide and the sodium hypochlorite in the mixture react, and in home use the sodium hydroxide component's potential for harming the eyes is poorly appreciated. Even water/sodium hypochlorite mixtures have been reported as bursting in storage, owing to the failure of the cap designed to vent gas slowly during the storage—a normal tendency may be accelerated by unusually hot weather. Vent caps should be checked with full personal protection, and the material should be stored at 15–18°C (59–64°F) and out of direct sunlight, which accelerates decomposition. The mixing of any household product with another should be attempted only after a thorough literature survey, which suggests that one should *not mix unless prepared for the consequences of unknown reactions.*

Rust Removers

Rust stains are effectively removed by various preparations containing oxalic acid, which, while toxic upon ingestion, do not seriously affect the skin if washed off promptly or adversely affect porcelain surfaces, such as in tubs or bowls. Another type of rust remover, sometimes packaged in an attractive squirt bottle, contains dilute hydrofluoric acid (HF). This is a poison that can quickly penetrate the skin and seek the bones, and though without initial pain, the resulting burns, which develop slowly, are painful and slow to heal. A spill of hydrofluoric acid must be treated with a calcium-containing compound and soda ash to precipitate the fluoride ion as harmless calcium fluoride and render a neutral pH. Extra care must be taken to avoid skin contact with this acid, as well as inhalation of the hydrogen fluoride gas. It is also highly corrosive to porcelain surfaces; this writer ruined a porcelain bathtub because he used the 10 percent commercial product without adequate attention to the time required for removal of the rust before the acid attacked the finish. But although HF is hardly a "safe" chemical to use without more precautions than normally taken with home application, it is still a valuable chemical.[8]

An interesting simple, inexpensive, and relatively safe "home" chemical operation for the cleaning of the copper bottoms of pots and utensils utilizes ordinary kitchen-strength (5 percent acetic acid) vinegar, and salt (sodium chloride). Rubbing this mixture on the pot with a cloth or paper towel will produce amazing results. Obviously the utensil should be thoroughly washed in water before use.

Paint and Paint Removers

Much interior home wall decorating is now done with water-based latex emulsions that are relatively harmless, but oil-based paints and enamels are often used for trim and for external application. Where solvents must be used as paint or varnish removers or as paint thinners, a thorough inquiry should be made into the specific hazards. If information is incomplete or not forthcoming, contact the National Paint and Coatings Association.[9] Adequate (which should be defined by the vendor or seller of the material) ventilation and precautions against fire should be taken as required. This is especially important where paint and varnish thinners and removers contain highly toxic and flammable solvents such as benzene, toluene, xylene, or methanol. The use of benzene in such applications is no longer condoned, but it is possible that old stocks still remain in some areas. Benzene is now officially listed as an OSHA carcinogen due to its action on the red marrow. Methanol produces serious damage to the optic nerve and is a violent poison if accidentally ingested. Some paints once contained lead pigments, but this has been outlawed in many cities and municipal areas. Care should be used to use nonlead paint on cribs and other surfaces where children may chew or eat flaked paint. (Called pica, this is a craving for unnatural foods, including flaked paint, dirt, stones, lead fishing sinkers, and other substances not intended for human consumption.) Since lead is a cumulative poison and has been linked to learning disabilities in children, its application in the home deserves serious review.[10]

Wood preservatives also may be a home hazard. After November 10, 1986, EPA regulations have restricted the sale of pentachlorophenol and creosote mixtures to certified pesticide applicators. Both materials are highly corrosive to the skin and eyes, and creosote is suspected of causing skin cancer in humans. It is classified by the EPA as mutagenic, as being able to change the genetic makeup of cells. Pentachlorophenol has been shown to be toxic to the fetus in laboratory animal studies and is considered a possible human carcinogen. Substitute preservatives for the home worker include tributyltinoxide and copper-8-quinolinolate. Both are safer and have not been linked to serious health problems to date.

No product, that has the potential for skin contact or inhalation exposure in use is completely free of problems for at least some people, since between 10 percent and 20 percent of the U.S. population is believed to suffer from allergies or other chronic diseases that may place them at risk upon exposure to the chemicals in such common household products as detergents, solvents, pesticides, polishes, disinfectants, as well as metals and rubber. Many chemicals are used in the home in the form of constituents of household products. For example, rugs are treated to prevent static or to delay deterioration, and furnace filteres are treated to reduce airborne bacteria. In 1981, the National Research Council issued a report on indoor air pollutants.[12-13]

Fuels

Many homemakers store small quantities of fuels of various types in their homes in addition to the more conventional fuels (natural gas and heating oil) used for home heating. Gasoline is widely used in power lawn mowers, snow throwers, blow torches, outboard boat motors, and camp lanterns, as well as in automobiles. Storage in a home or garage is unwise, since leakage of the container can cause a serious fire hazard that can go undetected for a long period before a stray ignition source produces a fire or explosion.[14]

Information available through local fire departments should be carefully followed. Needless to say, if any fuel (gasoline, oil, gas, wood, or charcoal) is burned without adequate air and enough ventilation to remove all smoke and combustion products, carbon monoxide and other gaseous products may be expected. *Gasoline, (either leaded or unleaded) should not be used for any purpose other than as a fuel* in a properly working system designed for its use, and *must never be used to light or rekindle a fire, such as an outdoor grill.* Storage should always be in approved metal safety containers with a flash arrester, not in plastic or glass containers. In addition, the recent revelations and animal investigations that raised serious questions as to the potential carcinogenic action of unleaded gasoline on humans deserve close attention over the next few years. Many service-station pump stands are already posted with this warning.[16]

Liquid propane torches have become very popular for home repairs to copper tubing and for other small heating and cutting purposes. When selecting such devices, be certain that they have been approved for safety by Underwriters' Laboratories (UL) or another recognized approval agency, and are kept in good condition and free from leaks, to prevent accidental ignition and explosions. Expended fuel cylinders should be buried to prevent refilling or careless disposal into a fire, where they may explode.[17]

The addition of small "lighters" using propane to the case of a digital wristwatch, which can be ignited by pressure on a small lever on the side of the watch, introduces still another potential fire hazard if not carefully controlled. Such watches, under the name of Protime wristflame piezo LCO watch-lighter, were being sold (December 1986) in California. No maker's name is on the carton, but they are made in Taiwan and claim "pat. published," as well as a statement of "no liability in case the product is misused."

For years, the use of kerosene, gasoline, or lighter fluid to kindle or "freshen" a fire, either in a fireplace, a stove, or an outdoor grill, has caused tragedy when unexpected ignition and flashback occur. In recent times, with the trend toward outdoor cooking, especially packaged charcoal lighter fluids have been made available for use on charcoal or wood-burning grills. These should *not* be used to "freshen" or "accelerate" a fire, since the volatility is high, and flashbacks resulting in explosions are to be expected. An aerosol sold as a "starting ether" has been marketed to aid in starting diesel or reluctant gasoline engines. A spray is directed into the air intake with the hope that ignition will take place in the cylinders, not outside them. This product contains diethyl ether, and is marked "extremely flammable," a classification that suggests it should be used only by persons thoroughly familiar with its hazards.

The vapors from all commonly used liquid fuels are heavier than air, and tend to accumulate in cellars, sumps, and other low areas, unless ventilation really is adequate (which, in fact, can only be determined with instrumentation not usually available in the average home). A spark from a starting relay or contact on an electric pump motor, light switch, hot water heater control or pilot light, domestic refrigerator or freezer starting relay, electric or gas clothes dryer—any of these may be an ignition source. Only natural gas and hydrogen are lighter than air, meaning that they will rise, and so monitoring for these two gases should be upward, in contrast to other fuel vapors. It should be noted that, although natural gas before ultimate distribution to home is odorized with a mercaptan, this is not always a reliable indicator, since many people have a poor sense of smell. Also, a mercaptan has been known to be less than adequate for this purpose, either as a result of improper injection or of condensation in very cold weather. In case of doubt, call the emergency number of your local gas supplier, available from telephone information or in the local telephone directory.

Incompatible chemicals should never be stored near each other, or where spills or other possible mixing can occur. Storage areas with really efficient ventilation, away from ignition sources, should be used for all fuels and other flammable materials—approved storage cabinets as certified by UL, Factory Mutual, or Factory Insurance Association are recommended, even for home use. An insurance carrier or local fire department should be able to supply details. Domestic household refrigerators are designed for the safe and proper storage of food, but they contain electrical contact ignition sources, both inside and outside the box, *that preclude their use to store flammable substances,* such as ether and other solvents, unless they have been properly modified by a skilled electrician to remove all ignition sources. When a refrigerator, freezer, oven, security safe, or other tightly closed cabinet is removed from service, especially at home or in a school, the door should be removed or rendered inoperable to prevent small children from climbing inside and closing the door (which cannot be opened from the inside), and being suffocated.

Another electrical/chemical hazard involves the "setting" or other deformation of electrical appliance cords when they are stored under pressure for long periods. In a recent incident in California, an expensive three-prong curling iron, shipped from France in a small, tightly wound condition, was being used properly, but when the iron was placed on the sink top, one of the curves from the compression in the lead-in electric wire forced the wire into contact with the hot element surface. A fire and eruption occurred, which would have been very serious had it happened while the iron was in contact with hair. Such devices are imported into the United States without any approval, such as the UL and other testing certification required of U.S. products.

Dyes

Home dyes are used to change the color of drapes, slip covers, clothing, and other textiles. Precautions against potential hazards, especially skin discoloration and possible adsorption of the dye by the skin, are usually supplied by the manufacturers, and should be properly observed. Although most benzidine- or congers-based dyes are now off the market, full information on all dyes should be available from the supplier or maker, and judgment as to necessary precautions to be applied should be made on the basis of the potential hazards.

Hair and Beauty Aids

The complex chemistry and "secret" formulations involved in chemicals for hair and beauty aids make these hazards difficulty to access. Certainly most beauty salons seem to be inadequately ventilated, and the operators seem not to care about their own or their clients' health and safety. Some years ago, NIOSH did a study on the health of beauty salon operators in Utah, but the report has never had wide circulation or been followed up to the writer's knowledge. Dermatitis has been reported from nail lacquer, permanent waving solutions, hair dyes and tints, lipsticks, and eye shadows, but data and concern are surprisingly limited. Very difficult to predict is the sensitization rections that may occur, in which a substanace, such as paraphenylenediamine hair dye, might also cause a cross-allergy to other substances, including aniline, benzocaine, sulphanamids, saccharin, azo dyes, and paraaminobenzoic acid, in some individuals. There are few cosmetics to which no one is allergic, although the sensitization risk may be relatively low. It is prudent, therefore, to inquire into the composition of preparations, both the vehicles and the active ingredients, and once an allergic reaction is noted, to avoid further exposures to the suspected agent in any form. It should be noted that an allergen is usually a protein, but it can be almost any substance in the environment, such as mold spores, plant pollens, animal dander, household dust, foods, dyes, plastics, and detergents, as well as cosmetics or drugs. For additional information about possible allergic reactions, a dermatologist should be consulted. Products "for professional use only" are often inadequately labeled.

Perfumes are very complex mixtures, and even domestic air-freshener perfumes may contain as many as 20 ingredients. The main skin hazards from perfumes are contact sensitization dermatitis, photosensitization, and pigmentation changes.

Of the three main classes of hair dyes—vegetable, metallic, and synthetic para-oxidation dyes—natural vegetable dyes are considered relatively harmless but synthetic organic and compound rinses may cause skin irritation. Metallic dyes, while staining the skin, are not likely to cause dermatitis. The synthetic para-oxidation dyes may cause contact sensitization, and may be highly damaging to the eyes. In all cases, the specific precautions recommended by the manufacturer should be followed to the letter, and a physician consulted at once if unusual effects are suspected or noted.

Solvent and Vapor Inhalation

Before the current interest in drugs (such as cocaine, marijuana, crack, and other street drugs, including angel dust and PCP), much publicity was given to the highly dangerous, practice, mainly by teenagers, of inhaling the vapors from plastic cement, model airplane glue, marking pens, typewriter correction fluids, and other volatile solvents. Benzene, toluene, xylene, the acetates, acetone, methyl ethyl ketone, and other solvents when inhaled produce euphoria or a sense of well-being. It is known that the inhalation of many other common solvents, such as chloroform, carbon tetrachloride, trichloroethylene, 1,1,1-trichloroethane, diethyl ether, and methyl chloride, can cause solvent addiction and ultimately injury to vital organs, including the liver and kidneys. The well-known synergistic reaction between carbon tetrachloride when inhaled following ingestion of alcoholic beverages great-ly enhances the toxicity of the carbon tetrachloride. Alcohol can have a "potentiat-ing" or escalating effect on tranquilizers, resulting in serious shock to the central nervous system.[18] (Questions about cocaine and its abuse can be answered by calling 800-COCAINE, a national treatment referral and information service of the Fair Oaks Hospital, 19 Prospect Street, Summit, NJ 07901.)

Home Fire Hazards

The average home has many substances that will either burn, melt, or decompose into toxic products. As Frank Brannigan, a fire protection engineer with dynamic delivery, has often pointed out, homes are built to burn as much as to live in. Wood, paper, and textiles will produce carbon dioxide and/or carbon monoxide, depending on conditions. Cellulose acetate and other esters at elevated temperatures will produce acidic products. Cooking, especially where oils, fats, and greases are allowed to overheat on a stove or in an oven, will burn or decompose into acrolein, carbon monoxide, and dense, highly odorous smoke. Even a few sausages or strips of bacon left in an overheated frying pan will produce sufficient volumes of toxic smoke to overcome persons who are caught without warning. Paraffin wax, used in home preserving and candle making, produces a smoky fire if overheated, as in an oven or stove. These examples suggest that a significant hazard in a home may be from fire gases or fire decomposition products, and even more complete evaluation of fire gases and smokes than those that have been made by the National Bureau of Standards, the University of Pittsburgh, Factory Mutual, and the National Research Council should be encouraged, and should include more impartial evaluation of plastics and building materials. A wider use of smoke detectors to alert home occupants to trouble before it becomes too late to evacuate and well-planned escape routes would greatly reduce the fatalities from even relatively minor fires, where the occupants were asleep or unable to move quickly enough. Once out of the house or apartment, the occupant should *not* reenter until the fire services declare it safe to do so without respiratory and other protective equipment.

If a home fire extinguisher is available, it should be used *only after* the fire department has been called and all personnel evacuated. In this connection, it is noted that over 20 years ago the pyrene or carbon tetrachloride-based extinguishers, as well as the chlorobromomethane extinguishers, were largely replaced, and now are no longer approved, due to their intrinsic toxicity, as well as the decomposition of the liquids into phosgene and other toxic gases. At one time, glass balls partly filled with approximately a quart of carbon tetrachloride, or CM_7, were sold widely for home extinguishers, but independent evaluation by the National Bureau of

Standards showed them to be relatively ineffective, and they are no longer approved. The newer agents, including carbon dioxide, dry chemicals, and the Halon extinguishers, are more effective as well as safer for home use. *No extinguisher, however, is a substitute for a prompt evacuation and call for the fire department.*

Miscellaneous Chemicals

Hundreds of other substances not previously considered in this chapter are used in home activities, in hobbies, or in small home industries and businesses. Many are so well established that, if the composition is known, precautions can be easily prescribed. Lye, used for opening plugged sink drains; sodium carbonate and trisodium phosphate mixtures, used in home cleaners; and hydrofluoric acid (mentioned previously) are examples. Acetic acid, at one strength (5 percent), is used as vinegar; at a higher strength, it is used as a photographic chemical. Antifreeze used in automobile cooling systems is *not* a beverage, but a toxic material, and should be kept away from children or anyone else who might drink it. The important consideration is to insist on knowing what precautions the maker recommends and to observe them to the letter. It is not possible for laws and "government" to protect us from ourselves; the initiative must come from within, and is based on the two elements of *knowledge* and *action*. Chemicals are neither good nor bad; they can serve a useful purpose if we use them properly and safely, and the responsibility for safe use and disposal must ultimately be that of the user.

The disposal aspect has been forcefully presented in a 36-page booklet[19] in which the whole subject is reviewed, including a section on "What to Do with Some Common Hazardous Wastes." This section, using symbols to illustrate the various possible disposal modes, discusses such items as automotive supplies, antifreeze coolant, windshield washer solution, engine degreaser, carburetor cleaner, chrome polish, car wax, and auto body filler. It also covers painting and decorating supplies, oil-based paint, alkyd enamel, epoxy enamel, varnish, other paints whose spills must be cleaned up with thinner, synthetic auto enamel, model airplane paint, paint stripper, brush cleaners, mercury batteries, fluorescent lamp ballast, broken smoke detectors, wood preservatives (with special attention to preservatives containing creosote or pentachlorophenol or arsenic), and wood that has been treated with preservative.

Glues and cements containing solvents other than water, are included as are asbestos, garden supplies (including pesticides, some of which are now labeled "Restricted Use Pesticide"—for professional licensed applicators); soil fumigants, including nematicides; fungicides; weed killers; molluscicides (snail and slug poison); rat, mouse, and gopher poison; cleaners; rust removers; aluminum cleaner; and swimming pool supplies. Described as well are toy chemistry sets, flea powder, ammunition, powder or primers, gun-cleaning solvent, antistatic brushes, photographic chemicals, photographic solutions,[20] ceramic glazes, acrylics, artists' oils, artists' mediums, thinners, fixatives, rubber cement thinner, fiberglass resins, epoxy resins, and aerosol cans of all types. Among common household items are food extracts and alcohol-containing liquids, housecleaning supplies, rug cleaners containing solvents, furniture polish containing solvent for wood floors, metal polish containing petroleum distillates, cleaners containing ammonia, laundry supplies including chlorine bleach, spot remover, moth balls (naphthalene), lighter fluid, lamp oil, shoe polish, and shoe dye.

Finally, the section reviews infectious wastes; medical supplies; expired prescriptions and other medicine; shampoo containing lindane (for head lice); mercury from broken thermometers; hearing-aid batteries; rubbing alcohol; cosmetics, including waving lotion in home permanents; relaxer in hair straighteners; depilatories; cuticle remover; perfume and cologne; aftershave and preshave for electric shavers; nail polish; nail-polish remover; cleaners for tub, tile, and shower stalls; disinfectants; and toilet-bowl cleaners.

In general, the approach is either to flush the material down the drain carefully with copious quantities of water, or to close it for delivery to a hazardous–waste disposal site by a competent person who knows and respects the hazards *(not a "trash collector")*. Under no circumstances should such items be discarded with ordinary trash or garbage. The cited references should be consulted for details, and, if the material is labeled with a precautionary label, the instructions should be followed to the letter.

Children are naturally curious. They touch, smell, and taste as a natural part of learning. Every home contains many products that make life easier and more pleasant, such as cleaning supplies, cosmetics, and medicines. Any of these products can poison a child who ingests or inhales it. Children should know that Mr. YUK means *NO*.

Based on long experience, the poison-control centers recommend that a special poison warning symbol, known as Mr. YUK, be attached to each dangerous product in the house. The labels, available from the local poison-control centers, contain a highly descriptive sketch of a face, with the telephone number of the local center. Among the substances the National Capital Poison Center at Georgetown Medical Center [phone (202) 265-3333] suggests be labeled with the Mr. YUK sticker are the following:

Acids	Copper and brass cleaners
Aerosols	Corn and wart remover
Ammonia	Dandruff shampoo
Antiseptics	Dishwasher detergents
Aspirin	Oven cleaner
Bathroom bowl cleaner	Paint thinner
Benzene	Pesticides
Bubble bath	Pine oil
Carbon tetrachloride	Drain cleaners
Cigarettes	Drugs
Cleaning fluids	Epoxy glue
Clinitest tablets	Eye makeup
Cologne	Furniture polish

Garden sprays
Gun cleaners
Hair dyes
Herbicides
Insecticides
Iodine
Kerosene
Mace chemical
Model cement
Nail polish
Nail-polish remover
Narcotics

Paint
Permanent-wave solution
Petroleum distillates
Rodenticides
Shaving lotion
Strychnine
Typewriter cleaner
Window-washing solvent
Silver polish
Turpentine
Vitamins

The poison-control centers recommend immediately calling a center in case a poisoning is suspected. *The phone number of the nearest center should be plainly posted near the phone.* In addition, the following additional suggestions are in order.

A bottle of ipecac (to induce vomiting) should be readily available in every home. Syrup of ipecac is a medicine for emergency use in poisoning. When given to a child or adult, it causes vomiting. Syrup of ipecac can be purchased in any drugstore and does not require a prescription. *Ipecac should never be given without calling the local poison-control center first, since in some poisonings vomiting is not indicated.* Poison-control staff members will give you clear directions for its use if it is necessary.

PESTICIDES

The increasing use of pesticides and other "lawn" chemicals in the home environment is another area of concern. New questions about lawn-maintenance chemicals have put the $1-billion-a-year service industry under increasing fire. Critics say too little is known about the potential damage to health and environmental safety from the 16,000 pesticide products approved for nonagricultural spraying to warrant their widespread use. In a recent lawsuit, a widow of an Arlington, Va.-based Naval lieutenant has blamed the 1982 death of her husband on Daconil, a fungicide that was sprayed on a golf course he frequented.[21–23]

CHRISTMAS TREE HAZARDS AND CONTROL

Although it is a seasonable operation, the serious question arises as to how properly to control combustibles, including trees, that are brought into a home for the holiday season. The most complete analysis we have seen to date is from the California State Fire Marshal.[24]

Fresh trees present no significant fire hazard. A "fresh" tree is one that has not lost an appreciable amount of its natural moisture (regardless of when it was cut). If a tree is kept from drying out (such as by keeping the cut trunk submerged in water), it can remain fresh and reasonably flame resistant during normal holiday use. However, when thoroughly dry, Christmas trees, especially Douglas firs, are without question the most flammable item to be found in the home. Once ignited, the speed and intensity of burning are extreme. A dry tree will appear to literally "explode" and be totally consumed, except for the trunk, in a matter of seconds. California regulations require Christmas trees to be "flameproofed" when placed in certain kinds of buildings (generally those used by the public). A growing number of local ordinances are extending that requirement to use in the home as well.

Treatment of Trees

In order to flameproof anything, it is essential to have a sufficient amount of effective flame-retardant chemical either into—or on the surface of—the material being treated. Since Christmas-tree needles are not absorbent, **the only effective type of treatment is the coating method**. To ensure that a chemical will effectively flameproof a Christmas tree, use a suffcient quantity of a product listed on the State Fire Marshal's (SFM) approved list.

Flocks that appear on this chemical list should be applied directly to untreated trees and not used after treatment with a clear chemical. An exception would be if the flock were used only as a light coating with the application and coverage less than that recommended by the manufacturer. In California, only SFM-approved products, applied by SFM-licensed applicators, may be used on trees that are required to be flameproofed.

Testing of Trees

The SFM's procedure for testing is to apply the fire-retardant solution to the branches of fresh Douglas fir, dry the sample for 30 days, and perform a simple ignition test with a small open flame. Even a totally inadequate treatment applied to a reasonably fresh tree will give the impression that the treatment has been effective. This is not valid. Attempts to flameproof Christmas trees with simple solutions of water-dissolved chemicals such as borax and boric acid, diammonium phosphate, or ammonium sulphate are completely useless since tree needles will not absorb these water-based solutions. Any source that recommends the use of common water mixed with chemicals for flameproofing Christmas trees is in error and should be ignored.

Inspection Procedures

The tree must have a tag showing it has received flame-retardant treatment. If done for a fee, such as on a tree lot, the firm must have a SFM registration and the tag must conform to SFM regulations, including the name of the chemical, the registration number of the chemical, the name of the applicator, the registration number of the applicator, and the date of treatment.

Examine the tree for adequacy of coverage. All areas, including the underside of the needles, must be treated. Clear coatings are harder to see, but still are readily detectable when properly applied. All approved products will work, but only if applied in sufficent amounts. This means a fairly heavy coating; any thin, barely visible coating, regardless of the product, is not likely to be adequate.

Cut off a small portion of a branch (4–6 inches long). Expose it directly to a 1½-inch flame, such as a wooden kitchen match or plumber's candle. After a few seconds of exposure, remove the flame. Although some brief afterflaming in the exposed area may occur, burning should not continue and spread into the unexposed part. Never test by applying a flame to the tree itself. This test discloses the degree of flame resistance (natural and/or induced) of the tree at the time.

To determine the adequacy of the treatment after the tree has become dry, accelerate the drying of the sample by placing it in an oven at 200°F for 45 minutes and repeat the test.

For additional details, and licensing requirements for applicators, contact the California Technical Services Division at (916) 427-4563, Office of the State Fire Marshal.

KEROSENE HEATERS

The introduction of kerosene heaters has introduced problems into the American home in that these heaters can be hazardous unless properly used and vented to remove combustion products. In some states, including California, the sale of unvented heaters designed for use inside the home is prohibited by Section 19881 of the Health and Safety Code, which states that no person shall sell, or offer for sale any new or used unvented heater, which is designed to be used inside any dwelling house or unit, with the exeption of an electric heater, or of decorative gas logs for use in a vented fireplace. Unvented fuel-burning room heaters shall not be installed, used, maintained, or permitted to exist in any Group 1 or 2 occupancy nor shall any such heater be installed in any building, whether as a new or as a replacement installation, unless permitted by this section of the law, but can still be sold for use outside the home and for use in other occupancies. The National Kerosene Heater Association has agreed to mark every heater or the boxes containing these heaters with a disclaimer stating "Unvented heaters may not be sold for use in residences in California." For information regarding other states, contact the local county council or city attorney or the National Kerosene Heater Association.[25]

DYES IN COSMETICS AND DRUGS

The Delaney Clause, passed in 1960 and named for then-Rep. James J. Delaney (D-N.Y.) bars the sale of a color additive that the Secretary of Health and Human Services has found to "induce cancer in man or animal". In August 1986, the FDA approved two dyes used in cosmetics and drugs—namely, Orange no. 17 and Red no. 19—which caused rodents to develop liver cancer. The FDA justified this action for external use because their carcinogenic risk for animals is not within the meaning of the Delaney Clause. A panel of Public Health Service scientists had calculated that the chances that Orange no. 17 would cause cancer in a person's lifetime is one in 19 billion and for Red no. 17 the risk is one in nine million.

Chemicals in cosmetics can also produce other problems, and may be primary irritants or sensitizing reactions (usually the latter). The most common sensitizers are paraphenylenediamine (a hair dye), nail polish, perfumes, eye makeup preparations, preservatives (parabens), and lanolin. Dermatitis due to cosmetics commonly affects the eyelids, neck, and ears, and the area chiefly involved may not be that to which the cosmetic was applied. Mild hair-dye dermatitis may initially affect the eyelids, while in the case of nail polish, the eyelids, neck, and face may show a reaction, sparing the nail areas. It should also be noted that nail polish and remover usually contain flammable solvents, such as acetone or related materials, and hence are a significant fire hazard as well.

Cosmetics most often associated with irritant reactions are antiperspirants, depilatories, and parmanent-wave preparations. The health effect on workers in hair parlors and salons has been studied in Utah, but the ventilation and materials used in beauty salons are subjects that seem to be neglected by the health professionals.

HOUSEHOLD CHEMICALS

Detergents and related cleaning compounds are a common cause of dermatitis. Many contain soap and synthetic detergents. When their cleaning and degreasing actions are noted, it is not surprising they can often directly penetrate the horny layer and defat the skin. The rash is usually persistent, and may continue for a long time in spite of treatment. Very few patients can avoid doing household washing, and even a slight contact may cause a condition to appear once the patient is sensitized.

The use of polishes and the wearing of rubber gloves can give rise to problems as well. About half the cases of contact dermatitis are on the hands; in industry, about 90 percent are on the hands.

PLANTS

Common plants responsible for dermatitis are primula, chrysanthemums, celery, tulips, and clematis. Daffodils and narcissi are the cause of many cases among workers with these flowers in the field.

MEDICINES

The following drugs when applied to the skin are often the cause of dermatitis: penicillin, streptomycin, antihistamines, the procaine series of local anaesthetics, neomycin, framycetin, and dequalinium chloride. In some cases, it may be impossible for the person to enter a room, a ward, or an operating room where particles of these drugs are in the atmosphere without developing an extremely itchy skin. Patch tests, in which a few drops of the suspected material are applied to the skin, covered with tape, and allowed to react for 48 hours, unless itching occurs before this time, are used to identify sensitizers causing allergic contact dermatitis. Positive reactions of an allergic nature include inflammation and usually result in papules or vesicles. If negative after 48 hours, they should be reexamined two days later. Some substances give positive patch tests only if the horny layer has been stripped from the area. A negative patch test reaction nearly always indicates an absence of allergic eczematous hypersensitivity to that particular substances.[27]

INCAPACITATING AGENTS

Incapacitating agents, designed to ward off a possible attack by a suspicious stranger, are finding wide use in the form of aerosol pens or containers, especially by women. Several chemicals are available, including MACE (long carried by mail carriers to ward off dog attacks) and the more recently developed Cap-Stun 2.

It is not clear whether these devices qualify under the regulations of the Federal Aviation Agency as "hazardous materials," but on a recent flight this observer noted three women (a passenger and two flight attendants) with the devices in the passenger cabin of a commercial DC-10. Whether these devices (which, like aerosols, can leak or otherwise by accidentally discharged) should be permitted on aircraft, buses, trains, and in other areas where people are limited in their ability to escape from exposure to the agent is not clear. It is suggested that persons carrying such devices should exercise extreme care to prevent accidental or casual discharge.

Even trace or small amounts of some materials in food may be of more significance than we realize. According to Dr. Johan Bjorksten, "The crucial role of aluminum in Alzheimer's disease, and particularly in senile dementia, has been reconfirmed. We are attempting to find those foods, and specifically those brands of foods, which have the lowest aluminum content." He said his research is the first step in developing a diet low in daily aluminum content for the general public. He and his colleagues already have performed more than 10,000 aluminum analyses of 3333 individual water and food samples from across the country at the Bjorksten Research Foundation in Houston, Texas. Of the water samples analyzed thus far, aluminum levels have ranged from as high as 5000 ppb to as low as 1 ppb. He noted that milk has been shown to be relatively low in aluminum, probably due to its high content of aluminum-eliminating calcium. However, soft drinks were found to contain from 60 to 1000 ppb of aluminum.

Of the foods tested, eggs showed nonexistent aluminum levels in the yolk, low levels in the albumin, and high levels in the shell. Calcium present in the shell, apparently limits the amount of aluminum passing into the albumin and yolk.

Many cheeses tested contained high levels of aluminum, which apparently were intentionally added during processing. Also, while some canned fruit (pears and peaches) showed low levels of aluminum, some fresh fruit and vegetables were found to have between 500 and 1000 ppb of aluminum.

Previous studies of dialysis patients, who lack natural defenses against aluminum entering the bloodstream, show that a large number eventually developed symptoms similar to those of Alzheimer's disease. "I believe that everything that has happened in these dialysis patients may eventually happen as well to healthy human beings once they've had adequate time to build up their aluminum levels," he said. Other studies have shown, he remarked, that animal life seems to go out of its way to avoid using aluminum anywhere in its metabolism "as if some hidden danger were lurking near it."

According to Dr. Bjorksten, aluminum is a suspect in diseases of aging because its small size enables the aluminum atom easily to penetrate almost anywhere, its high binding energy allows the aluminum atom to anchor itself in any position from which it cannot be dislodged by any force available to the organism, and the great stability of aluminum compounds causes them to increase at the expense of corresponding compounds of other metals.

With today's average diet yielding about 30 mg/day of aluminum, people begin getting senile at around 80 years. "By cutting that rate in half, it would take perhaps 14 more years of life for senility to set in," Dr. Bjorksten suggests.[28]

IRRADIATION OF FOODS

Irradiation of food promises considerable health as well as economic benefits. With some types of produce, it slows ripening, especially in tropical fruits. Exposing packages to 75 kilorads of radiation (the maximum allowed by law is 10 krads) can extend shelf time 25 percent.

Growers of mushrooms and asparagus, two highly perishable crops, are studying radiation.

Congress has allocated $10 million to the Department of energy to establish six irradiation demonstration facilities in farming regions around the United States.[29]

REFERENCES

1. Bretherick, *Handbook of Reactive Chemical Hazards*, 3rd ed., pp 873–877, Butterworths, London and Boston, 1985.

1a. Amateur rockets and motors made to accepted standards are available from Estes Industries, Penrose, CO 81240

2. M. Lukanov, "Bleaching and Bleaching Agents," *Encyclopaedia of Occupational Health and Safety*, 3rd rev. ed., International Labour Organization, Geneva, 1983.

3. V. J. Clancy, *Fire Hazards of Calcium Hypochlorite*, (*J. Hazardous Materials*), vol. 1, no. 1, 83–94, 1975.

4. Institute of Makers of Explosives, 1120 19th St., N.W., Washington, DC 20036.

5. Chemical Section, Fact Sheet, "Safety in the Use of Home Chemistry Sets," Stock no. 2500-2, 5C26209, National Safety Council, 444 N. Michigan Ave., Chicago, IL 60611.

6. J. Nichols, "Eye Safety in Chemical Operations," Chapter 26, pp. 573–1596, in H. H. Fawcett & W. S. Wood (eds.), *Safety and Accident Prevention in Chemical Operations,* 2nd ed., Wiley-Interscience, New York, 1982.

7. L. Bretherick, *Handbook of Reactive Chemical Hazards,* 3rd ed., pp. 939–1940, Butterworths, London and Boston, 1985.

8. D. A. Pipitone, *Safe Storage of Laboratory Chemicals,* pp. 96–97, Wiley-Interscience, New York, 1984.

9. National Paint and Coatings Asso., 1500 Rhode Island Ave., N.W., Washington, DC 20036.

10. Lead Industries Association, New York, NY 10017, or phone (212) 578-4750 for assistance regarding lead. Note also W. M. Bulkeley and D. Tracy, Lead-Paint Case May Stir Round of Product Suits, *Wall St. J.,* Nov. 18, 1987, 35.

11. Anon., *Indoor Pollutants,* National Academy Press, Washington, DC, 1981.

12. R. B. Gammage and S. V. Kaye, *Indoor Air and Human Health,* 430 pp., Lewis Publishers, Chelsea, Mich., 1985.

13. E. J. Calabrese, *Toxic Susceptibility: Male/Female Differences,* 336 pp., 1985; same author, *Age and Susceptibility to Toxic Substances,* 296 pp., 1986; Wiley-Interscience, New York.

14. Anon., "NFPA 101 Life Safety Code, 1988," National Fire Protection Association, Quincy, Mass.

15. Anon., *Fire and Smoke,* National Academy Press, Washington, D.C., 1986.

16. R. Lewis, *Toxicology of Selected Petroleum Hydrocarbons,* May 18, 1986; "Index and Abstracts for Reports and Other Publications," 1959–1985; H. Westberg and B. Lamb, "Human Exposures to Gasoline Vapors," Final Report, December 1985 by Health Effects Institute for API; H. N. MacFarland et al., "A Chronic Inhalation Study with Unleaded Gasoline Vapor," [reprint from *J. Am. Coll. Toxicol.,* **3,** No. 4, 231–248 (1984)]; S. Rappaport, S. Selvin, and M. Waters, "Gasoline Exposures in the Petroleum Industry, 1987," prepared for API by S. M. Rappaport and associates, available from American Petroleum Institute, 1220 L St., N.W., Washington, DC 20036.

17. Anon., *Handbook of Compressed Gases,* Reinhold, New York, 1988.

18. P. D. Hansten, *Drug Interactions,* 5th ed., Lea & Febiger, Philadelphia, Pa., 1985.

19. Anon., "Hazardous Wastes from Homes," 36 pp., Enterprise for Education, 1320A Santa Monica Mall, Santa Monica, CA 90401; note also video "Disposal of Household Chemicals," 20 minutes, loan from League of Women Voters, Washington, D.C., or local chapters, 1987.

20. Anon., "Disposing of Small Volumes of Photographic Processing Solutions," Eastman Kodak Co., 343 State St., Rochester, NY 14650.

21. Rachael Carson Council, Pesticides and Contract Lawn Maintenance, 8940 Jones Mill Rd., Chevy Chase, MD 20815.

22. Anon., Lawn Care Information Packet," Natural Resource Defense Council, Washington, D.C.

23. Anon., *Least Toxic Lawn Management, Common Sense Pest Control,* vol. 11, no. 2, spring 1986, S. Daar, Bio Integral Resource Center, Box 7414, Berkeley, CA 94707 (the Natural Resources Defense Council has an office at 122 East 42nd St., 45th Floor, New York, NY 10168. toll-free 1-800-648-NRDC for further information).

24. California State Fire Marshal, 7171 Bowling Drive, Suite 600, Sacramento, CA 95823.

25. National Kerosene Heater Association, 15 First American Center, 23rd Floor, Nashville, TN 37238; phone (615) 254-1961.

26. M. Mintz, "How Carcinogenic Dyes Got a Green Light," *Washington Post,* A25 (Feb. 27, 1987).

27. AMA, *Drug Evaluations,* 6th ed., 1650 pp, American Medical Association, Chicago, Ill., (Sept. 1986).

28. Anon., *Psychiatry '87,* **4** (June 1987) (published at P.O. Box 154, Mount Royal, NJ 08061); see also B. Meeham, and S. J. Meyer, "Is Your Child Taking Drugs?" *Readers Digest,* 55–59 (July 1986).

29. Anon., "Produce Freshness (by Radiation Treatment)," *Wall St. J.,* 23 (June 19, 1987).

SUGGESTED READINGS

Anon., "Repeated Oral Activated Charcoal in Acute Poisoning," *Lancet,* 1013–1015 (May 2, 1987).

Anon., "What To Do After An Accident. Claiming Compensation for Injury and Damage, and Coping with the After-Effects, 190 pp., consumers' Association, 14 Buckingham St., London WC2 N 6 DS, England, 1987.

Anon., "Questions and Answers, Protective Effect of Fabric Against Solar Radiation," *JAMA,* 106 (July 3, 1987).

Anon., "Rehabilitation Approaches to Drug and Alcohol Dependency," *Occu. Health Safety,* 91 (March 1985).

Anon., "The Great Soap Opera," *Consumer Repts.,* 423–426 (July 1987).

C. M. Ardies et al., "Effects of Exercise and Ethanol on Liver Mitochondrial Function," *Life Sci.,* 1052–1053 (March 16, 1987).

D. A. Brent et al., "Alcohol, Firearms and Suicide among Youth," *JAMA,* 3369–3372 (June 26, 1987).

B. G. Barley, "Stress and Disease," *Ladies' Home J.,* 38, 40, 132, 134 (May 1987).

C. E. Butterworth, Jr., *Nutritional Factors in the Induction and Maintenance of Malignancy,* 336 pp., Academic Press, Orlando, Fla., 1983.

A. Barber, "Anti-allergy Strategies: Love and Pollen Share the Air," *NIH Record,* National Institutes of Health, vol. 39, no. 9, 1, 2 (May 5, 1987).

Catalogue, *Technology for Survival,* Universal Electronics, 15015 Ventura Blvd., Sherman Oaks, CA 91403.

M. Diamond, *Fit for Life: A New Way of Eating,* 156 pp., Warner Books, New York, 1987.

P. J. Dyck et al., "Assessment of Nerve damage in the Feet of Long-Distance Runners," *Mayo Clinic Proc.,* **62,** No. 7, 568–1572 (July 1987).

L. Ember, Indoor Air Quality Program Set Up at EPA, *Chem. Eng. News,* 42 (July 20, 1987).

J. Elkington, *The Poisoned Womb: Human Reproduction in a Polluted World,* 255 pp., paper, Penguin Books, New York, 1985.

J. Fishman and B. Anrod, *Something's Got to Taste Good: The Cancer Patient's Cookbook,* 222 pp., Andrews and McMeel, 4400 Johnson Drive, Fairway, KS 66205, 1981.

A. M. Freedman, "Space-Age Savor: Flavor Specialists Strive for Better Microwave Foods," *Wall St. J.,* 17 (July 29, 1987).

R. Genders, *Cosmetics from the Earth—A Guide to Natural Beauty,* Alfred van der Marck, New York, 1985.

J. C. Giblin, *Milk: The Fight for Purity,* 106 pp., Thomas Y. Crowell, New York, 1986.

M. F. Gould, "Food Additives," *Lancet,* 1209 (May 23, 1987).

P. Johnson, *The Border War on Drugs,* Congress of the U.S. Office of Technology Assessment, OTA-0-336, Washington, D.C. (March 1987).

M. M. Jones et al, Chemistry & Society, 5th ed. Saunders College Pub., Holt, Rinehart & Winston, 15–45 Philadelphia, New York, and Chicago 1987.

A. P. Kaplan, *Allergy,* 718 pp., Churchill Livingstone, New York (distributed by Longman, White Plains, N.Y.), 1986.

W. E. M. Lands, *Fish and Human Health,* 170 pp., Academic Press, Orlando, Fla. (1986).

W. Mertz, *Trace Elements in Human and Animal Nutrition,* 5th ed., 460 pp., in two volumes, Academic Press, Orlando, Fla., 1987.

D. K. Pitts, "Cardovascular Effects of Cocaine in Anesthetized and Conscious Rats," *Life Sci.,* 1099–1112 (March 16, 1987).

W. H. J. Rogmans, "Prevention of Accidental Poisoning in Childhood," European Consumer Products Safety Association, The Hague, The Netherlands.

A. E. Slaby and P. L. McGuire, "Prevention of Child and Adolescent Suicide," *Psychiatry Lett.*, Fair Oaks Hospital, **IV,** issue 12, 65–74, (Dec. 1986) (Summit, N.J.).

W. J. Storck, "Demand for Home and Garden Pesticides Spurs New Products," *Chem. Eng. News,* 11–17 (April 6, 1987).

W. J. Storck, "Pesticides Growth Slows," *Chem & Engr. News,* 35–42 (Nov. 16, 1987).

A. P. Simopoulos, *Health Effects of Polyunsaturated Fatty Acids in Seafoods,* 458 pp., Academic Press, Orlando, Fla., 1986

A. J. Swallow, "Food Irradiation," *Lancet,* 1209 (May 23, 1987); also 810 (April 4, 1987), and 700 (March 21, 1987).

E. Tenner, "WARNING: Nature May Be Hazardous to Your Health," *Harvard Mag.*, **90,** No. 1, 34–38 (Sept.–Oct. 1987).

A. J. Vlitos, "Sugar and Health," *Lancet,* 918 (April 10, 1987).

J. M. Watson, *Solvent Abuse: the Adolescent Epidemic,* 234 pp., Croom Helm, London, England, 1986.

C. Welsh and B. Diffy, The Protection Against Solar Actinic Radiation Afforded by Common Clothing Fabrics, *Clin. Exp. Dermatol,* vol. 6, 577–82, 1981

F. L. Wiseman, Chemistry in the Modern World—Concepts and Applications, 495 pages, McGraw-Hill, New York 1985

Appendix: Controlled Substances (Drugs)

The drugs that come under the jurisdiction of the Controlled Substances Act in the United States are divided into five schedules. Listed below are some examples.

SCHEDULE I SUBSTANCES

The drugs in this schedule are those that have no accepted medical use in the United States and have a high abuse potential. Some examples are heroin, marijuana, LSD, peyote, mescaline, psilocybin, tetrahydrocannabinois, ketobemidone, levomoramide, racemoramide, benzylmorphine, dihydromorphine, nicocodeine, nicomorphine, methaqualone, and others.

SCHEDULE II SUBSTANCES

The drugs in this schedule have a high abuse potential with severe psychic or physical dependence liability. Schedule II controlled substances consist of certain narcotic, stimulant, and depressant drugs. Some examples of Schedule II narcotic controlled substances are opium, morphine, codeine, hydromorphone (Dilaudid), methadone (Dolophine), pantopon, meperidine (Demerol), cocaine, oxycodone (Percodan), anileridine (Leritine), and oxymorphone (Numorphan). Schedule II nonnarcotics are amphetamine (Benzedrine, Dexedrine) and methamphetamine (Desoxy), phenmetrazine (preludin), methylphenidate (Ritalin), amobarbital, pentobarbital, secobarbital, etorphine hydrochloride, diphenoxylate, and phencyclidine.

SCHEDULE III SUBSTANCES

The drugs in this schedule have an abuse potential less than those in Schedules I and II, and include compounds containing limited quantities of certain narcotic drugs, and nonnarcotic drugs such as derivatives of barbituric acid except those that are listed in another schedule, Glutethimide (Doriden), methyprylon (Noludar), chlorhexadol, sulfondiethylmethane, sulfonmethane, nalophine, benzphetamine, chlorphentemine, clortemine, mazindol, phendimetrazine, and paregoric.

SCHEDULE IV SUBSTANCES

The drugs in this schedule have an abuse potential less than those listed in Schedule III and include such drugs as barbital, phenobarbital, methylphenobarbital, chloral betaine (Beta Chlor), chloral hydrate, ethchlorvynol (Placidyl), ethinamate (Valmid), meprobamate (Equanil, Miltown), paraldehyde, methohexital, fenfluramine, diethylpropion, phentemine, chlordiazepoxide (Librium), diazepam (Valium), oxazepam (Serax), clorazepate (Tranxene), flurazepam (Dalmane), clonazepam (Clonopin), prazepam (Verstan), lorazepam (Ativan), mebutamate, and dextropropoxyphene (Darvon).

SCHEDULE V SUBSTANCES

The drugs in this schedule have an abuse potential less than those listed in Schedule IV and consist of preparations containing limited quantities of certain narcotic drugs, generally for antitussive and antidiarrheal purposes.

RETAIL DISTRIBUTION RESTRICTIONS FOR SCHEDULE V SUBSTANCES

Schedule V controlled substances or any controlled substance which is not a prescription item under the federal Food, Drug, and Cosmetic Act may be distributed without a prescription order at retail provided that such distribution is made only by a pharmacist and not by a nonpharmacist employee even if under the direct supervision of a pharmacist. However, after the pharmacist has fulfilled his or her professional and legal responsibilities, the actual cash, credit transaction, or delivery may be completed by a nonpharmacist. *Source:* Drug Enforcement Administration, Registration Unit ODRR, 1405 Eye Street, N.W., Washington, DC 20537. This administration is part of the U.S. Department of Justice.

16

Medical Care and Surveillance Program for Hazardous-Waste Workers

D. J. Kilian, Pamela Harris, and Susan Goddard

In many large industries, occupational health programs[1] for employees working with and around hazardous substances or physical forces have been developed into sophisticated models over the past 40 years. In many instances, they had a difficult beginning, but have evolved into impressive coordinated efforts involving management, safety professionals, industrial hygienists, and medical personnel. Many programs have progressed to medical surveillance, and epidemiologic and environmental studies that far outstrip health efforts in the private sector. The hazardous-waste industry is a relative newcomer to this area, with most responsible and well-organized companies being less than two decades old. Consequently, they do not have the experience and recognition of the problems that have existed since the beginning of the chemical, petrochemical, and petroleum industries. Time is required for companies to understand that these programs not only are good for their employees but are also are essential for the survival of the company. This is particularly true of the hazardous-waste industry, where litigation by employees and the community is abnormally high. The best legal defense for community challenges is a healthy, well-documented work force. In many cases, claims are made that have no reasonable scientific or medical justification, but a disturbing lack of 'no effect' health data leaves management in a difficult defense situation. Documentation of employee health status combined with an analysis of group data to be discussed later will provide substantial evidence that can be of great use and value to a company.

The older model health programs involving chemicals, radiation, or physical stresses practically always indicate knowledge of the specific agent involved along with the time and concentration of exposure. Furthermore, many times it is possible to search the literature for assistance regarding the human health effect from a particular health threat as well as animal toxicology studies or biochemical research. In the hazardous-waste industry, there is frequently a disturbing lack of ability to sort out exactly which chemical or dust is potentially a specific problem, as usually complex mixtures are involved.

Melius[2] concludes the following regarding medical monitoring of hazardous-waste workers: "Medical monitoring of these workers is problematic. While monitoring for the potential health effects of these multiple exposures may be useful, any attempt to monitor for possible health effects of all potential exposures could lead to a long array of medical tests. The utility and effectiveness of this approach is doubtful." We disagree with this conclusion, and feel that any hazardous-waste worker should have a complete medical workup designed to detect any effect from the complex mixtures that might be contacted. Federal law dictates that the generator provide a manifest to the disposer, so that the components of the mixture *are* known. Rapid access to a knowledgeable occupational physician is essential so that any unusual hazard (e.g., cyanide) can be monitored with urinary thiocyanate levels. In most instances, determination of the hazardous waste is very complex and often dictates the use of maximal personal protective equipment (see Chapter 11). This may be difficult to accomplish when the worker does not know what chemial is involved or its toxicological properties. Many times the assumption is made that the situation is not critical enough to require uncomfortable protective equipment. This is the main reason why the hazardous-waste industry must put great emphasis on good industrial hygiene programs and training in the proper use of personal protective equipment. Also, there must be good medical information about proper first aid after chemical exposure and the human health consequences of exposure to chemicals, hazardous dusts, radiation, biohazards or other potential problems in the workplace. Such audiovisual teaching talks[3] are available and are practical teaching tools for small or large groups of workers in this industry. Figure 16.1 is an example of a portion of such an audiovisual talk. Exposure to the training and written rules regarding the proper use of protective equipment must be documented by a signature from the employee. This provides great assistance in enforcing the rules, which should have discipline, including discharge for noncompliance.

Many hazardous-waste companies are facing difficult litigation in the negligence and intentional tort areas because the employee maintains that "nobody warned me about the hazards of the material. I was working with," or "nobody really made me wear a respirator." Because of the high rate of contracting certain jobs (many times the most disagreeable and hazardous), the litigation problems are magnified due to third-party involvement and the lack of spaces worker's compensation protection for the company. Most hazardous-waste workers have a wide variety of jobs to perform—each with its unique set of hazards—and this compounds the safety and personal protective equipment problems. The worker may be on heavy equipment preparing a secure landfill site (Figure 16.2), or processing chemicals into 55-gallon drums for storage into secure landfill sites (Figure 16.3). Since many waste-disposal

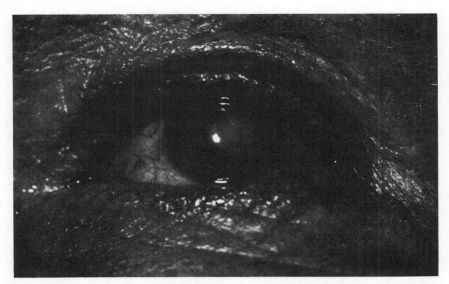

Figure 16.1. Permanent damage to corners of the eye from sodium hydroxide burn. Prompt and copious irrigation with plain water would have prevented this degree of injury. (Photo by D. J. Kilian.)

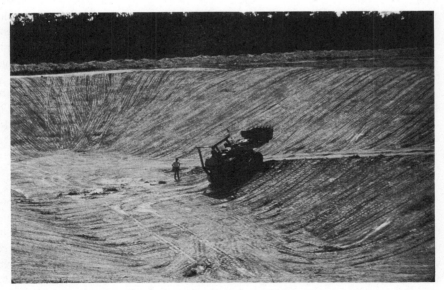

Figure 16.2. Hazardous-waste-site workers who operate heavy equipment in isolated locations may be required to take periodic health examinations. (Photo by D. J. Kilian.)

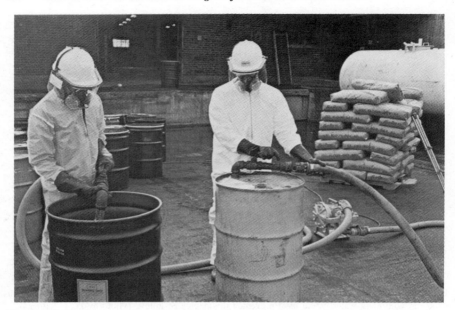

Figure 16.3. Proper protective equipment and periodic documentation of training is a must for hazardous-waste industry. (Photo by D. J. Kilian.)

sites operate on a 24-hour schedule, the worker may be required to put in long hours and be responsible for directing a newly arrived tank truck (Figure 16.4) to the proper off-loading site in the middle of the night. With the so many different jobs being performed, it is impossible at times to know what chemicals the employee is working around, and this dictates the need for proper personal protective gear and periodic medical surveillance.

However, this protective equipment can create problems of its own. Many waste sites are in the South, and during hot weather heat stress can be a real problem. It is essential to train these employees to recognize the early symptoms of heat exhaustion and to teach them the importance of maintaining proper hydration, as well as taking appropriate breaks to cool off. This worker profile illustrates the great need for as good as, or even better than, occupational health programs than the chemical industry now has in effect.

A superior occupational health program involves understanding and contributions from an informed management, industrial hygienists, safety engineers, training professionals, and medical personnel. The program must have the protection of the employee's health as its first priority, but it also can serve as a valuable resource in advising certain management functions, such as personnel, claims, line supervision, and the legal area. Preemployment and periodic medical exams should be performed, as well as, when indicated, biological monitoring. Because of the nature of the chemical worker's duties, industrial hygiene monitoring sometimes falls short of always being able to assure a safe work environment. Such monitoring is an

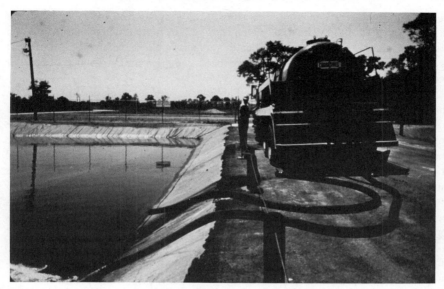

Figure 16.4. Many hazardous liquid wastes are brought to the processing site in a vacuum truck. The liquid will then be solidified and placed in a government-approved secure landfill. (Photo by D. J. Kilian.)

essential tool to evaluate an exposure and certainly should be done at each waste site.

Because of the mixed and frequently changing exposures, figures and statistics can be generated that may, in some instances, imply a false sense of security regarding environmental chemical hazards. Used properly, biological monitoring can be a valuable complement to industrial hygiene surveys. For example, blood leads, expired-air analyses, urinary metabolites, and other specialized tests not only give information on exposure but also on the accumulation of chemicals in the human body, along with levels that assist in evaluating the human health hazards. With some chemicals, environmental monitoring will yield the most important information. With other chemicals, biological monitoring is far superior. It takes a well-trained expert in occupational health to know which is more appropriate. Today many hazardous-waste companies do not recognize the need for this expertise, and are jeopardizing the health of their workers.

For several years, workers in the chemical industry have had their permissible chemical exposures regulated by federal (OSHA) and, in some instances, state or local standards. These were based primarily on the application and utilization of spaces of the threshold limit values (TLVs) and time-weighted averages (TWAs) of specific chemicals involved (see Chapter 8). Provisions were set in place for calculating allowable exposures when working more than an eight-hour day or when exposed to more than one chemical. It is difficult to apply these principles to a hazardous-waste worker because of the problems mentioned previously regarding mixed, and frequently changing, exposures. In this situation, it calls for innovative skills on the part of the industrial hygienist as well as more reliance on medical and biological monitoring. Long-range health studies should be established to prevent health effects that, unfortunately, have been rather common in the history of occupational medicine.

Medical surveillance is an integrated approach to evaluating not only the health status of the individual employee but of the entire work force as well. It requires a complete preemployment physical examination to determine the fitness of the applicant to perform the job, and also to serve as a baseline to detect early or subtle changes in a variety of health parameters so that corrective action can be instituted at an early stage to avoid permanent physical effects. This strategy requires a thorough hands-on physical examination by a qualified physician familiar with the work site and the materials handled. For example, it would not be wise to assign a person to a job involving asbestos disposal if that person had a prior history of asbestos exposure and also evidence of pleural plaques on preemployment X-rays.

As with the chemical industry, medical surveillance is important to the hazardous-waste industry because potential human health effects cannot be predicted by industrial hygiene monitoring alone. Medical monitoring as part of a medical surveillance program takes on even greater importance in light of the ever-changing environment in obtaining industrial hygiene data at a hazardous-waste facility. No industrial hygiene survey can reflect all of the potential exposure hazards at a site where exposures may change hourly. There are also problems with combined exposures, possible reactions between agents, and the expense of identifying all unknown chemicals in a sample. It must also be remembered that industrial hygiene monitoring measures only the *potential* exposures. If proper protective equipment is worn, an individual in a high-exposure area may have no health effects, but an individual who is more lax about self-protection may be at risk even though monitoring has identified his or her work site to be a low-exposure area.

Industrial hygiene data are a valuable part of a medical surveillance program. The survey data generated through an industrial hygiene program should be used to establish the parameters of the physical examination. Under the Occupational Safety and Health Act (PL 94-198 or OSHA), special kinds of medical testing and monitoring must be conducted when specific agents are identified in the workplace. These requirements for the hazardous-waste industry can be found in the OSHA "Standards for General Industry,"[8] as well as in 29 CFR, Part 1910, Hazardous Waste Operations and Emergency Response interim final rule, published in the *Federal Register,* **51,** No. 244, 45654–45675, (Dec. 19, 1986), which amends the OSHA standards for hazardous materials in Subpart H of 29 CFR Part 1910 by adding a new paragraph, 1910.120, containing employee protection requirements for workers engaged in hazardous-waste operations, including emergency response to hazardous substance incidents. Beyond the OSHA requirements, the presence, and therefore potential exposure, of certain agents warrants special medical monitoring because of the possibility of serious health effects and the importance of early detection.

The requirements of the physical examination are determined not only by OSHA standards, analysis of industrial hygiene data, potential exposures, and accepted medical practice, but also by the results of ongoing medical testing. If the results of an individual or a group indicate a problem, special testing may be required or additional tests may need to be added to the routine medical monitoring of the other personnel in the work force. For example, if the routine blood count reveals a low white count and the work site handles benzene, then repeated and additional hematological tests must be performed. Often it is wise to refer such an individual to a hematologist for a complete workup. Many times such investigations reveal a nonoccupational cause, but it is to the benefit of the company, as well as to the person, to discover health problems early and reduce insurance costs and loss of productivity.

The hazardous-waste industry cannot always rely on conventional testing measures. Heavy metal exposure is a good example. Metal exposure in the hazardous-waste industry may be from any one or combination of a large number of metals. The exposure is likely to be sporadic and may be the result of organic or inorganic forms of a metal. Analysis of the blood usually measures the metal that is absorbed and temporarily in circulation before deposition or excretion. Urinary analysis measures the metal that is absorbed but then excreted. Both of these conventional methods are exposure-time dependent. With a relatively constant exposure, such as might be found in a heavy-metal shelter, blood or urinary measures will probably be an accurate reflection of an individual's exposure. However, unless the tests are conducted at the correct time after a sporadic exposure, such as found in the hazardous-waste industry, measurements of metal levels may fail to detect an exposure problem. An additional consideration is the cost of conducting blood and/or urine analysis on five, six, or even seven different metals.

The hair is a tissue in which trace metals are bioaccumulated. The hair grows at approximately a centimeter a month. Therefore, a 3-cm length of hair analyzed for metals represents an average of three months of exposure. Because of the problems in standardizing preparation and analysis techniques, and disagreement concerning normal ranges of metals in the hair, hair analysis for heavy metal should be considered only as a screening tool. Hair analysis should not be used as a definite measure of abnormal body burden. If problems are identified through hair analysis, they should be investigated further using conventional medical testing methods. The analysis of the hair allows the quantification of several metals often at less than the cost of a single element analysis in the blood.[9,10] However, hair analysis has not gained the confidence of the majority of physicians because of its questionable accuracy and the exaggerated claims of some laboratories. Triple washing of the sample before analysis to eliminate external contamination can yield useful information, but the use must be decided on a case-by-case basis.

The recognition of the acquired immune deficiency syndrome (AIDS) and the resulting opportunistic diseases, such as cancer and fatal infections, has focused great attention on the immune system. Diagnostic tests for evaluation of the immune dysfunction have steadily evolved over the years and are at a stage where objective studies can be made. An example is the immune study done by the Mount Sinai

School of Medicine[11] on 45 Michigan farm residents who ingested food contaminated with polybrominated biphenyls (PBBs). When the results were compared with 46 nonexposed residents in Wisconsin, there was highly significant evidence of immune suppression when these diagnostic tests were utilized. A study in experimental animals[12] revealed that immune suppression can be produced in mice by doses of dioxin (TCDD) around 1 μg/kg body weight per week. This is a minuscule exposure, and since this material is easily absorbed through the skin or gastrointestinal tract, concern should be raised for workers exposed to this or similar material. Extrapolation of animal data to human significance is always difficult, but this work indicates that human exposure most certainly should be studied more intensely. For the past few years, the chemical and hazardous-waste industries have had many problems defending litigation where the claim has been made that the workplace has suppressed the immune system. At this point, there has not been enough human data developed with these tests to be certain of their significance, and several companies are undertaking good prospective immune studies to answer these questions.

For the most part, the specifics of the physical examination must be determined using industrial hygiene data and the past experiences of the chemical industry. There are little data in the literature that address the exposure-problem or health-effects issues in the hazardous-waste industry. Medical surveillance programs should include a full preemployment evaluation to assess an individual's capabilities and ensure proper placement. As important as establishing the person's health status, the preemployment examination also serves to document baseline data. This baseline profile is the point from which future health changes will be measured. Periodic examinations are also a part of an effective medical surveillance program. They provide early detection of health effects from exposure to chemical, biologic, or physical hazards. This early detection may prevent progression to a more serious disease state and be a flag to look for early problems in other workers. The time frame between periodic examinations (every six months, annually, once every two years) will depend on the types of work being performed and the kinds of exposures that can be expected. Time frames may also change based on the results of past examination. An effective medical surveillance program must always be flexible and capable of adjusting to changes.

A great deal of attention should be paid to the development of health-history questionnaires used in the hazardous-waste industry. The industry has the potential to handle materials that are known carcinogens, mutagens, and teratogens. A health-history questionnaire must thoroughly investigate past family health histories and the reproductive history of the worker and spouse. It should contain an exposure history (Chart 16.1) and attempt to examine life-style parameters. Parameters such as smoking, alcohol, and drug usage should be quantified whenever possible. The exposure history should contain questions concerning employment in specific industries, as well as exposure to specific chemicals. The completed questionnaire should be reviewed by the examining physician before the physical examination, and special tests should be added if indicated by questionnaire responses.

EXPOSURE HISTORY

Have you ever worked in or around a:	YES	NO	Have you ever worked with or been exposed to:	YES	NO		YES	NO
1. Chemical plant			26. Aldrin			51. Ethylene oxide		
2. Chemistry laboratory			27. Arsenic			52. Extreme heat or cold		
3. Coke oven			28. Asbestos			53. Heptachlor		
4. Construction			29. Benzene			54. Hexachlorobenzene		
5. Cotton, flax or hemp mill			30. Benzidine			55. Isocyanates (TDI, MDI)		
6. Electronics plant			31. Beryllium			56. Lead		
7. Farm			32. Bis chlormethyl ether			57. Loud or continuous noise		
8. Foundry			33. Cadmium			58. Mercury		
9. Hazardous waste industry			34. Carbon disulfide			59. Methylene chloride		
10. Hospital			35. Carbon tetrachloride			60. Microwaves, lasers		
11. Lumber mill			36. Chlorine			61. Nickel		
12. Metal production			37. Chlorodane			62. PCB's		
13. Mine			38. Chloroform			63. Pesticides, herbicides		
14. Nuclear industry			39. Chloroprene			64. Phenols		
15. Paper mill			40. Chromates			65. Phosgene		
16. Pharmaceutical			41. Chromic acid mist			66. Plastics		
17. Plastic production			42. Cutting oils			67. Radioative materials		
18. Pottery mill			43. DDT			68. Roofing materials		
19. Refinery			44. Dieldrin			69. Rubber		
20. Rubber processing plant			45. Dioxin			70. Silica		
21. Sand pit or quarry			46. Dust, coal			71. Solvents/degreasers		
22. Service station			47. Dust, sandblasting			72. Soots and tars		
23. Shipyard			48. Dust, other			73. Spray painting		
24. Smelter			49. Epoxy resins			74. Tri/per chloroethylene		
25. Waste industry			50. Ethylene dibromide			75. Vinyl chloride		

EXPLAIN ALL "YES" ANSWERS BY NUMBERS IN THE SPACE BELOW (GIVE APPROXIMATE DATES AND TOTAL NUMBER OF YEARS OF EXPOSURE). (PHYSICIAN: if assistance is required in interpreting exposure history information contact 713-670-7803.)

Chart 16.1. Form-questionnaire used to probe patient's occupational history.

As with many other industries, the hazardous-waste industry is faced with decisions concerning drug program/policy.[5] Drug testing is an emotional issue. It has raised concerns of possible violation of employee privacy and constitutional rights as well as concerns about accuracy and fairness. On the other side of the issue, the public has demanded that industries entrusted with the management of potentially dangerous materials ensure and insure the capability and safety of their employees. A President's Commission Report went so far as to call for widespread drug testing of all government employees.[6]

Before any company, regardless of the industry, implements a drug-testing program, many decisions must be made and a commitment given for a consistent program. A drug policy shoud be a safety and productive policy. Its purpose and plan should be to protect the safety of employees and the public. It is difficult to develop and enforce a business policy that is based on morality, or even legality. The policy should clearly state the company's plan and expectations. It should list prohibitive acts (e.g., possession, usage, selling, intoxication), where and when prohibition applies (e.g., on company time, property, vehicles, project sites), to which drugs and/or alcohol and to whom the policy applies (e.g. employees—full or part time, visitors, contractors, or vendors).

If the program includes drug screening, additional decisions are required. In general, there are three kinds of drug screening: preemployment, random, and probable cause. The courts have placed more restrictions on the testing of employees than on screening of jobs. Employers may establish freedom from use of illicit drugs as a condition of employment. Probable-cause testing, such as triggered by observation of unusual or unsafe behavior or an accident, is more likely to pass legal scrutiny than random testing done without regard to job performance. Private employers have greater rights to test current employees than do government employers. Other decisions necessary include which drugs to test for and the definition of a positive drug test. Some employers test only for illicit drugs, not prescription or over-the-counter medications. Not all employers test for marijuana. Urinary alcohol levels have little legal meaning. However, all states have a legal definition of alcohol impairment in blood concentrations. Urinary levels for drugs that define impairment do not exist so an employer must choose how a positive drug screen will be defined. Most laboratories report drugs such as cocaine, amphetamines, barbiturates, and opiates as detected or not detected. Marijuana is usually reported in nanograms of tetrahydrocannabinol (THC) per milliliter of urine. A physician or toxicologist can then advise as to what quantity of THC would be acceptable. Choosing a laboratory for drug screening must be done carefully. It should have a confirmation system to assure accuracy and minimize false positives. Analytical techniques should be state of the art. The laboratory should have a formal claim of custody procedure and be capable of litigation support.

It is important to inform all employees before a policy is put in place. Training front-line supervisors can actually be a more valuable tool than drug screening. Many companies also have employee assistance programs available to aid employees identified with drug or alcohol problems.

ANALYSIS OF MEDICAL SURVEILLANCE DATA

The data generated from a medical surveillance program must be in usable form. Though most hazardous-waste work forces are small, it is still difficult to control data adequately through paper files. Computerization of records offers more convenient storage and retrieval, and allows the statistical manipulation that would prove to be quite tedious if done by hand. There are several commercial computer software packages, which can be purchased, leased, or used through time-sharing agreements, that handle the kinds of information necessary for a medical surveillance program.[13] Computer programs can also be specifically written for a particular system or company. A computerized data base allows something as simple as an automated tick file, which gives the names of individuals who require an updated examination. Reports can be generated that identify and summarize problem areas that may have been missed using paper files. With some kinds of exposure, OSHA's record-keeping requirements are employment plus 30 years. Computer records are a much more efficient means of storing such bulk data. The computerized data base also allows correlation between work place exposures and health status, and makes group-trend analyses possible. Trend analysis, over time, on one individual can be conducted using paper files without a great deal of effort. Elevation of liver enzymes over the baseline for one worker over the course of employment can frequently provide clues of possible occupational etiology. However, group-trend analysis is a useful tool to identify shifts in the normal range for the whole work force and to activate remedial changes in the occupational environment before more serious health effects occur.

Many of the sophisticated (and very expensive) software packages for occupational health analysis require large mainframe computers that only large corporations have the resources to utilize. Intriguing software[14] for IBM PC (personal) computers has been developed that can allow smaller occupational medicine clinics rapidly to develop trend and group analysis of employee data. This is an important development as this is where most occupational medicine is practiced. Examples of the use of this software for trend analysis is demonstrated in Charts 16.2 and 16.3, to illustrate an organic lead exposure, and it reveals an upward shift of both urinary and blood lead values with time. Physicians rarely have the time to plot out such values manually, and an assistant can easily be trained to imput the data into the personal computer to assist the physician in evaluating possible changes in the work environment as reflected by the biological monitoring.

Visual computer-generated data on a hazardous-waste work force can be of great assistance to the responsible physician in evaluating any environmental or protective equipment changes that might affect the medical testing or the biological monitoring of organ system tests. This is well illustrated in scattergrams (Charts 16.4 and 16.5) of a work group that could have been exposed to organic lead. Each point on the scattergram would represent a separate determination of urinary or blood lead. It reveals not only an upward shift of composite values of the entire group but also a group relationship between the blood and urinary results. Chart 16.6 illustrates how group data generated on a personal computer can be useful to

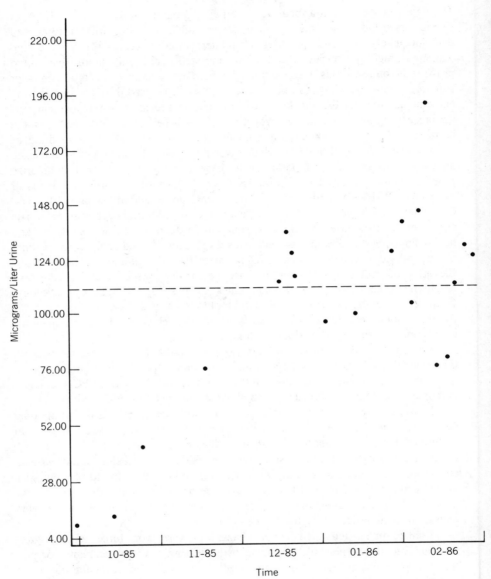

Chart 16.2. Organic lead values as reflected by urine lead levels in worker.

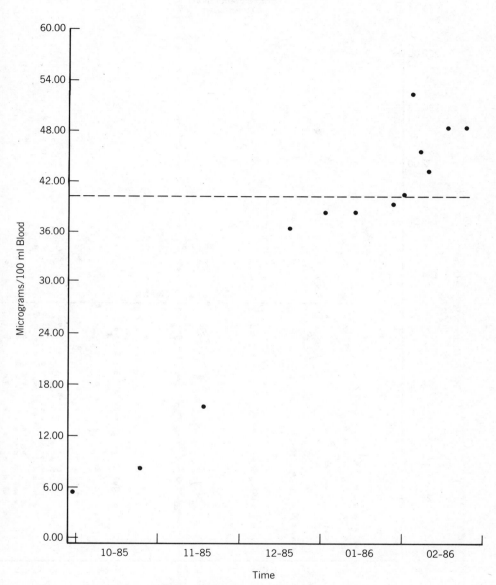

Chart 16.3. Organic lead levels as reflected in blood-level of worker.

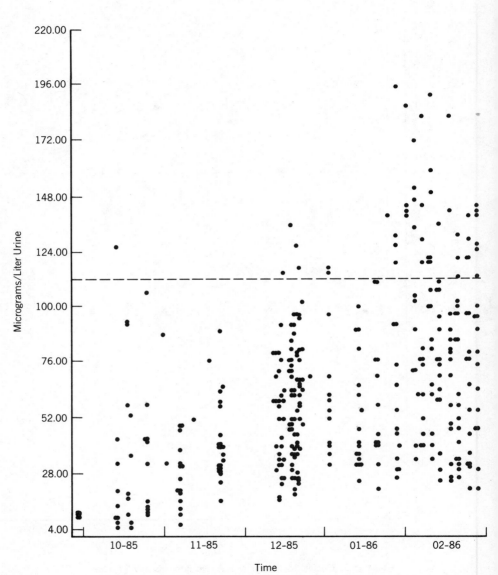

Chart 16.4. Scattergram of work group monitored for lead in urine.

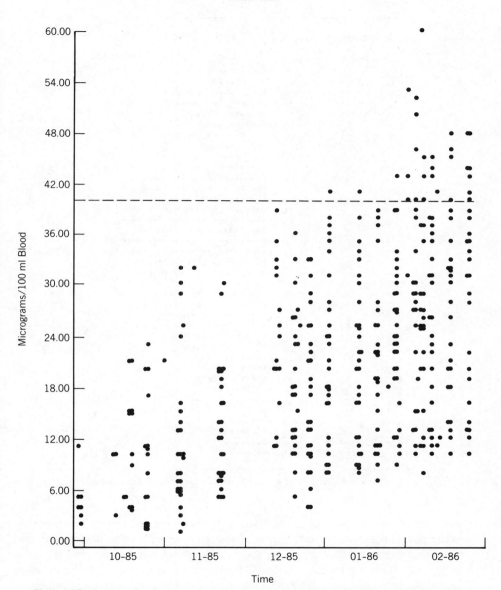

Chart 16.5. Scattergram of same work group shown in Chart 16.4, using urine as indicator of lead.

XYZ Corporation
SGPT

Six-month moving averages

Date—Range		Avg.	
11/81	4/82	31.87	**********************
12/81	5/82	31.81	**********************
1/82	6/82	32.00	**********************
2/82	7/82	28.11	******************
3/82	8/82	24.12	***************
4/82	9/82	21.75	*************
5/82	10/82	20.14	***********
6/82	11/82	20.33	************
7/82	12/82	21.00	************
8/82	1/83	23.00	**************
9/82	2/83	33.68	***********************
10/82	3/83	34.92	************************
11/82	4/83	34.92	************************
12/82	5/83	35.44	*************************
1/83	6/83	35.44	*************************
2/83	7/83	35.55	*************************
3/83	8/83	41.00	******************************
4/83	9/83	36.15	**************************
5/83	10/83	35.33	*************************
6/83	11/83	34.31	************************
7/83	12/83	32.40	**********************
8/83	1/84	37.64	***************************
9/83	2/84	31.71	**********************
10/83	3/84	31.15	*********************
11/83	4/84	29.18	*******************
12/83	5/84	28.59	*******************
1/84	6/84	27.24	*****************
2/84	7/84	22.47	**************
3/84	8/84	21.41	************
4/84	9/84	20.89	************
5/84	10/84	19.40	**********
6/84	11/84	16.50	********
7/84	12/84	17.92	*********
8/84	1/85	19.57	***********
9/84	2/85	18.93	**********
10/84	3/85	19.09	**********
11/84	4/85	19.40	**********

Chart 16.6. Printout of computerized data for study of clinical data.

evaluate the results of clinical chemistries, hematology, pulmonary functions, or other medical parameters that generate objective numbers. We have found that software programmed to analyze for six-month moving averages generate the most useful data. This chart utilizes the SGPT liver-enzyme test, which is one of the most useful to detect acute liver injury. An interesting improvement is noted in values for about eight months, and then a reversal that finally improved. One must interpret these results with caution, as such changes could be due to a high employee turnover rate, a possible influence from hepatitis in the community, or problems in managing a proper environmental or protective equipment program. However, it is a valuable tool to be used with discretion to correct some occupational-health problems. Chart 16.7 utilizes the white blood count, which could be useful in the

XYZ Corporation
WBC

Six-month moving averages

Date—Range		Avg.	
11/81	4/82	7.97	*************************
12/81	5/82	8.52	****************************
1/82	6/82	8.94	*****************************
2/82	7/82	9.02	******************************
3/82	8/82	8.98	*****************************
4/82	9/82	8.90	*****************************
5/82	10/82	8.73	****************************
6/82	11/82	7.95	************************
7/82	12/82	7.80	***********************
8/82	1/83	7.67	***********************
9/82	2/83	6.87	******************
10/82	3/83	7.10	*******************
11/82	4/83	7.10	*******************
12/82	5/83	6.96	******************
1/83	6/83	6.96	******************
2/83	7/83	6.97	******************
3/83	8/83	7.27	********************
4/83	9/83	7.44	*********************
5/83	10/83	7.47	*********************
6/83	11/83	7.82	***********************
7/83	12/83	7.49	*********************
8/83	1/84	7.32	********************
9/83	2/84	8.80	****************************
10/83	3/84	7.65	***********************
11/83	4/84	7.77	***********************
12/83	5/84	7.64	***********************
1/84	6/84	7.77	***********************
2/84	7/84	8.03	*************************
3/84	8/84	7.69	**********************
4/84	9/84	7.75	***********************
5/84	10/84	7.43	*********************
6/84	11/84	7.01	******************
7/84	12/84	7.48	*********************
8/84	1/85	6.55	****************
9/84	2/85	6.60	****************
10/84	3/85	6.51	****************
11/84	4/85	6.67	*****************

Chart 16.7. Printout of hematopoetic (blood) effect on workers exposed to benzene.

early detection of subtle changes indicative of hematopoetic effect of a group of workers exposed to benzene. One could use the platelet count or the mean corpuscular volume as a further refinement in early detection. These examples illustrate methodology that can be utilized to detect shifts within the normal range so that appropriate investigation can be instituted before serious health effects occur.

SUMMARY AND CONCLUSIONS

In the previous discussion, we described the difficult problems that the hazardous-waste industry faces in protecting the health of its employees. Because of the newness of its management structure, there is great difficulty in recognizing the need for sophisticated industrial hygiene and occupational medical programs. Most of the workers have had only a few years of service and the problem of long-term chronic diseases has yet to be faced. The turnover rate is high due to the unpleasant work involved, and this compounds the problem of assembling a good data base for epidemiology study. Legal defenses for alleged health effects are and will be difficult to undertake. Undoubtedly the driving force to improve the occupational-health programs will result from the litigation losses cutting sharply into the profit margin. It becomes obvious that those companies who recognize this fact early and take appropriate steps to establish a good occupational-health program will survive in this highly competitive industry.

We have outlined the steps necessary for an adequate program and indicated which phases are the most important. The cost of health professionals and medical diagnosis is high, but experience in the chemical industry has shown that these costs are essential for survival. It is imperative to recognize that the worker health problems in the hazardous-waste industry are formidable, but that implementation of the programs presented can ensure the maximum chance for a health worker. The lists in Appendix A, B, D, and E may suggest a starting point.

REFERENCES

1. B. D. D. Dinman, "Medical Aspects of the Occupational Environment," in *Industrial Environment—Its Evaluation and Control"*, National Institute of Occupational Safety and Health, U.S. Government Printing Office, Washington, D.C., 1973.

2. J. M. Melius, "Medical Surveillance for Hazardous Waste Workers," *J. Occup. Med.*, **28,** 679–684 (1986).

3. Medical Graphic Arts, Box 34, Lake Jackson, TX 77566.

4. "Standards and Guidelines for Cardiopulmonary Resuscitation (CPR) and Emergency Cardiac Care (ECC)." *JAMA*, **255,** No 21, (June 6, 1986).

5. N. Dunivant, "Drug Testing in Major U.S. Corporations—A Survey of the Fortune 500," Noel Dunivant and Associates: Raleigh, N.C., Oct. 1985.

6. "Report of the Presidential Commission on Organized Crime," p. 452. March 3, 1986.

7. T. J. Donegan et al., "Workplace Drug Testing," *The Legal Issues in Employee Testing and the Law*, Vol. 1, No. 3, November 1986.

8. "Occupational Safety and Health Administration Standards for General Industry," U.S. Department of Labor, OSHA Safety and Health Standards (29 CFR 1910), OSHA 2206 (revised Jan. 1, 1976, 649 pp.), U.S. Government Printing Office, Washington, D.C., or Commerce Clearing House, Inc., Chicago, Ill., Apr. 1, 1981.

9. D. W. Jenkins, "Toxic Trace Metals in Mammalian Hair and Nails," EPA-600/4-79-049, U.S. Environmental Protection Agency, Washington, D.C., Aug. 1979.

10. D. W. Jenkins, "Biological Monitoring of Toxic Trace Metals," Vol. 1, Biological Monitoring and Surveillance, EPA-600/3-80-089, U.S. Environmental Protection Agency, Washington, D.C., Sept. 1980.

11. J. G. Bekesi et al., "Immunologic Dysfunction Among PBB Exposed Michigan Daily Farmers," *Ann. N.Y. Acad. Sci.*, 320, 1979.

12. R. P. Sharma and P. J. Gehring, "Effects of 2,3,7,8-Tetrachlorodibenzo-p-dioxin (TCDD) on Splenic Lymphocyte Transformation in Mice after Single and Repeated Exposures," *Ann. N.Y. Acad. Sci.,* 320, 1978.

13. "Computer Systems Review," *Ind. Safe. Hyg. News,* 1–14 (Aug. 1983); see also G. I. Ouchi, *Personal Computers for Scientists—A Byte at a Time,* 276 pp., American Chemical Society, Washington, D.C., 1987.

14. Science Dynamics Corporation, P.O. Drawer 1787, Alvin, TX 77512.

SUGGESTED READINGS

Anon., "Occupational Diseases—A Guide to Their Recognition," DHEW (NIOSH) Publication No. 77-181, 1978.

Anon., "Dioxin Brief," Department of Community Health and Medical Care, St. Louis County, Missouri Division of Health, St. Louis, Mo., Jan. 18, 1983.

C. Ansberry, AIDS, Stirring Panic and Prejudice, Tests the Nation's Character, *Wall St. J.,* Nov. 13, 1987, 1, 6

C. R. Asfahl, *Industrial Safety and Health Management,* Prentice-Hall, Englewood Clifts, N.J., 1984.

Anon., "The Decision Against a Heart Drug," *Wall St. J.,* 22 (July 13, 1987).

S. S. Chissick and R. Derricot (eds.), *Asbestos: Applications and Hazards,* Vol. 1, 1979, Vol. 2, 1983, Wiley, Chichester, England, and New York.

S. S. Chissick and R. Derricott (eds.), *Occupational Health and Safety Management,* Wiley, Chichester, England, and New York, 1984.

R. A. F. Cox, *Offshore Medicine: Medical Care of Employees in the Offshore Oil Industry,* Springer-Verlag, New York, 1987.

G. W. Dawson and B. W. Mercer, *Hazardous Waste Management,* 532 pp., Wiley-Interscience, New York, 1986.

H. H. Fawcett and W. S. Wood (eds.), *Safety and Accident Prevention in Chemical Operations,* 2nd ed., 910 pp., Wiley-Interscience, New York, 1982.

V. Foa, E. A. Emmett, M. Maroni, and A. Colombi, *Occupational and Environmental Chemical Hazards: Cellular and Biochemical Indices for Monitoring Toxicity,* 558 pp., Wiley-Interscience, New York, 1987.

H. Freeman, Mental Health and the Environment, 469 pp., Churchill Livingstone, New York, 1984

J. M. Gould, "Environmental Abuse and Public Health," *Chem. Eng. Prog.,* 5 (July 1987).

M. H. Ho and H. Kenneth Dillon, *Biological Monitoring of Exposure to Chemicals, Organic Compounds,* 352 pp., Wiley-Interscience, New York, 1987.

J. A. Lee, The New Nurse In Industry, 110 pages, DHEW (NIOSH) Publication, No. 78-143, National Institute for Occupational Health and Safety, 1978.

ILO, *Encyclopaedia of Occupational Health and Safety,* 3rd rev. ed., in two volumes, 2538 pp., International Labour Organization, Geneva, Switzerland, or USILO Office, 1750 New York Ave., Washington, DC 20006, 1983.

S. L. Jacobs, "Industrial Hygienists Increase Firms Output and Efficiency," *Wall St. J.,* 33 (March 5, 1984).

M. Key and D. J. Kilian, "Counseling and Cancer Prevention Programs in Industry," in *Cancer Prevention in Clinical Medicine,* Raven Press, New York, 1983.

W. H. Lederer and R. J. Fensterheim (eds.), *Arsenic—Industrial, Biomedical, Environmental Perspectives,* Van Nostrand Reinhold, New York, 1984.

S. P. Levin and W. F. Martin, *Protecting Personnel at Hazardous Waste Sites,* 384 pp., Butterworth Publishers, Stoneham, Mass., 1984.

B. S. Levy and D. H. Wegman (eds.), *Occupational Health: Recognizing and Preventing Work-Related Diseases,* Little, Brown, Boston, 1984.

W. F. Martin, J. M. Lippit, and T. G. Prothero, *Hazardous Waste Handbook for Health and Safety,* 470 pp., Butterworth, Stoneham, Mass., 1984.

N. H. Proctor and J. P. Hughes, *Chemical Hazards of the Workplace,* 533 pp., J. B. Lippincott, Philadelphia and Toronto, 1978.

W. Rom (ed.), *Environmental and Occupational Medicine,* Little, Brown, Boston, 1983.

I. Rosenfeld, *Modern Prevention: The New Medicine,* 432 pp., Linden Press/Simon & Schuster, New York, 1986.

M. Rutter and R. R. Jones (eds.), *Lead versus Health: Sources and Effect of Low Level Lead Exposure,* Wiley, Chichester, England, 1983.

J. S. Sizer and B. S. Schindler, "In-house Medical Team Provides Emergency Response to Workers," *Occup. Health Safety,* 47–49 (June 1987).

R. E. Tucker, A. L. Young, and A. P. Gray, *Human and Environmental Risks of Chlorinated Dioxins and Related Compounds,* 823 pp., Plenum Press, New York and London, 1983.

17

Occupational Disease Awareness— The Teaching of Occupational Medicine in British and Irish Medical Schools

Ralph W. Fawcett

To deal with a problem properly, one must be aware of its existence. Awareness of occupational disease began centuries ago with observations of Hippocrates, Pliny the Elder, Paracelsus, and others, including the alchemists, who, in addition to seeking the Elixer of Life and the Philosopher's Stone, learned to their sorrow that certain substances, including lead, arsenic, and mercury, are toxic. In 1700, Ramazzini published *De Morbis artificum diatriba,* the first book that could be considered a complete treatise on occupational diseases. In the second edition, 1717, he discussed not only diseases resulting from excessive exposures to dusts and metal fumes, but also the effects of overexposure to several chemicals. As another important element in clinical evaluation, Ramazzini suggested that the examining physician ask one more question than those specified by Hippocrates, namely: "What is your occupation?" Unfortunately, even today, the question of occupation is often not routinely elaborated upon in medical history taking. Since a third of most patients' lives is spent at work, the potential impact of occupational effects, from either chronic or acute exposures, must be considered by the physician, no matter what his or her specialty.

In 1775, the London surgeon Percivall Pott recognized that cancer of the scrotum in chimney sweeps was an occupational disease. Three years later, rules requiring chimney sweeps to bathe daily were passed in Denmark, an early health measure that may have done more to prevent human cancer than the filing of reports by many research workers. Asbestos disease was first discovered at autopsy in London in 1899, and the beryllium disease from zinc beryllium silicate phosphors in the

1940s was first noted by a physician, as was the angiosarcoma of vinyl chloride monomer.[1]

Society eventually recognized the relationship betwen occupation and health, and, beginning in 1802, England passed a series of acts to protect workers, including the Health and Morals of Apprentices Act, establishing the first child-labor laws for cotton factories. It required, for example, the "washing down" of workplaces *twice a year*.

In Ireland, the Factory and Workshop Act of 1901, followed by the Irish Factory Act of 1955,[2] stipulated control measures to protect the workers' health.

In 1951, a British committee of inquiry chaired by Judge Dale considered comprehensive occupational-health provisions covering both industrial and nonindustrial occupations. Ten years later, the Council of the British Medical Association gave its opinion that sufficient evidence had accumulated for action, and the Parrett Committee endorced this view. A committee was organized, which produced the Robens Report in 1970–72, and eventually led to the passage of the comprehensive Health and Safety Act of 1974.[3] This act consolidated under the Health and Safety Executive the various directorates from previous laws, including the Factory Inspectorate, the Mines and Quarries Inspectorate, the Agriculture Safety Inspectorate, Radiochemical Inspections, and the Alkali and Clean Air Inspectorates. In addition to the main task of inspections, which are conducted on a frequency keyed to the perceived relative hazards of the industry, a wide variety of activities include investigations, research, and liaison with the legislators and with industry. The adversary relationship, often noted in legal manipulation in other countries, is largely lacking in the Irish and British programs, since regulations are usually agreed upon by all parties in advance of their promulgation, and enforced by persons with sufficient background information to ensure the *spirit* of the law. Simultaneously with the Health and Safety Act, the National Health Service created positions for specialists in environmental medicine to supplement the act with personnel needed to provide technical and medical input to the inspectors.

With the increased emphasis on health, as related to occupational exposures, it might be assumed that educational institutions would be acutely aware of the need for expanded training programs. A study in 1974 considered the role of occupational medicine in the 30 medical schools of the United Kingdom. The questionnaire inquired as to in what form instruction in occupational medicine was given, since suitable training might influence the career decisions of young graduates in entering this relatively new specialty of medicine.

Four schools—Dundee, Manchester, Newcastle, and the Welsh National—had departments of occupational medicine. Only seven of the 25 schools that replied allocate six or more hours to instruction in occupational medicine, while seven others gave from two to five hours to this subject. These numbers should be seen in the context of 1500–2000 contact hours in the clinical years of medical schools. Factory visits supplement formal instruction in some schools surveyed.[4]

In order to stimulate undergraduate student interest, Dr. Waldron has written *Lecture Notes on Occupational Medicine*,[5] in which he briefly describes and discusses the role of occupational diseases, the mechanism of action, the clinical features, and the treatment of common industrial toxicant exposures, such as lead, mercury, cadmium, beryllium, manganese, chromium, nickel, phosphorous and organo-phosphorous compounds, the organic compounds such as benzene and other cyclic compounds, the halogenated hydrocarbons, vinyl halides, the aromatic and aliphatic amines, nitro and phenolic compounds, and common pesticides. Industrial gases, such as carbon monoxide, carbon dioxide, hydrogen sulfide, phosgene, the oxides of nitrogen, arsine, phosphine, and the physiologically inert gases, such as nitrogen, argon, xenon, krypton, helium, hydrogen, and methane (the last two being highly flammable as fuels), and foreign-body granuloma, pulmonary edema, chemical pneumonitis, pneumoconiosis, and other lung involvements are considered. Diseases of the skin from occupational and natural agents, including skin sensitizers, are discussed. Poorly recognized but important agents are the dermatoses from certain imported woods. Physical hazards, including decompression sickness, heat, cold, occupational cataracts, shock (electrical and mechanical), miners' nystagmus, ionizing, and nonionizing radiation, noise, and infectious diseases, including serum hepatitis, anthrax, glanders, and Weil's disease (the last being an acute disease in human caused by infection with Leptospira icterohaemorrahagiae, found in rats and excreted by the rodent, making sewer workers, miners, bargemen, and workers in slaughterhouses and fish markets occupations at risk) are referenced.

With regard to postgraduate training, three universities (Manchester, Newcastle, and Dundee) offer training for a diploma in industrial hygiene. Diplomas in the Republic of Ireland and in the United Kingdom are granted by universities for academic achievement beyond the first professional degree, for example, the medical degree. They certify additional competence in a field, but do not require the many years of specialized training to become a member of a Royal College, such as the Royal College of Physicians (equivalent to the American Board of Internal Medicine).[6]

The London School of Hygiene and Tropical Medicine operates an institute of occupational health, which offers a course leading to a master of science in occupational medicine. This course requires nine months, but can also be taken over two years on a part-time basis. The institute also offers a three-month course for the D.I.H. (diploma in industrial health).

To assist on the graduate level, a more advanced text, *Occupational Health and Safety Concepts,* was recently published. In this book, Dr. Atherly introduces occupational health in terms of human safety, including an input–output model as a criterion for chemical-exposure evaluation. The role of the body's defenses against invasion from aerosols, stress, heat and cold, and metabolic transformation and conjugation is stressed. Modes of action, pathological processes, and diseases following harmful inputs are considered, with detailed examples of where control measures were not adequate until after serious exposures had occurred. The various strategies that can be employed to ensure the control of occupational exposures and diseases to an acceptable level are discussed in considerable detail, including in-depth analysis of the American and other TLVs and PELs. As part of these strategies, Dr. Atherley believes that all workers should be told something of the materials with which they come into contact, and not be left to find out for themselves, often at a higher risk and cost in both human health and economic terms than can be justified by the employee or the employer. (Note that this was written before the promulgation of the American OSHA Hazard Communication regulation, which requires material safety data sheets on every chemical in the workplace.)

As the environment becomes more complex, hazards may be introduced with little thought to their consequences. An interesting example is the changes occurring in offices. With the introduction of new technology (such as microprocessors, computers, visual display units or VDUs, reader units, new types of duplicating equipment, and related materials), offices are receiving long-overdue attention in terms of hazard control. The recently published booklet *Office Worker's Survival Handbook—A Guide to Fighting Health Hazards in the Office* illustrates the growing awareness and expanding scope of occupational health.[8] In addition, increased attention to indoor health hazards is bringing a new awareness of the problems of daily living.[9]

In conclusion, the United Kingdom and the Republic of Ireland are well aware of occupational disease and the control measures required to reduce the risks, but education and training in occupational medicine resulting in wide awareness and prevention before the fact have yet to be widely appreciated. The relatively recent interests of America are reflected by Appendices A, B, C, and E.

REFERENCES

1. C. E. Searle (ed.), *Chemical Carcinogens,* 2nd ed., in two volumes, ACS Mongraph 173, American Chemical Society, Washington, D.C., 1984; Hamilton and Hardy's *Industrial Toxicology,* A. J. Finkel (ed.), 4th ed. 446 pp., PSG Co., 1983.

2. "Factories Act of 1955," *Irish Law Times and Solicitors* J., **89,** 185 et seq. (1955).

3. For details of the major points of the British Health and Safety Act of 1974, see L. Bretherick (ed.), *Hazards in the Chemical Laboratory,* 4th ed., pp. 11–18, The Royal Society of Chemistry, London, 1986; see also other publications of the Health and Safety Executive, including: "Safety Representatives and Safety Committees' "Guidance Notes on Employer's Policy Statements for Health and Safety at Work, Advice to Employees, MHUDAS major hazard incident data service of H&S Executive (computerized).

4. H. A. Waldron, "Undergraduate Training in Occupational Medicine," *Lancet,* 277–278 (Aug. 3, 1974).

5. H. A. Waldron, *Lecture Notes on Occupational Medicine,* Blackwell Scientific Publications, Oxford, 1976.

6. Personal correspondence, H. A. Weldon to R. W. Fawcett, July 1, 1981.

7. G. R. C. Atherley, *Occupational Health and Safety Concepts—Chemical and Processing Hazards,* Applied Science Publishers, London, 1978.

8. M. Craig, *Office Worker's Survival Handbook: A Guide to Fighting Health Hazards in the Office,* BSSRS Publishing, London, 1981.

9. R. B. Gammage and S. V. Kaye, *Indoor Air and Human Health,* 430 pp., Lewis Publishers, Chelsea, Mich., 1985.

SUGGESTED READING

anon, "Early Detection of Occupational Diseases," 270 pp, World Health Organization, Switzerland, 1987

G. Hommel, "Handbuch der Gefahrlichen Guter (Handbook of Dangerous Goods)," 3 volumes, Springer-Verlag, Germany, 1987.

WHO/ILO "Multimedia Promotional Kit—Practical Guidelines for Reducing Drug and Alcohol Problems in the Workplace," World Health Organization, Switzerland, 1987

18

Superfund

Ronald D. Hill

In response to public concern over poor past disposal practices of hazardous wastes and the thousands of uncontrolled waste sites throughout the United States, in December 1980 Congress enacted the Comprehensive Environmental Response, Compensation and Liability Act, PL 96-510,[1] commonly known as CERCLA or Superfund. This Act was a result of the wide publicity that sites such as Love Canal, Valley of the Drums, and Stringfellow had received that made the public aware that uncontrolled hazardous-waste sites were either causing harm to the public health and environment or were a potential threat.

The Superfund Act was enacted in part because of the recognition that the Resource Conservation and Recovery Act, commonly referred to as RCRA or Solid Waste Act, provided a regulatory program for active hazardous-waste facilities but not inactive sites. Superfund afforded a federal response to the uncontrolled release of hazardous substances from a vessel or from any onshore or offshore facility. A key feature of the Act was the establishment of a trust fund to support the clean-up activities. This fund received $1.6 billion over a five-year period. The revenue was supported 87.5 percent by taxes on petroleum and chemical feedstock and 12.5 percent from a Treasury appropriation. This authority ran out in December 1985. After almost a year without new authority, extensive amendments, known as the Superfund Amendments and Reauthorization Act, P.L. 99-499,[2] called SARA, were adopted October 17, 1986. This Act established a new fund of $8.5 billion over a five-year period beginning January 1, 1987. The principal sources of revenue are a tax on petroleum, and on 42 listed chemicals, a broad-based corporate environmental tax, and appropriations from general revenues.

Although EPA has been severely criticized by Congress for lack of action in the cleanup of hazardous-waste sites, its record of activities during the first five years has been extensive.[3] A preliminary assessment of 20,023 sites was made. A total of

1477 sites was scored using the Hazardous Rating System to evaluate the health and environmental threat posed by the sites. The EPA placed 703 sites on the National Priority List (NPL) and 185 more sites were proposed for listing. Since this report, even more sites have been proposed. Some form of response action had been taken at 1174 sites and emergency response actions, often called removal actions, had been commenced at 808 sites. Of these sites, 611 had been financed by the government, 150 by the potentially responsible parties (PRP), and 47 by both the EPA and the PRPs. Remedial investigations and feasibility studies (RI/FS) were begun at 468 sites and long-term actions were completed at 14 NPL sites. The value of PRP response actions was estimated at $818 million.

OVERVIEW OF CERCLA AND SARA

As specified in its name, CERCLA is a very comprehensive law, directing the EPA, other federal agencies, and the states on how to collect and manage the "fund," conduct cleanups, and recover the costs of federally supported actions from the PRPs. The 1980 legislation established a fairly straightforward structure to attain these goals. The 1986 SARA amendments did not fundamentally alter the structure, but added far more detail than was present in the original law, as well as some additional requirements and provisions. In fact, the length of the amendments exceeded that of the original law.

The detailed new provisions speak of such issues as "how clean is clean," by defining cleanup standards and a preference for permanent-treatment on-site remedies. Deadlines with specific numbers of actions that must be taken for evaluating sites, placing them on the NPL, and undertaking response actions are included. Health-effects study requirements, applicable to every site on the NPL, were added. A new title was added on emergency planning and community right-to-know in response to concerns raised over catastrophic releases of toxic chemicals, as in the Bhopal, India, disaster where 2500 people were killed.

RELEASES, HAZARDOUS SUBSTANCES, REPORTABLE QUANTITIES

Section 103 of Superfund specifies that responsible parties must report to the federal government's National Response Center (800 424-8802) any spill or other release of a hazardous substance to the environment in a reportable quantity. Congress defines a "release" as any spill leaking, pumping, pouring, emitting, emptying, discharging, injecting, escaping, leaching, dumping, or disposing into the environment, including the abandonment or discharging of barrels, containers, and other closed receptacles containing any hazardous substance, pollutant, or contaminant.[2]

What is a "hazardous substance"? Superfund defines a "hazardous substance" as (1) any substance designated as a hazardous pollutant under Section 311 of the Clean Air Act; (2) any toxic pollutant listed under Section 307(a) of the Clean Water Act; (3) any hazardous air pollutant listed under Section 112 of the Clean Air Act;

(4) any hazardous waste under RACA; (5) any imminently hazardous chemical substance or mixture with regard to which the EPA Administrator has taken action under Section 7 of the Toxic Substance Control Act (TSCA); and (6) any substance designated as hazardous under Section 102 of Superfund. When all of these lists were combined into a "list of lists," 717 hazardous substances were identified.[4] The "list of lists" is presented in Appendix A.

The term "hazardous substance" does not include petroleum, natural gas, or synthetic gas of pipeline quality. In addition, certain solid wastes are suspended from regulation. These include solid waste from the extraction, beneficiation, and processing of ores and minerals, cement kiln dust, and waste generated from the combustion of coal or other fossil fuels.

Superfund also requires the EPA to establish regulations on "reportable quantities." This requirement establishes the quantity for each hazardous substance, the release of which shall be reported. "Reportable quantities" have been promulgated for 442 hazardous substances based on scientific criteria relating to the risk posed by a release of that substance (Appendix A).[4] The EPA is evaluating the remaining 275 hazardous substances for potential carcinogenicity and chronic toxicity. Until the EPA sets a reportable quantity for these substances, the quantity previously established under Section 311 of the Clean Water Act is used, or, if none exists, the reportable quantity is 1 pound.

The reportable quantities start at 1 pound for many substances and range up to 5000 pounds for substances such as chloroform, carbon tetrachloride, and hydrochloric acid. For mixtures and solutions, there is a "release" when a component hazardous substance is in the mixture or solution in its reportable quantity.

NATIONAL CONTINGENCY PLAN (NCP)

The cornerstone of the removal and remedial program of Superfund is the NCP. Section 105 of Superfund[1,2] specifies the content of this plan. The plan establishes the procedures, and standards, for responding to releases of hazardous substances, pollutants, and contaminants. In addition, it contains the NPL. This list indicates those sites that present the greatest danger to public health and welfare or the environment, and thus are eligible for cleanup action under Superfund. The NCP includes matters such as:

1. Methods for discovering and investigating facilities at which hazardous substances have been disposed of or otherwise came to be located.

2. Methods for evaluating, including analyses of relative cost, and remedying any releases or threats of releases from facilities that pose substantial danger to the public health or the environment.

3. Methods and criteria for determining the appropriate extent of removal, remedy, and other measures.

4. Appropriate roles and responsibilities for the federal, state, and local governments, and for interstate and nongovernmental entites in effectuating the plan.

5. A method for and assignment of responsibility for reporting the existence of such facilities that may be located on federally owned or controlled properties.

6. Criteria for determining priorities among releases or threatened releases throughout the United States (Hazard Ranking System—HRS).

The NCP was substantially revised and last reissued in November 1985.[5] SARA requires several changes in the NCP and a revised plan will be issued by the EPA in 1988.

There are seven phases for determining the appropriate response to a release of hazardous substances:

1. Discovery and notification.
2. Preliminary assessment and evaluation.
3. Removal actions.
4. Site evaluation and NPL determination.
5. Community relations.
6. Remedial action.
7. Documentation and cost recovery.

DISCOVERY AND NOTIFICATION

The response to a hazardous release starts when the EPA is informed that a release has occurred or is imminent. This notification can come from several sources, including a notification to the NRC; notification by the owners or operators of a facility; or investigations by state and federal government authorities. Over 25,000 sites have been identified in this manner.[3]

PRELIMINARY ASSESSMENT AND EVALUATION

A notification of a release will result in the EPA's undertaking a preliminary assessment ot evaluate the need for a "response action."

The assessment includes an evaluation of the magnitude of the hazard; the identification of any party or parties who are ready, willing, and able to undertake a response action; and an evaluation of whatever immediate removal is necessary. Readily available information and data are reviewed at this stage. Available records, photographs, etc., are collected and personal interviews are conducted. A perimeter inspection of the site to assess the potential for a release may also be taken.

The preliminary assessment will be terminated when it is determined that there has been no release; the released does not involve a hazardous substance, pollutant, or contaminant; the amount released does not require a federal response; a responsible party is providing an appropriate response; or the assessment is completed.

If the assessment includes the determination that a "removal action" is necessary, then the EPA is required to identify responsible parties and have them conduct a removal action or conduct the action themselves. If the assessment indicates a "remedial action" is necessary, then the procedures specified in the NCP for a remedial action is undertaken.

REMOVAL ACTIONS

Removal actions are undertaken when the EPA determines that there is a threat to public health or welfare or the environment. This determination is made after reviewing the following factors:

1. Is there an actual or potential exposure to hazardous substances or contaminants by nearby populations, animals, or food chains?
2. Is there an actual or potential contamination of drinking-water supplies or sensitive ecosystems?
3. Is there a hazardous substance or pollutant or contaminants in drums, barrels, tanks, or other bulk-storage containers that may pose a threat of release?
4. Is there a threat of fire or explosion?
5. Are there high levels of hazardous substances and soils that may migrate?
6. Are there weather conditions that may cause hazardous substances to migrate?

The purpose of a removal action is to abate, minimize, stabilize, mitigate, or eliminate a public health threat. In essence, a removal is usually a "Band-aid" action to abate the immediate threat of a hazardous waste to the public health or environment. It usually does not lead to a complete cleanup of a site. The complete cleanup follows the system described in the NCP.

Removal actions may include as simple an action as the installation of a security fence and warning signs to prevent access of humans and animals to the release or destruction of the waste on site, or the removal of the waste to approved RCRA facilities for treatment of disposal. Removal actions have included such activities as installation of drainage controls to prevent runoff of contaminated waters; capping of contaminated soils and sludges; segregation and storage of drummed wastes; removal of highly contaminated soils, sludges, or drums; provision of alternative water supplies; and incineration or treatment of waste on site.

SARA places a limit on removal actions of $2 million and/or the lapse of 12 months from the date of the initial removal, unless it is found that circumstances warrant continued action. Because of the "emergency" nature of removal actions, they are not required to comply with other federal, state, or local laws governing hazardous-waste disposal and treatment such as permit requirements. However, removal actions are required to the greatest extent practicable to meet or exceed applicable or relevant and appropriate federal public health and environmental requirements.

If the removal action does not sufficiently abate the trend, an orderly transition from a removal to a remedial action occurs. By mid-1986, the EPA had commenced removal actions at 808 sites.

SITE EVALUATION AND NATIONAL PRIORITY LIST

Those sites that the EPA decides warrant further evaluation after complection of a preliminary assessment undergo a site inspection (SI).[6] SIs generally include on-site and off-site observations and sampling to identify the presence of hazardous substances and to determine whether off-site migration has occurred. The SI should complete the collection of data so that an HRS scoring can take place.

The HRS is one of the most significant processes under Superfund because the decision to list or not list a particular site on the NPL is based on the HRS ranking. An HRS listing of a site assures evaluation of that site to determine the exact nature and extent of the risk that it presents and the most effective remediation alternative; that is, RI/FS process. Listing a site also means that federal fund money could be spent on the site and that PRPs will be identified for cleanup cost or action.

The HRS[7] evaluates relative risk among hazardous-waste sites. Risk is a composite measure of the probability and magnitude of adverse effects, and is specified in terms of what the risks are and who is at risk. In the first case, the concern is the "risk of" a release, exposure, health effect, and/or ecological damage. The second case is the "risk to" an individual, a population group, or an environmental resource. A hazardous-waste site usually poses a variety of risks to a variety of targets, and the HRS is intended to rank sites in terms of their overall relative risks to humans and the environment. A uniform application of the ranking system enables EPA to make a technical judgment regarding the potential hazards presented by a facility relative to other facilities. It does not address the feasibility, desirability, or degree of cleanup required.

The HRS assigns three scores to a hazardous facility:

S_M reflects the potential for harm to humans or the environment from migration of a hazardous substance away from the facility by routes involving ground water, surface water, or air. It is a composite of separate scores for each of the three routes.

S_{FE} reflects the potential for harm from substances that can explode or cause fires.

S_{DC} reflects the potential for harm from direct contact with hazardous substances at the facility (i.e., no migration need be involved).

The score for each hazard mode (migration, fire and explosion, and direct contact) or route is obtained by considering a set of factors that characterize the potential of the facility to cause harm (Table 18.1). Each factor is assigned a numerical value (on a scale of 0 to 3, 5, or 8) according to prescribed guidelines. This value is then multiplied by a weighting factor yielding the factor score. The factor scores are then combined: scores within a factor category are added; then the total scores for each factor category are multiplied together to develop a score for groundwater, surface water, air, fire and explosion, and direct contact.

In computing S_{FE}, S_{DC}, or an individual migration route score, the product of individual category scores is divided by the maximum possible score, and the resulting ratio is multiplied by 100. The last step puts the score on a scale of 0 to 100.

S_M is a composite of the scores for the three possible migration routes:

$$S_M = \frac{1}{1.73} \ \sqrt{S_{gw}^2 \ S_{sw}^2 \ S_a^2}$$

where
S_{gw} = groundwater route score
S_{sw} = surface route score
S_a = air-route score

The effect of this means of combining the route scores is to emphasize the primary (highest scoring) route in aggregating route scores while giving some additional consideration to the secondary or tertiary routes if they score high. The factor 1/1.73 is used simply for the purpose of reducing S_M scores to a 100-point scale.

The HRS does not quantify the probability of harm from a facility or the magnitude of the harm that could result, although the factors have been selected in order to approximate both those elements of risk. It is a procedure for ranking facilities in terms of the potential threat they pose by describing:

The manner in which the hazardous substances are contained;

The route by which they would be released;

The characteristics and amount of the harmful substances; and

The likely targets.

The multiplicative combination of factor category scores is an approximation of the more rigorous approach in which one would express the hazard posed by a facility as the product of the probability of a harmful occurrence and the magnitude of the potential damage.

The ranking of facilities nationally for remedial action will be based primarily on $S_M \cdot S_{FE}$ and S_{DC} may be used to identify facilities requiring emergency attention. Details on the calculation of HRS scores are presented in Ref. 7.

The Superfund amendments (SARA) required EPA, within 18 months after the enactment of the Act (October 17, 1986), to amend the HRS to assure, to the maximum extent feasible, that the hazard ranking system accurately assesses the relative degree of risk to human health and the environment posed by sites and facilities subject to review. The amended HRS should become effective within 24 months of the enactment or no later than October 1988.

As of June 1986,[8] 703 sites had been placed on the NPL and another 185 sites had been proposed (Figure 18.1). Table 18.2 presents a list of the NPL sites by state/territory. New Jersey, Michigan, New York, Pennsylvania, and California lead the list with 97, 66, 65, 65, and 61 sites respectively. Figure 18.2 and Table 18.3 show the type of activities at each of the 888 sites and Figure 18.3 shows the observed contamination.

TABLE 18.1. Of Comprehensive List to Rating Factors

Hazard Mode	Factor Category	Factors		
		Groundwater Route	Surface-Water Route	Air Route
Migration	Route characteristics	Depth to Aquifer of concern Net precipitation Permeability of unsaturated zone Physical state	Facility slope and intervening terrain One-year 24-hour rainfall Distance to nearest surface water Physical state	
	Containment	Containment	Containment	
	Waste characteristics	Toxicity/persistence Hazardous-waste quantity	Toxicity/persistence Hazardous-waste quantity	Reactivity/incompatibility Toxicity Hazardous-waste quantity
	Targets	Groundwater use Distance to nearest well/population served	Surface-water use Distance to sensitive environment Population served/distance to water intake downstream	Land use Population from within 4-mile radius Distance to sensitive environment

Fire and explosion	Containment	
	Containment	
	Waste characteristics	Direct evidence
		Ignitability
		Reactivity
		Incompatibility
		Hazardous-Waste Quantity
	Targets	Distances to nearest population
		Distance to nearest building
		Distance to nearest sensitive environment
		Land use
		Population within two-mile radius
		Number of buildings within two-mile radius
Direct contact	Observed incident	
	Accessibility	Accessibility of hazardous substances
	Containment	Containment
	Toxicity	Toxicity
	Targets	Population within one-mile radius
		Distance to critical habitat

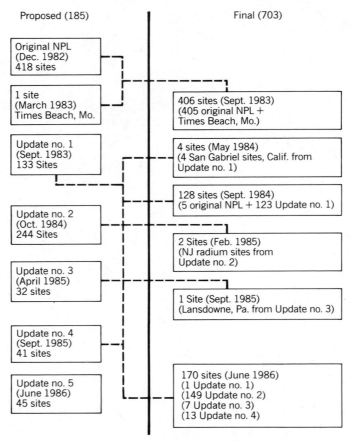

Figure 18.1. Development of NPL.

TABLE 18.2. Final and Proposed NPL Sites per State/Territory (by Total Sites) June 1986

State/Territory	Final NPL	Proposed* Nonfederal	Proposed* Federal	Proposed* Total
New Jersey	91	3	3	97
Michigan	56	10	0	66
New York	57	7	1	65
Pennsylvania	48	14	3	65
California	34	19	8	61
Florida	32	7	0	39
Minnesota	36	2	0	38
Ohio	27	3	0	30
Wisconsin	26	4	0	30
Indiana	23	5	0	28
Washington	19	3	6	28
Texas	21	3	2	26
Illinois	14	7	4	25

TABLE 18.2. (*Continued*)

State/Territory	Final NPL	Proposed* Nonfederal	Proposed* Federal	Total
Massachusetts	21	0	0	21
Missouri	12	3	2	17
Colorado	12	1	2	15
Delaware	9	4	1	14
Iowa	6	7	0	13
New Hamsphire	12	1	0	13
Virginia	7	5	1	13
South Carolina	10	2	0	12
Alabama	8	0	2	10
Kentucky	9	1	0	10
Utah	3	4	3	10
Arizona	5	4	0	9
Montana	7	2	0	9
Arkansas	7	1	0	8
Maryland	6	0	2	8
North Carolina	6	2	0	8
Puerto Rico	8	0	0	8
Rhode Island	8	0	0	8
Tennessee	7	0	1	8
Connecticut	6	1	0	7
Kansas	6	1	0	7
Louisiana	5	1	1	7
Maine	5	1	1	7
Hawaii	0	6	0	6
West Virginia	5	1	0	6
Georgia	3	1	1	5
Nebraska	2	2	1	5
Oklahoma	4	0	1	5
Oregon	4	0	1	5
Idaho	4	0	0	4
New Mexico	4	0	0	4
Mississippi	2	0	0	2
Vermont	2	0	0	2
Guam	1	0	0	1
North Dakota	1	0	0	1
South Dakota	1	0	0	1
Wyoming	1	0	0	1
Alaska	0	0	0	0
American Samoa	0	0	0	0
Commonwealth of Marianas	0	0	0	0
District of Columbia	0	0	0	0
Nevada	0	0	0	0
Trust territories	0	0	0	0
Virgin Islands	0	0	0	0
	703	138	47	888

*Includes 45 proposed update no. 5 sites, 28 proposed update no. 4 sites, 24 proposed update no. 3 sites, 86 proposed update no. 2 sites, two proposed update no. 1 sites.

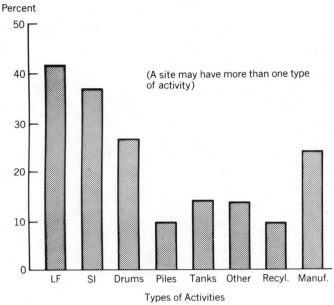

LF—Landfills
SI—Surface impoundments
Recyl. —Recycling/recovery, drum recycling, solvent recovery, waste-oil
processing, and battery recycling
Manuf. —Chemical/other manufacturing

Figure 18.2. Types of activities at 888 final and proposed NPL sites, June 1986.

TABLE 18.3. Types of Activities at 888 Final and Proposed NPL Sites in Order of Occurrence, June 1986

Surface impoundments	Tanks, below-ground	Battery recycling
Commercial/industrial landfills	Wood preserving	Surface mining sites
Containers/drums	Electroplating	Underground injection
Municipal landfills	Waste-oil processing	Drum recycling
Manufacturing other than chemical	Ore processing/refining	Road oil
Spills	Surface-water outfalls	Sand and gravel pits
Chemical processing/ manufacturing	Military ordnance	Sink holes
Leaking containers	Solvent recovery Open burning	Subsurface mining sites
Tanks, above-ground	Land farm/land treatment	Explosive disposal/ detonation
Waste piles	Incinerators	Laundry/dry cleaning
Groundwater plumes	Military testing/ maintenace	Tire storage/recycling

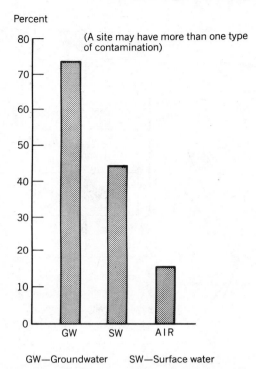

GW—Groundwater   SW—Surface water

Figure 18.3 Observed contamination at 888 final and proposed NPL sites, June 1986.

REMEDIAL INVESTIGATION/FEASIBILITY STUDY (RI/FS)

Once a site has been placed on the NPL, the EPA, a state, or the PRPs will conduct a remedial investigation (RI) and prepare a feasibility study (FS) leading to a remedial permanent remedy. The RI/FS is used by EPA to determine the nature and extent of the threat and to evaluate and select a remedy.

The remedial investigation emphasizes data collection and site characterization. Conducted concurrently with the feasibility study, the RI is the data-collection mechanism for the FS effort; this relationship is discussed later in this chapter. The RI also supports remedial-alternatives evaluation through bench and pilot studies. Figure 18.4 illustrates the RI process.

The initial activity in the RI is the scoping process. The scoping effort includes the collection and evaluation of existing data, identification of RI objectives, and the identification of general response actions for the FS. Data needs, preliminary plans, and investigation tasks are identified. The investigation scoping process may recur or be modified as more data are collected and site characterization becomes more complete.

The scoping process is critical to the development of a sampling plan and subsequent remedial investigation. This sampling plan describes the sampling

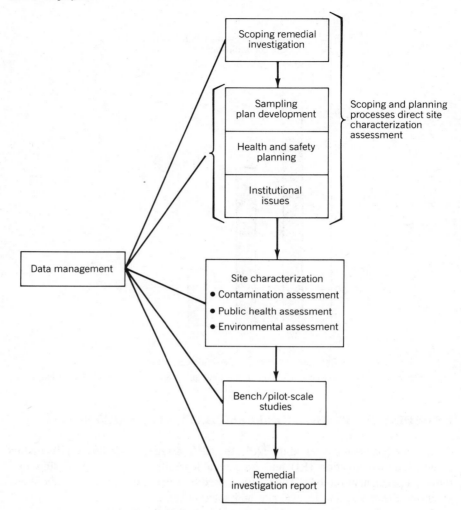

Figure 18.4. Remedial investigation process.

studies to be conducted, including sample types, analyses, and sampling locations and frequency. Planning needs such as sampling operational plans, materials, record keeping, sampling team personnel needs, and sampling procedures are also developed or identified for the investigation.

Associated with the scoping and sampling plan efforts are a variety of support actvities that may require the preparation of specific plans or implementation of specific procedures to supplement the remedial investigation and documentation of data. Specific plans may address data-management procedures, including quality-assurance/quality-control programs; may summarize health and safety planning requirements, including development of an overall health and safety program and a site-specific health and safety plan; and may review institutional issues arising from federal, state, and local regulations, policies, and guidelines that may affect the investigation.

Site characterization involves the collection and analysis of the data needed for the various types of assessments that are part of the investigation. Because site data and understanding vary, a multilevel approach to data collection is recommended. Each level differs in the scope of the activities. The three levels of data collection and site characterization efforts are:

LEVEL I—*Problem Identification and Scoping*. Existing site information is collected and evaluated to define the problem(s). This assessment is conducted for all sites and provides the basis for immediate mitigation actions for defining investigations needs in levels II and III. The data collected at this level are also used in identifying and analyzing remedial technologies.

LEVEL II—*Problem Quantification*. Specific site data are collected through sampling and field studies to characterize site problems and their dimensions more fully. Sufficient data should be collected to identify contaminants of concern to verify actual exposure pathways, and, in general, to characterize the site well enough to support, at a minimum, the screening of remedial technologies and alternataives.

LEVEL III—*Problem Quantification Detailed Investigation*. If level II data are insufficient, additional data are collected for use in a detailed analysis of remedial alternatives or in the selection of a cost-effective alternative.

The RI does not require that all three levels be completed; the process may terminate at any level provided that sufficient data have been obtained. For some sites, a level I study may furnish enough data for response decisions, particularly if a site has been well studied or the need for an immediate response is obvious. The investigation may end at level II if characterization data are sufficient to permit the selection of a response. Alternately, where level I analyses are sufficient to support FS decisions and a level II effort is not necessary, a level III study involving bench or pilot testing may be needed to select between alternatives or finalize a design. Thus, the investigation needs vary from site to site, and the levels of the RI must be appropriate to these needs.

Bench- or pilot-scale studies may be needed in the RI to obtain enough data to select a remedial alternative. The scope of bench and treatability, scale-up of innovative technologies, technology application issues, and evaluation of specific alternatives must be considered. Bench and pilot studies may also be conducted during remedial alternative design or construction more fully to evaluate specific requirements of the selected alternative; however, these studies are outside the RI and FS process. In general, bench-scale studies are appropriate for the RI stage while pilot-scale studies, if required, may be conducted during the final design.

Figure 18.5 depicts the concurrent activities associated with the RI and FS. The upper portion of the figure consists of two flowcharts illustrating the sequential, interdependent events associated with the RI/FS process. The lower portion is a tabulation of the tasks identified in the Model Statement of Work for the RI/FS.

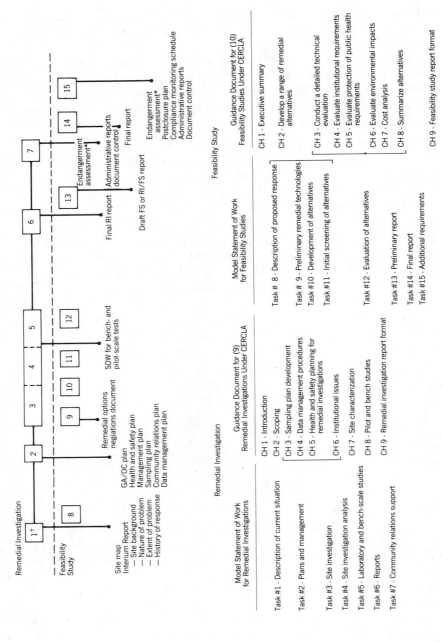

Figure 18.5. RI/FS process.

Remedial Investigation

Site map
Interium Report
— Site background
— Nature of problem
— Extent of problem
— History of response

GA/OC plan
Health and safety plan
Management plan
Sampling plan
Community relations plan
Data management plan

Remedial options
negiations document

SOW for bench- and
pilot-scale tests

Final RI report

Endangerment
assessment*
Administrative reports
document control

Draft FS or RI/FS report

Endangerment
assessment*
Postclosure plan
Compliance monitoring schedule
Administrative reports
Document control

Final report

Feasibility
Study

Remedial Investigation

Model Statement of Work
for Remedial Investigations

Task #1 - Description of current situation

Task #2 - Plans and management

Task #3 - Site investigation

Task #4 - Site investigation analysis

Task #5 - Laboratory and bench-scale studies

Task #6 - Reports

Task #7 - Community relations support

Guidance Document for (9)
Remedial Investigations Under CERCLA

CH 1 - Introduction

CH 2 - Scoping
CH 3 - Sampling plan development
CH 4 - Data management procedures
CH 5 - Health and safety planning for
remedial investigations
CH 6 - Institutional issues
CH 7 - Site characterization

CH 8 - Pilot and bench studies

CH 9 - Remedial investigation report format

Feasibility Study

Model Statement of Work
for Feasibility Studies

Task # 8 - Description of proposed response

Task # 9 - Preliminary remedial technologies
Task #10 - Development of alternatives
Task #11 - Initial screening of alternatives

Task #12 - Evaluation of alternatives

Task #13 - Preliminary report

Task #14 - Final report
Task #15 - Additional requirements

Guidance Document for (10)
Feasibility Studies Under CERCLA

CH 1 - Executive summary

CH 2 - Develop a range of remedial
alternatives

CH 3 - Conduct a detailed technical
evaluation
CH 4 - Evaluate institutional requirements
CH 5 - Evaluate protection of public health
requirements
CH 6 - Evaluate environmental impacts
CH 7 - Cost analysis
CH 8 - Summarize alternatives

CH 9 - Feasibility study report format

† Numbers in the boxes refer to tasks described in the Model Statement of Work for RI/FS under CERCLA Guidance issued February 1985.
See Appendix A.
* Endangerment assessments may be prepared at any point in the RI/FS process in support of enforcement actions.

This Model Statement of Work sets forth the tasks that a contractor will perform in conducting a government-led RI/FS. The lower portion of Figure 18.5 also identifies the chapters in the "Remedial Investigation and Feasibility Study Guidance Documents"[9] that the EPA has produced.

The vertical lines on the chart indicate some of the plans, reports, or milestones recommended in the RI/FS guidance. These connectors and the listings below them illustrate the integration of the RI/FS process.

The feasibility study process is outlined in Figure 18.6. The first step of the

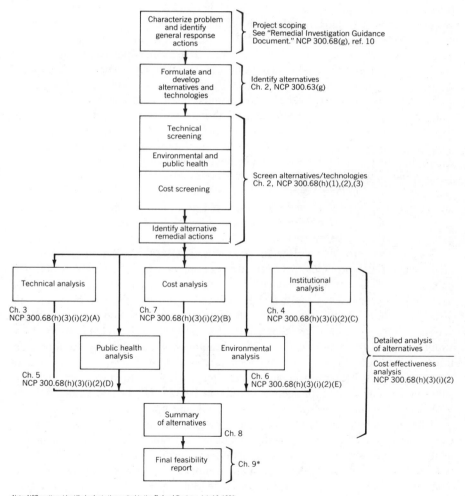

Note: NCP sections identified refer to those cited in the *Federal Register,* July 16, 1982.
*Not specified sections of the NCP.

Figure 18.6. Feasibility study process.

study, defining the objectives of the action and broadly developing response actions, should be performed as a refinement to project scoping during the remedial investigation and should be summarized in the final RI report. There may be modification of this scoping as data are collected or as the general response actions are more fully developed during the FS stage. The remedial alternatives developed at this point are general response actions that broadly define the nature of the response. In general, they should address whether source control measures designed to prevent or minimize migration of hazardous substances from the source and/or measures designed to mitigate the effect of contamination that has migrated into the environment are necessary, and what phasing of these measures may be necessary.

The next step in the process is the development of specific alternatives within the general response categories. First, the technologies within the categories are screened for their technical applicability to the site. Technologies considered technically appropriate are then combined to form operable units that address one or more aspects of the identified site problems. These operable units may then be combined to form alternatives addressing the complete site. The alternatives are then screened on the basis of public-health, environmental, and cost concerns.

The next five activities make up the detailed analysis of alternatives, which is necessary to provide the decision maker with information for selecting the alternative that is cost-effective. These activities include the engineering analysis of the alternatives in terms of constructability and reliability to ensure the implementability of the selected remedial action; an evaluation of institutional requirements such as compliance with other federal and state environmental statutes and community relations; an evaluation of public-health protection requirements that must be met; an evaluation of environmental effects of the action; and a detailed cost analysis.

A major issue in all remedial actions is "how clean is clean," that is, to what extent should a site be cleaned up?

Congress has provided a clear directive in SARA for the selection of a remedial plan. Section 121 provides that "remedial actions in which treatment which permanently and significantly reduces the volume, toxicity, or mobility of the hazardous substances . . . are to be preferred," and that off-site transport and disposal without treatment is the least favored method of completing remedial actions. This provision was adopted to discourage untreated land disposal, or simply moving waste from one location to another without reducing the long-term threat. To underscore the fact that treatment is preferred over land disposal or containment, the EPA must review a site every five years to ensure that the final solution continues to be protective of human health and the environment if the remedial action involves leaving the hazardous substances at the site.

If hazardous substances (or pollutants or contaminants) will remain at the site (i.e., on-site remedies), the remedial action must result in a level or standard of control for the substance that at least attains the legally applicable standards, requirements, or criteria under federal environmental laws (including the Resource Conservation and Recovery Act, the Toxic Substances Control Act, the Safe Drinking Water Act, the Clean Air Act, and the Clean Water Act) or state environmental or facility siting laws that are more stringent than federal standards. If land disposal is chosen as part of the remedial action for on-site remedies, any state standard that would effectively result in a statewide prohibition of the land disposal shall not apply except in certain narrowly defined circumstances. No federal, state, or local permit is required for actions taken entirely on site, if the remedial action is carried out in compliance with the cleanup standards.

If an off-site remedy is chosen, the hazardous substances must be transferred to a facility that is operating in compliance with a RCRA or other federal permit. The substances can only be sent to a land disposal facility if (1) the unit to which the substances will be sent is not releasing any hazardous wastes into the groundwater, surface water, or soil, and (2) any releases from other units at the facility are being controlled by a corrective-action program.

There are six statutory exceptions to the new requirement that the remedial action meet the applicable or relevant environmental standards and criteria. These include cases where the remedial action is only part of a larger action that will attain the applicable levels when completed; compliance would result in greater risk; compliance is technically impracticable; the remedial action selected will attain a standard of performance that is equivalent to the required standard; the state standard at issue has not been consistently applied within the state; and in the case of a remedial action under Section 104 using the Fund, a remedial action that complies with the standard will not provide an appropriate balance between the need for protection of public health and the environment and the monies' availability in the Fund.

As of late 1986, the EPA had initiated 489 RI/FSs. SARA established a mandatory time schedule for the EPA to conduct RI/FSs in the future. Within three years, 275 RI/FSs must be initiated and within five years a total of 650 RI/FSs must be initiated.

The RI/FSs conducted to date have provided some valuable information on Superfund site characteristics. Table 18.4 lists the substances most frequently found at sites.

TABLE 18.4. Substances Most Frequently Found at Superfund Sites

Substance Name	Site Frequency
Trichloroethylene (TCE)	297
1,1,2-Trichloroethylene	297
Lead (Pb)	273
Toluene	235
Benzene	204
Chloroform	179
Polychlorinated biphenyls, NOS	159
1,1,2,2,-Tetrachloroethene	145
Zinc and compounds, NOS (Zn)	137
1,1,1-trichloroethane	137
Cadmium (Cd)	132
Arsenic (As)	127

(continued)

TABLE 18.4. *(Continued)*

Substance Name	Site Frequency
Chromium and Compounds, NOS (Cr)	125
Phenol	124
Ethylbenzene	106
Xylene	106
1,2-Trans-dichloroethylene	104
Copper and compounds, NOS (Cu)	98
Methylene Chloride	93
Chromium	80
1,1-Dichloroethane	75
Mercury (Hg)	75
Cyanides (soluble salts), NOS	74
1,1-Dichloroethene	71
Vinylchloride	65
Carbon tetrachloride	63
Chlorobenzene	62
1,2-Dichloroethane	61
Nickel and compounds, NOS (Ni)	59
Heavy metals, NOS	57
Pentachlorophenol (PCP)	52
Naphthalene	45
Trichloroethane, NOS	40
Methyl ethyl ketone	39
Volatile organics, NOS	34
Manganese and compounds, NOS (Mn)	29
Iron and compounds, NOS (Fe)	28
Barium	28
Acetone	27
Chromium, hexavalent	26
Arsenic and compounds, NOS (As)	25
Dichloroethylene, NOS	25
Phenanthrene	25
Benzo A pyrene	25
1,1,2-Trichloroethane	24
Anthracene	21
Styrene	21
Pyrene	21
Creosote	21
DDT	21
Sulfuric acid	20
Selenium	20
Lindane	20
Tetrachloroethane, NOS	19
1,1,2,2-Tetrachloroethane	19
Waste oils/sludges	19
Bis (2-ethylhexyl)phthalate	18
Acid, NOS	18

TABLE 18.4. *(Continued)*

Substance Name	Site Frequency
Fluorene, NOS	17
Benzo (J,K)fluorene	17
Radium and compounds, NOS (Ra)	16
Ethyl chloride	16
Aluminum and compounds, NOS (Al)	14
Dichloroethane, NOS	14
Trichlorofluoromethane	14
Dichlorobenzene, NOS	13
Uranium and compounds, NOS (U)	13
Acenapthene	13
Trinitrotoluene (TNT)	13
Chlordane	13
Radon and compounds, NOS (Rn)	12
Cis-1,2,dichloroethene	12
Cis-1,2-dichloroethylene	12
Cis-dichloroethylene	12
1,2-dichloroethylene	12
Asbestos	12
Tribromomethane	12
Antimony and compounds, NOS (Sb)	11
Hydrocarbons, NOS	11
Chloromethane	11
Di-n-butyl-phthalate	11
Hexachlorobenzene	11
Tetrahydrofuran(I)	11
DDE	10
Dioxin	10
Ammonia	10
Dieldrin	10
Chrysene	10
Cresols	9
2,4-Dinitrotoluene	9
Hexachlorocyclopentadiene (C56)	9
Methyl isobutyl ketone	9
Waste solvents	9

RECORD OF DECISION

Once the RI/FS process is complete, the EPA selects a response action. The agency is required to establish an administrative record called Record of Decision, or ROD, in support of the selection of a response action. The ROD serves as a basis for judicial review of agency action and must be available to the public. Public participation must take place in the development of the ROD. The EPA is required to publish a notice and analysis of a proposed plan and allow the opportunity for comments and public meetings. It also requires the final plan to be published and made available to the public before a remedial action is begun, along with a response to significant comments, criticisms, and new data. The EPA is also required to publish an explanation of any part of the completed remedial action that differs from the final plan.

As of June 1986, 126 RODS or enforcement decision documents (EDD) had been signed.

REMEDIAL ACTIONS

By the end of 1986, the EPA had completed 14 remedial actions (RA) and another 103 had been initiated. SARA mandates that 175 new RAs be initiated during the first three years after enactment and an additional 200 RAs be initiated during the fourth and fifth year after enactment.

Management techniques for hazardous wastes found at Superfund sites may be grouped into two broad categories—land disposal (either on site or off site) and use of technologies that permanently reduce or destroy the hazardous character of the waste. In general, land disposal was used more frequently than other management techniques in the first five years of Superfund, because, for many waste types, this is typically less expensive than technologies that change the nature of the waste. As a result, hazardous-waste management at Superfund sites has frequently relied on relatively inexpensive land disposal. This reliance has limited the development and use of typically more expensive options. The heavy reliance on land disposal of hazardous wastes is illustrated in Figure 18.7. This figure summarizes a review of remedial activities at 51 NPL sites, which revealed that on-site land disposal, including capping and on-site land filling, was used at 52 percent of the sites and off-site land disposal was used at 54 percent of the sites.

Concern over the long-term reliability of land-based disposal practices prompted Congress to direct the EPA to give preference to providing treatment that permanently and significantly reduces the volume, toxicity, or mobility of the hazardous substance. Since technology is not readily available for many Superfund problems, SARA authorized a research, development, and demonstration program. The EPA established the Superfund Innovative Technology Evaluation (SITE) program to find better solutions to hazardous-waste cleanup.[11] As part of the SITE program, the EPA is planning to evaluate the most promising new technologies in several demonstration projects each year at Superfund sites across the nation. Testing may involve only one technology at a site or a set of them at various stages of the cleanup investigation. The EPA will choose the specific Superfund sites after a nationwide search that will match the effectiveness and compatibility of various technologies with specific wastes and conditions at the selected sites (see Figures 18.8 and 18.9). Appendices A, B, C, D, and E project the current concern for prompt and proper enforcement of SARA.

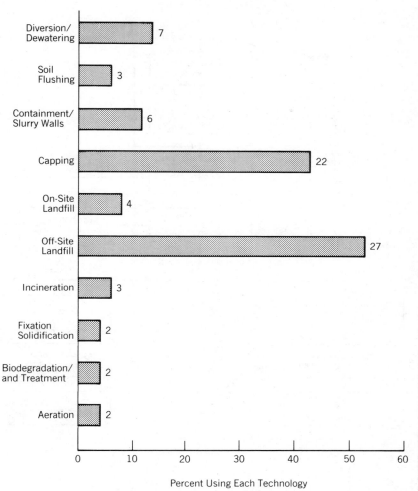

Percent Using Each Technology

Figure 18.7. Sites using each treatment technology.

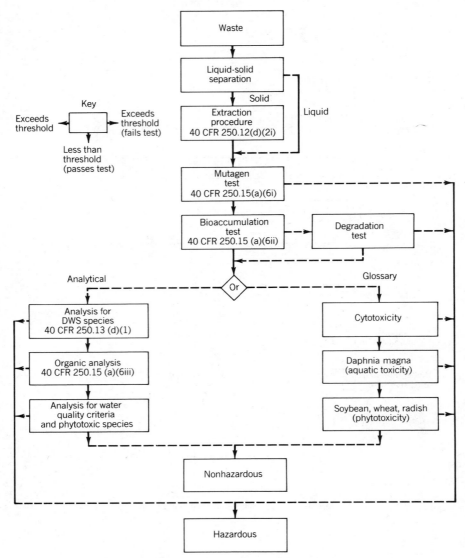

Figure 18.8. Protocol for classification of hazardous wastes.

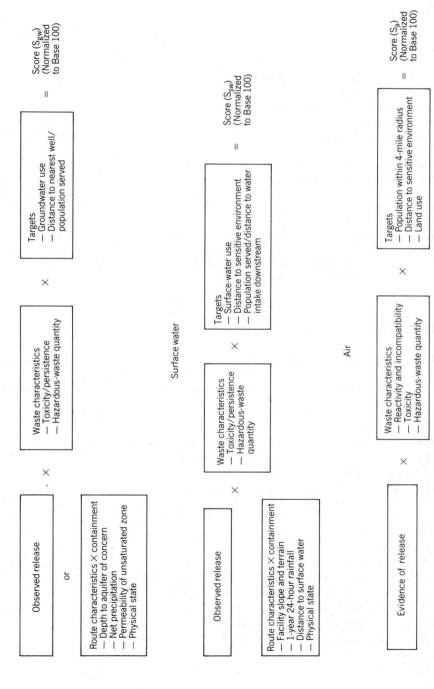

Figure 18.9. Environmental Protection Agency hazard-ranking system.

305

REFERENCES

1. Comprehensive Environmental Response, Compensation and Liability Act, PL 96-510, Washington, D.C., Dec. 1980.
2. Superfund Amendments and Reauthorization Act, PL 99-499, Washington, D.C., Oct. 17, 1986.
3. "U.S. EPA, The Superfund Progress Report," Washington, D.C., Nov. 1986.
4. *Federal Register,* **51,** No. 188, 34534–34549 (Sept. 29, 1986).
5. *Federal Register,* **50,** 47912, (Nov. 20, 1985).
6. A. D. Zuras; F. J. Priznar, and C. S. Parrish, "The National Priorities List Process," *Proceedings: Management of Uncontrolled Hazardous Waste Sites,* Hazardous Materials Control Research Institute, Silver Spring, Md., Nov. 1985.
7. EPA, "Uncontrolled Hazardous Waste Site Ranking System—A User's Manual," HW-10, U.S. Environmental Protection Agency, Washington, D.C., 1984.
8. "National Priorities List Fact Book—June 1986," EPA, HW-7.3, Washington, D.C., June 1986.
9. "Guidance on Remedial Investigations Under CERCLA," EPA, EPA/540/G-85/002, Cincinnati, Ohio, June 1985.
10. "Guidance on Feasibility Studies Under CERCLA," EPA, EPA/540/G-85/003, Cincinnati, Ohio, June 1985.
11. "Superfund Innovative Technology Evaluation (SITE) Strategy and Program Plan," EPA, EPA/540/G-86/001, Washington, D.C., Dec. 1986.

SUGGESTED READINGS

J. M. Bass, W. J. Lyman, and J. P. Tratnyek, "Assessment of Synthetic Membrane Successes and Failures at Waste Storage and Disposal Sites," EPA 600/S2-85/100, 6 pp., 1985.

G. W. Dawson and B. W. Mercer, *Hazardous Waste Management,* 532 pp., Wiley-Interscience, New York, 1986.

Superfund Technology Reports

"Slurry Trench Construction for Pollution Migration Control." EPA/540/2-84/001

"Case Studies of Remedial Response at Hazardous Waste Sites." Vol. I, EPA/540/2-84/002

"Case Studies 1–23: Remedial Response at Hazardous Waste Sites." Vol. II, EPA/540/2-84/002B

"Review of In-Place Treatment Techniques for Contaminated Surface Soils." Vol. I, "Technical Evaluation," EPA/540/2-84/003A

"Review of In-Place Treatment Techniques for Contaminated Surface Soils." Vol. 2, Background Information for In Situ Treatment," EPA/540/2-84/003B

"Modeling Remedial Actions at Uncontrolled Hazardous Waste Sites," EPA/540/2-85/001

"Covers for Uncontrolled Hazardous Waste Sites," EPA/540/2-85/002

"Guidance on Remedial Investigations Under CERCLA," EPA/G-85/002

"Guidance on Feasibility Studies Under CERCLA," EPA/G-85/003

"Handbook: Dust Control at Hazardous Waste Sites," EPA/540/2-85/003

"Leachate Plume Management," EPA/540/2-85/004

"Handbook: Remedial Action at Waste Disposal Sites" (revised), EPA/625/6-85/006

"Handbook for Stabilization/Solidification of Hazardous Waste," EPA/540/2-86/001

"Systems to Accelerated In Situ Stabilization of Waste Deposits," EPA/540/2-86/002

"Mobile Treatment Technologies for Superfund Wastes," EPA/540/2-86/003F

"Superfund Treatment Technologies: A Vendor Inventory," EPA/540/2-86/004F

"Superfund Innovative Technology Evaluation (SITE) Strategy and Program Plan," EPA/540/G-86/001

For Ordering Information Contact: ORD Publications, EPA, 26 W. St. Clair St., Cincinnati, OH 45268; (513) 569-7562.

19

Prevention and Control of Oil and Hazardous-Material Spills

Roy W. Hann, Jr.

In the minutes or hours after a spill of oil or a hazardous material, a decision maker can save or cost the employer the value of his or her salary for a lifetime. This sobering thought should make an individual in a management position in government or industry become intensely interested in preventing an event from happening or in carrying out proper contingency planning to assure a proper response to those spills that do occur.

This chapter focuses on the interrelated process of preventing and dealing with oil and hazardous-material spills. Records indicate that the problem of spillage and response is a significant one that needs to be reduced with regard to the number and magnitude of spills and warrants the development of the expertise and plans effectively to control the spills that do occur.

Unfortunately, observations made by the author at spill sites over the past decade, coupled with experience and knowledge shared by others, indicate that the record of responses to spills leaves much to be desired. Past failures in response need to be overcome by proper contingency planning, including, in particular, site-specific planning, resource acquisition, and timely spill response; use of appropriate technology; use of appropriate response organizations; and the provision of effective technical support.

This chapter is designed to help the administrator, engineer, or designated spill-response manager achieve the fundamental knowledge to develop or review spill contingency plans and their response activities.

To initiate the discussion, it is appropriate to consider spills in the context of the overall hazardous-material scenario. Figure 19.1 is a hazardous-material diagram developed by the author.

The top portion indicates that nonhazardous raw materials are transformed into

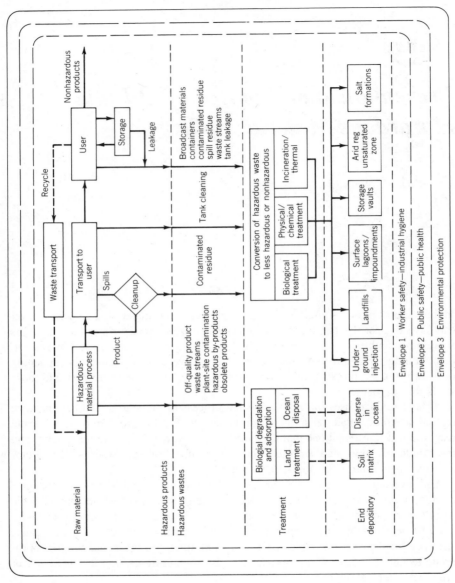

Figure 19.1. Hazardous-material diagram.

useful hazardous products in a manufacturing process and that this processing may generate hazardous-waste streams. These wastes result when hazardous products or their hazardous manufacturing by-products are mixed with air, water, soil, or other nonhazardous substances. These wastes are shown on the diagram crossing the boundary from hazardous products to hazardous wastes (i.e., below the dotted boundary).

Continuing across the top of the diagram, the hazardous product is shipped by pipeline, tanker, freighter, barge, railroad car, or truck, to the ultimate user of the product. While in the transportation mode (or storage mode prior to use), the product may be spilled as a result of collision, operating error, vandalism, tank leakage, or an act of God. If recovered in "pure" form, the material may be returned to the normal flow stream: however, if the material is contaminated by or contaminates air, water, soil, or another material, it becomes a hazardous waste and crosses the dotted line into the hazardous-waste arena.

The users of the hazardous products utilize them in a wide variety of ways. Some hazardous substances, such as pesticides and herbicides, are disseminated widely in the environment to accomplish their purpose; some hazardous materials are transformed into nonhazardous materials, such as plastics or fabrics; but some by-products, spills, effluents from processes, contaminated containers, etc., lead to waste materials and again cross the dotted line into the hazardous-waste category. A small fraction of waste materials is recycled back to original suppliers for reprocessing and use (e.g., dry-cleaning solvent).

Surrounding this waste-product/waste-material system are three envelopes. The first is the worker safety (e.g., industrial hygiene) envelope. The second is the human population–public health envelope, and the third is the environmental system envelope. These envelopes are useful in evaluating the roles of different governmental organizations relating to hazardous materials, in interrelating with appropriate discipline fields, and in determining which environmental system is appropriate in a given situation.

Spills, whether accidental or intentional, or acute or chronic, are a significant part of the overall hazardous-material process. They are particularly significant because of the sudden and often unexpected exposure of the spilled material to the affected environmental system and the human and other living resources that may unexpectedly be exposed.

In this chapter, we will deal with aspects of oil and hazardous-material spills up through the point where the contaminated material has been collected and delivered to a formal hazardous-waste treatment and disposal facility. In other words, the treatment and depository activities shown below the two lower dotted lines in Figure 19.1 are considered to be the purview of other chapters.

We are concerned with spills of oil and hazardous materials because they can cause harm to workers (envelope 1, Figure 19.1), to the public (envelope 2, Figure 19.1), or to the environmental system (envelope 3, Figure 19.1), and because of the economic cost to the spiller, third-party interests such as fisheries and other businesses, and to the public.

INTERRELATIONSHIP OF RISK ASSESSMENT, PREVENTION PLANNING, CONTINGENCY PLANNING, AND MITIGATION

Figure 19.2 presents a general probability-of-harm equation that shows how the probability of harm is a product of the collective probabilities of several components. Also shown (row 1) are the roles of statistical evaluation and logical comparison in evaluating past probabilities of the subcategories and predicting likely probabilities of future spills as the result of similar or altered behaviors or operations in the future. Row 2 shows how preventative planning can be applied to each of the individual probability categories to reduce the individual probabilities. Note that prevention planning can reduce all of the probability elements.

Row 3 on the diagram shows how contingency planning can reduce the probability of harm, but only in the last two categories, which apply after the spill has occurred. Row 4 shows how remedial action, in the form of damage assessment, mitigation, and compensation, can help overcome the spill harm but only after it has occurred (last column).

This equation and related discussion show how risk assessment, prevention planning, and contingency planning and remedial actions are all interrelated as components of the spill scenario. Although this chapter will focus most intently on prevention planning, contingency planning, response, and remedial action, the evaluation of spill statistics is an essential part of environmental impact assessment and is in the approval process for projects with spill potential.

PREVENTION PLANNING

The second row in Figure 19.1 depicts the role of prevention planning in altering the various probabilities in the probability-of-harm equation. Prevention planning is the dominant process in reducing each of the risk elements.

Figure 19.3 depicts graphically the author's portrayal of the prevention process or cycle. The first step in the process is to have a proper design and construction criterion, which, when properly executed, will yield a well-designed and constructed ship, barge, pipeline, railcar, vehicle, or other component operating on a properly designed waterway, railroad, highway, right-of-way, etc.

The second step is to have proper maintenance and operating procedures, including emergency response actions, which are to be followed to ensure that the ship, barge, pipeline, vehicle, or facility is properly maintained and operated in a manner to avoid mechanical and operational failures.

The third step is to provide proper training to the various personnel to carry out the design, construction, maintenance, and operational criteria needed to operate the systems correctly and safely. This training may be in the form of specialized direct training or by requiring licensing, registration, or certification as indications of professional competence. The author is reminded of the fiery collision of the freighter *Mimosa* and the tanker *Berman Agate* off Galveston, Texas, in 1979, in which investigation indicated that both captains had fraudulent licenses.

$$P_{(harm)} = P_{(accident)} * P_{(release)} * P_{(reaching\ damagable\ environmental\ feature)} * P_{(damage\ to\ features)}$$

Likelihood of harm caused by an oil spill

	A $P_{(accident)}$	B $P_{(release)}$	C $P_{(reaching\ damagable\ environmental\ feature)}$	D $P_{(damage\ to\ features)}$
1 Statistical evaluation and logical comparison	Ship and pipeline safety statistics	Ship and pipeline spill statistics	Spill transport statistics or mathematical models	Spill cleanup statistics and reporting
2 Prevention planning	Prevention planning systems design RE: Accident system location relative to danger	Prevention planning system design RE: Release	Prevention planning system location relative to environment vulnerability	Defensive protection of vulnerable environment
3 Contingency planning			Contingency planning and response	Contingency planning and response
4 Remedial actions				Damage assessment Mitigation Compensation

Figure 19.2. Probability-of-harm equation.

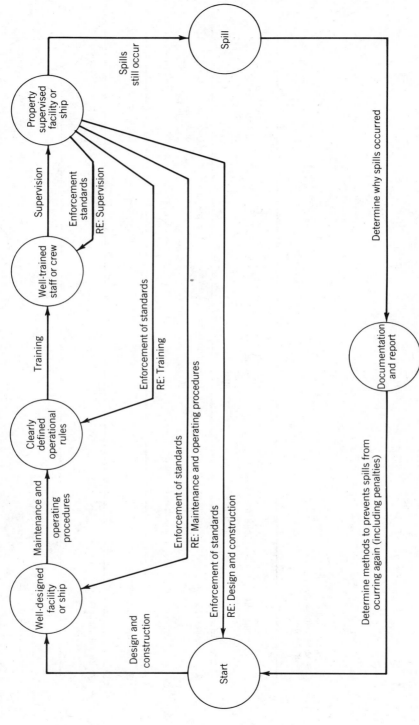

Figure 19.3. Oil and hazardous-material spill—prevention plan cycle.

The fourth step in the prevention process is the task of supervising the first three steps by the operating entity to see that the system operates as it should.

The final step recognizes the reality that enforcement, either internal or external, is necessary to assure compliance in each of the initial four steps of the prevention cycle. This enforcement may be in the form of plan review, construction certification, periodic maintenance and other inspections, policing of operations, examination and verification of training, and evaluation of supervision methods through environmental audits or other review processes.

It is well recognized that "prevention" is not perfect and collisions or other accidents from a variety of causes lead to spills and impact. This triggers the bottom half of the cycle, which involves determining where the top half of the cycle went wrong and developing the corrections to the system to avoid repetition of the bad event.

To return to the probability-of-harm diagram, Figure 19.1, it is suggested in element B2 that prevention planning be used to avoid an accident that may lead to a spill. This may be accomplished by establishing shipping lanes, setting speed limits, installing navigational aids, furnishing vessel escort for a ship, providing deeper burial or better location marking for a pipeline, and so on.

The second probability component of the probability-of-harm diagram is the probability of release, which is also limited by prevention (element B2). The chance of loss is reduced through providing defensive space or thicker hulls in a ship or barge; retaining empty storage space in which to store cargo from a damaged tank, and having pumping systems to do so; furnishing control and shutdown systems, extensive valving, thicker pipe, encasement, sumps, and other design features in a pipeline, and the like.

The prevention component of the third part of the probability-of-harm equation (element B3) involves keeping a leaked material from reaching a sensitive environment or economic system. These prevention methods may include relocating the shipping lane or pipeline to a greater distance from a sensitive environment; using a retaining boom around a ship; building a dike around a tank or tank farm, or building dams and special structures in a creek. The basic concept from radiation protection of time, distance, and shielding is appropriate: time to permit response, distance to minimize likelihood of contact, and shielding with booms, barriers, dams, and so on, to prevent the spilled material from getting to the vulnerable system.

The prevention of the final component of the probability-of-harm equation (element B4) involves prevention of damage from the spilled material by protection barriers (for protection as opposed to containment), including dams and booms; provision for flooding of marsh areas or beaches; provision for removing fish, mariculture organisms, or livestock; and provision for dispersing the spill from the surface into the water column so it moves with the current. These activities can be likened to the evacuation and property-protection activities that take place before a hurricane.

Prevention becomes even more important when the chance of effectively dealing with a spill event does not exist or is reduced. For example, greater safety factors and greater emphasis on quality assurance are required for nuclear systems or hazardous materials such as chlorine. Similarly, in a developing country where response capability for oil spills does not exist in the absence of specialized equipment and resources, greater emphasis needs to be placed on avoiding the spill in the first place.

CONTINGENCY PLANNING OVERVIEW

Recognizing that prevention is not always successful, the focus shifts to contingency planning to deal with the spill or other calamity. It should be noted that oil and hazardous-material response contingency planning only assists in limiting the last two elements of the probability-of-harm equation.

Figure 19.4 shows the contingency planning cycle as envisioned by the author. It involves seven steps in a continuing cyclic process. The initial step is the development of an administrative contingency plan. This plan establishes overview responsibility and authority, and generally provides for notification and fulfillment of other legal requirements. A given administrative plan interacts with other industrial and national, state, and local government administrative contingency plans, and should be consistent with them. A number of the detailed components of the contingency planning steps are presented in Table 19.1.

Unfortunately, for many organizations, the contingency planning process stops with the creation of the administrative plan document, which may be placed on a shelf to gather dust. Thus, when the spill occurs, the contingency plan shifts through the short-circuit loop shown in Figure 19.4 to the assembly of response elements and initiation of detailed response planning after the spill rather than before it.

In the author's opinion, the most important, and most often neglected, aspects of contingency planning are the second and third phases of the contingency planning process, which encompass site-specific planning and the acquisition of resources to be prepared to deal with a spill. These two components, which are described more fully in Table 19.1, are coupled with the administrative plan to make up the prespill activities. Often the prespill planning group is different from the actual response group for an industrial organization.

Site-specific planning involves careful evaluation of the type of incident that can happen to a facility, waterway, pipeline, ship, and so forth, and determination of what response would be needed to deal with the expected incident.

The next phase is the acquisition of the resources needed to deal with the incident. This may mean training response personnel in both administrative and line responses, obtaining specialized spill-control equipment and supplies, negotiating contracts with spill-control contractors, carrying out scientific and engineering studies, and building storage facilities, end anchorages, and temporary contaminated-material storage areas.

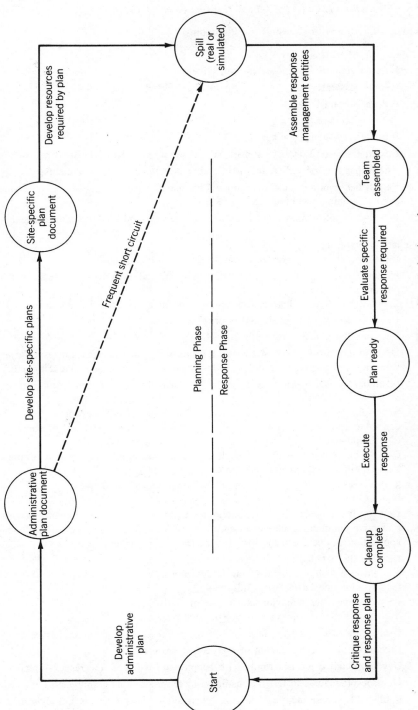

Figure 19.4. Oil and hazardous-material spill—contingency planning cycle.

Spill
(real or
simulated)

Develop resources
required by plan

Assemble response
management entities

Team
assembled

Site-specific
plan
document

Evaluate specific
response required

Frequent short circuit

Develop site-specific plans

Planning Phase

Response Phase

Plan ready

Administrative
plan document

Execute
response

Develop
administrative
plan

Cleanup
complete

Critique response
and response plan

Start

TABLE 19.1. Steps to Contingency Planning

Develop administration plan

1. Defined authority, purpose, and objectives.
2. Establishes policy.
3. Assigns responsibility.
4. Delegates authority.
5. Provides financial resources.
6. Designates institutional, personnel, and material resources to be used in response.
7. Establishes role of spiller, industry, and/or government or governments.
8. Establishes common or core resources for use of subentity plans (i.e., equipment, supply, training programs, etc.).
9. Establishes notification procedures for management and government agencies.

Site-specific planning

1. Develop local site version of administrative plan components.
2. Evaluate resources to be protected: Environmental systems—estuaries, marshes, breeding grounds, etc.
   Economic systems—Beaches, aquaculture, resort areas, fisheries, marinas
3. Develop the response goals and priority of action.
4. Determine mechanism for initiating action.
5. Develop the framework of authority, responsibility, and hierarchy of response to be followed in the area (i.e., spiller, industry group, government, contractor, etc.).
6. Inventory the various resources available to deal with the expected problem:
   a. Laws
   b. Agreements
   c. Management structure
   d. Communications
   e. Specialized equipment and supplies
   f. Traditional equipment and supplies
   g. Money
   h. Land
   i. Engineering plans
   j. Response personnel
   k. Technical assistance personnel
   l. Construction
   m. Background studies (environmental, etc.)
   n. Logistical support
7. Develop the detailed response strategy for control, including equipment placement, protective booming, containment and removal locations, removal devices, chemical application devices, and the like, for the expected problem.
8. Develop the detailed technical response strategy to:
   a. Provide technical input to the design process.
   b. Provide needed technical information.
   c. Document the behavior and impact of spills.
   d. Assess the damage caused by spill and response.
9. Evaluate needed resources in excess of those already available (see item 6).
10. Develop a plan of acquisition of the needed resources.
11. Develop detailed job descriptions for people who will staff the response team.
12. Develop procedures to test the readiness of the plan or its components.
13. Publish the plan for the use of those involved and for outside review and suggestion for improvement.

TABLE 19.1. (*Continued*)

Develop resources required by the plans
1. Acquire specialized equipment and supply resources.
2. Develop institutional arrangements.
3. Train personnel.
4. Carry out background engineering and scientific studies.
5. Build specialized defenses:
   a. Storage
   b. Deployment
   c. Anchorages
   d. Pooling areas
   e. Disposal areas

Assemble response management entities
1. Assemble cleanup line management staff.
2. Assemble technical assistance staff.

Evaluate specific response required
1. Determine material or materials spilled or in imminent danger of spill or flotation.
2. Evaluate spill nature, size, and potential impact.
3. Evaluate resource levels needed.
4. Evaluate source of resources to be used (hierarchy of response levels to be used) for cleanup.
5. Evaluate additional technical response resources.

Carry out response
1. Carry out containment, removal, disposal, and/or dispersion in accordance with plans.
2. Carry out documentation of spill according to technical assistance plan.
3. Carry out damage assessment according to technical assistance plan.

Critique response and response plan
1. Evaluate the effectiveness of the spill-control response.
2. Evaluate the effectiveness of the technical response.
3. Evaluate the effectiveness of the previous contingency plan.
4. Make recommendations for future plan revisions and responses.

In recommending site-specific contingency planning, the author is always envious of the fire-protection field, where insurance companies, through their rate-setting mechanism, are able to make sure that communities have site-specific plans. The insurance companies require (1) water distribution systems that can provide the needed water flows through a required number of hydrants to potential fire sites, (2) fire departments with the necessary equipment and trained personnel, and (3) site-specific plans that tell the fire fighters where to attach their hoses to fight a fire at a specific location, such as the local shopping center, hospital, or high school.

Fire fighting, like oil-spill control, allows time for only minor fine tuning of the plan after the alarm bell rings. After the spill alarm bell sounds, the contingency plan shifts from the *planning mode* to the *response mode*. First the response team management is assembled. It modifies previous plans (if they exist) to adjust to the actual incident and takes the steps to put the response to the incident in motion. The response is then carried out. The response may range from simply hiring a contractor to clean up a small spill to the six-month, 10,000-man effort expended on the Amoco Cadiz oil spill in France.

The final step of the contingency planning cycle is the evaluation of the response in order to improve the contingency plan and future responses.

In the probability-of-harm equation, it is indicated that effective contingency planning can reduce the likelihood of the oil or hazardous material reaching an endangered target (element C3) by providing for containment and removal of the spilled material en route from the spill to the impact zone, or by dispersing the oil or hazardous material into the water body and transferring the impact from a coastal-boundary impact to a water-mass impact.

The plan can also be effective in removing the oil from the first environmental system affected and thus preventing it from reaching another, perhaps more sensitive, system. This is particularly true in beach cleanup where the main goal is to stabilize and remove oil from the ecosystem rather than reclaim the beach.

Contingency planning can also result in reducing the harm upon impact by providing for defensive protection of endangered systems (interacts with prevention), such as removing and stockpiling beach sand and harvesting and transplanting marine life, and the use of proper cleanup methods that minimize harm to the environment (e.g., fast response on beaches to minimize sand removal, marsh cleanup that does not disturb root systems and yet prevents smothering, etc.).

Contingency Planning in the Prespill Mode

One of the major problems with the development and maintenance of effective contingency plans is that few organizations choose to invest major resources in disaster planning activities unless forced to do so by government agencies, insurance companies, or external environmental action groups.

The author believes that major enterprises with spill potential should maintain ongoing contingency planning activities. These activities may or may not involve personnel who will have a direct responsibility in the event of a spill.

Figure 19.5 is a diagram showing responsibilities for a cooperative staff or contingency planning group during nonresponse periods. These duties focus on prevention, administrative contingency plan development, site-specific planning, and resource acquisition.

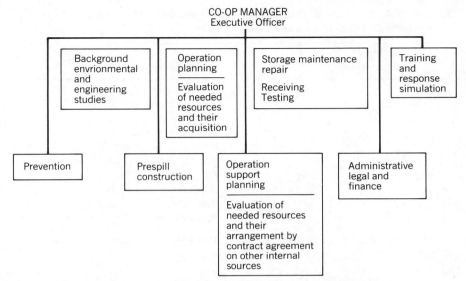

Figure 19.5. Responsibilities of cooperative staff during nonresponse periods.

RESPONSE DECISIONS

A key responsibility of those responding to spills is the recognition that those often involved in the operational aspects of oil and hazardous-material spills are not aware of the environmental characteristics and environmental sensitivity of the environmental systems that may be affected. This can lead to the use of response technology that is inappropriate because it will not work in the atmospheric, aquatic, or terrestrial systems involved, or will cause unnecessary or unacceptable harm to the living systems or economic enterprises affected by the spill.

On a large offshore oil spill, there may be time to bring both operational and technical resources together. In reality, however, this needed input will only be gained by including technical components in preplanning activities, such as providing background studies of topography, winds, currents, and living resources; preparing specialized reports, charts, and diagrams for response personnel; and training response personnel to use the prepared material effectively and to seek supporting professional guidance in spill situations.

Table 19.2 is a vulnerability index developed by Hayes and Gundlock, which has often been used to classify coastal environmental systems with regard to oil spills. Table 19.3 is a related table developed by the author that rates coastal environmental systems in terms of how easily or readily oil may be removed from them.

Use of Table 19.3 information to temper Table 19.2 information is needed for a rational response strategy. For example, Table 19.2 would appropriately indicate that a beach with fine-grained sand has a low vulnerability to oil-spill damage; however, beach cleanup on fine-grained sand is of very high priority because oil

TABLE 19.2. Summary of Coastal Shoreline Systems in Order of Increasing Vulnerability to Oil-Spill Damage

Vulnerability Index	Shoreline Type
1	Exposed rocky headlands
2	Eroding wave-cut platforms
3	Fine-grained-sand beaches
4	Coarse-grained-sand beaches
5	Exposed, compacted tidal flats
6	Mixed sand and gravel beaches
7	Gravel beaches
8	Sheltered rocky coasts
9	Sheltered tidal
10	Salt marshes

Source: "Vulnerability of Coastal Environments to Oil Spill Impacts," Gundlock and Hayes.

TABLE 19.3. Spilled Oil Removability Index (Lowest Number = Best Removal)

1. Oil or mousse trapped in quiescent areas where it is consolidated by current, wind, booms and where it can be removed by vacuum trucks or shore-operated skimmers from a water surface.
2. Mousse on the surface of gently sloping hard-packed beaches.
3. Consolidated oil or mousse removed by vessel-operated or dynamic skimmers.
4. Oil on the surface or uniformly soaked into the surface of gently sloping hard-packed beaches.
5. Oil trapped in pools in marshes or rocks accessible to externally located vacuum systems.
6. Heavy oil concentrations floating loose on the water and removed by skimmer systems.
7. Oil or mousse on the surface of irregular or low-load bearing-capacity beaches that must be removed by manual or semimanual method.
8. Oil or mousse in marsh or mangrove areas where water flushing to collection point is possible and water access for logistical support is available.
9. Oil or mousse in inaccessible marsh or rocky areas where logistics are expensive and removal is by hand, such as by dipping or using absorbents.
10. Removal of buried oil on beaches where clean overburden material must be removed by hand to get to the heavily oiled layers of sand and mousse.
11. Oil or mousse in vegetation where removal of oil requires removal of the vegetation, such as seaweed, marsh grass, or trash.
12. Light concentrations of oil on the water surface.
13. Removal of the oil-contaminated layer on mud flats or marshes by scraping, skimming off the contaminated layer, or dredging.

can be effectively removed from the beaches, thus preventing it from refloating and being carried to other coastal systems where cleanup is more difficult or costly.

RESPONSE RESOURCES

A wide range of response resources is available for dealing with oil and hazardous-material spills. Figure 19.6 is a matrix of response research organization and capabilities. The depth of resources needed will vary with the size, geographic zone of impact, and complexity of a spill. Furthermore, the level of capability of the response resource will vary among geographical areas and with the capability and interest of local and state governments.

Cooperatives as a Unique Response Resource

A very valuable and unique resource for oil and hazardous-material spills response is the cooperative organization.

Oil-spill cooperatives tend to fall into three classifications:

1. The true industry cooperative
2. Industry and government cooperative
3. Equipment cooperatives

The true cooperative is essentially industry sponsored based on an acceptable distribution-of-cost basis. The cooperative will purchase and maintain a core of response equipment either at a central site or at members' facilities. The cooperative organization will hire a core staff to administer cooperative activities, maintain the common equipment resource, carry out site-specific contingency planning in conjunction with member companies, develop and participate in training activities with member company personnel, and develop logistical and other supporting resources from industry and government to call in as needed. In the response mode, the cooperative may either direct and participate in the response or participate as a resource under a member company's response plan and organization. A typical cooperative of this type is the Clean Seas Cooperative in Santa Barbara, Calif.

The industry–government cooperative is essentially a true cooperative but with a major participation by local government. It is prevalent where industry and government consider the prevention and control of spills a joint responsibility The Corpus Christi Area Oil Spill Control Association in Corpus Christi, Texas, is typical of the industry–government cooperative. In this cooperative, costs are borne equally by industry and government, and each has committed personnel resources to back up cooperative and contract personnel as needed.

The equipment cooperative is the cooperative acquisition and maintenance of an equipment pool available to member companies. When a spill occurs, the equipment is merely made available to the company responsible for the spill to be used by company or contractor personnel. The Clean Gulf Cooperative, which serves the

CAPABILITY

		Oil/Hazardous-Material Spill Cleanup									Technical Assistance/ Documentation				
	Source	Organized manpower	Oil/haz.-mat. spill equipment	Oil & haz.-mat. spill supplies	Contingency public works equipment	Vacuum trucks & tank trucks	Vessels	Aircraft/helicopters	Manpower logistics	Other	Oil & haz.-mat. spill specialists	Engineering manpower	Scientific manpower	Legal manpower	Financial management
Industry	Company resources	x	x	x					x	x	x	x	x	x	x
Industry	Cooperative resources	x	x	x		x	x		x		x				
Contractors & Suppliers	Oil & haz.-mat. spill contractors	x	x	x		x	x		x		x				
Contractors & Suppliers	Construction contractors	x			x										
Contractors & Suppliers	Oil & haz.-mat. industry service contr.	x			x	x	x	x	x						
Contractors & Suppliers	Oil & haz.-mat. spill suppliers		x	x											
Consultants & Academic Organizations	Oil & haz.-mat. spill consultants										x	x		x	
Consultants & Academic Organizations	Environmental consultants												x		
Consultants & Academic Organizations	Universities										x				
Consultants & Academic Organizations	Research organizations										x	x	x		
Local/State Government	Public works transportation	x			x			x							
Local/State Government	Fire/police	x	x								x				
Local/State Government	Port authorities						x								
National Government	Navy/Coast Guard	x	x					x	x	x	x				
National Government	Army	x			x				x	x					
National Government	EPA	x	x						x	x	x		x		
National Government	Public works	x			x					x					

Figure 19.6. Response resource organization matrix.

offshore oil industry on the U.S. coast of the Gulf of Mexico, is a typical equipment cooperative.

A different type of cooperative is a hazardous-material manufacturing industry cooperative to respond in the event that one of the producing companies has a spill. The Chlorine Institute, which provides emergency technical information and responds to chlorine spills, is typical of this type of cooperative.

Cooperatives can be valuable, capable, and economical resources for oil and hazardous-material response. The reader is cautioned, however, that along with the many capable cooperatives are a large number of "paper tiger" cooperatives, which were created to give an appearance of response capability when in fact they are merely mutual-aid entities with little true response capability.

CONTINGENCY PLANNING: RESPONSE MODES

The response needed to respond to a spill will vary based on many factors. It may range from a fire department hazardous-material response team responding to a leaking 55-gallon drum in a highway tractor-trailer to the 10,000-man, six-month response to the Amoco Cadiz oil spill in France. Only those responsible for the contingency planning for a company, facility, port, region, city, and so on, or their consultants can adequately determine the type and magnitude of event that must be considered. Then the appropriate sophistication of response may be determined. A typical response structure for a major oil spill on water is shown in Figure 19.7.

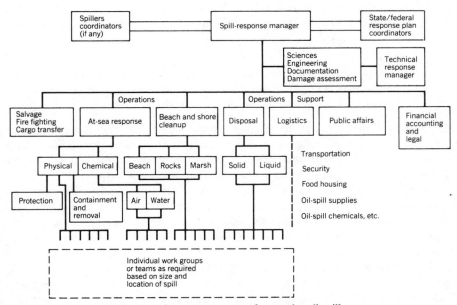

Figure 19.7. Typical response structure for a major oil spill on water.

The diagram interacts with the activities of a spill-response manager with management personnel of the spilling entity; federal, state, and local on-scene coordinators; a technical response manager and science and engineering support staff; direct operational entities to carry out the spill cleanup; and the operation's support components groups to handle logistic, public affairs, financial, legal, and related activities. These five major components that are interacting with the spill-response manager can be expanded or contracted as necessary according to spill size and complexity.

The author chooses to emphasize the title of spill-response manager to differentiate the individual responsible for actual cleanup from the legal term "on-scene coordinator" or "OSC," which designates the federal government person in charge under the U.S. Federal Water Pollution Control Act. On a federally funded spill response, the spill-response manager and the on-scene coordinator may be the same person.

RESPONSE PRIORITIES

In the hectic minutes and hours after a spill occurs, the most important task for those in charge is to initiate response activities in proper sequence according to reasonable priorities. For example, health and safety and stopping the spill take initial priority over cleanup and bird-reclamation activities. Table 19.4 shows typical response priorities for hazardous-material and oil spills. The primary differences between hazardous-material spills and oil spills are:

1. Hazard to workers and public—hazardous-material spills generally pose greater risk to response personnel and the public than do oil spills.

2. Scale—oil spills generally involve more material than hazardous-material spills.

3. Liability—the greatest financial risk in hazardous-material spills is related to avoiding harm to personnel and the public where the greatest cost associated with oil spills is generally related to oil-removal activities.

In Table 19.4, the first two steps relating to hazardous-material spills require careful evaluation and consideration. This is particularly the case when materials that are spilled or are in danger of spillage, reaction, explosion, fire, and so on, are unknown or are in proximity to others that may interreact.

In most oil-spill situations, however, the products being handled and their properties are well known and personnel can generally move with the most expeditious speed possible to stop the release and limit the spread of the oil. By moving swiftly, overall economic cost and environmental damage can be greatly reduced.

For oil spills, the need to respond quickly often creates the need for a quick-acting first-strike capability, which may then be replaced by slower-acting resources that will carry out the main mass as part of the response. Figure 19.8 presents this concept in a major spill where local cooperative, oil company resources, and local government agency and public works agency resources respond initially and are

TABLE 19.4. Response Priorities

Hazardous-Material Spill (Careful Evaluation)	Oil Spill (Speed)
1. Location and notification	1. Location and notification
2. Determination of spilled material or materials and other materials in proximity	2. Spilled material generally identified by contingency plan or operating document
3. Evaluation of safety considerations of entry	3. Evaluate any special personnel or public dangers such as high LEL readings, low O_2 readings, or H_2S
4. Rescue and safety actions	4. Rescue and safety if needed near the spill source
5. Stop source	5. Stop source of spill
6. Protective	6. Protective
7. Contain spilled material	7. Contain spilled material
8. Prevent spilled material from creating human exposure and reaching sensitive environments	8. Prevent spilled material from reaching sensitive environment
9. Remove spilled hazardous material and contaminated water, soil, and other materials	9. Remove spilled oil and contaminated materials
10. Transport hazardous-waste material to hazardous-waste-treatment facility	10. Transport oil and contaminated materials to reclamation, treatment, and disposal facilities
11. Restore damaged environmental system	11. Restore damaged environmental system
12. Carry out mitigation, damage assessment, and compensation activities	12. Carry out mitigation, damage assessment, and compensation activities
13. Documentation of all aspects of the spill and response	13. Documentation of all aspects of the spill and response

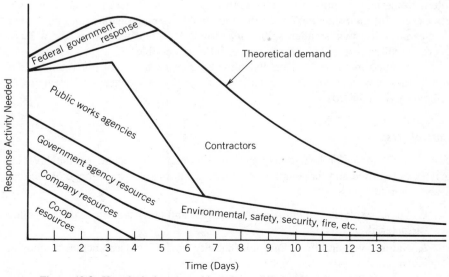

Figure 19.8. Hypothetical response hierarchy at different times in a spill response.

replaced with more appropriate agency and contractor resources for longer-term activities. The early responders return to their normal nonemergency duties as soon as relief capability is developed.

SPECIAL ITEMS RELATING TO OIL-SPILL RESPONSE

Reasonableness of Response

In the United States, the public, through its action groups and local and state governments, determines the sophistication with which contingency planning and spill-response preparation are carried out and to what extent cleanup activities are carried out.

In California, for example, the public has demanded and received effective contingency planning, an effective group of well-equipped oil-spill-control cooperatives, and a high level of cleanup.

In Texas, however, only in the environmentally sensitive resort-oriented Corpus Christi area is there a truly effective oil-spill-control cooperative, and in general site-specific contingency planning, response preparation, and execution are well below California levels.

In the international arena, an interesting phenomenon exists, which the author calls the "standard of reasonableness." International spill response on major spills is overseen by international insurance interests on behalf of ship and cargo owners. The level to which response activities are carried out appears to be governed by a standard of reasonableness determined by a country's everyday cleanup activity for local spills; for example, if a nation insists on high standards for cleanup of its everyday spills, then it can expect and will be given a high level of cleanup on international tanker spills. Countries such as the United States, France, and Japan can expect this high standard. If, on the other hand, a smaller nation does not bother to clean up its own smaller spills, its standard of reasonableness for a large international spill is either "zero" or "as little as possible."

The implied message is clear: Establish an internal policy of high standards if you expect those coming from outside your country to finance spill cleanups to achieve high standards.

Cost of Response

The cost of an oil or hazardous-material response will depend on the level of personnel required and the length of cleanup, according to a wide range of factors. These include:

1. Toxic, explosive, flammability, reactive, and other properties of the spilled material
2. Nature, vulnerability, and "cleanability" of the environmental system in which the spill takes place
3. Training level and experience of response personnel

4. Characteristics of the spilled material with regard to its spread into the environment

5. Properties of the material with regard to containability and the effectiveness of removal technology

6. Level of mechanization available in terms of oil and hazardous-material spill-control equipment, fire-fighting equipment, and public works equipment

7. Season of year and weather conditions during the spill

8. Speed and effectiveness of response

9. Extent of impact in terms of length of stream, volume of soil, area of spread, or other appropriate units

10. "Reasonableness" of cleanup or level of cleanup required

11. Natural rate of loss of spilled material into the environment

12. Cost for treatment and disposal of removed materials

13. Cost of mitigation, damage assessment, and compensation

For coastal oil spills, the author determined the cost of cleanup for a quality spill response to be between five and 10 times the value of the spilled oil when oil was $40 per barrel, and 10 to 20 times the value of the spilled oil when the value of oil was $20 per barrel. Thus a spill of 7000 barrels of crude oil (i.e., approximately 1000 metric tons) would have a value of $140,000 and a coastal (or river) cleanup could be expected to cost in the range of $1.4 million to $2.8 million.

A common failing in spill response is to underestimate the spill cost and resource requirement and thus escalate the ultimate cost by underspending for a competent and adequate response in the critical early stages and then have to pay a longer-term higher cost to remedy the effect of the inadequate early response. The author has yet to see too much early response that would lead to an ultimate higher cost.

The best way to minimize cost is to invest in proper contingency planning. Then a proper plan is executed by qualified personnel who are operating under pre-executed agreements, and so on.

TECHNICAL ASPECTS OF SPILL RESPONSES

Response Resources

Response resources for oil and hazardous-material response can generally be divided into two major groups: traditional resources, including emergency, construction, industrial, and maritime and farm equipment; and specialized resources, including oil and hazardous-material equipment and supplies.

Traditional Resources

Traditional resources are the backbone of many oil and hazardous-material responses because they are available when specialized resources may not be. Or as the old saying goes, "When war comes, you fight it with the weapons available, not those you would like to have."

In countries that have not yet developed specialized resources, the traditional resources are often the only ones available. Indeed, when initial spill-control expenditures are made, they should be for equipment that improves the capability of traditional resources rather than for exotic spill-response equipment.

Traditional resources include (but are not limited to):

Emergency resources
    Fire engines
    Ambulances
    Emergency communication networks
Construction/industrial resources
    Heavy equipment
    Bulldozers
    Front-end loaders
    Backhoes
    Graders
    Scrapers
    Cranes
Transportation equipment
    Tank trucks
    Vacuum trucks
    Railroad cars
    Dump trucks
Farm equipment
    Tractors
    PTO pumps
    Sprayers
    Vacuum wagons
    Disks
Maritime equipment
    Tankers
    Barges
    Tugs
    Work boats
    Salvage equipment
    Pumps
Other
    Water-well drilling equipment
    Pumping systems
    Cleaning equipment
    Shovels, buckets, other hand tools
    Laboratory analysis equipment

Specialized Resources

These resources are those specifically designed to deal with oil and hazardous-material spills. They may range from simple containment booms to elaborate trailer-mounted incinerators and unit processes to deal with hazardous-material spills. A typical list follows.

Booms and Barriers. A wide variety of floating barriers are manufactured of different sizes, shapes, and materials to contain spilled materials, divert spilled material, or exclude spilled materials from sensitive areas.

Skimmers. A wide range of skimmers use one or more of such processes as weirs, oliaphilic drums, belts or ropes, inclined planes, vortexes, or suction to remove oil or hazardous materials from the water surface for transport to receiving facilities.

Sorbents. Absorbent or adsorbent materials selectively absorb oil or hazardous materials for removal and disposal. These sorbents are made from a wide range of natural and manufactured materials.

Chemicals. Specialized chemicals are used to disburse oil and hazardous materials after surface tension and thus spreading, make and break emulsions, and neutralize or alter hazardous materials.

Chemical Spreading Equipment. A wide range of chemical spreading equipment, ranging from hand sprayers and truck sprayers to vessel and aircraft spraying equipment, dispense the special chemicals.

Storage Facilities. Emergency storage facilities, range from fast erecting tanks to rubber and plastic pillows and liners for pits and reservoirs.

Special Treatment Units. A wide variety of special treatment units have been developed (but not widely distributed) for oil–water separation, chemical processing, incineration, and the like.

Instrumentation/Safety Equipment. A wide range of safety equipment in the form of breathing equipment, protective clothing, protective footwear, and so on, is needed, particularly for hazardous-material spills. Similarly, a wide range of analysis equipment, including explosion meters, gas-measuring equipment, and organic vapor analyzers, is needed to measure hazard characteristics.

Unit Operations and Processes. The traditional and specialized resources are utilized together to achieve components of the cleanup process. The terms "unit operations" and "unit processes" are borrowed from chemical and environmental engineering to describe the collection of the individual unit operations (single activities) into unit processes (groups of activities) to achieve a purpose in the cleanup operation.

Figure 19.9 illustrates a group of unit processes to carry out the major activities of a coastal oil-spill response. The diagram includes several basic processes to collect the oil from different environmental systems: the initial transportation step to move the material to interim storage facilities, a secondary transportation from interim storage, and the ultimate disposal activities of oil recovery, treatment processes, and final disposal.

Figure 19.10 shows a detailed diagram of one of the basic processes in Figure 19.9, specifically, the process to remove oil from the water surface at the shoreline. This diagram indicates the linkage of the individual unit operations.

This concept of unit operations and processes can be expanded to any spill-response activity using traditional and specialized resources.

Special Response Technology

Space limitations prevent a detailed presentation of oil-spill-control technology using traditional and specialized resources. The technologies correspond to the priority of response items in Table 19.4. The reader who is interested in pursuing response technology in greater depth is encourged to focus on the following topics.

1. Boom characteristics and fundamentals of angle deployment to prevent entrainment
2. Booming strategy for containment, diversion, and exclusion objectives
3. Boom anchorage and tending
4. Selection of skimmers for different situations

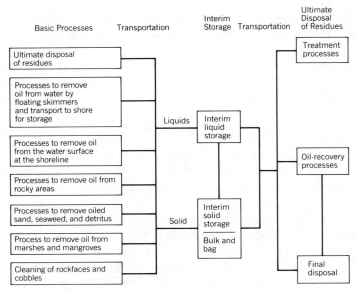

Figure 19.9. Oil-spill coastal cleanup: interrelationship of unit processes.

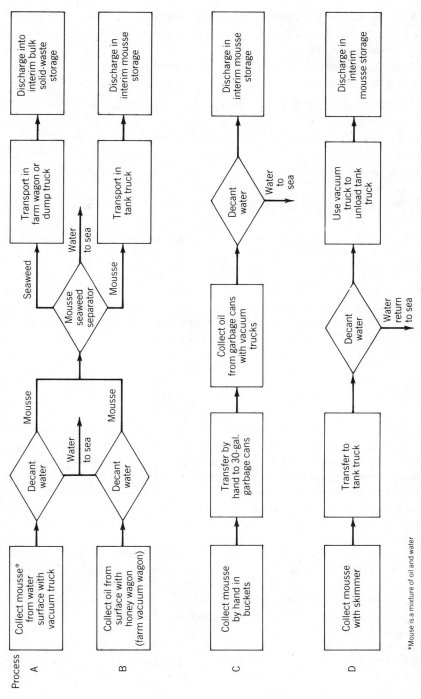

Process

A

B

C

D

Collect mousse* from water surface with vacuum truck

Collect oil from surface with honey wagon (farm vacuum wagon)

Collect mousse by hand in buckets

Collect mousse with skimmer

Decant water → Water to sea

Decant water

Transfer by hand to 30-gal. garbage cans

Transfer to tank truck

Decant water → Water return to sea

Mousse

Mousse

Mousse seaweed separator → Water to sea

Collect oil from garbage cans with vacuum trucks

Use vacuum truck to unload tank truck

Seaweed

Mousse

Decant water → Water to sea

Transport in farm wagon or dump truck

Transport in tank truck

Discharge into interim bulk solid-waste storage

Discharge in interim mousse storage

Discharge in interim mousse storage

Discharge in interim mousse storage

*Mouse is a mixture of oil and water

Figure 19.10. Unit process. Removal of mousse from water surface to interim storage (Amoco Cadiz spill).

5. Establishment of logistical chains for skimmed oil
6. Use of sorbent materials for removal, polishing-treatment, safety, and cleanup activities
7. Philosophical and technical considerations of chemical use
8. Chemical application and chemical logistical considerations
9. Use of overflow and underflow dams to retain floating and sinking materials for removal
10. Removal technologies for beaches, rocky areas, and marshes
11. Characteristics of spills to groundwater systems and removal technologies
12. In situ treatment technologies for oil and hazardous-material components in soil
13. Methods for constructing temporary storage for liquid and solid spill residues
14. The role of technical response activities in providing engineering and scientific information before, during, and after a spill.
15. Evaluation of logistical requirements for specific spill responses
16. Determination of the characteristics and use of personnel protection devices
17. Determination of instrumentation used in oil and hazardous-material spill situations to measure environmental parameters, characteristics, and transport of spilled materials and environmental risk

SUMMARY

Basic elements of the prevention and control of oil and hazardous-material spills have been presented and inter-related with the probability-of-harm equation for evaluating environmental risk. A major focus was in the elements of contingency planning and related spill-response organizations. The need for the often-neglected steps of site-specific planning and resource acquisition was emphasized.

Special emphasis was placed on making response decisions based on environmental considerations, evaluating response resources, and using cooperative resources.

In considering response activities, an inter-related priority table of typical response priorities was presented for both hazardous-material spills and for oil spills.

Special lessons relating to reasonableness of response and cost of response were presented to aid the responder in making judgement decisions.

Technical aspects of the response were presented in the form of traditional and specialized resources and the reader was shown how these resources can be linked through unit operations and processes to apply them to the needs of spill response.

SUGGESTED READINGS

R. L. Berglund and G. M. Whipple, "Predictive Modeling of Organic Air Emissions," *Chemical Engineering Progress,* **83**(11), 46–54 (Nov. 1987).

C. D. McAuliffe, "Measuring Hydrocarbons in Water," *Chemical Engineering Progress,* **83**(11), 40–45 (Nov. 1987).

J. M. Neff, "Biological Effects of Oil in the Marine Environment," *Chemical Engineering Progress,* **83**(11), 27–33 (Nov. 1987).

J. O. Stull, "Protective Suits for Chemical Spill Inspection," *Chemical Engineering Progress,* **83**(11), 34–39 (Nov. 1987).

20

Vapor Suppression by Aqueous Foams

Edward C. Norman

The use of aqueous fire-fighting foams for vapor suppression in no-fire situations is well known. Standard practice in the case of unignited spills of flammable liquids is to apply fire-fighting foam. The blanket of foam suppresses the release of vapors from the spill, thereby preventing the vapor concentration over the spill from reaching its lower explosive limit. This use is estimated to account for as much as 40 percent of all sales of fire-fighting foam.

Fire-fighting foams have also been used, at least experimentally, for vapor suppression on spills of a variety of materials that would not be classified as fuels. These materials include chlorine, anhydrous ammonia, sulfur trioxide, and oleum. The efficacy of fire-fighting foams has been somewhat limited in this use because of the instability of these foams to extremes of pH and their relatively rapid drainage rate.

Foam-generating equipment that is used in fire protection also is generally unsuitable for use with hazardous materials. When fighting a fire, it is necessary to have foam nozzles that will project the foam a reasonable distance so that the fire fighter can stand back from the fire and its radiant heat. Nozzle range and foam-making ability are a trade-off situation. There is a fixed quantity of energy available at the nozzle in the form of foam-solution pressure. This energy may be used either to make good, slow-draining foam or to project the stream long distances. It cannot do both at the same time. Foam nozzles are usually compromised in favor of range over foam-making ability.

Another factor is expansion ratio. As will be seen later, it is desirable for vapor-suppression use to have an expansion ratio in the area of 30 to 1 to 50 to 1. Foam with this expansion ratio, being very light, cannot be projected as far as the low-expansion (ratio of about 8 to 1) foam used for fire fighting.

Range is not a consideration in hazardous-material-spill situations. Since there is no radiant heat, a nozzle operator with proper personal protection equipment can stand close to the spill. Therefore, it is possible to design equipment for this purpose that maximizes foam-making ability.

Special foam concentrates have been developed for use on those hazardous materials that produce large changes in pH. These concentrates are designed to produce exceptionally stable slow-draining foam that is not destroyed by the dissolution in the foam of high- or low-pH materials. Materials that do not product a significant pH change, such as low boiling organic chemicals, may be suppressed with the foam produced by alcohol-resistant AFFF fire-fighting foam, assuming that the foam is generated by equipment that is designed to maximize foam-making ability.

MECHANISMS

The mechanisms of suppression of vapors by foam vary somewhat, depending upon the hazardous material involved. For the purpose of discussion of these mechanisms, hazardous materials have been divided into three categories: fuming acids, volatile organics, and volatile inorganics.

Fuming acids include not only those materials that are acids in their own right, such as hydrochloric and nitric acids, but also materials that react with water to form acids, such as titanium tetrachloride, chlorosilanes, or sulfur trioxide, The foam has three basic functions regarding these materials. It provides a physical barrier to vapor release, it absorbs the vapors being given off by the spill, and drainage from the foam dilutes and/or hydrolyzes the spilled materials, rendering them nonfuming. In the cases of oleum, sulfur trioxide, and titanium tetrachloride, a stratification occurs that aids in suppression.

Oleum is a solution of sulfur trioxide in sulfuric acid. Therefore, oleum and sulfur trioxide may be considered the same chemical for purposes of discussion. Spills of sulfur trioxide or oleum produce large quantities of dense smoke. This smoke is composed of droplets of sulfuric acid formed by the reaction of sulfur trioxide with atmospheric moisture:

$$SO_3 + H_2O \rightarrow H_2SO_4$$

When foam is applied to a spill, this reaction takes place at the interface between the foam and the spill. The sulfuric acid formed is less dense than oleum or sulfur trioxide, so that it forms a layer on top of the spill. This layer then becomes a reaction zone, with sulfur trioxide being added from the spill, and water, in the form of foam solution, being added from the foam. This forms more sulfuric acid, making the layer thicker (see Figures 20.1 to 20.4). Eventually, by making repeated foam applications, the entire spill can be converted to sulfuric acid, which is nonfuming.

Titanium tetrachloride reacts with water by a two-step reaction:

$$TiCl_4 + H_2O \rightarrow TiOCl_2 + 2HCl \tag{1}$$
$$TiCl_2 + H_2O \rightarrow TiOCl_2 + 2HCl \tag{2}$$

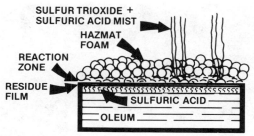

Figure 20.1. Suppression of oleum reactivity using hazmat foam. (Courtesy National Foam, Lionville, Pa.)

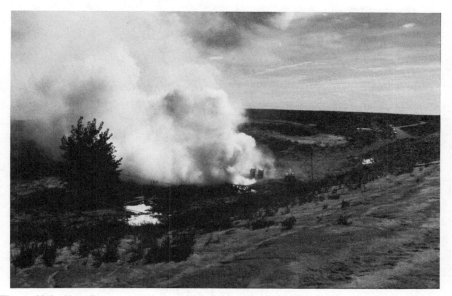

Figure 20.2. Sixty-five percent oleum spill before application of foam. (Courtesy National Foam, Lionville, Pa.)

When there is an excess of $TiCl_4$ present, only step 1 takes place. When there is an excess of water present, both steps take place. When $TiCl_4$ vapor is released to the atmosphere, there is sufficient moisture in the air to carry out both steps. Therefore, $TiCl_4$ spills generate large white clouds containing particulate TiO_2 and copious amounts of HCl.

Foam application to a $TiCl_4$ spills produces a situation at the interface where there is an excess of $TiCl_4$. Consequently, a large amount of $TiOCl_2$ is formed. This is a solid that forms a porous raft that floats on the $TiCl_4$.

As foam drainage trickles through this raft, it becomes a reaction zone, with $TiOCl_2$ being converted to TiO_2 and HCl at the top and $TiCl_4$ being converted to $TiOCl_2$ at the bottom. The HCl evolved is absorbed by the foam. Continued foam

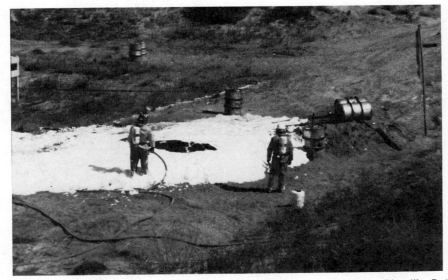

Figure 20.3. Same oleum spill after application of foam. (Courtesy National Foam, Lionville, Pa.)

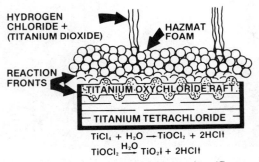

Figure 20.4. Hazmat foam mitigates titanium tetrachloride reaction. (Courtesy National Foam, Lionville, Pa.)

application will eventually result in a pool of aqueous HCl containing particulate TiO_2.

In both of these cases, plain water cannot be used, because it cannot be applied gently enough to avoid disruption of the reaction zone. If the reaction zone is disrupted, the hydrolysis of the spill becomes violent, and large quantities of vapor are emitted.

Application of foam to other fuming acids, such as hydrofluoric, nitric, or hydrochloric acid, provides a convenient means slowly to dilute the spill to a nonfuming form, while suppressing and absorbing the emission of fumes. In one actual incident, a special acid-stable foam (National Foam's Hazmat NF No. 2) was applied to a spill of a mixture of 70 percent hydrofluoric acid and 40° Baume (62 percent) nitric acid. The foam completely suppressed the emission of fumes, permitting the spill to be neutralized with lime slurry poured through the foam blanket.

Similarly, spills of such materials as chlorosilanes and thionyl chloride, which emit hydrochloric acid on hydrolysis, can be controlled by application of a blanket of acid-resistant foam. The drainage from the foam slowly hydrolyzes the spilled material while preventing emission of hydrochloric acid vapor.

Volatile organics include such materials as ethylene oxide, vinyl chloride, methyl and ethyl mercaptan, and other organic chemicals that boil at or below ambient temperature. As these materials are similar in chemical nature to the higher boiling organics, which are easily suppressed with fire-fighting foams, it is possible to suppress these low boilers with the same foams. Because the boiling points of these materials are below the temperature of the foam solution, best results are obtained by using foam-generating equipment that produces high-quality slow-draining foam. Foam quality may be enhanced by proportioning the foam concentrate at higher than the nominal percentage. For example, a foam concentrate intended for proportioning at 6 percent in fire situations could be proportioned at 8–10 percent for maximum performance.

The best foam concentrate for this use is alcohol-resistant AFFF, which is offered by most suppliers of foam concentrates. Alcohol-resistant AFFF is, by its nature, slow draining, and is not subject to destruction by polar materials.

The action of the foam on volatile organics is that of physical suppression and absorption of vapor. Physical suppression is enhanced in most cases by the formation of an ice layer at the foam/spill interface. The foam blanket also insulates the spill, preventing transfer of heat from solar radiation and the ambient air to the spill.

Volatile inorganics are inorganic chemicals other than fuming acids that emit vapor when spilled. Examples are anydrous ammonia, chlorine, hydrazine, and bromine. The use of the appropriate acid- or alkali-resistant foam suppresses the release of vapors by the same mechanisms as in the case of volatile organics. As in all other cases, it is vital to use the proper foam-generating equipment.

EQUIPMENT

Two functions are required of the equipment—proportioning and foam generation. Proportioning is the process of mixing the foam concentrate with water in the proper proportion. Proportioning devices suitable for use with fire-fighting foams are also suitable for use with the special foams used on hazardous-materials spills. Detailed description of these devices is beyond the scope of this chapter, as there is a wide range available. They may be as simple as a venturi-type in-line inductor or as complex as a balanced-pressure fixed proportioning system. Choice of the proper device will be dictated by the size and nature of the hazard and the water pressure available.

There are several types of foam-generating equipment in use by the fire service.

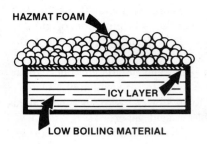

Figure 20.5. Vapor suppression of low boiling chemical using midexpansion hazmat foam permits immediate control of vaporization. (Courtesy National Foam, Lionville, Pa.)

Not all of them are suitable for hazardous-material spill use, as foam quality is not critical in fire-suppression situations. These devices can be generally classified as low-expansion, medium-expansion, and high-expansion generators.

Low-expansion devices are the most common. They include air-aspirating foam nozzles, foam chambers, foam–water sprinklers, nonaspirating foam nozzles, and conventional sprinklers. The only low-expansion devices suitable for use in spills control are air-aspirating devices. Nozzles designed for use with protein foam are preferred, as they produce higher quality foam than that generated by "all-purpose" or AFFF nozzles. Low-expansion nozzles should be used only with alcohol-resistant AFFF. Best results with the special acid- or alkali-resistant foams are obtained with medium-expansion equipment.

Medium-expansion foam-generation equipment (Figure 20.5) produces foam with expansion ratios ranging from 25 to 1 to 200 to 1. This type of equipment is commonly used for fire fighting in Europe, but has not been widely adopted by U.S. fire departments. However, medium-expansion generators are available in the United States from Angus, Feecon, MSA, National Foam, and Rockwood.

High-expansion generators produce foam with expansion ratios between 200 to 1 and 1000 to 1. While there is no performance barrier to using high-expansion ratios on hazardous-material spills, foams at these expansion ratios are easily disrupted by wind and are generally not suitable for outdoor use. Also, in those applications where the foam has a diluting or hydrolyzing effect, the low water content in high-expansion foams will make the spill-control process a lengthy proposition.

TEST RESULTS

Prior to 1987, there were few test reports available on experiments with the use of foam on hazardous-material spills, and most of these dealt with laboratory-scale spills. National Foam conducted a series of large-scale outdoor tests in 1987, the results of which were presented to the American Institute of Chemical Engineers meeting in August 1986, and will be published by the AIChE.

Two test methods were used. On fuming acids, which emit visible vapors, foam was applied to 50–70-gallon spills in a 50-square-foot pan and the results observed visually. The test procedure is as follows:

The chemical is transferred from drums to the pan. Foam is then applied and the timer started. The foam blanket is maintained by reapplications, if necessary, until the vapor release is reduced to occasional small "puffs" through the foam blanket. The time required from the start of foam application to attain this condition is recorded as "control time."

A weighed 50-square-foot pan was used for volatile organics and volatile inorganics, with the evaporation rate being recorded both with and without foam. The percentage mitigation was calculated as follows:

$$\text{Evaporation rate} = \frac{\text{Original weight} - \text{Final weight}}{\text{Time} \times \text{Area}} = \text{pounds/minute/square foot}$$

$$\text{Mitigation percent} = \frac{\begin{array}{c}\text{Evaporation rate} \\ \text{(no foam)}\end{array} - \begin{array}{c}\text{Evaporation rate} \\ \text{(with foam)}\end{array}}{\begin{array}{c}\text{Evaporation rate} \\ \text{(no foam)}\end{array}} \times 100$$

TABLE 20.1

Chemical	Foam Concentrate	Foam Expansion Ratio	Results
35 percent oleum	Hazmat NF no. 2[a]	48:1	Control time[d] < 1 min.
65 percent oleum	Hazmat NF no. 2	48:1	Control time[d] 5 min. 20 sec.
Sulfur trioxide	Hazmat NF no. 2	48:1	Control time[d] 4 min. 30 sec.
Chlorosulfonic acid	Hazmat NF no. 2	48:1	No control[d]
Titanium tetrachloride	Hazmat NF no. 2	48:1	Control time[d] 1 min. 40 sec.
Ethylene oxide	Universal[b]	7.5:1	Mitigation[e] > 80 percent
Vinyl chloride	Universal	9.4:1	Mitigation[e] 65–80 percent
Methyl mercaptan	Universal	9.4:1	Mitigation[e] > 80 percent
Anhydrous ammonia	Hazmat NF no. 1[c]	48:1	Mitigation[e] > 75 percent

[a]Acid-resistant foam.
[b]Alcohol-resistant AFFF.
[c]Alkali-resistant foam.
[d]Visual observation method—see text.
[e]Weight pan method—see text.

Example: Four hundred pounds of chemical is added to a 50-square-foot pan. After 30 minutes, 250 pounds remains. The pan is recharged to bring the weight up to 400 pounds and foam is applied. Thirty minutes after foam application, 350 pounds of chemical remains after allowing for the weight of the foam.

$$\text{Evaporation rate (no foam)} = \frac{400 - 250}{30 \times 50} = 0.1 \text{ pound/minute/square foot}$$

$$\text{Evaporation rate (with foam)} = \frac{400 - 350}{30 \times 50} = 0.0333$$

$$\text{Mitigation percent} = \frac{0.1 - 0.033}{0.1} \times 100 = 67 \text{ percent}$$

SUMMARY

Aqueous foams can be used effectively to suppress vapor release from spills of many hazardous materials. For best results, it is important to use a foam concentrate that is resistant to the spilled material. Foam-generating equipment should be of a type that produces a stable, slow-draining foam. Expansion ratios of more than 30 to 1 are desirable for use on water-reactive materials. Foams with expansion ratios of 8 to 1 or higher can be used on materials that are water reactive. Foam application may be expected to reduce the rate of vapor emission from a spill by 75 percent or more. Repeated foam applications to water-reactive or water-soluble materials will dilute and/or hydrolyze the spilled material to make it nonfuming.

21

Innovative On-Site Treatment/Destruction Technologies for Remediation of Contaminated Sites

Masood Ghassemi

It is now widely recognized that the traditional approaches to the cleanup of contaminated sites consisting of site isolation and/or excavation and redisposal in landbased containment systems do not provide the desired long-term environmental protection. Waste treatment and destruction can provide a more permanent solution and are now being actively evaluated as alternatives to waste relocation and site isolation. Treatment/destruction can be carried out on site (in situ or in mobile units) or at off-site facilities, with the former offering the advantage of eliminating risks associated with waste transportation to off-site locations.

Seven in situ and four above-ground mobile-site cleanup technologies are reviewed from the standpoint of operating principle, state of development, reported experience, and application requirements. The in situ technologies discussed are bioreclamation, soil vapor extraction, air stripping, steam/hot air stripping, immobilization, soil washing, and vitrification. Three high-temperature destruction systems, one low-temperature stripping, and a soil-washing system are reviewed as examples of innovative technologies for mobile system applications.

At present, there are a number of impediments to rapid commercialization and widespread use of the new technologies. Two key areas relate to the current lack of (1) reliable cost and performance data on candidate technologies and (2) streamlined procedures to facilitate acquisition of necessary permits. These issues are being addressed by the EPA through its Superfund Innovative Technology Evaluation (SITE) initiative and by various regulatory agencies through an examination of ways to faciliate permits.

Technologies that have been considered or used in the past for mitigating problems at contaminated sites have emphasized site isolation using physical barriers and/or removal of contaminated soil and waste for disposal at off-site land-based disposal facilities.[1,2] According to the EPA, of a total of 66 Record of Decisions (ROD) approved in fiscal year 1985 by the agency for remedial action at Superfund sites, 54 percent included off-site disposal of wastes as an element of the remedial action; on-site land filling (i.e., construction of an on-site containment facility or disposal cell to contain wastes) and site capping (i.e., construction of a synthetic, soil, or clay cap at the site to reduce infiltration into the waste) were involved in 42 percent of the cases.[3]

There is a substantial amount of uncertainty regarding the effectiveness of the currently available land-based containment and disposal technologies to provide long-term environmental protection. This recognition of the questionable long-term effectiveness of the existing land-disposal and containment methods has promoted considerable interest in developing, testing, and commercializing remediation technologies that provide for treatment or destruction of the waste. Waste treatment and destruction can be carried out on site or at off-site facilities, with the on-site treatment offering the advantage of eliminating the risks associated with waste transportation to off-site locations.

This chapter reviews some of the promising treatment/destruction technologies that have been tested or are under development for on-site remediation at contaminated sites. For discussion purposes, on-site remediation technologies have been grouped into two categories: in situ technologies and above-ground technologies. Some technologies discussed under the in situ category require above-ground processing of the material resulting from in situ treatment. The discussion of technologies is preceded by a review of some of the limitations of the heretofore widely used land-based containment systems and a discussion of certain recent regulatory developments that place restrictions on the use of land-based systems and promote alternatives to land disposal.

LAND-BASED CONTAINMENT SYSTEMS

Landfills and Surface Impoundments

Land-based containment systems such as landfills and surface impoundments have been widely used for waste disposal. For example, according to recent EPA estimates,[4] there are more than 180,000 active surface impoundments in the United States. Many of the currently active landfills and surface impoundments were placed in service at a time when there were no regulations in effect to govern their siting, design, and construction and to require performance monitoring and reporting. Because of this, and the then lack of full appreciation of the potential consequences of facility failure, there have been numerous cases of containment system failure due to poor siting and inadequate design, construction, operation, and maintenance practices. Because many of these facilities contain hazardous wastes and are located over usable waters, some site failures have resulted in or present a threat of groundwater contamination. A number of these facilities are now on the National Priority List for remediation under the Superfund program.

Landfills and surface impoundments rely on natural or manufactured liners and caps to contain the waste and present physical barriers against migration of waste constituents away from and infiltration of surface water or groundwater into the disposal site. Thus, siting in suitable geological formations, use of properly designed and constructed liners and caps, and installation of reliable leak-detection and groundwater-monitoring systems would be the key requirements for developing adequate land-based containment systems and protecting groundwater resources. The EPA and many of the states have developed guidelines and regulations governing the design, construction, operation, and monitoring of land-based containment systems. Some of the standards and guidelines appear overly conservative, reflecting attempts to compensate for the many existing technical uncertainties and the lack of long-term performance data from actual facilities that comply with the recommended standards. Thus, under Sections 3004(o) and 3015 of the Resource Conservation and Recovery Act (RCRA), as amended by the Hazardous and Solid Waste Amendments (HSWA) of 1984, certain landfills and surface impoundments are required to have "two or more liners and a leachate collection system above [in the case of a landfill] and between such liners." Guidelines that have been drafted by EPA pursuant to this HSWA requirement recommend use of two liners and leachate-collection and leak-detection systems.[5] Figure 21.1 is a schematic drawing of a cross section of multilayer cap and liner systems for landfills and surface impoundments.

The stringencies in the regulations and the redundancies in the recommended designs have been justified on the basis of the experience that indicate that (1) even some well-designed facilities that have used the state-of-the-art technologies have failed, (2) geological deposits that are relied upon to provide protection against groundwater contamination are often discontinuous and cannot eliminate the potential for lateral and vertical migration of waste, and (3) when damage occurs, the cost of cleanup can be very high.

In establishing the technical data base for developing regulatory guidelines, design and construction standards, and monitoring and reporting requirements for land-based hazardous-waste containment systems, the EPA has sponsored a number of studies in recent years where case-study-type information has been collected on existing facilities and perspectives of facility owners/operators, design engineers, construction contractors, and state and local regulatory agencies have been solicited on ways to ensure the long-term effectiveness of containment systems. These studies have indicated the following.[6–10]

The requirements for developing successful containment systems include adequate site investigation, good project planning during the design and construction phase, and rigorous execution of a comprehensive quality assurance/quality control (QA/QC) program. Problems resulting from inadequate site investigation and poor design and construction practices cannot be fully and permanently corrected through piecemeal remedies applied as the problem surface.

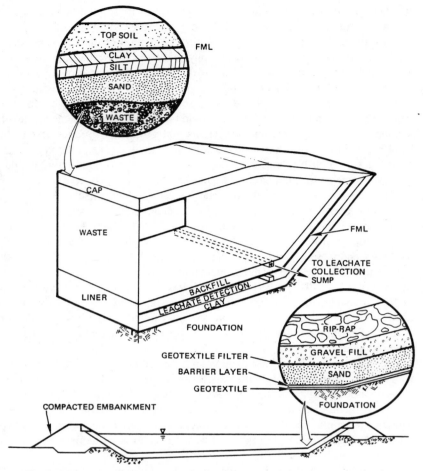

Figure 21.1. Liner and cap systems for landfills and surface impoundments.

Construction supervision and inspection by competent and conscientious inspectors to ensure adherence to recommended specifications and rigorous documentation and record keeping are cornerstones of an effective QA/QC program. The program should cover all steps (i.e., planning, design, construction, etc.) leading to the development of a completed facility and should encompass all system elements, support facilities, operations, and corrective measures (i.e., monitoring, leak detection subdrains, repairs, etc.).

QA/QC programs for facilities lined with flexible membrane liners should emphasize liner–waste compatibility as a criterion for liner selection, proper installation procedures (particularly in the seaming step), and the use of protective cover (especially when the liner would be exposed to severe stresses of the elements).

Even though waste–liner compatibility tests provide valuable data for selecting a suitable liner, the characteristics of the waste that will come into contact with the liner are often not known at the time of design and the characteristics may change during site operation, requiring periodic reexamination of the compatability issue.

Subdrain leak detectors, which permit direct observation, have merits over monitoring wells (or other indirect methods) by allowing more rapid detection of failure, permitting monitoring over a relatively large area under the liner, and yielding more reliable results. Unless groundwater monitoring is relatively comprehensive and is tailored to the specific hydrogeological and other features of a site, it may prove inadequate in providing a true picture of the background conditions and changes in water quality.

Even if a leak is detected, it is very difficult to pinpoint its exact location in an in-service liner; the repair of in-service liners is very complex and can be very costly depending on the accessability of the liner and the amount of waste that must be removed to obtain access to the liner.

The EPA has published a number of guidance and technical resource documents covering the latest technologies for design and construction of land-based containment systems. (Some examples are cited as Refs. 5, 11, and 12). Based on the information provided in these documents, it appears that the technology and know-how currently exist for constructing and installing effective land-based containment systems. In actual practice, however, the best technology and know-how have not often been and may not always be utilized, as evidenced by many documented cases of site failure. A recent assessment of flexible membrane liners (FML) successes and failures at waste storage and disposal sites identified 12 "failures" at 10 sites, based on data provided by five vendors for 27 case-study facilities selected by the vendors.[13] At four or five of these facilities, groundwater contamination apparently resulted from the failures. The following were identified as contributing factors, if not causes, for the failures[13]:

Failures to control the operations (at an operating site) so as to safeguard the liner.

Poor (or inadequate) design work.

Failure to use an independent, qualified design engineer.

Poor (or inadequate) installation work.

Poor (or inadequate) communication and cooperation between companies working on an installation job.

The use of untrained and/or poorly supervised installers.

Failure to conduct (or adequately conduct) waste–liner compatibility tests.

Adverse weather conditions during installation.

Use of old dump site, with contaminated soil, as site for lined facility.

Selection of companies (for liner job) by processes that did not help ensure good material and workmanship would result.

Selection of liner material by processes not involving detailed bid specifications (prepared by design engineer, not liner manufacturer).

Facility age (more failures were associated with the older sites).

The completion of a major containment system involves many steps and requires a range of expertise and inputs from many participants. In the absence of a comprehensive quality-assurance program, many opportunities exist for inadvertent mistakes and underestimation of the complexities of the job requirements, and this can lead to inadequacies and site failures. Some examples of the many problems that must be addressed and applicable preventive and corrective measures are listed in Table 21.1. EPA recently published a "Technical Guidance Document"[12] presenting guidance for preparing a site-specific construction quality assurance plan for a land disposal facility. The guidance describes considerations that EPA believes can ensure that a completed facility has been constructed to meet or exceed all design criteria, plans, and specifications.

TABLE 21.1. Examples of Liner and Cover Systems Problems and Applicable Preventive and Corrective Measures[7]

General problem areas (both clay and FML):	
Poorly written and difficult-to-read specifications and guidelines	Requiring (educating) designers and suppliers to write lucid and easy-to-follow specifications
Inadequate QA/QC	Developing and implementing adequate QA/QC at all steps of design, construction, installation, and operation of facility
Liner-waste/leachate incompatibility	Selection of suitable liner based on literature data, manufacturer's information, actual or estimated waste characteristics, and liner-waste compatibility tests
Locating leaks	Use of methods (some still in developmental stage) for leak detection. Examples: water balance for surface impoundments, electrical conductivity method, use of observation wells, groundwater monitoring, and visual inspection of caps
Facility foundation (both clay and FML):	
Compaction to less than the required density (resulting possibly in later differential settlement which can introduce stresses in the overlying liner)	Use of the state-of-the-art earthwork techniques/practices and an adequate QC to ensure that such practices are actually utilized
Permitting the foundation to develop a moisture condition that is incompatibile with subsequent liner placement steps	Same as above

TABLE 21.1 (*Continued*)

Problem	Preventive/Corrective Measures
Inadequate surface finishing to reduce the potential for liner puncture (this is generally a concern for the FML only)	Same as above
Inadequate sterilization of the foundation soils to suppress the growth of vegetation that can potentially penetrate the liner	Same as the above

Clay liner and caps:

Problem	Preventive/Corrective Measures
Where in situ clays are involved, failing to detect and remove discontinuities such as sand or silt lenses, roots, and rocks, from the clay	Detailed soil investigations to determine the applicability of overexcavation and recompaction of clay
Where recompacted emplaced soil liners are used, inadequate protection of stockpile from contamination	Covering stockpiles (or seeding for lengthy storage), inspection to detect and remove contaminants, and adjustment of moisture content
Failing to attain the desired permeability that generally results from the difficulty of ensuring that conditions in the field closely meet those specified in the design specifications	Use of laboratory permeability tests for general guidance during final design in conjunction with field permeability tests on individual lifts and the completed liner for construction verification
Cracking, particularly by dessication, between the time that the liner is completed and when it is backfilled or put directly back into service	Inspection of moisture content, destruction of large clay clods during construction; immediately after installation, placement of backfill, synthetic material, or fluid over the liner
Flextural cracking of the cap during installation due to the operation of heavy equipment on spongy waste	Placement of additional lifts on as-needed basis; reducing sponginess of waste fill by mixing soil or granular waste into soft wastes or reducing thickness of wastes containing soft wastes

FML liners and caps:

Problem	Preventive/Corrective Measures
Damage to liner material due to exposure to adverse weather, vandalism, and repeated folding and unfolding	Storing liner material in a secure area, reducing time between delivery and placement of liner, avoiding unnecessary folding/unfolding, and inspecting materials
Placement of panels in a wrong configuration (e.g., seams on side slopes oriented parallel rather than correctly perpendicular to the side)	Identification of panels by number at manufacture and fabrication and strict adherence to design specifications
Placements that bridge a gap between two surfaces (e.g., at penetrations)	Ensuring complete liner contact with supporting soil and proper subgrade compaction around appurtenances

(continued)

TABLE 21.1 *(Continued)*

Problem	Preventive/Corrective Measures
Improper anchoring (e.g., backfilling anchor trenches before seaming is completed)	Anchoring panel edges with sandbags before seaming, careful operation of equipment during anchor trench backfilling
Improper timing (e.g., placement during inclement weather, including windy conditions)	Avoiding installation during inclement weather and effective QA to assure this; patching and seaming to correct most wind-related damage
Placement of the liner with little clearance between it and the leachate collection pipes. This is often unavoidable per the requirements of the leachate collection system, but any ruptured pipe could potentially puncture the liner	Careful placement and compaction of drainage beds
Inadequate seams resulting from use of inadequate seaming techniques, seaming during adverse weather conditions, seaming with inadequate materials, seaming new material to old liner material, and not paying special attention to seaming around penetrations	Strict adherence to the seaming procedures (e.g., time and amount of solvents, pressure applied to seams, etc.) recommended for the specific liner material at hand; use of experienced installers (at least at the foreman level); installation during suitable weather conditions
	Removal of slacks and wrinkles, except those included intentionally to allow for thermal expansion and contraction
	Allowing enough time for the completed seam to develop strength before loading
	Giving special attention to making connections between the liner and structures
	Taking special precautions when new cap material is seamed to old liner material (e.g., ensuring that the bottom liner and caps are compatible when seamed, removing the surface cure from the bottom liner using solvents and scrubbers, and repairing damage that the bottom liner suffers when it is uncovered
Mechanial damage to liner during placement of backfill	Use of minimum soil lift of 12–18 inches; careful operation of equipment on backfill, specify maximum weight to be driven on liner; use of temporary ramps for equipment to drive the disposal unit on and off

The documented inadequacies of many existing containment systems and the potential difficulties in implementing the guidelines and recommendations that reflect the best available technologies can be attributed to several factors, most important among which are the following.

The high cost associated with the implementation of necessary site investigations and the state-of-the-art design, construction, and operating practices.

Lack of technical resources on the part of some consulting engineering firms, construction contractors, and liner manufacturing, fabricating, and installing companies to fully understand, appreciate, and implement the many critical requirements for developing adequate containment systems.

Lack of knowledge by uninformed customers and the prevalent business practice of securing engineering, construction, and liner installation services largely on the basis of costs.

The heretofore lack of stringent regulations and the often inadequate resources of the regulatory agencies to develop and enforce technically defensible regulations within very stringent time frames specified in various laws and court rulings.

Even if the present practices could produce reliable and cost-effective containment systems, such systems at best can be viewed as an interim solution whereby the problem of hazardous-waste management is merely transferred to new locations and/or future generations. It is because of this and the other considerations discussed above that attention is now being directed at finding more permanent solutions to waste-management problems through such options as waste minimization, treatment, and destruction.

Cutoff Walls and Bottom Barriers

Use of landfills and surface impoundments in connection with site remediation requires that the waste, contaminated soil, or groundwater be excavated/removed and transferred to such facilities. Alternatively, the contamination can be isolated or contained in place by constructing low-permeability subsurface barriers that completely or partially surround the contaminated area. Such barriers provide for containment of contaminated groundwater, diversion of uncontaminated groundwater around a contaminated area, and lowering the groundwater table inside the isolated area. The most commonly used types of subsurface barriers (or cutoff walls) are cement-bentonite and soil-bentonite slurry walls or trenches, grout curtains, and sheet piles. Slurry walls have been installed to retard the movement of groundwater or leachate at numerous waste sites. Significant recent advances in the capacity of excavating equipment and refinements in techniques have lowered the cost of slurry walls and this has contributed to their increased acceptance and use.[14] Slurry walls are constructed by excavating a trench of desired configuration using a soil or cement, bentonite, and water mixture to support the sides. The trench is then backfilled with material having far less permeability than the original or the surrounding soil.

The cutoff walls in general are not impermeable, and some leakage through them is inevitable. A second limitation is that exposure to the wastes at some sites may cause increases in wall permeability. Certain chemicals have been shown to have pronounced effects on both bentonite and Portland cement, and even brief exposure of some walls to high-strength leachates can seriously threaten their integrity.[15] Engineering case studies at two Superfund sites (the Stringfellow site in southern California and the Sylvester site near the New Hampshire/Massachusetts border) have indicated the difficulty of containing hazardous waste with grout curtains and slurry walls.[16] The use of cutoff walls primarily constitutes an interim measure of groundwater protection while the source of contamination is being eliminated or the contaminated groundwater is being remediated in situ or pumped out for treatment in surface facilities. Although cutoff walls have been used as groundwater barriers in the construction industry for decades, their use in pollution control is fairly new and long-term performance data are not available in site-cleanup applications.

Several concepts have been proposed for in-place construction of bottom barriers at uncontrolled hazardous-waste sites, including existing landfills that, because of poor siting or liner failure, are contaminating the groundwater or threatening to contaminate the groundwater. These bottom sealing concepts rely on the drilling technology and the grouting practice that have been used in the oil and gas industry and for construction-site dewatering and construction structural support. Systems proposed include directional drilling, pancake slurry jetting, jet grouting, hydrofracing, block displacement, and chemical mixing/sediment solidification.[17] Of these, the block displacement is the only approach known to have been attempted in the context of an uncontrolled chemical dump site.[17] The technique involves injecting a barrier material through bore holes a few meters apart. Continuous pumping of the slurry under pressure produces a large uplift force against the bottom of the block and results in a vertical displacement proportional to the volume of the slurry pumped. Based on the bore-hole spacing used at the EPA-sponsored demonstration project in Jacksonville, Fla., approximately 155 bore holes would be needed for each acre of the contaminated site.[17]

Under EPA sponsorship, field tests were recently conducted with two chemical grouts to determine if a continuous impermeable seal could be developed by injecting grout into coarse-grained soils.[18] Acrylate and sodium silicate grouts were injected into separate 2- by 4-meter test beds of medium sand at a 30–50-cm depth using a maximum hole spacing of 40 cm (center to center) to produce a panlike layer of grout. While some silicate grout bulbs coalesced, there were significant gaps in the grout layer and shrinkage of grout produced nonuniform cementing. The acrylate grout flowed to the bottom of the sand bed and did not produce grout bulbs. In a larger field test, 30 percent sodium silicate was injected at a 2.44-meter depth in fine sand using injection holes on 1.52-meter centers. Significant problems were noted when the pools were excavated. The pods were not symmetrical and ungrouted areas were present between pods. Pockets of coarse sand in the finer sand were not cemented although they had been filled with grout. Roots and rootlet holes in the cemented sand were not sealed. Data from the field tests thus indicated that conventional injection of chemical grouts did not produce an impervious seal and that other techniques may be needed to obtain a useful seal.

The above-cited field evaluations of chemical grout injection techniques were conducted at test sites that did not contain hazardous wastes. The use of chemical grouts under waste sites (or around contaminated areas in the form of grout curtains), however, requires careful consideration of interfering reactions from waste, contaminated soil, or groundwater. Testing of grouts on a laboratory scale has shown that solutions simulating wastes in groundwater can seriously alter the gelling time of the grouts or can completely inhibit gellation.[19] In 20-day waste-exposure tests, silicate grout and Portland cement grouts showed less interaction with the waste than urethane and acrylate grouts. Silicate grout was attacked and dissolved by sodium hydroxide. Several companies now market proprietary chemical formulations for fixation and solidification of wastes and contaminated soils and claim a very high degree of stability for the products. A field demonstration program is planned to evaluate the effectiveness of one such fixation formulation in an in situ application at a site in Florida using advanced Japanese ground engineering technologies for boring and injection and mixing of fixation chemicals.

According to the above discussion, a significant amount of developmental work is needed in order to transform the proposed bottom-sealing concepts into commercially viable technologies for site remediation.

REGULATORY CONSIDERATIONS

Land-Disposal Restrictions

In recent years, a number of laws have been enacted and regulations promulgated on both the federal and state levels placing some severe restrictions on land disposal of hazardous wastes while at the same time bringing additional waste generators (e.g., the "small quantity generators") and waste quantities (e.g., from cleanup of uncontrolled hazardous-waste sites) under regulation. Because of these regulatory restrictions and requirements (see Table 21.2 for pertinent provisions of the 1984 Hazardous and Solid Waste Amendments) and the growing public opposition to siting new land-disposal facilities, there has been a significant rise in the cost of land disposal and a scarcity of available commercial disposal sites. Not only are land-disposal facilities that meet the stringent requirements for siting, design, construction, monitoring, and plans and financial assurace for closure and postclosure care in short supply, but their continued use poses potential liabilities for waste producers. By law waste producers can be held responsible for their hazardous wastes indefinitely, whether they dispose of the wastes on their own facilities or in off-site commercial facilities via contract service.

The disposal of wastes in land-based facilities cannot ever be eliminated completely, as there will always be a need to dispose of certain troublesome wastes and residues that are not amenable to destruction or further treatment and material

TABLE 21.2. Some Provisions of the 1984 Hazardous and Solid Waste Amendments (HSWA) Affecting Land Disposal of Hazardous Wastes

"Banned wastes"

The land disposal of hazardous wastes must be banned unless EPA determines that the prohibition of one or more methods of land disposal is not required in order to protect human health and the environment. A method of land disposal may not be determined to be protective of the health and the environment unless a petitioner demonstrates that there will be no migration from the disposal unit as long as the waste remains hazardous.

EPA must promulgate regulations specifying levels or methods of treatment, if any, which substantially diminish the toxicity of the waste or substantially reduce the likelihood of migration of hazardous constituents from the wastes such that threats to human health and the environment are minimized. "Otherwise banned" wastes so treated are exempt from the ban.

Other than disposal in injection wells, EPA must decide whether to ban the land disposal of dioxins and solvents within 24 months of enactment, and eight months later, the "California wastes." The decision whether to ban these wastes from injection wells must be made within 45 months of enactment. Within 24 months of enactment, EPA must publish a schedule for determining whether to ban the land disposal of "listed" hazardous wastes. (*Note:* On November 7, 1986, EPA published final rules prohibiting land disposal of wastes containing dioxin and 21 solvents, unless they have been treated to reduce toxicity.)

Liquids in landfills

Within six months of enactment, the landfilling of bulk or noncontainerized liquids is prohibited. Within 12 months, the disposal of nonhazardous liquids is prohibited in "Subtitle C" facilities unless the only reasonable alternative is disposal in a non-Subtitle C landfill or unlined surface impoundment that contains or may contain hazardous waste, and such disposal may not endanger a drinking water supply. Within 15 months of enactment, EPA must promulgate regulations that minimize the landfilling of containerized hazardous liquids, and prohibit the landfilling of liquids absorbed in materials that biodegrade or release liquids when compressed.

Retrofitting of surface impoundments

Per specified compliance dates and subject to certain exemptions, "interim status" impoundments must either comply with the double-liner, leachate collection, and groundwater monitoring requirements described below or stop receiving, storing, or treating hazardous waste.

Storage of banned wastes

Surface impoundments that store or treat hazardous waste banned from land disposal units must (a) remove hazardous treatment residues within one year of the waste's placement in the impoundment, (b) unless it meets the conditions for exemption from retrofitting requirements, comply with the requirements for new impoundments described below, and (c) be solely for the purpose of accumulating sufficient quantities to facilitate proper subsequent management.

Minimum technology standards for new land-disposal facilities

A landfill unit or impoundment for which a "Part B" permit application has not been received by the date of enactment must have a double liner with leachate collection system (for landfills) and between the liners and monitor groundwater.

TABLE 21.2 (*Continued*)

Waste minimization
After September 1, 1985, manifests must contain a generator certification that the volume and/or quantity and the toxicity of the waste has been reduced to the maximum degree economically practicable, and the method used to manage the waste minimizes risk to the extent possible. Biennial reports must indicate efforts to reduce waste volume and the reduction actually achieved. After September 1, 1985, as a condition for an on-site permit, the generator must certify at least annually that efforts have been undertaken to reduce waste volume and that reduction has actually been achieved. By October 1, 1986, EPA must submit a report to Congress on the feasibility of establishing waste minimization regulations. (*Note:* EPA has now submitted its report to Congress, indicating that it has no immediate plans to impose a regulatory program to force industry to reduce waste generated. EPA, however, plans a series of actions over the next few years to help increased minimization. These include[20]: development of nonbinding guidance on what practices constitute waste minimization; development of new biennial report data sheets for more accurate and consistent data collection; continued research and development activities on waste audits and technology transfer documents; and incorporation of waste minimization reporting in premanufacture notices under the Toxic Substances Control Act.)

---

recovery. At the present time, disposal in the state-of-the-art land-based containment systems continues to remain a very practical and economically viable option for management of certain waste streams, such as concentrated inorganic sludges and the residues from waste incineration. The current regulatory strategy for hazardous-waste management thus emphasizes efforts to reduce dependence on land-disposal methods by minimizing the amount of waste that would be destined for land disposal. This strategy, which is reflected in various provisions of the 1984 Hazardous and Solid Waste Amendments (see Table 21.2), emphasizes source controls to reduce the amount of wastes produced, waste separation and concentration to reduce volume, waste utilization through exchange and energy and material recovery, and waste treatment and destruction.

Site-Cleanup Technology Selection Under CERCLA

Prior to the enactment of the Superfund Amendments and Reauthorization Act of 1986 (SARA), the evaluation, selection, and use of cleanup measures at Superfund sites conformed to the National Contingency Plan (NCP), which had been developed pursuant to the requirements of the Comprehensive Environmental Response, Compensation, and Liability Act of 1980 (CERCLA or Superfund Act). NCP established protocols for conducting remedial investigations (RI) and feasibility studies (FS) as steps in the determination of suitable cleanup remedies. The RI process consists of (1) collection and analysis of data on waste characteristics, their hazards, and routes of exposure; and (2) assembling of data on treatability of wastes and performance of treatment processes, as necessary. In the FS process, a number of potential remedial alternatives are developed and screened, and the most promising subset of alternatives is evaluated against a range of factors and compared against one another. The detailed analysis of alternatives, which is the basis for selection of a site-cleanup remedy, include the following.

Refinement and specification of alternatives in detail, with emphasis on use of established technology.

Detailed costs estimation, including operation and maintenance costs, and distribution of costs over time.

Evaluation in terms of engineering implementation, reliability, and constructability.

An assessment of the extent to which the alternative is expected effectively to prevent, mitigate, or minimize threats to and provide adequate protection of public health and welfare and the environment.

Although the NCP states that the "innovative or advanced technology shall, as appropriate, be evaluated as an alternative to conventional technology," many of the waste-treatment and destruction technologies, particularly the innovative ones, do not meet the "proven-technology" and "cost-effectiveness" criteria for application to site cleanup and hence have been rejected in favor of land-based disposal methods that are considered to be both proven and cost-effective. This assertion regarding land-based disposal systems has, of course, been questioned by many, who point to the numerous documented cases of failure. These critics[1,16,21] argue that if the analysis of remediation costs includes the costs for implementation of a comprehensive QA/QC program, which is required to ensure adequate performance, and/or the cost of corrective action associated with the failure of disposal methods, then treatment and destruction methods that provide more permanent remedies may, in fact, prove the most cost-effective solution in the long term.

Emphasis on Innovative Technologies Under SARA

While retaining the basic protocol and framework for technology screening and selection of remedies for Superfund sites, SARA adds some new features and emphasis. The most significant emphasis is on risk reduction through destruction or detoxification of hazardous waste by employing treatment technologies that reduce toxicity, mobility, or volume rather than protection achieved through prevention of exposure (e.g., via site isolation and pollution containment). SARA requires that the EPA select a remedy that utilizes permanent solutions and alternative treatment and resource-recovery technologies to the maximum extent practicable.

Pending the upcoming revision of the NCP, EPA has published interim guidance regarding implementation of SARA provisions for selection of site-cleanup remedies.[22] The proposed remedy selection process under SARA is depicted in Figure 21.2. The initial screening of the alternatives (FS phase II) is based on the consideration of the effectiveness, cost, and implementability of each remedy. Although cost will continue to be an important factor in comparing alternatives that produce similar results, it cannot be used to discriminate between treatment and nontreatment alternatives. According to the interim guidelines, innovative technologies should be carried through the screening if there is reasonable belief that they offer potential for better treatment performance or implementability, few or lesser adverse effects than other available approaches, or lower costs than demonstrated technologies. As noted previously and shown in Figure 21.2, the selection of a remedy for a site should consider not only cost-effectiveness but also, to the maximum extent practicable, utilization of permanent solutions and alternative treatment and resource-recovery technologies.

Superfund Innovative Technology Evaluation (SITE) Program

To promote development and use of alternative or innovative site-cleanup technologies, SARA authorizes an expenditure of $98 million over five years (1987–1991) for the purposes of carrying out the applied research, development, and demonstration support programs. Pursuant to this authorization, EPA is currently engaged in an initiative called the Superfund Innovative Technology Evaluation (SITE) program. The objective of the SITE program is to demonstrate, evaluate, and report on competitively selected commercially developed technologies that are applicable to onsite or off-site cleanup of hazardous-substance spills and releases at Superfund sites. Under the current plans, the demonstration testing and evaluation of each selected technology will be carried out as a cooperative effort between EPA and the developer of the technology.[23] Both EPA and the developer will contribute funds and personnel to the project. In general, the developer of the technology will contribute the demonstration part while EPA will contribute to the evaluation part of the project. In addition, EPA intends to provide third-party contractors and consultants to perform portions of work under the EPA-contributed evaluation part of the project.

Each year for the next several years, EPA plans to issue solicitations for demonstrating technologies under the SITE program. Each solicitation is expected to result in the implementation of approximately 10 demonstration projects. According to the EPA SITE Strategy Program Plan,[24] the demonstration program will emphasize technologies that are designed to treat Superfund waste for which treatment options need to be identified and developed. These high-priority wastes include the following: (1) wastes that are difficult to treat, that is, for which few or no treatment options are currently available, or the options are very expensive; (2) wastes that frequently are found at Superfund sites and in large volumes (particularly contaminated soils); (3) waste with a large potential for creating adverse health and/or environmental effects; and (4) wastes projected to be restricted by EPA from land disposal in the near future. The technologies will also meet one or more of the following criteria[24]:

Provides a permanent solution (i.e., destroys the contaminants or significantly reduces their toxicity, mobility, volume, or a combination thereof).

Can be used on site as opposed to requiring costly transport of waste (although off-site technologies will also be considered).

Has significantly lower cost than current methods.

Has significantly better performance than the current methods (e.g., provides better treatment or destruction and is easier to operate).

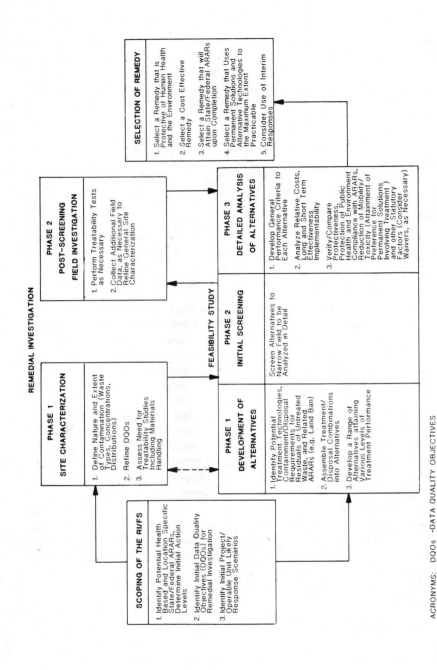

REMEDIAL INVESTIGATION

PHASE 1 SITE CHARACTERIZATION

1. Define Nature and Extent of Contamination (Waste Types, Concentrations, Distributions)
2. Refine DQOs
3. Assess Need for Treatability Studies Including Materials Handling

PHASE 2 POST-SCREENING FIELD INVESTIGATION

1. Perform Treatability Tests as Necessary
2. Collect Additional Field Data, as Necessary to Refine General Site Characterization

SELECTION OF REMEDY

1. Select a Remedy that is Protective of Human Health and the Environment
2. Select a Cost Effective Remedy
3. Select a Remedy that will Attain State/Federal ARARs upon Completion
4. Select a Remedy that Uses Permanent Solutions and Alternative Technologies to the Maximum Extent Practicable
5. Consider Use of Interim Responses

SCOPING OF THE RI/FS

1. Identify Potential Health Based and Location Specific State/Federal ARARs, Determine Initial Action Levels
2. Identify Initial Data Quality Objectives (DQOs) for Remedial Investigation
3. Identify Initial Project/ Operable Unit Likely Response Scenarios

FEASIBILITY STUDY

PHASE 1 DEVELOPMENT OF ALTERNATIVES

1. Identify Potential Treatment Technologies, Containment/Disposal Requirements for Residuals of Untreated Waste, and Related ARARs (e.g. Land Ban)
2. Assemble Treatment/ Disposal Combinations into Alternatives
3. Develop a Range of Alternatives attaining Various Levels of Treatment Performance

PHASE 2 INITIAL SCREENING

Screen Alternatives to Narrow Field to be Analyzed in Detail

PHASE 3 DETAILED ANALYSIS OF ALTERNATIVES

1. Develop General Performance Criteria to Each Alternative
2. Analyze Relative Costs, Long and Short Term Effectiveness, Implementability
3. Verify/Compare Protectiveness, Protection of Public Health and Environment Compliance with ARARs, Reduction of Mobility/ Toxicity (Attainment of Preference for Permanent Solutions Involving Treatment and other Statutory Factors (Consider Waivers, as Necessary)

ACRONYMS: DQOs – DATA QUALITY OBJECTIVES
ARARs – APPLICABLE OR RELEVENT AND APPROPRIATE REQUIREMENTS

Figure 21.2. Proposed remedy-selection process under SARA.

360

Produces emissions, effluents, and/or residues that are easy to manage from the environmental, cost, and health standpoints.

Is easy and safe to operate.

The first SITE program solicitation ("SITE-001") was issued by EPA in March 1986.[23] Twenty proposals were received representing the following technologies[25]:

ten incineration/thermal

three biological treatment

two containerization

one solidification/stabilization

one in situ vapor extraction

one chemical detoxification

one robotics

one vapor condensation

SITE proposals were evaluated according to the following criteria[25]:

Technology is applicable to problems at Superfund sites and represents an alternative to land-based technologies.

Technology is innovative.

Full-scale unit of demonstratable size capable of generating representative cost and operational data will be demonstrated.

Treatment unit is constructed and fully operational or expected in the near future.

Previous relevant test data indicate successful performance.

Based on the above evaluation criteria, the technologies listed in Table 21.3 have been selected for field evaluation.[26] Five of the technologies listed are discussed in some detail later in this chapter.

Once the technologies have been selected, the various EPA regions are to nominate sites for technology demonstration. EPA will then select site(s) based on matching characteristics of a site with those required by the technologies. Based on current schedules, the actual demonstration projects could begin in nine to 12 months.[26] EPA is currently evaluating proposals it has received for securing services of two SITE evaluation contractors (SEC) to assist EPA in the testing and evaluation of the selected technologies.[27]

As a result of the second round of SITE program solicitation (RFP SITE-002), EPA has received 23 additional proposals for technology demonstration.[26] These proposals are currently under evaluation and about 10 of them will be selected for field demonstration.

Site remediation technology development efforts are also ongoing or planned by the private sector as well as certain other agencies of the U.S. government. In response to CERCLA/SARA, the Department of the Navy is currently evaluating cost-effective technologies that address inactive disposal sites, leaking underground storage tanks, and spills. Input to this technology evaluation has been solicited from

TABLE 21.3. Technologies Selected for Demonstration Under the First Round of SITE Programs[26]

Technology	Developer	Technology Description
Biological degradation of organic contaminants	Detox Industries, Inc., Houston, Texas	Biodegradation of contaminants in water, sludge, and/or soil using special microorganism cultures and proprietary ingredients.
Circulating Bed Combustor (CBC)[a]	GA Technologies, San Diego, Calif (Technology now owned and marketed by Ogden Environmental Services, San Diego)	Destruction of contaminants in a fluidized bed; higher gas velocity through combustion chamber and recycling of fines allow for improved performance over conventional fluidized beds.
Electric Pyrolyzer*	Westinghouse Waste Technology Services Division	Rapid transfer of energy (supplied by electricity) to waste causes dissociation of organic molecules to individual atoms. Resultant products are clean off gas and a vitrified solid.
Fluidized Bed thermal combustion	Waste-Tech Services, Golden, Colo.	Special fluidized bed system design, including a secondary reaction chamber and ionizing wet scrubber; Operating temperatures can vary from 600°C to 1200°C.
Incinetron hazardous-waste destruction system, pure oxygen burner	Advanced Combustion Technologies, Inc., Norcross, Ga.	Pure oxygen in combination with air and natural gas combusted to destroy liquid hazardous waste. Use of pure oxygen allows temperature of up to 4500°F compared with conventional burners that have maximum temperatures of 2400°F. Advanced injection and mixing concepts are employed.
Shirco Infrared System*	Shirco Infrared Systems, Inc., Dallas, Texas	Waste material is exposed to infrared radiation as it is moved on a conveyor belt through the heating chamber. Exhaust gases pass through a secondary incineration chamber before discharge.

Technology	Company	Description
"Chloranan 20" solidification process	Hazcon, Inc., Katy, Texas	"Chloranan 20" is mixed with the organic waste stream and a cementatious product (fly ash, cement, kiln dust, etc.). The proprietary compound "neutralizes"/encapsulates organic molecules and renders them ineffective in retarding or inhibiting solidification. The hardened product can be handled with a forklift. The field blending unit is totally enclosed.
Pyroplasma system	Westinghouse Plasma Systems, Madison, Pa.	Pyrolysis of waste in a plasma field. Electric arc used to produce plasma at temperatures between 5000°C and 15,000°C. Chemicals in the waste are broken down to their atomic state in an oxygen-deficient atmosphere. The plasma torch is a vital feature of the system.
Vacuum Extraction*	Terra Vac, San Juan, Puerto Rico	Removal of volatile contaminants from in-place soil by application of vacuum through extraction wells.
Basic extraction sludge technology (BEST)	Resource Conservation Company, Bellevue, Wash.	A solvent-extraction-type process for dewatering or deoiling hazardous sludges and contaminated soil. Wastes are separated into three fractions: dischargeable water, reusable organics/oil, and oil-free soilds.
HWT chemical fixation process*	International Waste Technologies, Wichita, Kans.	A fixation/solidification process using proprietary formulations. Suitable for both organic and inorganic wastes.

*Example technologies discussed in more detail in this chapter.

the commercial/industrial sector.[28] These solicitations are expected to result in contracts for commercial systems for both immediate operational application and test and evaluation of innovative and emerging new systems that are considered to have potential applications for Navy specific problems.

Impediments to Use of Innovative Technologies

Despite recognition by EPA and the Congress that alternatives to the site-isolation and land-based containment systems must be developed and used for cleanup of contaminated sites, there are a number of informational, institutional, and regulatory impediments to the commercial development and use of innovative technologies.[29] Informational impediments are primarily associated with the current unavailability of sufficient, and independently verified, cost and performance data for many of the proposed innovative technologies. A major objective of the EPA SITE program is to overcome this impediment by developing reliable data on the technologies covered. Institutional impediments relate to the potential lack of sufficient liability insurance for technology developers, an interpretation of the term "cost-effectiveness" that can continue to encourage selection of traditional containment systems, and the general preference of the communities surrounding the Superfund sites for remedial alternatives that remove the waste from their area. Although some of these constraints can be addressed through development and dissemenation of technical information on technology capabilities, limitations, costs, etc., institutional impediments are generally outside the regulatory arena and the SITE program.

Regulatory impediments to the use of innovative technologies include the array of permits that are required and the very slow nature of the permit review process. The SITE program is a new program and policies and procedures have not yet been developed, especially at the state and local levels, to readily accommodate demonstration or full-scale use of innovative cleanup technologies. On the federal level, EPA has set up task forces and policy groups to identify key regulatory constraints and develop policies and procedures for overcoming these constraints through streamlining the permitting, financial assurance, and delisting of treatment residues as required under RCRA. An example of such ongoing groups is the Mobile Treatment Task Force, which is investigating impediments and issues concerning the use of mobile treatment units at Superfund sites.[29]

IN SITU TECHNOLOGIES

Overview of Limitations and Capabilities

In situ technologies are generally based on technologies that have been developed and are used in conventional water and wastewater treatment and in mining, oil and gas, and chemical process industries. These technologies use biological, chemical, physical, or thermal methods to degrade, detoxify, extract, or immobilize contaminants in place. The success of in situ treatment would thus depend to a great extent on the availability of equipment and procedures capable of delivering, distributing, mixing through, and recovering the excess treatment agents or process residues at a reasonable fast rate. Although a number of delivery and recovery systems have been proposed, the techniques have not generally been adequately evaluated in remedial action applications under a range of field conditions. Treatment agents such as ambient or heated air, steam, or solutions containing surfactants, chelating agents, bioactive materials, oxidizing/reducing chemicals, and the like can be delivered to the subsurface via gravity (e.g., flooding, ponding, or surface seepage) or via forced systems such as injection wells. Recovering the unused treatment agents and by-products can again be via gravity (e.g., open ditches and trenches and porous drains) or forced or vacuum systems (e.g., well points, induced draft fans, and underdrain collection pipes).

Although the proposed material-delivery and -recovery systems have not been fully tested (at least under the range of conditions encountered at contaminated sites), purely technical considerations and the limited data from research and development projects and from actual site cleanup involving decontamination of spill-impacted soils and groundwaters indicate considerable difficulty in a large-scale field application. These difficulties stem from several sources, including the following:

Nonhomogeneity and variable properties of the waste/soil media through which the treatment agents must be moved, which can give rise to channeling and nonuniform or incomplete treatment.

Slow treatment rate due to slow rate of fluid flow, especially in low-permeability media or where treatment can result in the formation of precipitates or biological deposits.

Potential for spread of contamination and the requirement for containment of the treatment agents and the reaction products within the target zone.

With some exceptions, the proposed in situ technologies do not provide for continuous monitoring at the treatment zone so that adjustments to treatment conditions can be implemented as the treatment progresses. Also, except for cases of spills involving single or few known chemicals, contaminants found at uncontrolled sites are complex mixtures of many chemicals. It would thus be very difficult, if not impossible, to formulate an all-encompassing treatment condition (and treatment agent) to achieve removal, detoxification, etc., of all contaminants present at a site. Some in situ treatment systems (e.g., soil washing) can produce a large volume of process wastewater that must be treated for material recovery or detoxification prior to reuse or disposal.

On the bright side, in situ technologies offer a number of advantages over on-site or off-site above-ground treatment. The most important of these are:

Eliminates safety, environmental, and the public health risks associated with excavation, transportation, storage, and handling of hazardous materials.*

Does not require additional land area for treatment systems (e.g., as would be needed in land spreading for biotreatment).

In the absence of excavation, there should not be a significant increase in soil volume after treatment and hence a need for additional disposal capacity.

Decontaminated soil is left in place (i.e., it does not have to be taken to another place for disposal).

In general, successful application of in situ treatment requires a good knowledge of subsurface characteristics, including the vertical and horizontal distribution of contaminants. Some in situ treatment systems by themselves do not constitute complete treatment and can best be used as an element of the total site remediation program. In selecting an in situ treatment system for a site, the capabilities and requirements of the technology must be matched against site-specific conditions and the remediation objective.

Representative In Situ Technologies

To illustrate the capabilities and limitations of the in situ technologies, seven such technologies are briefly reviewed here. These technologies along with their operating principles and certain desirable features and limitations, are listed in Table 21.4.

BIORECLAMATION

Provided that the contaminants are biodegradable and are not present at toxic levels, and that proper conditions exist or can be developed in the subsurface that promote biological activity, bioreclamation can be a very effective, low-cost, and safe method for soil and groundwater decontamination. This technology relies on the concept of stimulating the indigenous subsurface microbial population, or special cultures of microorganisms that would be introduced to the subsurface, to degrade the organic contaminants to inert or less harmful end products. Although in situ biodegradation can take place under both aerobic and anaerobic environments, the aerobic systems are preferred because they are faster, are more controllable, and can bring about a more complete degradation of contaminants.

Enhancing the biological activity in the subsurface may require pH adjustment and/or addition of oxygen and supplemental nutrients such as nitrogen, phosphorus, and trace metals, and sometimes organic carbon. The optimum treatment conditions

---

* A Superfund site in southern California previously received refinery and oil and gas exploration wastes. The wastes at this site now are reported to contain a high concentration of volatile sulfur compounds, including pockets of sulfur dioxide gas. Because the site is essentially in a residential area, control of air pollution is a major consideration in the evaluation of remedial action alternatives for this site. Proposed site remediation systems that require waste excavation feature the use of large pressurized tents that would cover active excavation areas and use of foams and plastic sheets to cover waste during storage and transportation.

TABLE 21.4. In Situ Remediation Technologies

Principle/Description	Desirable Features	Limitations
Bioreclamation Degradation of organic contaminants to inert or less harmful products via action of suitable microorganisms that are developed in or added to contaminated soil or groundwater. Oxygen and nutrients are added to the system to support biological growth.	Simple, low-cost, and safe method Effectiveness demonstrated to more than 30 organic spill sites	Generally limited to applications involving localized groundwater contamination (organic spills) Not applicable where the contaminants are refractory or are present at toxic levels pH-adjusting chemicals, oxygen, and nutrients may have to be provided Effective, proven method for uniform distribution of oxygen and nutrients in the subsurface (especially to great depths) does not exist Channeling and uneven treatment may result due to nonhomogeneity of soil and/or formation of precipitates and biological deposits For contaminated soils, the application seems to be limited to permeable soils (requires hydraulic conductivities perhaps exceeding 10^{-3} to 10^{-2} cm/sec) Difficult to monitor or control.
Soil Vapor Extraction Application of vacuum to the subsurface to remove volatile contaminants. The vacuum may be applied through vertical extraction wells (low water tables) or horizontal extraction systems (high water table). The extracted air may require treatment before discharge to the atmosphere	Simple, possibly low-cost, and safe method (with proper controls) Has been used in full-scale applications Can treat significant soil depths in the unsaturated zone Has been used to remove chemical spills before reaching groundwater	Applicability limited to cases involving volatile compounds; low groundwater table, and loose sandy formations Proper location and design of wells require good knowledge of subsurface characteristics Channeling and uneven treatment may result due to nonhomogeneity of the subsurface

TABLE 21.4. (*Continued*)

Principle/Description	Desirable Features	Limitations
		Not recommended for low hydraulic conductivity soils (requires conductivities perhaps exceeding 10^{-3} to 10^{-2} cm/sec)
		Difficult to monitor or control treatment progress and completeness
		Limited field experience and operating data available
		Treatment rate can be very slow
Air Stripping Forcing clean air into the soil through injection wells and withdrawal of contaminated air through extraction wells. The contaminated air is either discharged to an emission-control system or is vented to the atmosphere	Has been tested on a pilot scale Simple, possibly low-cost, and safe (with proper controls (method	Same as those listed for soil vapor extraction
Steam/Hot Air Stripping Injection of steam and/or hot air into the subsurface to remove volatile contaminants. Off gas collected at the surface or through extraction wells for above-ground processing. One system, known as the detoxifier, uses a novel adaptation of the drilling technology for in situ steam injection and mixing	For the detoxifier: Equipment design permits thorough in situ mixing and hence uniform treatment On-line monitoring allows good process control and adjustment of treatment conditions to achieve desired level of cleanup Closed loop and mobile nature of operation System field demonstrated in an application involving decontamination of soil contaminated with hydrocarbons	Treatment depth possibly limited Limited field experience available Better understanding is needed of the behavior of the steam and of contaminant distribution among various phases Potential for groundwater pollution exists

Immobilization		
Rendering contaminants in soil/waste less mobile by addition of physical or chemical agents that react with or encapsulate contaminants	Both organic and inorganic wastes can be handled with new proprietary formulations	System for in situ delivery and mixing of chemicals not field demonstrated Difficult to assess long-term effectiveness based on short-term leaching tests
Soil Washing		
Flushing or rinsing of contaminants from soil using suitable solutions (e.g., surfactants or chelating agents). Treatment solutions can be delivered and collected via gravity or forced systems	Can potentially provide for recovery of chemicals in cases involving spills of individual chemicals	System primarily conceptual and essentially no field experience or operating data available Not feasible when complex wastes containing a range of contaminants with different solubility characteristics are involved Difficult to limit reactions to target contaminants Channeling and uneven treatment may result due to nonhomogeneity of the subsurface Treatment rate can be very slow Difficult to monitor and control treatment progress and completeness Difficult to meet current requirements for residual levels in the treated soil Recovered solutions can be very dilute and large in volume and hence costly to treat and dispose of
Vitrification		
A soil-melting technology whereby electric current is passed between eletrodes placed in the ground. The soil and inorganic contaminants are converted to a stable glass. The organic contaminants are pyrolyzed and the pyrolysis products are combusted. Process off gas is collected under a hood and treated before discharge	The product glass is very stable and leach resistant Considerable data from bench-, engineering-, and large-scale tests available System ready for deployment at sites contaminated with metals and inorganics	Limited data for cases involving organic contamination Many of the tests conducted to date have been in connection with radioactive-waste management Available process and emissions control information must be verified in actual application to contaminated sites

and supplementary nutrient requirements can be established through bench-scale studies prior to implementing a field program. In general, pH values between 6.5 and 8.5, temperatures between 85°F and 95°F, and a ratio of organic carbon to available nitrogen and phosphorus (i.e., C:N:P) of 300 to 15 to 1 are considered suitable for biological activity. Considerable work has been carried out and are in progress to develop bacterial strains and enzymes most suitable for degrading specific contaminants. Detox Industries (Houston, Texas) has reportedly developed and used a bacterial culture that effectively degrades high levels of PCBs in soils, sludges, and aqueous wastes. In a demonstration test in a bioreactor, PCB levels of 2000 ppm in sludge and 44,000 and 29,000 ppb in the aqueous phase were reduced to 4 ppm overall in less than four months.[30]

When the contamination in the subsurface is limited to the soil in the unsaturated zone, the need for oxygen (for aerobic bacteria) and water restricts the use of in situ biological treatment to near-surface contamination. However, when the groundwater is also contaminated, or any contamination resulting from the treatment of the overlying soil can be contained, soil and groundwater decontamination can be carried out simultaneously by recirculating the groundwater using a system of injection/percolation and extraction wells. As shown in Figure 21.3, the required supplementary nutrients and pH adjusting chemicals are added to the water for delivery to the subsurface.

In situ bioreclamation has some distinct advantages over the conventional "pump-and-treat" methods that involve pumping the groundwater to the surface for treatment in above-ground units.[32] First, because the active treatment zone is in the subsurface, in situ biodegradation has the potential to treat both the contaminant in the groundwater and the contaminants sorbed to the soil matrix. Second, in situ

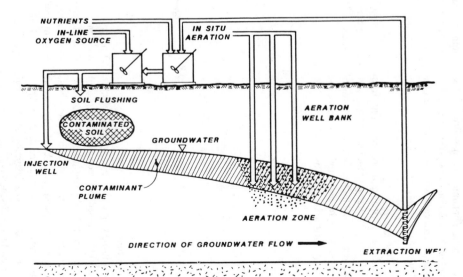

Figure 21.3. Bioreclamation technology for contaminated soil and groundwater.

biodegration requires minimal equipment, that is, that associated with pumping, nutrient mixing and injection, and oxygen addition. Pump-and-treat systems would be more expensive because of the cost of the above-ground equipment.

In situ bioreclamation has been successfully used in several applications, involving cleanup of spill-impacted soils and groundwater.[33,34] These applications, however, have generally involved single contaminants or simple mixtures of contaminants and relatively small areas or zones of contamination. The first field demonstration of technology at a waste-disposal site involving a complex mixture of both organic and inorganic wastes was recently completed at Kelly Air Force Base (AFB), Texas.[32] The site originally was used as a disposal pit for chromium sludges and other electroplating wastes. Prior to closure in 1966, it had been used as a chemical evaporation pit for chlorinated solvents, creosols, chlorobenzenes, and waste oils. The site was selected for the project because it offered a number of advantages with respect to demonstrating in situ biodegradation, namely, the presence of a highly adaptive and substantial microbial population, location in an area with a near-optimum soil and groundwater temperatures, presence of a perched aquifer not used for drinking water, and the biodegradable nature of the organic contaminants present at the site. A very small portion of the site (about 60 feet in diameter) was used for the demonstration project.

The design of the treatment system and selection of the operating conditions at the Kelly AFB site were based on results of geological investigation and site characterization, determination of the contamination profile, microbial investigation, and biodegradability studies. The system used to circulate groundwater within the treatment area consisted of nine 4-inch-diameter pumping wells and four 6-inch-diameter injection wells. One up-gradient and two down-gradient monitoring wells were also used to determine any effects of the system outside the perimeter of the treatment area. The saturated zone within the treatment area was at a depth of 15 to 20 feet below the land surface. The nutrient solutions used consisted of chloride, nitrogen, and phosphorus. Hydrogen peroxide addition was used as the method for providing oxygen to the subsurface.

The system at Kelly AFB was operated and monitored from June 1985 to February 1986. The results from the demonstration project indicated a need for additional studies and demonstration works to develop the technology as a viable method for application to large sites with a range of hydrogeological and contaminant characteristics. In the demonstration project, the total concentration of perchlorethylene (PCE) and trichloroethylene (TCE) in-site groundwater decreased from 4.0 to 0.93 ppm, while the concentration of trans-1,2-dichloroethylene (a decomposition product of PCE and TCE) increased from 0.03 to 1.4 ppm. Mobilization of heavy metals (antimony, lead, arsenic, cadmium, silver, and thallium) from soil was indicated but was not detected in the groundwater. However, heavy metals were found in sediments deposited in several surface pipes. The introduction of nutrients and hydrogen peroxide to the system resulted in an almost immediate and significant decrease in permeability and heavy precipitation of calcium phosphate.

The costs for treating the Kelly AFB site were $36 per ton of contaminated soil, with analytical costs accounting for 25 percent of this cost. Based on results from the demonstration project, it was concluded that in situ treatment can be performed for $50 to $100 per ton of contaminated soil for a typical site, and this would be less than the typical cost for removal and redisposal of soils.

Soil Vapor Extraction

Volatile organic compounds (VOCs) in the soil can be removed by application of vacuum or injection of ambient air or steam/hot air into the subsurface. In vapor extraction systems, vacuum is applied to extraction wells to induce a flow of clean air from the atmosphere into the subsurface. The vacuum not only draws vapors from the unsaturated zone, but also decreases the pressure in the soil voids, thereby releasing additional VOCs. System performance can be enhanced by placing appropriately designed air inlets at strategical locations. The extraction wells are connected to the suction side of a positive displacement blower through a surface collection manifold. Typical blowers have ratings of 100–1000 cfm, at vacuum ratings of up to 10 inches Hg gage; ratings of the electric drive motors are 10 hp or less.[35] Depending on its VOC concentration, the extracted gas is then either directly discharged to the atmosphere or processed for VOC removal (e.g., via vapor-phase-activated carbon adsorption) prior to discharge. At one industrial installation, where the initial VOC extraction rate was over 200 pounds/day, the extracted gas was conveniently and inexpensively disposed of by piping the gas to the combustion air intake of a nearby boiler that was in continuous operation.[35]

Vapor extraction and air stripping (discussed below) are best suited for cleanup of the contamination in the unsaturated zone in relatively permeable formations. Where the soil contamination extends to the groundwater table, the screened sections of the extraction wells should be extended to just above the surface of the groundwater table. If the groundwater is at a shallow depth, or if contamination is confined to the near-surface soils, horizontal extraction wells, consisting of per-forated pipes buried in trenches, should be used. The greatest application of the VOC extraction systems appears to be in containing the spread of contamination in the soil in cases typically stemming from surface spills or leaks from underground storage tanks and pipes. Removal of contaminant from the overlying soil can be a very cost-effective source-control method for preventing release or further release of contaminants to the groundwater. In cases where aquifer contamination has already occurred, VOC extraction from soil should not be viewed as a complete remedial program, but only as an element of such a program.

Several successful full-scale applications of the vapor extraction technology have been reported in the literature.[35,36] Terra Vac Inc., San Juan, Puerto Rico, has used soil vapor extraction for monitoring leaks from underground storage tanks and for removal and recovery of a range of volatile compounds, including solvents, from contaminated sites.[36,37] Extraction wells as deep as 300 feet have been installed. Based on these applications, the radius of influence of the negative pressure applied to the extraction wells has been estimated to generally extend outward from the wells 10 to 40 feet, depending on the soil conditions. The extracted gas typically passes through separator tanks, condensers, or afterburners to either recover or destroy VOCs.

In one soil vapor extraction application involving soils contaminated with spent 1,1,1-trichloroethane (TCA), over three years of operation resulted in the removal of over 12,000 pounds of VOCs.[35] During this time, the concentration of TCA in the extracted gas has decreased from more than 2000 ppm to about 50 ppm. It is expected that the system will be continued in operation until the total concentration of VOCs in the extracted gas is approximately 20 ppm. The soils at this site are predominantly alluvial clayey silts and sands that are considered relatively impervious. With the particular well design, a vacuum of about 3 inches Hg was generally sufficient to induce 100 cfm of air through the soil.

Many factors must be considered in evaluating the applicability of the vapor extraction system to a particular site. These include[35]; characteristics of the contaminants, primarily from a volatility viewpoint; the extent of dispersion of VOCs in the soil; characteristics of the soil from the standpoint of permeability and uniformity; emissions-control requirements; schedule for cleanup; and site factors such as location, distance to the water table, and physical constraints. A vapor extraction system would be especially attractive for sites that are located in highly developed areas and/or in cases where the contamination is spread to adjacent properties or underneath buildings. In these situations, a remedial option involving excavation and removal of contaminated soil may be impractical or very costly.

The cost to install and operate a vapor extraction system would be highly site specific. A complete blower assembly can be purchased for less than $5000.[35] However, this may represent only a small fraction of the total project cost, which would typically include costs associated with the initial engineering and subsurface site characterization studies, permissions, emissions control, performance monitoring, and installation of system appurtenances such as piping, valving, and instrumentation. Some cost-saving possibilities, which should be examined during project planning, include the use of existing or planned groundwater monitoring wells as part of the extraction wells, completing the soil borings used in site characterization as air inlet or extraction wells, and disposal of extracted gas via combustion in existing boilers.[35] The cost for sampling and analysis of the extracted gas to monitor and evaluate system performance is the major element of the operating cost. Except for routine data recording, inspection, and servicing, soil vapor extraction systems will normally operate continuously and unattended.

As noted above, many site-specific factors must be considered in evaluating the suitability and cost of a vapor extraction system for use at a particular site. Because of this, it has been recommended that before a full-scale system is installed, a partial system be installed and operated on a short-term basis to determine whether a full-scale system is feasible and to establish criteria for the design of the full-scale system.[35] To provide flexibility in operation, large sites should be divided into smaller areas, each with its own independent extraction system. The discharge side of the blowers for the individual systems can then be connected to a common header pipe that would discharge to the emission control system for the site.

Air Stripping

In this process, the passive air inlets in the vapor extraction system are converted into active air-injection wells through which clean air is mechanically injected into the soil and forced to travel through the soil, volatizing trapped VOCs. As in the vapor extraction system, the contaminated air is withdrawn from the soil and either vented to an emission-control system or the atmosphere, depending on VOC concentration. As shown in Figure 21.4, separate blower and manifold systems are used for air injection and extraction. All vents are installed to the lowest depth of the contaminated zone, but above the groundwater table. Both series of vents are perforated and grouted along predetermined lengths to reduce short-circuiting and loss of the injected air to the ground surface. To achieve flow containment, extraction wells are generally placed on the perimeter of the area being treated, surrounding the injection wells that would be located in the middle.

The U.S. Army Toxic and Hazardous Materials Agency recently conducted a 14-week pilot-scale field demonstration program to evaluate the feasibility of the air-stripping system for remediation of VOC-contaminated soils.[38,39] Based on information from previous subsurface soil and contaminant characterization studies, two areas within the contaminated site, representing low and high VOC levels, were selected for the demonstration project. (Borings in the test plots had generally encountered sandy materials with traces of silt and gravel.) Two distinctly different pilot systems were installed to test several designs and performance variables. The study focused on the removal of trichloroethylene (TCE) as an indicator of VOC contamination. To prevent freeze-up in subzero conditions, the injection air for both systems was preheated to 45–55°F. The injection and extraction wells consisted of 20-foot, 3-inch PVC pipes, assembled in 5-foot sections. The injection and extraction pipes were slotted (slot size of 0.06 inch.) in the bottom 15-foot and 5-foot sections respectively. The injection vent pipes were left open at the base, whereas the extraction pipes were capped at the base. The annular space outside the PVC casing was packed with gravel along the slotted interval, and the solid-wall intervals with a cement/bentonite grout. The extraction air from each pilot system was passed through canisters of activated carbon before discharge to the atmosphere. Other features of the two systems and the results obtained are summarized in Table 21.5. A schematic of the vent pipe and manifold system layout is shown in Figure 21.5.

The pilot study demonstrated the effectiveness of in situ air stripping in removing TCE and other solvents from porous soils. The carbon adsorption system also proved effective in removing TCE, other chlorinated solvents, and PCB from the extracted gas. Preliminary estimates based on the soil and contamination conditions at the test site indicated a remediation cost of $15–$20 per cubic yard of contaminated soil. Based on the pilot study results and the consideration that the treatment of the effluent air can account for up to 50 percent of the total cost, an estimate of $15–$30 per pound of removed VOC has been considered reasonable, with the higher estimate representing treatment of the extracted air by carbon adsorption.[39]

As with vapor extraction, in situ air stripping would find greatest applicability to sites that contain primarily volatile contaminants in loose sandy soils well above the groundwater table.

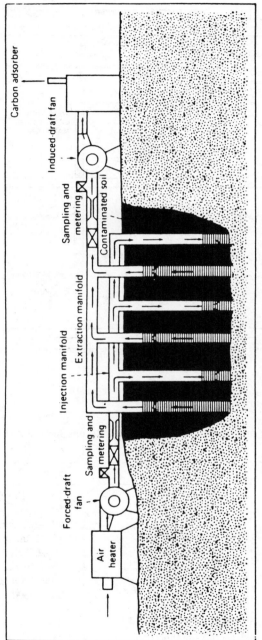

Figure 21.4. Air stripping for removal of volatile organic compounds.

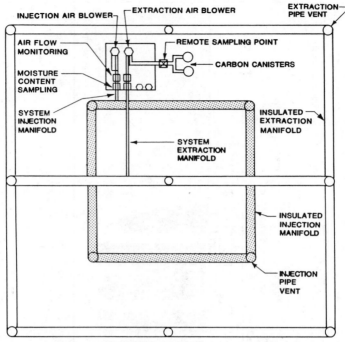

Figure 21.5. Vent pipe and manifold system layout for the in situ air stripping demonstration project.

TABLE 21.5. Design and Operating Features and Results for the Air-Stripping Pilot Systems[38,39]

Parameter	System 1	System 2
Test-plot size	50 × 50 ft	100 × 100 ft
Vent-pipe spacing	20 ft	50 ft
Extraction flow rate	40–55 cfm	200–220 cfm
Extraction vacuum	0.5–1.3 in. w.g.	17–20 in. w.g.
Injection flow rate	55–60 cfm	46–223 cfm
Injection pressure	0.9–1.4 in. w.g.	10–11.9 in. w.g.
Pretest soil TCE	<0.05–2.3 mg/kg	0.06–4000 mg/kg
Post-test soil TCE	0.05–4.9 mg/kg	0.06–5000 mg/kg
Pretest soil moisture	3–13%	3–13%
Post-test soil moisture	1–36%	2.2–12.5%
TCE removal in 14 weeks	1 kg/8000 ft^3 soil	730 kg/50,000 ft^3 soil
Iniitial off gas TCE	30–70 ppm	250–300 ppm
Final off gas TCE	<5000 ppb in 10 wks	250–300 ppm during test
TCE removed, calculated	75% of initial	25% of initial

STEAM STRIPPING

The volatilization of the hydrocarbon contaminants in the soil can be facilitated by application of heat in the form of steam. Steam can be delivered to the subsurface through injection wells or by use of special drilling and subsurface injection equipment. The excess steam (i.e., the steam that is not condensed in the soil) is collected at the surface or in a network of extraction wells. This excess steam, which contains the VOCs removed from the soil, can then be treated in an above-ground facility before discharge or recycling.

The behavior of steam in the soil and the partitioning of contaminants between the solid, liquid, and vapor phases appear to be very complex and affected by many factors, including porosity, permeability, initial moisture content, and other characteristics of the soil; volatility, concentration, and solubility of contaminants; steam pressure and injection rate; and characteristics of the injection and extraction system used.

Some fundamental analysis and testing of steam condensation, movement, and contaminant stripping have been carried out by Heijmans Milieutechniek B.V. in the Netherlands.[40] These studies indicate that for an initial soil moisture content of 0–300 kg/m^3, 50–100 kg of steam would condense in a cubic meter of soil. In a soil with a permeability of 10^{-3} cm/sec and a water content of 100 kg/m^3, it has been shown that it takes about 20 minutes for the condensation front to travel a radial distance of 1 meter from the injection point. Steam stripping tests have indicated effective removal of a range of contaminants from several types of soil. Tests conducted at a former manufactured-gas plant site indicated complete removal (i.e., to below detection level) of the following contaminants from the indicated initial levels: benzene (55 mg/kg), toluene (15 mg/kg), xylene and ethylbenzene (2–4 mg/kg), and phenol (30 mg/kg). The soil at this site consisted of "rough, sandy" material containing a contaminant layer between 1.8 and 2.6 meters below the land surface. Tests at other sites have indicated similar removal effectiveness for other contaminants, including naphthalene, polycyclic aromatic hydrocarbons, and organic bromide compounds. All tests were conducted under a 2-meter by 2-meter "vacuum bell" (a shroud connected to the inlet side of a blower) with four lances for injection of steam into the subsurface.

A very innovative application of in situ steam stripping, including a system for processing and recycling of the extracted gas in a closed-loop operation, was recently demonstrated in the United States at a 10,000-square-foot site in southern California.[41] The system, known as the "In Situ Detoxifier," is patented and is marketed in the United States by Toxic Treatments (USA) Inc. of San Mateo, Calif. The soil at the demonstration site was contaminated with petroleum hydrocarbons from leaking undergound fuel-storage tanks, with total petroleum hydrocarbon concentration levels in the top 25 feet of soil generally in the 100- to 1000-ppm range. One segment of the site had total hydrocarbon concentration values in excess of 15,000 ppm.

In addition to steam injection capability, the Detoxifier can deliver to and mix with the subsurface soil other treatment agents in liquid, vapor, powder, or slurry form. Thus, potentially a range of in situ treatment methods can be implemented, including solidification/stabilization, oxidation/reduction, neutralization, and air stripping. A brief description of the In Situ Detoxifier is given below. More detailed descriptions of the Detoxifier and its capabilities are contained in ref. 41 and 42.

The Detoxifier, shown in Figure 21.6, is a completely mobile system that would be taken from site to site for in situ remediation. The heart of the system is the "process tower," which is essentially a drilling and treatment agent dispensing system, capable of penetrating the soil/waste deposit to depths of 25 feet or more. The process tower consists of two cutter/mixer bits connected to separate, hollow Kelly bars. The bits overlap and rotate in opposite directions. The rotating action provides for simultaneous cutting and mixing of the soil/waste material. Treatment agents are conveyed through the Kelly bars and ejected through feed jets and orifices to the mixing area. A rectangular shroud covers the mixing area to minimize dust generation and capture gas and vapor released during subsurface generation. The captured off gas is treated in a process train and recycled to the treatment zone. The off gas from the shroud is monitored continuously (e.g., for total hydrocarbons using a flame ionization detector). The output is used to adjust the treatment conditions, including the length of treatment, to achieve desired treatment objectives.

In actual site cleanup, the treatment of an area is on a block-by-block basis. For example, the area to be treated is divided into rows of blocks, with the process tower moved to an adjacent block after the treatment of a block is completed. Each bit assembly is capable of drilling a hole 4.5 feet in diameter. To cover all the areas to be treated, the shroud is positioned with about 10 percent overlap of the grid cells. With this overlap, the effective treatment area per block is about 24 square feet.

At the southern California demonstration site, a mixture of hot air and steam was used for stripping. For some blocks, an oxidizing solution was also included in the mixture. The off gas from the shroud, which contained the exit air, steam, and volatilized hydrocarbons, was cooled and passed through a scrubbing system (to remove particulates), a refrigeration system (to condense and remove excess moisture), and an activated carbon adsorption system (to remove hydrocarbons). Following carbon adsorption, the gas was compressed, reheated, and recycled to the treatment zone through the two Kelly bars in the process tower.

The southern California project was the first full-scale demonstration of the Detoxifier technology. The key aims of the project were to:

Demonstrate the capability of the equipment to dispense steam, hot air, and liquid remediation agents at desired depth, to provide good mixing of the treatment agents with the soil, and to recover contaminants (i.e., hydrocarbons).

Evaluate the adequacy of the various components of the off-gas treatment train under a range of loading conditions.

Identify and provide the data base for any needed design improvements to the process tower and various components of the off-gas treatment train.

Inasmuch as the above objectives were achieved, the demonstration project was considered a success. The results indicated that by adjusting the treatment con-

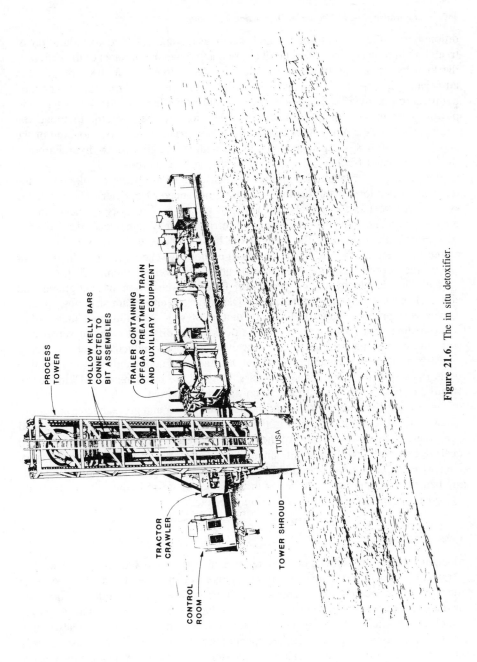

PROCESS
TOWER

HOLLOW KELLY BARS
CONNECTED TO
BIT ASSEMBLIES

TRAILER CONTAINING
OFFGAS TREATMENT TRAIN
AND AUXILIARY EQUIPMENT

TRACTOR
CRAWLER

CONTROL
ROOM

TOWER SHROUD

TTUSA

Figure 21.6. The in situ detoxifier.

ditions (i.e., the amounts of air and steam used, and the rate and duration of treatment in terms of speed and number of up and down movements of the drill bit), the total hydrocarbons in the soil could be reduced to less than 100 ppm via hot air/steam stripping. The result also indicated that off gas monitoring via on-line total hydrocarbon analysis can provide a reasonably accurate basis for assessing completeness of in situ treatment and hence decision by the operator to move the equipment to a new block. One key problem area was the quick overloading of the carbon adsorption system when treating soils with very high levels of hydrocarbons. This necessitated frequent replacement of the carbon charge.

Based on the demonstration project results, designs are being developed by the technology vendor for fabrication of a more advanced Detoxifier. The advanced system will be more compact and will incorporate several improvements in the off-gas treatment train, including use of a refrigeration system ahead of the carbon adsorption unit to remove the bulk of the hydrocarbons from the scrubbed gas, thereby prolonging the life of the activated carbon. A schematic flow diagram for one of the several designs under consideration is shown in Figure 21.7.

With the development and successful field demonstration of equipment and approaches such as those featured in the Detoxifier, in situ steam stripping appears to be a very promising approach to remediation of VOC-contaminated sites. Additional testing under a range of site conditions (e.g., different types of subsurface soils and contamination conditions), however, must be conducted to enable better assessment of system capabilities and potential areas of applicability and to develop basis for cost estimating. Fundamental studies of the mechanism and kinetics of steam stripping in the subsurface, such as those reported by Hilberts,[40] must be expanded to include an evaluation of the potential for air and groundwater pollution, spread/dilution of contamination in the subsurface via reposition of the volatilized compounds, and characteristics of the treated soil (e.g., from the standpoint of load bearing capacity) and their significance in subsequent use of the rehabilitated land. Under EPA sponsorship, Drexel University (Philadelphia, Pa.) is currently conducting bench-scale parametric studies of the behavior of steam in the soil as a function of soil type, moisture content, injection rate, etc.[43]

IMMOBILIZATION

Contaminants in the soil can be rendered less mobile by the addition of physical or chemical agents. For example, many heavy metals can be rendered less mobile by the addition of precipitating agents such as lime or limestone, sorptive agents such as clay or agricultural products and by-products (e.g., straw, sawdust, bark), solidification/encapsulation agents such as Portland cement, or strongly adsorptive complexing agents (e.g., tetraethylenepentamine, or Tetrine. "Tetrine" is the trade name for a series of organic chelating, sequestering, and complexing agents consisting of ethylenediaminetetraacetic acid (EDTA) and its salts.]

Most commercial immobilization systems do not provide complete control or a very high degree of long-term effectiveness due to compositional changes that may be brought about by microbial or chemical action in the disposal environment.

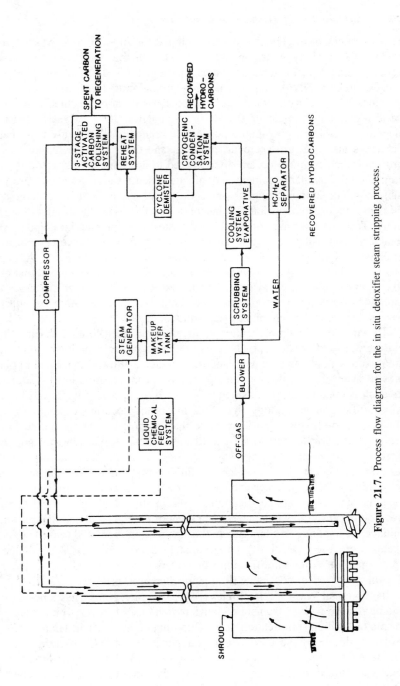

Figure 21.7. Process flow diagram for the in situ detoxifier steam stripping process.

These systems have generally been developed for application to waste slurries and sludges (particularly, heavy metal sludges) with the objective of improving the handling and leaching characteristics of the wastes destined for land disposal. Processing generally takes place in above-ground units (e.g., in drums or tanks) or in ponds. Proprietary methods and chemical formulations, which contain as their basic ingredients cement or silicate-based materials (e.g., fly ash, blast furnace slag, or other readily available pozzolanic compounds), are used. Silicate-based processes also use lime, cement, gypsum, and other suitable setting agents. The procedure and formulation are often altered to accommodate specific wastes. The commercially available cement and silicate-based fixation processes are generally ineffective in immobilizing organics or when wastes contain certain nontarget inorganic or organic substances that may interfere with the immobilization reactions. Tests with a range of hazardous wastes at a commercial disposal site have indicated that volatile organic compounds can have an adverse impact on the effectiveness of several commercial immobilization processes.[44] A number of processes using organic polymeric compounds have been developed that are effective in encapsulating excavated or drummed wastes.[45] Similar processes and formulations have not generally been available for encapsulation of bulk organic wastes or large volumes of in-place soil.

To date, in situ immobilization application has been limited to cases involving closure of liquid or slurry ponds. Large volumes of low-reactivity, solid chemicals are mixed with the pond content and the product is allowed to remain in place. The present state of technology limits application of in situ mixing to the treatment of low-solids-content slurries or sludges.[46] Enrico, Inc. (Amarillo, Texas) has reported an solidification technology that will impart load-bearing capacity to industrial sludges in ponds, pits, and lagoons so that the sludges can be buried in place or removed and transported to off-site disposal sites. In one reported application,[47] Enrico's "injector/mixer" system was used to inject and thoroughly mix the solidification agent into the sludge and fluids remaining in two PCB impoundments after sludge dewatering. The additive reportedly solidified the sludge into a material meeting the following specifications[47]: minimum 150 lb/ft^2 loading capacity, no free liquid, no slump when placed on a sheet of plexiglass at a 45-degree angle, and suitable for handling in a landfill. In this application, over 600 tons of solidification agents were used to solidify approximately 2200 cubic yards of sludge over a 13-day period. After solidification, the material was removed and transported to a landfill approved to accept PCB-contaminated wastes.

International Waste Technologies (IWT), Wichita, Kans., has reportedly formed a joint venture with Mitsubishi of Japan to demonstrate a very innovative approach to in situ fixation/solidifcation at a PCB-contaminated site in Hialeah, Fla.[48] The project, which will be carried out under the EPA SITE program, will employ Japanese advanced construction equipment (the "JST" method and the "Tone BW" long wall drill, describe later) to inject and mix with soil certain proprietary fixation chemicals that have been developed by IWT. The plan calls for surrounding the contaminated area with a wall of overlapping columns of low-permeability material (see Figure 21.8). The contaminated area will then be treated by drilling columns to

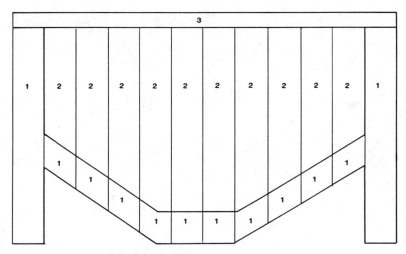

1. HIGHLY IMPERMEABLE BARRIER INJECTION
2. TREATMENT IN CONTAMINATED ZONES
3. SURFACE TREATMENT

Figure 21.8. Profile view of treatment plan for in situ containment and stabilization at the demonstration project site in Florida.

a point below the contaminated zone, injecting chemicals to create a low-permeability barrier for a few feet, and treating the soil with fixation chemicals above the barrier. The overlapping pattern that will be used within the treatment zone is shown in Figure 21.9. The results will be total encapsulation of the contaminated area.

The JST method is a soil-consolidation method consisting of installation of two liquid paths in the rod of an earth auger, supply of fixation ingredients under low pressure by the respective pumps, and intermixing of these liquids by mixing auger head for rapid fixation.[49] The basic procedure, illustrated in Figure 21.10, involves driving a bore hole with a special auger to the prescribed depth, allowing the contaminated soil to remain in the bore hole. Fixation chemicals are then injected and mixed with the soil as the auger is rotated and retracted. Fixation chemicals are added as two separate solutions that are mixed after they leave the auger head, thereby preventing the mixture from hardening inside the equipment. An alternative method is to inject one liquid while boring and another liquid during retraction.

The "Tone BW" long wall drill (Figure 21.11) was designed for the construction of cement-bentonite slurry cutoff walls. The unit, described in more detail in ref. 49 and 50, consists of a boring head that includes five in-line drill bits powered by electric motors and suspended by steel cable from a derrick. The submersible electric motors provide the rotational motion and the required torque to the spindles of multiple drill bits through reduction gears and transmission arrangement. Cuttings are removed by a suction pump set on the ground through a reverse circulation line together with stabilizing solution. A cross section of a typical trench cut by the

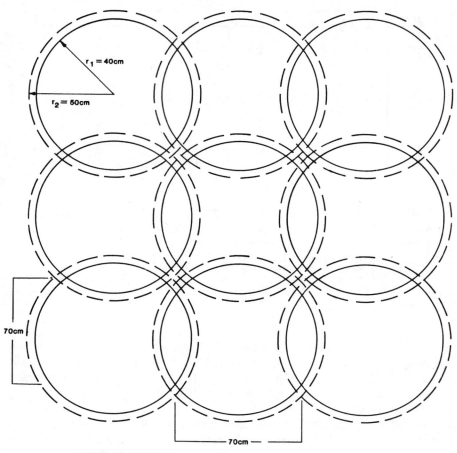

r₁ = RADIUS OF BLADES

r₂ = EXTENDED ZONE OF MIXING

Figure 21.9. Top view of treatment of columns done by JST methods.

drill is shown in Figure 21.12. The overlapping circles can be converted to flat walls by the addition of a side-cutter assembly. Overlapped circles are recommended for cutoff walls because the absence of side cutters enables greater speed and requires less maintenance. Typical trenches using the long wall drill are constructed up to 165 feet deep; specialized drills are available for constructing trenches to 425 feet deep.

The fixation chemical proposed for use at the demonstration site in Florida is IWT's proprietary formulation HWT-20, which will be applied to soil at a level of 300 lb/ton of soil.[49] According to IWT, HWT compounds are inorganic polymers that react with the target contaminants to form a crystalline polymer network. The

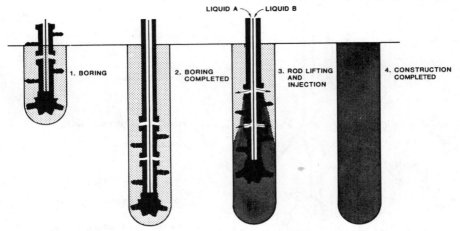

Figure 21.10. In situ fixation and solidification with the JST method.

reaction is considered to proceed in two phases. The first phase involves fast reactions that alter the chemical structure of the organic and inorganic constituents of the waste through a variety of mechanisms including ion exchange and substitution reactions. The second phase generates a macromolecular network in a much slower reaction. During the second phase, the physical characteristics of the treated waste change from sol to gel to crystalline, inorganic polymer. The bonding characteristics and durability of the structure can be varied to suit particular waste situations and desired leaching standards.

According to IWT,[49] a variety of organic and inorganic wastes have been effectively stabilized by treatment with HWT-20 formulation. For example, the results shown in Table 21.6 are reported for treatment of an API separator bottoms (24.9 percent oil and grease content) with 15–25 percent by weight of the fixation agent.

The demonstration project in Florida will involve treatment of approximately 7000 cubic yards of contaminated soil.[51] Maximum PCB concentration in the soil is 6000 ppm. The soil profile from the ground surface down consists of 4–5 feet of sand, 4–5 feet of water, 4–5 feet of limestone, and quartz sand.

SOIL WASHING

Techniques such as those used in solution mining and mineral extraction have been proposed for removal of contaminants from in-place soil.[52] Extractant fluids such as water or solutions containing surfactants or chelating agents can be delivered to the subsurface via gravity using such systems as flooding, surface seepage, and ponding, or via forced systems using injection wells or specialized equipment such those described for fixation/solidification or steam stripping, which can also provide for

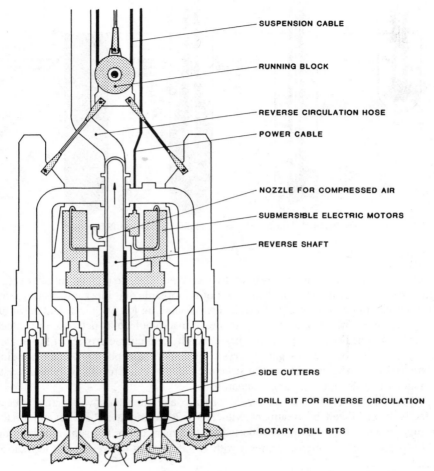

SUSPENSION CABLE

RUNNING BLOCK

REVERSE CIRCULATION HOSE

POWER CABLE

NOZZLE FOR COMPRESSED AIR

SUBMERSIBLE ELECTRIC MOTORS

REVERSE SHAFT

SIDE CUTTERS

DRILL BIT FOR REVERSE CIRCULATION

ROTARY DRILL BITS

Figure 21.11. Tone BW long wall drill.

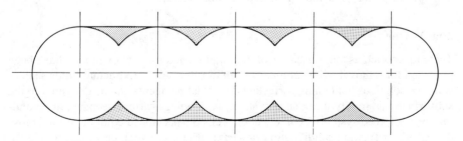

Figure 21.12. Cross section of trench cut by Tone BW long wall drill.

TABLE 21.6 Treatment of an API Separator Bottoms with Fixation Agent

Compound	Concentration in Waste, (ppm)	Leach Value (ppm)
Chromium	630	0.03–0.04
Lead	250–332	0.05
Ethylbenzene	10	ND
m-Xylene	40	ND
o- and p-xylene	43	ND
Anthracene	19	ND
Crysene	29	ND
Methylnaphthalene	170–470	ND
Naphthalene	13–93	ND
Phenanthrene	110–206	ND

Note: Leach value determined using "toxicity characteristic leaching procedure" (TCLP); ND indicates not detected at a detection limit of 100 ppb

the in situ mixing of the reagents with the soil. Unused treatment chemicals and reagents can then be collected via gravity (e.g., using porous drains, trenches, and open ditches) or forced systems such as well points.

Much of the soil-washing research and development and demonstration work[53–55] has been in connection with above-ground processing of excavated soil and development of systems and equipment for soil handling and extractant processing. The emphasis has been on applications to emergency chemical spills and recovery of the spilled chemicals. The results reported indicate that while the concept of soil washing remains a valid one, a large number of problems can be anticipated in a field application (in situ or above ground). These include the loss of extractants in side reactions, less than quantitative recovery of the excess chemicals, generation of a large volume of a dilute waste requiring treatment for material recovery prior to recycling or disposal, incomplete and nonuniform treatment due to soil heterogeneity, and slow processing rate. The in situ application is further complicated by the extreme difficulty in monitoring and controlling the treatment progress, potential for the spread of contamination to clean areas through redeposition of extracted contaminants, and potential for groundwater contamination.

In situ soil washing would find its greatest site remediation application in cases where the soil contaminant(s) can be extracted with a single extractant fluid. For example, soils contaminated with heavy metals or with petroleum hydrocarbons can be decontaminated by washing with an aqueous solution containing chelating agents or surfactants respectively. To date, in situ soil washing has only been used in laboratory and small-scale field pilot tests.[55] As with all in situ treatment systems, proper design and operation of a soil-washing system require a good knowledge of the subsurface characteristics, including vertical and horizontal distribution of the contamination.

VITRIFICATION

In situ vitrification (ISV) is a thermal treatment/destruction process that converts contaminated soil into a chemically inert, stable glass and crystalline product. The process was originally developed for the U.S. Department of Energy (DOE) for management of radioactive wastes. Battelle, Northwest Laboratories (Richland, Wash.), the developer of the process, has an exclusive license from DOE to apply the technology to the management of nonradioactive hazardous wastes.[56] Toward that end, Battelle is developing and demonstrating the technology for specific hazardous chemical waste types through the stage of full-scale demonstration. Once a demonstration has been successfully completed, Battelle intends to sublicense the technology to other companies to perform commercial remediation for that waste type. The company expects to perform three to five demonstrations on various wastes during the next three years.[56]

ISV technology has been selected for independent evaluation under the second round of the EPA SITE solicitation program.[56] For its work on the ISV technology, Battelle was the recipient of a 1986 National Society of Professional Engineers (NSPE) award for Outstanding Engineering Achievements.[57] NSPE awards recognize technological originality and innovation, importance to industrial development, application of known and new engineering principles, and fulfillment of human and social needs.

The ISV process is illustrated in Figure 21.13. The process principle and sequence are described by Battelle as follows.[58] A square array of four electrodes is inserted into the ground to the desired treatment depth. Because the soil is not electrically conductive once the moisture has been driven off, a conductive mixture of flaked graphite and glass frit is placed among the electrodes to act as the starter path. An electrical potential is applied to the electrodes, which establishes an electric current in the starter path. The resulting power heats the starter path and surrounding soil up to 3600°F, well above the initial melting temperature or fusion temperature of soils (normally between 2000 and 2500°F). The graphite starter path

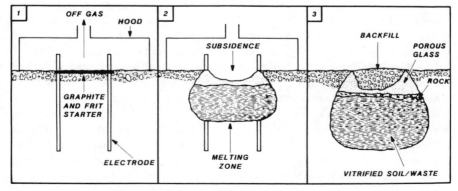

Figure 21.13. In situ vitrification process sequence.

is eventually consumed by oxidation and the current is transferred to the molten soil, which is now electrically conductive. As the vitrified zone grows, it incorporates nonvolatile elements and destroys organic components by pyrolysis. The pyrolysis products migrate to the surface of the vitrified zone, where they combust in the presence of oxygen. A hood placed over the processing area provides for collection of the combustion gases, which are drawn into the off-gas treatment system.

During the melting procedure, the power to the system is maintained at sufficient levels to compensate for the heat losses from the surface and to the surrounding soil. As the melt grows in size, the resistance of the melt decreases, making it necessary to adjust the voltage/current to the electrodes in order to maintain a constant power. This is done by adjusting the tap position on the primary power supply to the electrode. (There are 14 effective taps that permit adjusting the voltage from a maximum of 4000 volts to a minimum of 400 volts per phase and the current from a minimum of 400 amperes to a maximum of 4000 amperes per phase.) The electrical power for the system is either brought in or generated on site using diesel generators.

The large-scale process equipment and field setup for ISV are shown in Figure 21.14. Except for the off-gas hood and the connecting lines, which are transported to the site on flat-bed trailers and assembled at the job site, all components are contained in three transportable trailers. These are the off-gas-treatment, process-support, and process-control trailers. The process off gas is cooled, scrubbed, and filtered in the off-gas-treatment trailer before discharge to the atmosphere. The process-support trailer contains the glycol cooling system that interfaces with the scrub solution in the off-gas-treatment trailer and extracts and rejects to the atmosphere the heat removed from the process off gas. The monitoring and process control are done from the process-control trailer.

As shown in Figure 21.14, site cleanup with the ISV technology is on a block-by-block basis. The three processing trailers would be typically coupled together and moved from one block to another as a unit. The hood would be moved

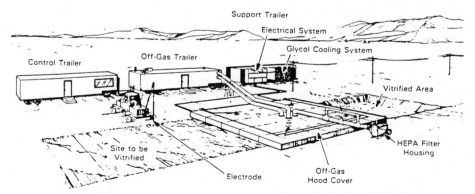

Figure 21.14. Large-scale process equipment and setup for in situ vitrification.

from one position to the next with a crane. Moving from one position to another takes about 16 hours, which can also allow time for routine equipment maintenance. A large-scale ISV would be capable of processing an average of 3 to 5 tons of soil per hour. On the average, processing at one processing position would be completed in about 150–200 hours, depending on the treatment depth and the electrode spacing. For processing to depths of 50 feet, single processing operations can run in the range of 300–400 hours and result in a vitrified mass of greater than 1000 tons. The cost of ISV for large-scale site cleanup involving contaminated soils is estimated at $100–$250 per ton.

To date, some 43 bench-, engineering-, pilot-, and large-scale tests have been conducted in support of ISV technology development and commercialization. These tests, which have been largely with actual or simulated radioactive wastes, are characterized in Table 21.6. The tests have established outstanding ISV product characteristics from the standpoint of leaching and long-term durability, a very low release rate for the inorganic contaminants from the system, and a very high destruction/removal efficiency (DRE) for organic contaminants. The virtified products have been subjected to a variety of leach tests, including the EPA's Extraction Procedure Toxicity (EP Toxicity) and Toxic Characteristic Leach Tests (TCLP). These tests show a uniformly low leach rate for heavy metals of about 1×10^{-4} lb/ft^2/day or lower.

The retention factor, defined as the ratio of the initial concentration of an element in the waste (or in the off gas) to the concentration of the element exiting the melt (or the off-gas treatment system), has been measured for a number of elements. The results indicate that the retention factor for the melt increases significantly with the increase in the treatment depth. The presence of combustibles can provide a path to the surface by entraining the metals in the combustion products or pyrolytic gases. The closer the combustibles are to the surface, the more likely it is that the entrained material will not be retained in the melt and will have to be removed by the off-gas scrubbing system. However, even with the very volatile elements and shallow treatment depths, retention factors of at least 100 in the melt can be obtained with the use of a meter of clean overburden. Retention factors obtained in the pilot-scale tests for several elements are shown in Table 21.8 for both the melt and the off-gas treatment system. These data, which also provide an indication of the amount of material that would be captured in the off-gas scrub solution requiring treatment

TABLE 21.7 In Situ Vitrification Test System Characteristics[58]

System, Scale	Power, kW	Electrode Spacing, Feet	Vitrified Mass per Setting	Number of Tests
Bench	10	0.36	2–5 pounds	4
Engineering	30	0.75–1.2	0.05–1 ton	25
Pilot	500	4.0	10–50 tons	14
Large	3750	11.5–18.0	400–800 tons	4

TABLE 21.8 Retention Factors for Metals in the In Situ Vitrification Process[58]

Type of Metal	Soil	Off Gas	Combination
Particulates:			
Sr, Pu, U, La, Nd	10^5	10^5	10^{10}
Semivolatiles:			
Co, Cs, Sb, Te, Mo	10^2	10^4	10^6
Volatiles:			
Cd, Pb	2–10	10^4	10^5

before disposal, show an overall system retention factor of 10^5 to 10^{10} for the elements tested.

Bench- and engineering-scale tests have been conducted with soils contaminated with PCBs and electroplating sludges, or containing buried containers of solid or liquid combustible organics. These tests indicate a very high destruction and removal efficiency (DRE) for the organics, and that the DRE can be further enhanced by the addition of a layer of clean soil. Under sponsorship of the Electric Power Research Institute (Palo Alto, Calif.), an engineering-scale test was conducted using soils contaminated with PCBs.[59] The tests showed a DRE of greater than 99.5 percent in the melt. The small release in the process off gas (about 0.05 percent) was effectively retained in the off-gas treatment system (a dual activated carbon filter), yielding an overall system DRE of >99.9999 percent. Limited amounts of PCBs (0–0.7 ppm) were detected in the surrounding soil and none were found in the vitrified block, indicating that migration away from the vitrification zone would not be a significant concern.

Detailed cost analyses have been carried out for the ISV process. The amount of moisture in the soil and the cost of electricity have been identified as the two factors that most significantly affect the total cost. The calculated costs for treating saturated and dry contaminated soils and a wet industrial sludge are plotted in Figure 21.15 as a function of the local electric rate. As shown there, the maximum cost for all three cases occurs at an electric rate of 0.0825 cent/kWh, beyond which the use of a portable diesel generator for power is recommended.

Engineering analyses have been conducted of the applicability and limitations of the ISV process for application to a range of waste and site characteristics. The analyses indicate that, except for the effect on cost, the ISV process can be implemented at sites with high groundwater tables, as long as the rate of recharge does not exceed the vitrification rate. The melt typically proceeds at a rate of about 3–6 in./hr. Thus, soils with permeabilities in the range of 10^{-5}–10^{-9} cm/sec can be vitrified even in the presence of groundwater in the water table, without taking steps to lower the water table or to install underground barriers.

Based on the existing data base and experience, the ISV technology appears to be ready for deployment at sites where the soil is contaminated with heavy metals and inorganics. Considerably fewer test details are available to assess applicability to sites containing a range of organic contaminants.

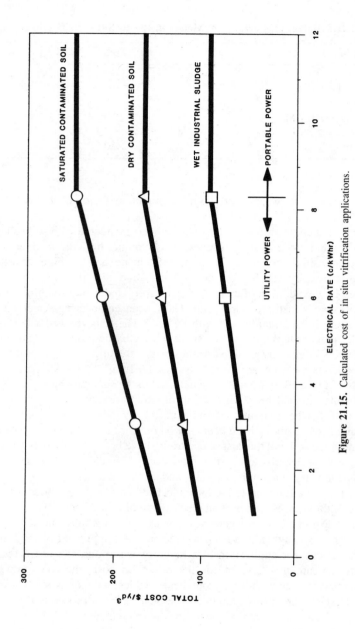

Figure 21.15. Calculated cost of in situ vitrification applications.

ABOVE-GROUND, ON-SITE TECHNOLOGIES

Mobile Treatment Systems

Bringing systems for the treatment/destruction of the wastes to the contaminated sites eliminates the health and safety risks that would otherwise be associated with the transportation of the wastes to off-site treatment/destruction facilities. Because site remediation is generally a temporary activity, on-site processing of wastes and contaminated soils in mobile or transportable systems, which can be taken from site to site, becomes economically attractive. Although systems such as land farming, which would not involve treatment in mobile units, could be used at certain sites, air-pollution considerations, large land area requirements, and the refractory and toxic nature of wastes at many sites preclude their widespread use at uncontrolled hazardous-waste sites. Land farming is also viewed more as a conventional rather than an innovative technology and hence is not included in the discussion in this chapter. Also not discussed here are systems such as air/steam stripping or activated carbon adsorption for treatment of contaminated groundwater; such systems have been successfully used at a number of locations throughout the country (e.g., in Battle Creek, Mich., and in Tacoma, Wash., where the water supply wells were contaminated with chlorinated solvents[60–66]).

Mobile or transportable treatment units (TTUs) have been widely used for processing water for potable use and sewage and industrial wastewaters for pollution control. The feasibility of using a range of water and wastewater treatment technologies in a TTU for the management of concentrated wastewaters at uncontrolled hazardous-waste sites and of spill-impacted waters in emergency response situations have been evaluated for EPA.[63,64] The types of TTU systems that have been or are being developed by the EPA for emergency response include[65]:

A carbon adsorption/sand filter system

A rotary kiln incineration system

An in situ containment/treatment unit (ISCTU)

A soil-washer system

An activated carbon regeneration system

A flocculation-sedimentation system

A reverse osmosis (RO) treatment system

An independent physical/chemical (IPC) wastewater treatment system

The TTU equipment is usually mounted on one or more trailers or housed in trucks that are taken to sites as complete, fully operational systems or is transported to sites largely as unassembled components that are assembled or connected at the site. Because of over-the-road transportation restrictions, TTUs are generally smaller and have somewhat different configurations than conventional equipment used in permanent structures. To provide flexibility, a concept of modular construction reportedly has been featured in one incineration system, which consists of a number of interchangeable modules designed to handle different types and forms of wastes.[66] The modular design also allows construction of relatively large plants, thereby overcoming the size limitation of the conventional TTUs.

A recent business review of TTU technologies indicates that a large number of vendors offer such systems and capabilities.[67] The majority of these systems, however, are for conventional waste-management applications. At this time, only a few vendors offer systems that are specifically designed for or have been tested in site remediation applications. With some exceptions, most systems do not represent true innovations in concept, method, equipment, or approach, but are merely new applications of existing technologies and practices. In general, very little cost and performance data are available for applications involving actual site cleanup. Also, the performance claims and cost data that have been provided by some vendors have not been independently verified.

The potentially significant role that TTUs can play in solving the nation's hazardous-waste management problems, including the cleanup of contaminated sites, is now well recognized and has been discussed at a number of recent professional meetings and industry forums.[68] Recommendations have been developed on strategies to address many regulatory, information, and institutional issues that can act as impediments to the use of TTUs. The most important of these issues appears to be related to regulatory permitting and permit requirements. An administrative mechanism has not yet been established for issuing TTU permits. The State of California currently requires the submission of an "operation plan" for statewide use of a TTU, and a site-specific "certification application" for use of the unit at a specific site. The operation plan is essentially a modified version of the RCRA "Part B" permit application for hazardous-waste management facilities. Because of limited personnel at the regulatory agencies, the processing of the many permit applications that are being received is expected to be very slow.

The EPA SITE program and the reauthorization and increased funding for the Superfund program have generated a tremendous amount of interest in the use of TTUs for site cleanup. The EPA Office of Solid Waste and Emergency Response recently published a compendium that discusses the capabilities and limitations of five broad treatment categories for use in mobile systems to treat wastes at Superfund sites.[65] The five categories are thermal treatment, immobilization, chemical treatment, physical treatment, and biological treatment. The specific technologies covered and the status of the TTUs using those technologies are listed in Table 21.9. Summary information for mobile thermal treatment systems is given in Table 21.10.

The Illinois Environmental Protection Agency (IEPA) is currently involved in a pioneering and unique program that solicits (and indirectly promotes) qualified contractors who will agree to own and operate the so-called "Transportable Thermal Destruction Unit" (TTDU).[69] In September 1985, IEPA issued a request for statements of qualifications for cleanup of two contaminated sites, one involving PCB contamination of soil. Of the nine proposed TTDUs, one was selected for implementation in 1987. The selected TTDU employs rotary kiln technology for waste destruction.

TABLE 21.9. Treatment Technologies and Status of Mobile Systems[65]

Technology	Status
Incineration:	
Rotary kiln	Commercial
Liquid injection	Commercial
Fluidized bed/circulating bed	Pilot
Infrared	Pilot
Pyrolysis:	
Plasma arc	Pilot
Electric pyrolyzer	Pilot
Immobilization:	
Cement based	Commercial
Fly ash or lime based	Commercial
Asphalt based	Pilot
Chemical treatment:	
Oxidation-reduction	Commercial
Neutralization	Commercial
Precipitation	Commercial
Dechlorination	Commercial
Physical treatment:	
Distillation	Commercial
Steam stripping	Commercial
Phase separation	Commercial
Air stripping	Commercial
Activated carbon	Commercial
Clarification	Commercial
Evaporation	Commercial
Soil washing	Pilot
Filtration	Commercial
Ion exchange	Commercial
Membrane separation	Pilot
Biological treatment:	
Aerobic	Commercial
Anaerobic	Commercial

Example Mobile Treatment Systems

To illustrate the applicability of mobile systems to the processing of soils and wastes at contaminated sites, three high-temperature destruction systems, one low-temperature thermal stripping system, and a soil-washing system are discussed here. The thermal technologies reviewed are the Westinghouse Electric Pyrolyzer, the Ogden Environmental Services' Circulating Bed Combustor, and the Shirco infrared system.

Adequate data from actual site remediation applications are currently unavailable to provide a reliable data base for developing cost estimates for site cleanup using

TABLE 21.10. Mobile Thermal Treatment Systems[65]

Company	Technology	Waste Types Handled	Mobile System Status	Capacity
DETOXCO	Rotary kiln	Combustible wastes; soils contaminated with combustibles	Demonstration-scale system operating	3000 lb/hr soil
ENSCO Environmental Services	Rotary kiln	Organic-contaminated solids, liquid, sludges, soil; organics include PCBs, dioxin	Full-scale system operating	35 MM Btu/hr 10,000 lb/hr soil 600-lb/hr hydrocarbons
GA Technologies, Inc.[a]	Circulating fluidized bed	Organic-contaminated solids, liquids, sludges, soil	Mobile system under design	9 MM Btu/hr 10,000 lb/hr soil 600 lb/hr hydrocarbons
J. H. Huber Corporation	Advanced electric reactor	Organic-contaminated solids, liquid, soil; organics include PCBs, dioxin, chemical warfare agents	Pilot-scale system operating	3000 lb/hr
Modar, Inc.	Supercritical water oxidation	Organic-contaminated liquids	Pilot-scale system operating	30 gal/day or organic material in an aqueous solution containing 1–100% organics
Shirco Infrared Systems, Inc.[a]	Infrared incineration	Organic-contaminated solids, sludges, soil; organics include PCBs, dioxin, explosives	Pilot-scale system operating	100 lb/hr
Waste-Tech Services, Inc.	Fluidized bed	Organic-contaminated solids, liquids, sludges, soil	Demonstration-scale operating	Not available
Westinghouse Plasma Systems	Plasma arc	Organic-contaminated liquids	Pilot-scale system constructed	60 gal/hr
Winston Technology	Rotary kiln	Organic-contaminated liquids, solids, sludges, soil; organics include PCBs	Full-scale systems constructed	8 MM Btu/hr
Zimpro, Inc.	Wet-air oxidation	Organic-contaminated liquids, sludges	Full-scale system operating	600 gal/hr

[a]See text for discussion and updated information on these technologies

TTUs. The cost, however, would be expected to be highly site specific. Budgetary estimates provided by vendors indicate a cost of $100–$400 per ton for thermal destruction systems.

THE WESTINGHOUSE ELECTRIC PYROLYZER

The Pyrolyzer is a mobile thermal destruction system for treatment of soils, solids, and sludges contaminated with organic hazardous wastes. The process has been selected by EPA for independent evaluation under the SITE program. Development testing of a 5-ton/day prototype unit has been completed using nonhazardous, surrogate waste materials.[70] The unit is currently being modified so that it will be useful at commercial sites. A 20-ton/day unit has been constructed in California and is being readied for use at an actual hazardous-waste site. In addition, a 100-ton/day unit is under construction and should be available for use in 1988.[71] The 20-ton/day system is mounted on two 40-foot trailers, one housing the power supply and the other containing the process equipment.

The heart of the process is a pyrolysis unit that uses electric energy to achieve temperatures in the vicinity of 3000°F. Liquids, gases, or solids of different compositions can be fed to the Pyrolyzer with appropriate adjustment of the processing rate. The environment in the reactor is largely free of oxygen, thus precluding combustion reactions and the concomitant generation of products of incomplete combustion. The high temperature in the reactor is sufficient to melt most materials, including dirt, thus creating a molten bath or melt.

A process flow diagram for the Pyrolyzer is shown in Figure 21.16. Technical brochures provided by Westinghouse provide the following process description.[71] The waste material is first sent to a material separation system (a bar screen). Here, particles larger than 4 inches are removed, reduced in size, and recycled to the bar screen. The waste particles smaller than 4 inches are fed via bucket conveyor through a rotolock valve to the reactor. Inside the reactor, the inorganic solids melt, liquids vaporize, and organic materials dissociate into atoms. Large particles fall into the molten pool at the bottom of the reactor where metals (specific gravity >3) settle to the bottom. Aluminates, silicates, and other siliceous components form a vitreous melt with a specific gravity of <2 that floats on top of the molten metal pool and whose surface remains exposed to the environment of the reaction chamber.

The pyrolysis reactions convert organics to carbon monoxide, hydrogen, and carbon. Sulfur and halogens in the original feed are released into the gas phase as corresponding hydrogen compounds. The gases generated are drawn off the reactor into a cooling and cleanup system. The cleanup system consists of a cyclone, a baghouse, and an acid gas scrubber. The gases are drawn from the reactor through the cleanup train by an induction fan, which maintains the reactor at a slightly negative pressure. The gases can then be recycled to the reactor or the gas cleaning train, or discharged to the stack. The gas recycle feature thus allows for a multipass processing of the vapor phase, which gives direct control of vapor-phase residence time. Particles carried over or formed in the gas cleanup train are collected in the

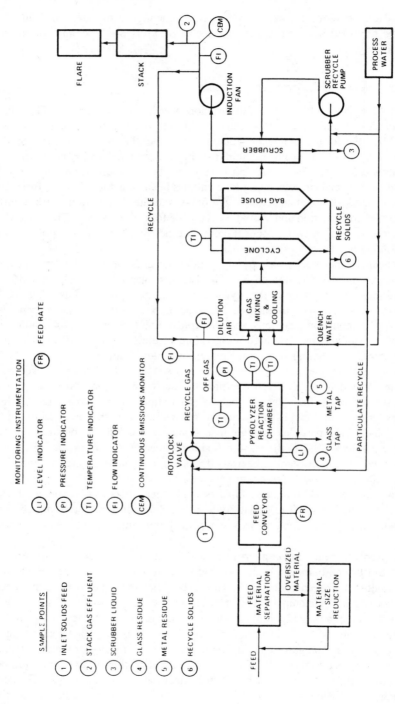

Figure 21.16. Electric Pyrolyzer process flow diagram, sample points, and monitoring implementation.

cyclone and baghouse and can be recycled to the reactor. The scrubber water will contain salts and particulates and may be discharged to the sewer after sampling. The molten material is tapped from two levels in the reactor. The upper tap will remove the siliceous phase and the lower tap will remove the metal phase (if any). The melt is quenched by water as it leaves the tap trench. The cooled residue will be collected in suitable containers or otherwise stored on site.

The Pyrolyzer has no requirements for oxygen or auxiliary fuel. It requires electric power (480 volts, three-phase), water, and sanitary sewer hookup. The unit reportedly generates less off gas and is much more economical to operate than conventional incinerators. The vitrified, glassy residues that are produced have superior leach-resistant characteristics and may be declared inert for delisting purposes.

CIRCULATING BED COMBUSTOR (CBC)

The CBC is a fluidized bed incineration system developed by GA Technologies (San Diego, Calif.). The technology is now owned and marketed by Ogden Environmental Services, Inc. (San Diego). The CBC technology was originally developed for use in power generation. There are now over 25 CBCs operating worldwide on low-grade fuels.[74] The use of the CBC for hazardous-waste incineration represents a new application of a commercial technology. A 2 million Btu/hr stationary pilot plant has been operated in San Diego, where test burns have been conducted on a range of wastes and contaminated soils. Destruction/removal efficiencies (DRE) of 99.9999 percent and 99.992 percent have been reported with PCB- and pentachlorophenol-contaminated soils (10,000 ppm PCBs and 136 ppm PCP) respectively.[72] The company has submitted proposals to undertake site remediation at a number of contaminated sites in California and in other states. The CBC has been selected for independent evaluation by the EPA under the SITE program. A 10-million-Btu/hr transportable unit capable of handling 75 to 100 tons/day of contaminated soil is currently under construction and should be available for field demonstration sometime in 1988.[73] Very preliminary costs provided by the vendor indicate soil treatment costs ranging from $100/ton to $400/ton, depending on the nature of contamination and the volume of the material to be processed.[72]

A schematic diagram of the CBC is shown in Figure 21.17. It is a fluidized bed system operated with an "expanded" bed to increase combustion efficiency. A bed of sand sits on a support plate within a vertical reactor. Hot air is injected beneath the sand bed. The physical action of the hot bed stream percolating through the sand bed (which can be from 24 to 48 inches deep, in a reactor from 3 to over 12 feet in diameter) creates the appearance of a fluid in the reactor. The top of the sand bed undulates in apparent fluid motion. Within the bed, the hot air imparts a high degree of agitation throughout the sand. Therefore, conditions for effective combustion are present: air, heat (the hot air stream), and a high degree of turbulence. the air velocity through the bed is maintained at a relatively high value (normally in excess of 10 ft/sec). At this high velocity, the bed sand, as well as other materials within the bed, will be elutriated into the gas stream. A cyclone separator at the exit of the

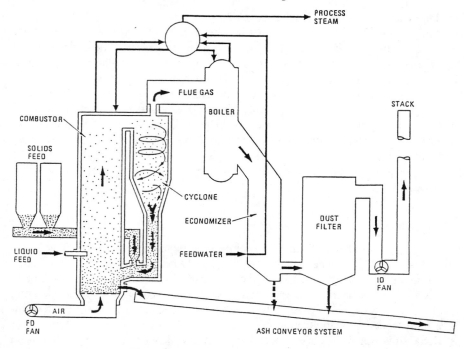

Figure 21.17. The circulating bed combustor.

reactor captures most solids within the gas stream and injects them back into the sand bed. The waste materials fed to the CBC are normally injected into, and the residues are removed from, the cyclone return loop. The residence time of the solids within the reactor is controlled by controlling the rate of residue discharge from the cyclone return loop. Through the recirculation feature of this process, the solids can be retained in the system for fractions of a minute or for over half an hour, until the residual organic content is reduced satisfactorily (or is eliminated). Pilot tests have indicated that organics destruction in the off gas is effective in proportion to destruction of the organics in the residuals, without the use of an afterburner.

Another important feature of the CBC is its ability to feed limestone (or other alkali) into the sand bed. The presence of an alkali will help neutralize the acidic component(s) present in the waste or generated as result of combustion. A conventional wet scrubbing system is used to treat the off gas prior to discharge to the atmosphere. The discharge to the reactor and the residues are removed from the cyclone return loop. The temperature within the CBC reactor is relatively low (normally in the range of 1400°F to 1600°F). The ability to recycle waste through the reactor allows the use of lower temperatures. Rather than raise the temperature within the reactor, additional residence time is provided. This translates to less fuel usage, less danger of creating fusion within the bed, and less corrosion problems when handling wastes and contaminated soils containing or generating acidic compounds.

As with all fluidized bed systems, the CBC requires feed preparation for size reduction. A waste size of less than 1 inch in diameter is desired. Therefore, application to soils containing rocks, clumps, and other large discarded objects would require feed pretreatment.

SHIRCO INFRARED SYSTEM

Shirco Infrared Systems, Inc. (Dallas, Texas) markets an infrared incineration system for destruction of hazardous wastes. The company has a portable pilot test unit that it has used to evelute process applicability to a variety of waste types. The pilot test unit can process 30–100 lb/hr of feed material, depending on waste properties and process requirements.

The Shirco incinerator features infrared lamps (powered by electricity) that heat the waste as it travels through the treating chamber on a woven metal alloy conveyor belt. The heating, which can produce temperatures ranging from 500°F to 1850°F, and the long residence time (10–180 minutes), can result in the volatilization and destruction of organics. The off gases are burned in a propane-fired secondary chamber that is designed to operate at temperatures in the 1000–2300°F range with a 2.2-second gas residence time and using up to 100 percent excess air. Exhaust gases leaving the secondary chamber pass through a venturi scrubber prior to atmospheric discharge.

Figure 21.18 depicts one of several possible configurations of a typical infrared waste-disposal system. Descriptions of the system components identified in the figure are given in Table 21.11.

The Shirco technology has been successfully tested in several applications involving contaminated soils. For example, in Times Beach, Mo., the pilot unit was used to treat dioxin-contaminated soils containing 260 ppb of 2,3,7,8-tetrachlorodibenzo-p-dioxin (TCDD). In these tests, the dioxin in the treated soil was below the detection limit of 0.038 ppb. Tests on the particulate emission samples indicated a dioxin removal and destruction efficiency of 99.999997 percent.[76]

Shirco has received orders for several 100-ton/day units from hazardous-waste management companies.[75,76] One such unit has been delivered to Haztech (Decatur, Ga.) and is currently being used at a Superfund site in Braden, Fla. The soil at this site is contaminated with PCBs, hydrocarbons, and heavy metals. Deliveries were scheduled for three other units in 1987—one for use at a steel mill site in Indian Town, Fla., where the soil is contaminated with PCBs. Shirco has announced designs of two new systems: a 5- to 25-ton/day mobile unit and a 400-ton/day transportable unit.[75] The small mobile system is for use at very small waste sites or environmentally threatening emergencies such as accidental spills, train derailments, or explosions. The 400-ton/day transportable unit is a larger version of Shirco's 100-ton/day mobile system and will be for use at very large sites, containing more than 100,000 tons of wastes.

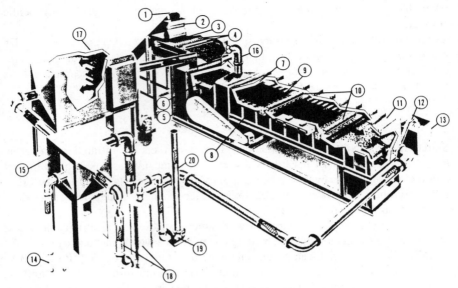

Figure 21.18. Shirco infrared incineration system.

The Shirco system should be capable of handling most types of solid, liquid, and gaseous wastes. Wastes containing less than 22 percent solids and those containing solids that cannot be ground or shredded to a maximum size of 1–1½ inches cannot be properly processed by this system.[65]

LOW-TEMPERATURE THERMAL STRIPPING

Volatile contaminants in the soil can be removed by aeration using ambient or heated air. Spills-impacted granular soils containing trichloroethylene (TCE) and other VOCs reportedly have been treated successfully using the Royer Model 365 soil shredder. This shredder is a mobile unit and is used as follows.[77] After the soil is loaded into the receiving hopper of the shredder, it is carried to the top of a flighted conveyor where it cascades onto the shredding belt, The high-speed shredding belt churns and tosses the material while closely spaced rows of tempered steel shredding cleats on the belt produce a continuous raking action to shred and aerate the soil. Only particles of preselected size are discharged through the adjustable, variable-sweep fingers while oversize clods are forced back for further processing. Nonshreddable material, such as sticks, stones, metals, and glass, are automatically rejected from the end product and discharged through a trash chute away from the shredded material. The overall VOC removal efficiency can be increased by increasing the number of passes through the shredder.

Aeration/shredding is a slow process and merely transfers the VOCs from the soil

TABLE 21.11. Components of the SHIRCO Infrared Incineration System[76]

No.*	Component	Description
1	Feed system	Material may be fed to the incinerator by a conveyor, overhead hopper, drum shredder, or other method
2	Rotary air-lock	Minimizes air infiltration into the system
3	Metering conveyor	Synchronized with the incinerator belt to feed the material at the desired rate
4	Spreading/leveling devices	Material spread to the width of the incinerator and leveled to the optimum process thickness
5	Feed module	Containing conveyor drive, access door, and observation sightglass
6	Incinerator conveyor	Woven metal alloy belt conveying material through the chamber at the desired rate
7	Fiber blanket insulation	Allows for rapid heating and cooling of the incinerator
8	Heating modules	Contains the incinerator heating elements and rotary rakes. The number of modules is determined by the desired process feed rate and material composition
9	Electrical infrared heating elements	Consists of silicon carbide rods, located above the conveyor belt to heat the material directly with radiant energy. The heating elements have a greater than 99% efficiency and can be adjusted for temperature control
10	Rotary rakes	To gently stir the material for maximum exposure to air and infrared energy
11	Discharge module	Contains the discharge hopper, access doors, and sight glasses. The processed materials leaves the incinerator at this point
12	Ash discharge system	Prevents air infiltration and delivers ash/processed material to receiving containers
13	Receptacle	For ash/processed material
14	Blower	Supplies combustion air to the system
15	Air preheater	An energy-recovery device
16	Furnace exhaust	Insulated with fiber blanket
17	Secondary process chamber	Provides residence time, turbulence, and supplemental energy, if required, to destroy gaseous volatiles from the incinerator
18	Scrubbing system	Selected for individual process requirements
19	Blower and damper	Controls sytem draft
20	Exhaust stack	Provided with sample ports

*The numbers refer to the system components shown in Figure 21.18.

to the air. The rate of volatilization can be increased and air-pollution problems can be controlled, however, by using preheated air for aeration and conducting the operation in a closed system equipped with an off-gas treatment system. Such a system has been developed and pilot tested in the field by the U.S. Army Toxic and Hazardous Materials Agency.[39,78]

Figure 21.19 is a schematic diagram of the low-temperature thermal stripping process. In this system, contaminated soil is fed into a "thermal processor" similar to the units that are commonly used in industry to heat or dry bulk solids, slurries, pastes, or viscous liquids. The processor is essentially an indirect heat exchanger consisting of a parallel double-screw mechanism housed in a jacketed trough. The screw shafts and flights, as well as the trough, are hollow to allow for the circulation of heating fluid (i.e., hot oil). The temperature of the heating oil is controlled from ambient to a maximum of 600°F by an electric-resistance heater. Preheated air is introduced to the thermal processor as a carrier gas to enhance volatilization and to remove VOCs. The off gas passes through an afterburner, where the VOCs are destroyed at 1832°F with a residence time of greater than two seconds.

Results from the pilot-plant test runs indicate that low-temperature thermal processing is an effective means for removing VOCs from soil. In a 22-day test,

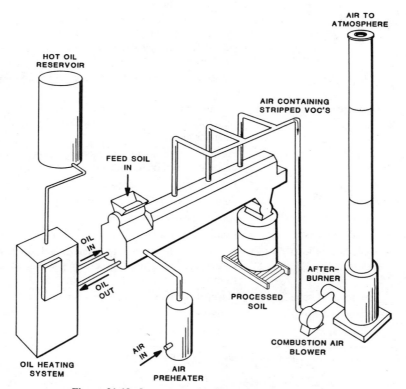

Figure 21.19. Low-temperature thermal processing system.

more than 15,000 pounds of soil containing up to 20,000 ppm VOC (primarily in the form of dichloroethylene, trichloroethylene, and tetrachloroethylene) were treated. The results indicated greater than 99.99 percent VOC removal and no detectable VOCs in the stack gas.[72] In the pilot-plant tests, the soil discharge temperature ranged from 120°F to 300°F, the air inlet temperature was 190°F, and the conveyor temperature ranged from 210°F to 570°F.

Because of the low temperature of the operation, the auxiliary fuel requirements for the low-temperature thermal processing would be significantly lower than incineration processes that operate at much higher temperatures. This would be an important consideration when a large volume of soil must be processed. The low operating temperature can also be a limitation since the system would not be suitable for applications involving less volatile organic compounds. To achieve effective heat transfer and VOC removal, considerable feed pretreatment would also be required to break up clumps and remove rocks and other large objects. The process cost thus appears to be highly dependent on the characteristics of the feed material and the pretreatment required. Considerable additional testing would be needed to evaluate the applicability and cost for processing soils with a range of characteristics and to develop a basis for the design of full-scale units.

SOIL WASHING/EXTRACTION

The Release Control Branch of the EPA's Hazardous Waste Engineering Research Laboratory has supported a program aimed at developing a mobile system for extracting spilled hazardous materials from excavated soils.[54] Based on laboratory evaluation of techniques for scrubbing or cleaning soils contaminated with hazardous materials, a full-scale prototype unit has been constructed for the extraction of hazardous materials from spill-contaminated soils.[79] The system will (1) treat excavated contaminated soil, (2) return the treated soil to the site, (3) separate the extracted hazardous materials from the washing fluid for further processing and/or disposal, and (4) decontaminate process fluids before recirculation or final disposal. A process flow diagram for the EPA soil scrubber is shown in Figure 21.20.

The EPA soil washer utilizes conventional equipment for scrubbing, size reduction, washing, and dewatering of soils. The process sequence includes initial removal of oversized chunks (>2.5 cm), water knife scrubbing to deconsolidate the remaining soil matrix and to strip any contaminant loosely adsorbed on the solids (>2 mm) or held in the void spaces of the soil, and four-stage countercurrent extraction coupled with hydrocyclone separation after each extraction step to separate the solids (<2 mm) from the liquid. Froth flotation is used to give maximum mixing of extractant and soil in each stage. The overhead extract (mostly sorbent) from the first-state extractor hydrocyclone contains the highest level of dissolved or dispersed contaminants and fines. This extract must be clarified and then treated before it is recycled. The aqueous washing fluid may contain additives such as acids, alkalis, detergents, and selected organic solvents to enhance soil decontami-

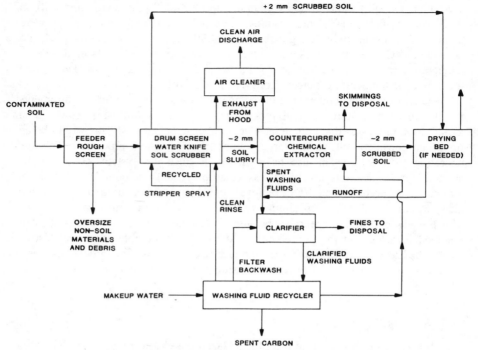

Figure 21.20. Process flow scheme for the EPA soil scrubber.

nation. The nominal processing rate will be 3.2 cubic meters (4 cubic yards) of contaminated soil per hour when the soil particles are primarily less than 2 mm in size and up to 14.4 cubic meters (18 cubic yards) per hour for soils of larger average particle size.

The complete system for soil washing requires auxiliary equipment for processing wastewater for recycling and, under certain circumstances, a system for the confinement, collection, and treatment of released gases and mists. Treatment residues consist of skimmings from froth flotation, fine particles discharged with the used washing fluids, and spent carbon. The principal limiting constraint on the treatability of soil is clay content, since breaking down and efficiently treating consolidated clays is impractical or not economically attractive.

The EPA prototype soil washer is now available for field use. EPA plans to demonstrate the material segregation capability of the system at a PCB contamination site in Missouri.[80] Separation of fines, which contain the bulk of the PCBs, would reduce the volume of the material that must be disposed of by incineration. The countercurrent washing capability of the system is to be tested in an application involving soils contaminated with phenols, based on laboratory tests that indicate water scrubbing should result in about 98 percent removal of the phenols.[80]

As noted in the discussion of the in situ system, soil washing would probably be of limited applicability in site cleanup service where a range of contaminants and soil characteristics is encountered. Laboratory and field tests indicate that while certain contaminants such as simple phenols can be readily extracted from both organic and inorganic soils, other contaminants (e.g., PCBs and arsenic) cling tenaciously to the soils and are released less readily into the washing fluids.[54] At a battery-dumping pit in Leeds, Ala., the leaching of lead-contaminated soil (47,000 ppm lead) with a 2 percent aqueous solution of EDTA resulted in a residual lead level of 80 ppm in the soil. Despite this high extraction efficiency, the soil washing was considered unacceptable as the treated soil did not meet the target cleanup goal of 5 ppm residual lead in the soil.[80] Soil washing for lead removal at this site was conducted in a closed-loop operation; the extracted lead was removed by sulfide precipitation and the regenrated EDTA solution was recycled. Soil washing was also considered for the cleanup of lead-contaminated soils at Lee's Farm, a former battery manufacturing site in Wisconsin.[81] Sulfide precipitation and electrolysis were considered feasible for the removal of lead from the EDTA extraction solution.

REFERENCES

1. J. s. Hirschhorn, "Selecting Site Cleanup Technology: A Case Study," *Proceedings, 6th National Conference on Management of Uncontrolled Hazardous Waste Sites,* Washington, D.C., November 4–6, 1985, pp. 311–313.

2. *Remedial Response at Hazardous Waste Sites: Summary Report,* (EPA-540/2-84-002a) and *Case Studies 1–23* (EPA-540/2-84-002b), March 1984.

3. *Record of Decision (ROD) Annual Report, FY '85,* Hazardous Site Control Division, U.S. Environmental Protection Agency, Washington, D.C., June 1986.

4. *Surface Impoundment Assessment National Report,* U.S. Environmental Protection Agency, Office of Drinking Water, Washington, D.C., EPA 570/9-83-002, Dec. 1983.

5. *Draft Minimum Technology Guidance on Double Liner Systems for Landfills and Surface Impoundments: Design, Construction and Operation,* U.S. Environmental Protection Agency, Office of Solid Waste, Dec. 19, 1984.

6. M. Ghassemi et al., *Assessment of Technology for Constructing and Installing Cover and Bottom Liner Systems for Hazardous Waste Facilities; Vol. I, Data Base Development: Perspectives of Industry Experts, State Regulators, and Owners and Operators, and Vol. II, Technical Analysis,* Final Report, prepared by TRW, Inc., for EPA under Contract no. 68-02-3174, Work Assignment 109, Apr. (Vol. II) and May (Vol. I), 1983.

7. M. Ghassemi et al., *Assessment of Hazardous Waste Surface Impoundment Technology: Case Studies and Perspectives of Experts,* EPA-600/S2-84-173, Jan. 1985 (NTIS PB85-117059).

8. M. Ghassemi et al., *Leachate Collection and Gas Migration and Emission Problems at Landfills and Surface Impoundments,* EPA-600/S2-86-017, Feb. 1986 (NTIS PB86-16104/AS).

9. M. Ghassemi and M. Haro, *ASCE J. Environ. Eng.,* **111,** 602 (1985).

10. M. Ghassemi, *ASCE J. Environ. Eng.,* **112,** 613 (1986).

11. *Lining of Waste Impoundment and Disposal Facilities,* EPA Office of Solid Waste and Emergency Response, SW-870, March 1983.

12. *Technical Guidance Document: Construction Quality Assurance for Hazardous Waste Land Disposal Facilities,* EPA/530-SW-86-031, Oct. 1986.

13. J. M. Bass et al., "Assessment of Synthetic Membrane Successes and Failures at Waste Storage and Disposal Sites," *Proceedings, 11th Annual Research Symposium on Land Disposal of Hazardous Waste,* EPA/600/9-85/013, Apr. 1985, p. 262.

14. C. R. Ryan, "Slurry Cutoff Walls: Applications in the Control of Hazardous Wastes," in A. J. Johnson et al. (eds.), *Hydraulic Barriers in Soil and Rock,* ASTM STP 874,, American Society for Testing and Materials, Philadelphia, 1985, pp. 9–23.

15. *Slurry Trench Construction for Pollution Migration Control,* EPA-540/2-84-001, Feb. 1984.

16. G. J. Trezek, *J. Hazard. Waste Hazard. Mat.,* **3**, 281 (1986).

17. W. Grube, "Bottom Barriers at Hazardous Waste Sites," EPA/Dept. of Army Barrier Workshop, A. W. Breidenbach Environmental Research Center, Cincinnati, Ohio, Sept. 7–8, 1983.

18. J. H. May, "Evaluation of Chemical Grout Injection Techniques for Hazardous Waste Containment," *Proceedings, 11th Annual Research Symposium on Land Disposal of Hazardous Waste,* EPA/600/9-85/013, Apr. 1985, pp. 8–18.

19. P. G. Malone et al., "Development of Methods for In Situ Hazardous Waste Stabilization by Injection Grouting," *Proceedings, 10th Annual Research Symposium on Land Disposal of Hazardous Waste,* EPA-600/9-84-007, Apr. 1984, pp. 33–42.

20. *Minimization of Hazardous Waste,* EPA Report to Congress, released Oct. 30, 1986; in *Focus,* a publication of the Hazardous Materials Control Research Institute, Silver Spring, Md., Dec. 1986, p. 4.

21. J. S. Hirschhorn, *J. Hazard. Waste Hazard. Mats.,* **3**, (1986).

22. *Interim Guidance on Superfund Selection of Remedy,* EPA Office of Solid Waste and Emergency Response, Directive no. 9355.0-19, Dec. 24, 1986.

23. RFP SITE-001, "Demonstration of Innovative Technologies for Site Cleanup," EPA Hazardous Waste Engineering Research Laboratory, Cincinnati, Ohio, March 17, 1986.

24. *SITE Strategy and Program Plan,* EPA/540/g-86/001, Office of Solid Waste and Emergency Response, Directive no. 9380.2-3, Dec. 1986.

25. "Fact Sheet for Status of Proposals for Superfund Innovative Technology Evaluation (SITE) Demonstration Program," RFP SITE-001, SITE Program Implementation, EPA Hazardous Waste Engineering Research Laboratory, Cincinnati, Ohio, July 3, 1986.

26. Information provided by Ronald D. Hill, EPA Hazardous Waste Engineering Research Laboratory, Cincinnati, Ohio, March 23, 1987.

27. "Technical Support Services for the Superfund Innovative Technology Evaluation Program," *Commerce Bus. Daily,* Issue PSA-9138, 1 (July 24, 1986).

28. "Hazardous Waste Cleanup Remedial Measure Technologies," *Commerce Bus. Daily,* 10 (Nov. 10, 1986).

29. R. D. Hill et al., "Superfund Innovative Technology Evaluation Program," *Proceedings, 7th National Conference on Management of Uncontrolled Hazardous Waste Sites,* Washington, D.C., Dec. 1–3, 1986, pp. 356–360.

30. Information provided by Thomas Darda, Detox Industries, Houston, Texas, June 23, 1986.

31. *Handbook for Remedial Action at Waste Disposal Sites* (revised), EPA/625/6-85/006, Cincinnati, Ohio, Oct. 1985.

32. R. S. Wetzel et al., "Effectiveness of In Situ Biological Treatment of Contaminated Groundwater and Soils at Kelly Air Force Base, Texas," *Proceedings, National Conference on Hazardous Wastes and Hazardous Materials,* Washington, D.C., March 16–18, 1987, sponsored by EPA et al., pp. 123–128.

33. P. E. Flathman and J. A. Caplan, "Biological Cleanup of Chemical Spills," paper presented at the the HAZMACON 85 Conference, Oakland, Calif., Apr. 23–25, 1985, sponsored by the Association of Bay Area Governments. Oakland, Calif.

34. J. A. Caplan, "In Situ Biodegradation of Methylethyl Ketone in Soil and Ground Water," paper presented at the HAZMACON 86 Conference, Anaheim, Calif., Apr. 29–May 1, 1986, sponsored by the Association of Bay Area Governments, Oakland, Calif.

35. M. B. Bennedsen et al., "Use of Vapor Extraction Systems for In Situ Removal of Volatile Organic Compounds from Soil," *Proceedings, National Conference on Hazardous Wastes and Hazardous Materials,* Washington, D.C., March 16–18, 1987, sponsored by EPA et al., pp. 92–95.

36. J. C. Agrelot et al., "Vacuum: Defense System for Ground Water VOC Contamination," paper presented at the Fifth National Symposium on Aquifer Restoration and Ground Water Monitoring, National Water Well Association, Columbus, Ohio, May 21–24, 1985.

37. J. J. Malot, "Unsaturated Zone Monitoring and Recovery of Underground Contamination," paper presented at the Fifth National Symposium on Aquifer Restoration and Ground Water Monitoring, National Water Well Association, Columbus, Ohio, May 21–24, 1985.

38. G. H. Anastos et al., *In Situ Air Stripping of Soils Pilot Study,* U.S. Army Toxic and Hazardous Materials Agency, Report AMXTH-TE-TR-85025, Aberdeen Proving Ground (Edgewood Area), Ma., Oct. 1985.

39. D. L. Koltuniak, "In-Situ Air Stripping Cleans Contaminated Soil," *Chem. Eng.* 30–31 (Aug. 18, 1986).

40. B. Hilberts, "In Situ Steam Stripping," in J. W. Assink and W. J. Van Den Brink (eds.), "Contaminated Soil," *Proceedings, First International TNO Conference on Contaminated Soil,* Utrecht, The Netherlands, Nov. 11–15, 1985, Martinus Nijhoff Publishers, Dordrecht, The Netherlands, pp. 680–687.

41. M. Ghassemi et al., *Evaluation of ATW-Calweld In Situ Treatment System,* final report submitted by CH2M HILL to Toxic Treatments (USA) Inc., San Mateo, Calif., Nov. 1986.

42. M. Ghassemi, "Innovative In Situ Treatment Technologies for Treatment of Contaminated Sites," paper accepted for publication in the *Journal of Hazardous Materials, 1987.*

43. Information provided by Dr. Arthur D. Lord, Physics Department, Drexel University, Philadelphia, Pa., Apr. 7, 1987.

44. J. H. Kyle et al., "The Effect of Volatile Organic Compounds on the Ability of Solidification\Stabilization Technologies to Attenuate Mobile Pollutants," *Proceedings, National Conference on Hazardous Wastes and Hazardous Materials,* Washington, D.C., March 16–18, 1987, sponsored by EPA et al., pp. 152–157.

45. M. D. Shaw, "Macroencapsulation: New Technology Provides Innovative Alternatives for Hazardous Materials Storage, Transportation, Treatment, and Disposal," *Proceedings, National Conference on Hazardous Wastes and Hazardous Materials,* Washington, D.C., March 16–18, 1987, pp. 96–100.

46. M. J. Cullinane, "Stabilization/Solidification of Hazardous Wastes," *Proceedings, National Conference on Hazardous Wastes and Hazardous Materials,* Washington, D.C., March 16–18, 1987, sponsored by EPA et al., pp. 167–168.

47. R. L. Smith et al., "In Situ Solidification/Fixation of Industrial Wastes," *Proceedings, 6th National Conference on Management of Uncontrolled Hazardous Wastes,* Washington, D.C., Nov. 4–6, 1985 pp. 231–233.

48. "IWT, Mitsubishi Form Joint Venture to Clean Site Using Chemical Fixation," *HazTech News,* **1,** 161 (Nov. 20, 1986).

49. "Presentation of the HWT Chemical Fixation Technology and Japanese In-Place Treatment Equipment," International Waste Technologies, Wichita, Kan.

50. "New Technology Available for In Situ Soil Treatment," in *The Hazardous Waste Consultant,* McCoy & Assoc., Lakewood, Colo., 1-1-1-6, (Jan./Feb. 1987).

51. Information provided by Jefferey P. Newton, President, International Waste Technologies, Wichita, Kans., Jan. 27, 1987.

52. K. Wagner and Z. Kosin, "In Situ Treatment," *Proceedings, 6th National Conference on Management of Uncontrolled Hazardous Waste Sites,* Washington, D.C., Nov. 4–6, 1985., pp. 221–230.

53. W. D. Ellis et al., "Treatment of Soil Contaminated with Heavy Metals," *Proceedings, 12th Annual Research Symposium on Land Disposal, Remedial Action, Incineration, and Treatment of Hazardous Waste,* Cincinnati, Ohio, Apr. 21–24, 1986, EPA/600/9-86/022, Aug. 1986, pp. 201–209.

54. R. Scholz, and J. Milanowski, *Mobile System for Extracting Spilled Hazardous Materials from Excavated Soils,* EPA-600/S2-83-100, Dec. 1983.

55. J. Nash and R. P. Traver, "Field Evaluation of In Situ Washing of Contaminated Soils with Water/Surfactants," *Proceedings, 12th Annual Research Symposium; Land Disposal, Remedial Action, Incineration, and Treatment of Hazardous Waste,* Cincinnati, Ohio, Apr. 21–23, 1986, EPA/600/9-86/022, Aug. 1986, pp. 208–217.

56. Information provided by James E. Hansen, Manager ISV Technology Transfer and Commercialization, Battelle, Northwest Laboratories, Richland, Wash., March 26 and Apr. 8, 1987.

57. *Environmental Science and Technology,* **21,** 317 (1987).

58. V. F. Fitzpatrick et al., *In Situ Vitrification: A Candidate Process for In Situ Destruction of Hazardous Waste,* Battelle, Northwest Laboratories, Richland, Wash., Report PNL-SA-14065, presented at the Seventh Superfund Conference, Washington, D.C., Dec. 1–3, 1986.

59. C. L. Timmerman, *In Situ Vitrification of PCB-Contaminated Soils,* Final Report prepared by Battelle, Northwest Laboratories, Richland, Wash., for the Electric Power Research Institute, Palo Alto, Calif., Research Project 1263-24, Oct. 1986.

60. *Superfund Record of Decision: Verona Well Field, MI (Second Remedial Action, 08/12/85),* Environmental Protection Agency, Office of Emergency and Remedial Response, EPA/ROD/RO5-85/020, Aug. 1985.

61. W. D. Byers, "Response to Solvent-Contaminated Groundwater, a Case History," paper presented at the ISA Pacific Northwest Instrumentation '86 Conference and Exhibit, Portland, Oreg., Apr. 8–10, 1986.

62. W. D. Byers and C. M. Morton, "Removing VOCs from Groundwater: Pilot, Scale-up, and Operating Experience," *Envir. Prog.,* **4,** 112 (1985).

63. M. Ghassemi et al., *Feasibility of Commercialized Water Treatment Techniques for Concentrated Waste Spills,* EPA-600/7-81-025 (NTIS Publication no. PB 82-108-440), July 1981.

64. M. Ghassemi et al., "Comparative Evaluation of Processes for the Treatment of Concentrated Wastewaters at Uncontrolled Hazardous Waste Sites," paper presented at the EPA National Conference on Management of Uncontrolled Hazardous Waste Sites," paper presented at the EPA National Conference on Management of Uncontrolled Hazardous Waste Sites, Washington, D.C., Oct. 15–17, 1980.

65. *Mobile Treatment Technologies for Superfund Wastes,* Environmental Protection Agency, Office of Emergency and Remedial Response, EPA 540/2-86/003(f), Sept. 1986.

66. *Chemical Engineering,* 9 (March 16, 1987).

67. D. Duxbury, *Transportable Treatment Technologies, a Business Review,* The Center for Environmental Management, Tufts University, Medford, Mass., July 1986.

68. *National Hazardous Forum on Transportable Treatment Units, February 26–28, 1986, and April 8–10, 1986,* The Center for Environmental Management, Tufts University, Medford, Mass., July 1986.

69. J. F. Frank and R. Kuykendall, "Illinois Plans for Onsite Incineration of Hazardous Waste," Illinois Environmental Protection Agency, Springfield.

70. "Westinghouse Chosen for SITE," *World Wastes,* 13 (Jan. 1987).

71. Information provided by Robert Reed, Regional Sales Manager, Environmental Technology Division, Westinghouse Electric Corporation, Madison, Pa., Apr. 8 and 10, 1987.

72. "A Guide to Innovative Thermal Hazardous Waste Treatment Processes," in *The Hazardous Waste Consultant,* McCoy & Assoc., Lakewood, Colo., **4,** 4-1–4-39 (May/June 1986).

73. Information provided by Harold R. Diot, Ogden Environmental Services, Inc., San Diego, Calif., Apr. 1, 1987.

74. H. M. Freeman, *Innovative Thermal Hazardous Waste Treatment Processes,* EPA/600/2-85-049, Apr. 1985 (NTIS Publication no. PB85-192847).

75. *Hotline,* **1** (March 1987) (Hotline is a publication of Shirco Infrared Systems, Inc., Dallas, Texas).

76. Information provided by James B. Fowler, Vice-President, Shirco Infrared Systems, Inc., Dallas, Texas, Apr. 6, 1987.

77. S. E. Johnson et al., "On-site Removal of Volatile Organic Contaminants from Soils, Two Case Studies," *Proceedings, 3rd Annual Eastern Regional Ground Water Conference,* Springfield, Mass., July 28–30, 1986, pp. 585–599, sponsored by the National Water Well Association et al.

78. N. P. McDevitt et al., *Installation Restoration General Technology Development, Task 11: Pilot-scale Investigation of Low Temperature Thermal Stripping of Volatile Organic Compounds (VOCs) from Soil; Volume 1, Technical Report, and Volume 2, Appendices,* U.S. Army Toxic and Hazardous Materials Agency, Aberdeen Proving Ground, Ma., Report no. AMXTH-TE-CR-86074, June 1986.

79. "Mobile System for Extracting Spilled Hazardous Materials from Soil," EPA Fact Sheet, EPA Hazardous Waste Engineering Research Laboratory, Release Control Branch, Edison, N.J., Sept., 1985.

80. Information provided by Richard P. Traver, Release Control Branch, EPA Hazardous Waste Research Laboratory, Edison, N.J., Apr. 6, 1987.

81. C. Castle et al., "Research and Development of a Soil Washing System for Use at Superfund Sites," *Proceedings, 6th National Conference on Management of Uncontrolled Hazardous Waste Sites,* Washington, D.C., Nov. 4–6, 1985, pp. 452–455.

SUGGESTED READINGS

Anon., "Three Plans for Love Canal Cleanup Proposed by EPA," *L.A. Times,* Part I, 17 (June 25, 1987).

B. J. Barfield, R. C. Warner, and C. T. Haan, *Applied Hydrology and Sedimentology for Disturbed Areas,* 603 pp., Oklahoma Technical Press, Stillwater, 1981.

R. L. Berglund AND G. M. Whipple, "Predictive Modeling of Organic Emissions," *Chem. Engineering Progress,* Vol. 83, No. 11, Nov. 1987, 46–54.

J. M. Forseth and P. Kmet, "Flexible Membrane Liners for Solid and Hazardous Waste Landfills—A State-of-the-Art Review," 29 pp., University of Wisconsin Extension, Madison, Wis., 1983.

A. DuPont, "Lime Treatment of liquid Waste Containing Heavy Metals," *Pollution Eng.,* 84–88 (Apr. 1987).

J. P. Giaroud, "Synthetic Pond Liner Assessment," 56 pp., report prepared for Battelle, Pacific Northwest Laboratories, Woodward-Clyde Consultants, Chicago, Ill., 1983.

K. Schneider, "Radioactive Waste Is Turned into a Fertilizer in Oklahoma," *New York Times,* A1, B5 (Nov. 16, 1987).

L. Theodore and J. Reynolds, *Introduction to Hazardous Waste Incineration,* 750 pp., Wiley-Interscience, New York, 1987.

22
Social Dimensions of Facility Siting

Audrey Armour

Reduction, recycling, reuse, and recovery are clearly the cornerstones of an effective waste-management program. But regardless of how well the four R's are implemented, there will always be a need to dispose of wastes in an environmentally safe manner. The development of new and better waste-management facilities is a critical component of any waste-management strategy. It is also likely to be the most contentious. Proposals to site such facilities, especially ones involving hazardous wastes, are generally met with strong public opposition and many have failed to pass the "public acceptance" test.

The "not-in-my-backyard" (NIMBY) syndrome has become a convenient catch phrase to explain the problems proponents face in siting waste-management facilities. There is no denying that the syndrome exists—there are those who simply do not want such facilities in their area. But public resistance to siting proposals is far more complicated than the NIMBY explanation suggests. The way out of the current dilemma of facility siting is coming to depend more and more on understanding and being responsive to the full complexity of public concerns.

PUBLIC OPPOSITION: A MANIFESTATION OF SOCIAL TRENDS

Siting controversies are not new. Facility proponents and planners have experienced public opposition many times in the past. But the conflict that surrounds siting proposals today is significantly different from what it used to be. What is most apparent is that the range of concerns on the public's agenda has broadened considerably. Opposition to hazardous-waste management facilities is not the classic case of industry versus environmentalists.[1] The issues often extend well beyond traditional environmental ones to include:

1. Quality-of-life issues (such as disruption of way of life, loss of community character, interference with use and enjoyment of property, increased stress and anxiety, loss of community cohesion).

2. Sociopolitical issues (including equity, accountability of public officials, role of scientists and technocrats in decision-making processes, access to information, regulating of the regulators).

3. Moral and ethical issues (in particular, the issue of individual moral rights to protect oneself and one's family or community against harm versus one's social obligation to act in the general public interest).

What makes these issues so hard to deal with is that the concerns that underlie them are rooted in and reinforced by a set of broad social forces or factors. These include the following.

Factor one—the legacy of the environmental movement. The public is much more informed about the scientific and technical aspects of environmental issues then ever before. The proliferation of environmental study courses in our schools, continuous mass media coverage of environmental issues, and the appearance of various popular-science magazines on newsstands, are all contributing to an ongoing education process. As a result, people are much less intimidated by technical expertise. They are becoming much more capable of challenging scientific findings.

Factor two—science anxiety. Greater exposure to environmental issses has contributed to greater anxiety regarding science and technology. "Science anxiety" has been defined as a "state of nerves related to the multiple dilemmas associated with the siting of nuclear power plants, the disposal of radioactive and toxic wastes, the mysterious goings-on in genetic engineering . . . repeated scares about drug and pesticide safety, contradictory findings about cancer-producing elements in food processing and packaging, and ill-advised pronouncements on all sorts of scientific matters by scientists with name-recognition who venture outside their fields of expertise."[2] The pervasiveness of such problems and the nagging sense that things are somehow getting out of control are contributing to a kind of schizophrenia about science. It is regarded with both awe and contempt. At the very least, it can be said that there is less complacency about its continued contribution to social well-being.

Factor three—the growing "health" consciousness. Over the past decade, there has been a deepening of public concern about health and life-style issues. The ecological problems of the '60s have become much more meaningful in the perceived threat of health risks associated with many proposed projects. This quality-of-life concern is reinforced by the strong promotion in our society of fitness and positive life-style change. Concern about personal safety and well-being provides strong motivation for becoming an active and vocal participant in public decision-making processes, especially those involving the siting of facilities regarded as hazardous.

Factor four—loss of trust in proponents and regulators. In conjunction with the above factors, there has been a corresponding and mounting distrust of facility managers and regulators. Media exposure of irresponsible industrial environmental management practices has reinforced public scepticism and belief in human frailty.

The common expectation is that facility operators will fall down on the job, that they will take shortcuts and break the rules if it means saving time or money, or that over time they will become complacent and sloppy on the job.[3] Government officials in particular have lost credibility with the public, which tends to see them as being unwilling to question the fallibility of technical analyses, overly concerned with economic interests, and blinded by short-term political gains. As a result, potentially affected publics are less willing to assume that their interests are being safeguarded and to defer to authority than they once were.[4–7]

As a backdrop to these social forces, there are three additional sources of unease: the unprecedented rate of technological change, the explosion of information availability, and the rapid shifting of social values and life-style aspirations. When all seven forces are combined, it becomes obvious that the current strong public resistance to facility-siting proposals has arisen in a social context that is in the throes of fundamental, widespread disturbing change. NIMBY represents, in effect, a logical response to two profound social "crises": a crisis of transformation (anxiety about our ability to adapt to and cope with rapid change) and a crisis of confidence (anxiety about our ability to manage risk, uncertainty, and complexity). Each crisis reinforces the other and together they result in an undercurrent of stress that quite naturally seeks a focus in particular issues.

It is not surprising, then, that when a specific focus is provided, as in the case of a proposal to site a hazardous-waste-management facility, the stress and anxiety spill over onto the agenda. The proposed facility is associated with all the worst that is known about modern-day environmental problems. Family and community are perceived as being intruded upon by a threatening, outside force and the need becomes strong to maintain some measure of control over events affecting one's quality of life. Issues become framed in terms of perceived threats to family safety, economic security, way of life or life-style, and community character and cohesion.[6,8–10] And concern naturally centers on how decisions will be made—the factors that will be taken into account, the extent to which citizens will be involved, and whether the process will be fair and the final decision and equitable one.[3,5]

When these expectations are not met, public controversy usually results.

RESOLVING PUBLIC ACCEPTANCE ISSUES

Over the past 20 years, methods of site selection have evolved from rather crude site-screening approaches to very systematic and highly technical procedures. For major facilities, the state of the art has become so sophisticated that it could be said that "a new discipline has grown up." Yet, despite these advances, siting methodologies remain weak in one crucial dimension—they often fail to take full account of social concerns and to reconcile legitimate, competing interests. Inadequate attention to the "soft" issues involved in th siting of waste-management facilities—issues relating to quality of life, perceived inequities, and distrust of proponents and regulators—more often than not accounts for siting failures.

At present, any new technology or facility has to pass at least three "acceptance" tests:

1. It has to be scientifically, technically, and economically acceptable; that is, it has to be feasible.

2. It has to be legally or administratively acceptable; that is, it has to meet specified regulations and policies.

3. It has to be publicly acceptable; that is, it has to be justified and rationalized to the various potentially affected interests as being responsive to their concerns.

It used to be that public acceptability equated with scientific/technical and legal/administrative acceptability. That is no longer the case. The main implication of the social forces discussed above is that gaining public acceptance now depends to a considerable degree on incorporating into the siting process an element of accommodation to the broader underlying anxieties that fuel siting controversies. More specifically, it means accepting the need on the part of potentially affected publics to question a technology's full implications and appropriateness, the fallibility of scientific and technical studies, and the reliability and trustworthiness of project proponents and government regulators. It also means accepting the demand that environmental and social factors be given equal consideration with economic and technical concerns, that potentially affected publics have full access to information, and that they be actively involved in all stages of the planning and decision process.

It follows that "public acceptance" involves both substantive and procedural issues. This distinction is an important one. The former focuses on outcomes, the net social value of the proposed facility. Unfortunately, there are few generally accepted standards by which to measure this. In a pluralistic society, there are many social values, and the attitudes, preferences, and priorities that help to shape them are constantly shifting. What this means is that substantive issues have to be negotiated with affected interests to ensure that studies undertaken encompass the full range of public concerns and reflect relevant social values. It also means that the process of dealing with such issues is one of continual renegotiation. It is unrealistic, in other words, to expect the substantive issues to be "finally resolved" at some point. Their inherent nature is such that they change with time and place.

Procedural issues are different. They have to do with "rights" to "fair" and "equitable" treatment. Debate is likely to center on the scope of technical analyses (what factors are relevant and should be taken into account?), the validity of different kinds of information inputs (what emphasis should be given to "expert" versus "lay" knowledge and judgments?), and the accessibility of the process to public involvement (what constitutes full opportunity for participation?).

Of the two kinds of issues, the resolution of procedural issues is probably the more important in terms of public acceptance. Affected publics that feel that they have not been given the opportunity to be fully informed, to have their concerns listened to, and to exercise their basic democratic rights are not very likely to accept recommendations and decisions resulting from public review processes, regardless of how substantive such decisions may be.[1-13] Of course, it is always possible to impose a project on a local area despite public dissatisfaction with the way in which the process was conducted, but not without significant ramifications. A process that fosters rather than alleviates fear and anxiety can poison the ongoing relationship that has to exist among citizens, facility proponents, and government regulators over the lifetime of the project. It can make the siting of the next facility all the more difficult.

Each community will differ in its perceptions of and responses to a specific siting proposal, depending on how informed local citizenry are about waste-management issues, their past experience with such facilities and with government regulatory processes, and their socioeconomic status, degree of satisfaction with quality of life in their community, and life plans. Gaining a sound understanding at the outset of the attitudes and values that will likely influence the willingness of a specific community to accept a hazardous-waste management facility is essential to effective facility siting. A skillful diagnosis must be made of the local context—public attitudes, local issues and associated interests, and preferred decision-making processes—so that a siting process that is responsive to local concerns can be designed. General siting methodologies must be tailored to suit the particular sociopolitical characteristics of the context within which they will be applied. Experience suggests that this tailoring is best done in consultation with the potentially affected parties.

Finally, in determining how to proceed, it is important to recognize that the issue is not one of general public acceptance, but rather the acceptability of the facility proposal to the various publics that perceive themselves to be potentially affected. Everyone talks about "the public interest" and "public acceptance," but when it comes to "going public" with a proposal, there are many, often competing, interests vying for attention in the decision process. Each must be given its due. All concerns must be recognized as legitimate and responded to accordingly. This point is particularly relevant when it comes to addressing social impact concerns. Impact studies have long been regarded as superficial in their assessment of the implications of proposed facilities for people and their day-to-day quality of life. Comparatively, social impacts, if addressed at all, have tended to be given far less attention than natural environment and economic impacts.[14] It is this inattention that has resulted in numerous cases of failed siting attempts. Social issues often drive the process and can be a key determinant of the outcome of siting efforts.

CONCLUSION

Minimizing unnecessary social conflict and avoiding unduly protracted siting processes while at the same time achieving environmentally sound and equitable siting decisions present a formidable challenge. To meet it, careful attention must be given to the social dimensions of facility siting. The "hard sell," going public only after technical studies have been initiated or completed, relying on scientific analysis and the force of fact to win the day, and leaving it to the public hearing process to resolve sociopolitical issues are the kinds of strategies that have proved to be ineffective.[6,9,15-17] They inhibit the interpersonal exchange of feelings, thoughts, and information so vital to the resolution of siting conflicts and they generate unproductive adversarial stances—the staking out of extreme positions, the selective treatment of facts, exaggerated claims, and defense by ridicule tactics.

Changes are needed in the way in which the public is involved in the siting process and its concerns are addressed. Strategies that acknowledge the legitimacy of competing perspectives and aim to foster a spirit of cooperation are an important key to resolving public acceptance issues. Lists of hazardous chemicals that are an important component in hazardous waste sites may be used as a starting point in such understanding and eventual public acceptance. (See Appendices A, B, D, and E.)

REFERENCES

R. Collins, et al. 1985. "Locally Unwanted Land Use and Community Reaction." in Institute for Environmental Negotiation, *Not-In-My-Backyard! Community Reaction to Locally Unwanted Land Use.*, The Institute, Charlottesville, Va. 1985.

Robert J. Moolenaar, "New Scientific Issues," in Sandra Panem (ed.), *Public Policy, Science, and Environmental Risk,* The Brookings Institute, Washington, D.C., 1983.

Brad Franklin, *Social Considerations Relative to the Siting of Low Level Radioactive Waste Disposal Facilities in Canada,* Atomic Energy of Canada Ltd., Ottawa, Ont., 1986.

Audrey Armour (ed.), *The Not-In-My-Backyard Syndrome, Symposium Proceedings,* York University, Faculty of Environmental Studies, North York, Ont., 1983.

Felicity Edwards and Natalia Krawetz, *Air Toxics: A Sociopolitical Issue,* Krawetz and MacDonald Research Management, Edmonton, Alta., 1985.

E. Peelle and R. Ellis, "Hazardous Waste Management Outlook: Are There Ways Out of the "Not-In-My-Backyard" Impasses?" *Forum for Applied Research and Public Policy,* Sept. 1987.

Jerome Ravetz, "Scientific Uncertainty Looms Large Over Environmental Policymakers," *Transatlantic Perspectives* **11**, 10–12 (1984).

Armour and Associates and Institute of Environmental Research Inc., *Social Impact Assessment of Landfill Siting Options,* Regional Municipality of Peel, Brampton, Ont., 1986.

Natalia Krawetz, *Hazardous Waste Management: A Review of Social Concerns and Aspects of Public Involvement,* Alberta Environment, Research Secretariat, Edmonton, Alta., 1979.

Bryant Wedge, "The NIMBY Complex. Some Psychological Considerations," in Institute for Environmental Negotiation, *Not-In-My-Backyard! Community Reaction to Locally Unwanted Land Use.* University of Virginia, Charlottesville, 1985.

Tom Connolly, "The Hearing Process: A Help or a Hindrance?" in Audrey Armour (ed.), *The Not-In-My-Backyard Syndrome. Symposium Proceedings.* York University, Faculty of Environmental Studies, North York, Ont., 1983.

Pat Hayes, 1983. "Perspectives on NIMBY: Views from the Front Line," in Audrey Armour (ed.), *The Not-In-My-Backyard Syndrome. Symposium Proceedings.* York University, Faculty of Environmental Studies, North York, Ont., 1983.

Barry Sadler, *Project Assessment, Procedural Fairness, and the Public Interest,* Federal Environmental Assessment Review Office, Ottawa, Ont., 1983.

Reg Lang, and Audrey Armour, *The Assessment and Review of Social Impacts,* Federal Environmental Assessment Review Office, Ottawa, Ont., 1981.

Richard Ellis, and J. Desinger, "Project Outcomes Correlate with Public Participation Variables," *J. Water Pollution Cont. Fed.,* 1564–1567, 1981.

Institute of Environmental Research, *The Design of a Public Consultation Program for Hazardous Waste Management Facilities,* Toronto, IER Inc., 1979.

Roger E. Kasperson, et al., 1980. "Public Opposition to Nuclear Energy: Retrospect and Prospect, *Sci. Technol. Human Values* **5,** 11–23 (1980).

23

What We Learned from the Rhine

Howard H. Fawcett

In the beginning, when God created heaven, earth, and water, (all, we assume, of pristine purity), He made a serious mistake by creating Adam and Eve. They and their virtually limitless offspring have contributed both human and technical violations to the "real world," and today environmentalists claim that only one "virgin" (uncontaminated) river exists—the Franklin River in Tasmania. The desire by some to dam and otherwise downgrade the virgin status of this river has received wide attention.[1]

Dr. Werner Stumm has pointed out that the ratio of pollutant fluxes to natural fluxes increases with the increasing activity of civilization. The quality of water bodies (streams, rivers, ponds, lakes, and oceans) reflects the range of human activity, not only the technical (chemical, steel, petroleum, and other works), but also the sewage and other disposed wastes and discards. As noted in Table 12.1, the Rhine River serves a high population density, which, in turn, reflects the "background" pollution.[2]

Until relatively recent times, most wastes were predominately catabolic (excreta of humans and animals and other biogenic components). Now more and more waste consists of discards of modern industrial society (such as synthetic chemicals, mining products, by-products of fossil-fuel combustion and energy production, metals, oxides of sulfur, nitrogen, heat, and radioactive isotopes). Chemical wastes should be viewed as major environmental and human problems unless properly controlled, but should be seen as supplements to other wastes, runoff from agriculture, and the natural processes that have polluted the environment for many centuries. This is especially obvious in a river basin where the landscape is dotted with reminders of Roman and Middle Ages civilizations, as well as large numbers and types of barges and boats carrying chemicals, petroleum, and petrochemicals, dry cargo, and other varied commodities in large amounts, to say nothing of the extensive agricultural activity, including vineyards and other crops.

TABLE 23.1. Comparison of Loading (Pollution) Parameters of Some Rivers

River and Population Density (Inhabitants/km^2)	Inhabitants per Runoff (per m^3 sec. $^{-1}$)	Gross National Product for Unit Flow ($/m^3)
Rhine (140)	15,000	3.4
Danube (83)	10,400	1.1
Ohio (76)	5,800	1.3
Mississippi (19)	3,300	0.75
All world's rivers (27)	3,000	0.15
All U.S. rivers (28)	4,200	1.0
All European rivers (66)	6,500	—

Source: W. Stumm and J. J. Morgan, *Aquatic Chemistry,* 2nd ed., p. 692, Wiley-Interscience, New York, 1981.

On October 28, 1986, the Sandoz facility at Schweizerhalle (near Basel on the Rhine) was routinely inspected by fire-prevention expert Hans Waeckerlig. He found that everything was in order, including warehouse 956. On October 31, between 10.08 and 10.11 p.m., the security officer on duty completed one of his rounds in the warehouse without having found anything unusual to report.

On November 1, at 00.19 hours, the fire alarm was raised almost simultaneously by a police patrol and Sandoz safety personnel. Warehouse 956 was already ablaze and the fire had spread so rapidly that the 10 fire brigades with 160 men were able to do little more than ensure that it did not engulf neighboring buildings. Their attempts to extinguish the fire with foam were ineffective and water had to be used. The volume required proved too great for the capacity of the catch basins, or bund; as a result, several hundred thousand liters of this water drained into the nearby Rhine. Unfortunately, it was by then contaminated by the chemical and agrochemical substances that had been stored in the warehouse. No lives were lost, but these relatively few minutes saw the start of a major catastrophe with tragic consequences for the environment.

Warehouse 956, which was 295 by 164 feet in size, was built in 1968. It was originally used to store plant and equipment, but in 1979, after inspection by competent authorities, was approved for the storage of chemicals and agrochemicals with a fire point in excess of 21°C. At the time of the fire, it contained approximately 1000 metric tons of agrochemical products and 300 tons of formulation auxiliaries and other chemicals. These were of varying degrees of toxicity and were responsible for killing large numbers of fish in the Rhine. The most lethal substances involved were mercury compounds. The warehouse was equipped with the proper fire-prevention aids, such as hand-held and larger extinguishers, water hydrants, and fire-detection devices and alarm systems.

(The foregoing description of the chronolgy of events and of warehouse 956 was presented at a Sandoz press conference on November 21, 1986, in Basel.)

National and international authorities (Basel is at the junction of France, Germany, and Switzerland) took steps to monitor the effect of the fire on the air, the river, and the groundwater. With regard to harmful effects on human beings, the investigators and examinations performed in the weeks after the accident failed to reveal any cases of even the lowest grade of intoxication among either the firefighting personnel or the general population. Three reports published subsequently, including one by the Federal Office of Health (May 1987), have excluded the likelihood of long-term effects on the health of the local population.

As far as the Rhine is concerned, both its fauna and its flora have suffered over a length of about 250 kilometers (155 miles). On the other hand, the river's microbiota (i.e., its microscopic flora and funda) appears to have remained sufficiently intact to maintain its selfcleaning capacity, although it could be years before the water regains its prefire status. The values for noxious substances in the river are currently not elevated and the restrictions imposed on use of the water have now been lifted. Groundwater contamination was localized and only slight, and no further damage is expected on the basis of what is known about the hydrogeological conditions.

Nineteen of the products stored in the warehouse were agrochemicals. The total amount of chemicals stored was 1351 metric tons (1 metric ton equals 2200 pounds), of which 987 tons were agro products and 364 tons were formulation auxiliaries and other chemicals. At a press conference on November 21, 1986, Sandoz itemized these, with the amounts stored as of that date.

Organophosphates/insecticides, 859 tons stored: The various active substances, of moderate to high toxicity, are noncarcinogenic and nontetraogenic. Organophosphates are chemically and biologically degradable. They do not become concentrated at any point in the food chain. They are toxic to fish. In agricultural practice, they are applied in amounts of 200–500 g/ha as insecticides. They are registered and used on a worldwide basis.

Urea Derivative Metoxuron; 12 tons stored: The active substance is virtually nontoxic, is nontoxic to fish, and is biologically as well as chemically degradable. In agricultural practice, the product is applied in amounts of 2–4 kg/ha for weed control. It is also used worldwide.

Nitrocresol Derivative DNOC/Herbicide, 73 tons stored: the active substance is toxic, and is toxic to fish. It is degradable. It is used for weed control in amounts of approximately 10 1/ha on a worldwide basis.

Oxazolidin fungicide, 26 tons stored: The active substance is of low toxicity and is nontoxic to fish. It is biologically and chemically degradable. Concentration in the food chain does not occur. It is used for repeated application in amounts of 200 g/ha. It is used worldwide.

Organic Mercury Compounds, 11 tons stored: Aqueous concentrations of ethoxyethyl mercury hydroxide and phenyl mercury acetate. This corresponds to 2.6 tons of mercury. These substances are highly toxic. Sandoz has since discontinued the production of pesticides containing mercury. Other agrochemicals (active substances):

1.9 tons endosulfan
180 kg tetradifon
158 kg captafol
720 kg zineb
30 kg scillirosid
13 kg zinc phosphide
(These compounds are of low to high toxicity and of varying degradability.)
Diluents, Adjuvants, Other Chemicals, 364 tons: these are relatively nontoxic and of varying degradability.

The cleanup work at the site of the fire was completed on January 22, 1987. The debris of the fire, packed into about 250 truck dump bodies, 17 railway cars, and over 6000 drums, was stored in intermediate facilities located within the Sandoz works at Schweizerhalle. Adequate disposal possibilities were sought, depending on the type of material (wood, steel, contruction debris, chemical waste) and degree of its contamination. Once the necessary permission of the authorities was received, complete disposal of all these materials required several months.

According to the findings of an initial inventory of the Ecosystem Rhine of the Swiss Federal Institute for Water Resources and Water Pollution Control (EAWAG), the microbiology of the Rhine has remained to the extent that bacterial self-cleansing of the river is possible.

After the removal of the toxic substances deposited on the bed of the Rhine down river from the outlet at Schweizerhalle, which has completed on December 19, 1986, a partial restoration of life in the river with invertebrate animals may be expected early this year. This would create the conditions for restocking the Rhine with fish.

Although no indications of a long-term danger to the health of the general population are known so far, the question of health is being pursued further. The so-called filter project also is part of this study, that is, chemical-analytical and toxicological analyses are being made of the residue obtained from protective mask filters and filters of air-conditioning units.

Thus far, 460 claims for damages have been presented, and approximately two-thirds of these have been settled.

Of paramount consideration is the prevention of future fires. To achieve this, better protection of the plant facility from the outside and reduction of potential hazards inside are the stated objectives. The surveillance of the area and its plant has been generally strengthened, particularly at night and over the weekend, including patrols of all warehouses every two hours; fences have been strengthened and made more secure; and a floodlighting system has been installed along the edge of the wood adjoining the plant.

The potential hazards have been reduced by reducing the quantities stored; the maximum quantity permitted per warehouse bay has been reduced by a factor of as much as four, and stocks of agrochemicals will be cut by a third. In addition, a more detailed classification of materials has been developed to ensure that no 'incompatible' or reactive materials are stored together. The former criteria used only four classes, namely, fire promoting, inflammable, explosive, and water sensitive; the new system will use 10 categories for separation of materials.

Two substances are no longer used in the manufacturing processes at the plant, mercury and phosgene. Dyestuffs have been reviewed according to the criteria of risk, toxicity, ecology, hygiene, and cost-effectiveness, and the production of about 100 dyestuffs has been discontinued.

The range of agrochemicals is also being reviewed according to their usefulness to agriculture, toxicity, combustibility, and cost-effectiveness, and the production of pesticides and insecticides at the Schweizerhalle works has been reduced by more than 60 percent.

The attempts to minimize or eliminate future fire damage have been studied in the context of shortening intervention time (using an improved alarm system), automatic fire alarms, and additional use of sprinklers where indicated. Fire-fighting water will be prevented from entering the Rhine by a more adequate water-retention system. A provisional system incorporates two tanks having a total capacity of 15,000 cubic meters (3.9 million gallons). The definitive system will include two catch basins of 15,000 and 2500 cubic meters respectively.

The warehouse inventory is kept up to date, and every week, on Thursday night, updated stock lists are printed out for all warehouses and immediately sent to the fire department, the safety service, and the warehouse management from Sandoz's mainframe computer.

To restore the fish and related aquatic life in the Rhine, Sandoz is working with the fishing interests on the Upper Rhine to develop a restocking hatchery for young fish (Rhine trout), and with the Baden-Wurttemberg on its eel-restocking project.

In addition to discovering the necessity of following in great detail every chemical from the "cradle to grave" (purchasing to ultimate disposal), the lesson that a warehouse can be a major hazard, often overlooked by regulatory and safety personnel in favor of the dynamics of material handling, processing, and packaging, to say nothing of hazardous-materials transport, is worthy of note by all who use or handle chemicals. In addition, at the annual general meeting of shareholders on May 5, 1987, Dr. Marc Moret, chair of the board and chief executive officer of Sandoz, introduced some philosophical perspective that could be useful:

> When men's best-laid schemes are thwarted by tragic events, questions as to how and why are generally in vain, because there are no answers. Nevertheless, I feel it is appropriate that I should offer this particular audience some thoughts on the subject of Schweizerhalle, six months after.
>
> The tremendous pace of technological progress in recent years has made considerable demands on the ability of our generation to adapt. We have had to come to terms with a new world, we have learned to think in new concepts. All this, as little as 40 years ago, seemed to lie several centuries ahead. In the process we have rediscovered what it means to be afraid. We all claim to be in favor of progress, but sometimes the worrying question nags us, whether things have not in fact gone too far. Like a child seeing piles of presents under the Christmas tree, we can't

help wondering whether all these things are really intended for us, whether we are really entitled to them. These and other questions suddenly surfaced as a result of the fire of 1 November 1986. Emotions were aroused which had to find release. Among the inhabitants of the area most directly affected, this took the form of anger at the awful stench and fear awakened by the wailing of sirens. And it is a well-known fact that when fear is great, the worst always seems more imminent than a turn for the better . . .

The most pressing of these problems at the moment, six months after the event, is the loss of confidence in the ability of the chemical industry in general and of Sandoz in particular to keep the risks inherent in its activities within limits which man and the environment can reasonably be expected to tolerate. Were we to have to operate in the future without the public's trusts, both parties would be permanently the poorer. The economy would also suffer and it is therefore both our duty and our desire to regain the trust we have lost . . .

In seeking to achieve the objective of restoration of confidence, there is little to be gained by railing against progress in general and "chemistry" in particular. The solution lies in greater responsibility in exploiting the potential of chemistry. By this I mean first and foremost the more rapid development of products and protection processes which have less impact on the environment. I say more rapid development to emphasize the fact that this is not something completely new. It is simply that we have intensified our efforts and tightened up our guidelines since "Schweizerhalle." Standards have become more rigorous and our decision-making now has a prominent ethical component. More than ever before we shall weigh up the pros and cons as between benefits and potential dangers, and if necessary, ignore purely economic considerations. This applies to all levels of our operations and has already resulted in the dropping of certain products and the discontinuation of research in certain areas. In the future only chemical compounds which give absolutely no cause for concern as regards toxicity and mutagenicity will stand any chance of further development, regardless of how original they might be. The same applies to that other major hurdle in the product development process, the method of manufacture. If safety problems cannot be satisfactorily solved, projects will be abandoned even at this stage.

Our commitment to more "responsible" chemistry is also reflected in the orientation of our research. As you know, we are very much involved in the development of biological insecticides and currently occupy a leading position in this field. This involvement began as long ago as the seventies and has been maintained in spite of slow market acceptance. Also, within the framework of integrated crop protection, our seed research teams have been developing disease- and pest-resistant strains which require little or no chemical treatment. Our pharmaceutical research effort is also playing its part by developing drugs with a more favorable benefit/adverse effect relation . . .

We are not simply flirting with actions which are in practice superficial and cosmetic in order to win back the trust I mentioned earlier. We are setting ourselves measurably higher professional, technological and commercial standards, and we are doing so in the knowledge that we can count on the unreserved support of more than 42,000 Sandoz employees throughout the world. This will ensure perpetuation of the proud tradition of Sandoz. The accident of Schweizerhalle has become a challenge for us all.

To summarize, the incident of November 1, 1986, has had far-reaching consequences, especially as it relates to rethinking the priorities and procedures of a major company. We know it was not "fatal" to the Rhine (this writer observed live fish of considerable size being pulled from the Rhine on May 1–4 in the vicinity of Basel). However, like Bhopal, Chernobyl, and Miamisburg, a new respect for the interaction between chemicals, people, and the environment has been raised, and, like Creation itself, will, it is hoped, be more completely understood with the passage of time, and perhaps meditation. One example of the American attempt is reflected by the regulation of discharge of 63 chemicals (see Appendix E).

REFERENCES

1. C. B. Patterson, "A Walk and Ride on the Wild Side," *Nat'l Geographic Mag.*, **163**, No. 5, 676–693 (May 1983).
2. Personal conversations with Prof. W. Stumm at the EAWAC (Swiss Federal Institute for Water Resources and Water Pollution Control), Dubendorf, Switzerland (near Zurich); also W. Stumm and J. J. Morgan, *Aquatic Chemistry, An Introduction Emphasizing Chemical Equilibria in Natural Waters,* 2nd ed., Wiley/Interscience, New York, 1981; W. Stumm, R. Schwarzenbach, and L. Sigg, "From Environmental Analytical Chemistry to Ecotoxicology—A Plea for More Concepts and Less Monitoring and Testing," *Angew. Chem. Int. Ed. Engl.* **22**, 380–389 (1983).

SUGGESTED READING

Erster Zwischenbericht an die Regierung Des Katons Basel-Landschaft uber Bestandesaufnahme, Oekologische Beurteilung, Empfohlene Massnahmen and Absichten Fuer Weiter Unterschungen Nach Dem Schadenfall Sandoz, Auftrag Nr. 4727, Berichtsperiode 12, November bis 12, Dezember 1986, Eidgenossische Technischne Hoch-Schulen, EAWAG, Dubendorf, Dez. 12, 1986, 70 pp. with additions and photos (German).

Hazardous Materials Spill Conference: Preparedness, Prevention, Control and Cleanup of Releases, May 5–8, 1986, St. Louis, Mo., 565 pp., Government Institutes, Inc., 966 Hungerford Drive, #24, Rockville, MD 20850.

R. Helmer, "Approaches to Hazardous Wastes Management," 15 pp., World Health Organization, Room L-120, CH-1211, Geneva 27, Switzerland; See also New Books, Environmental Engineering, World Health Organization, and Pollution and Health, International Collaboration in Monitoring, 22 pp., 1986.

P. L. Layman, "Rhine Spills Force Rethinking of Potential for Chemical Pollution," *Chem. Evg. News,* 7–11 (Feb. 23, 1987).

S. O. Rohmann and N. Lilienthal, *Tracing A River's Toxic Pollution,* 209 pp., Inform, 381 Park Avenue South, New York, 1987.

Sandoz, Press Office material, "Corporate Affairs and Business Economics," Basel, Switzerland, 1987.

I. M. Suffet and M. Malaiyandi, *Organic Pollutants in Water: Sampling, Analysis, and Toxicity Testing,* Advances in Chemistry Series 214, 797 pp., American Chemical Society, Washington, D.C., 1987.

24

The Design of Safe Means for Transport of Dangerous Goods: An Underdeveloped Area?

J. C. Astro and J. van der Schaaf

The transport of dangerous goods is regulated in order to prevent, as far as possible, loss of life or injury to persons, loss of or damage to the means of transport or property surrounding the means of transport, or contamination of the environment. The main outline of regulation should be to restrain as much as possible specific risks connected to the handling and transport of dangerous goods. Primarily, regulation is a matter of safety and protection. International uniform regulation serves also to facilitate international and intermodal transport.

The scope of this chapter is to make a plea for taking the safety of the transport process of dangerous goods as an integral system, or, in other words, to give full consideration to the safety of the total chain of activities from filling to discharging. This means the safety of filling and discharging of packages, tanks, etc.; the loading and unloading of these packages, tanks, etc., on or off the means of transport; and the different modes under normal and accidental conditions that might appear during transport, including the possible effect on the environment. There is a need for such an approach because of the diversity of regulations, for instance, concerning filling and discharging and for operation and handling of such means of transport, and the international regulations governing the various modes of transport.

For example, in general no requirements are given for safe loading and unloading of dangerous goods in the IMDG Code; this is left to the national governments. But

---

The views expressed in this chapter are those of the authors and do not necessarily represent the official view of the Ministry of Transport and Public Works, The Netherlands.

it may be clear that, for example, facilities on tanks for dangerous goods for tie-down and for safe loading and unloading on or from a vessel are part of one general safety concept. There also is the need to deal with the safety of activities that have to be undertaken to cope with accidental situations such as fire or collision.

The safety of all the parts of the transport process should be integrated in one design concept. Therefore, the starting points for design have to be formulated. Of course, a lot of experience is already incorporated in the existing means of transport, and also stringent requirements concerning the safe transport of dangerous goods are in practice. But the idea to consider an overall safety concept has not been elaborated into an equivalent level in all modes.

This chapter can give a start to an exchange of views about the safety of means of transport for dangerous goods in all possible situations. First of all, starting points for design or a program of standards have to be formulated. To demonstrate the preferable approach for a safe means of transport, it is the authors' opinion that these starting points for design are to be set on the basis of a risk analysis of all the risks involved in the entire chain, from filling with a dangerous substance, and the process of handling, operation, and transport, even in accidental situations, up to discharging.

At this stage, some explanatory remarks are in order.

Starting points for a safe design have to be based on a systematic approach to all possible situations that might occur with the means of transport. Thus, starting points for design are the basis for design criteria. Design criteria describe the practical design and its plan of execution. They are set out in recommendations, regulations, or technical codes. They can be given as, for example, a set of performance tests representative of normal or deviating from normal conditions of transport (see packagings and IBCs) or as a set of design requirements (see tank containers). The latter show their value in practice and are adapted on the basis of experience. For instance, the requirements for seagoing vessels for bulk cargoes of dangerous goods are already stringent (see the Bulk Chemical Code and the Gas Carrier Code), but they only consider the design of the vessel, and as far as the vessel is concerned, safety during filling or discharging. This seems to be practical, but is it enough? There also are design criteria for systems to be used for signaling, alarms, and fire extinguishing, as well as a system for inspection and certification. These items guarantee a certain level of safety.

To handle a dangerous substance, it has to be locked in a package or tank, or the like. The word "confinement" will be used as a general concept of separating the goods from the surroundings.

AN EXAMPLE OF AN APPROACH

Chemical plants are designed after a thorough process development from laboratory scale (Figure 24.1) via pilot plant (Figure 24.2) to definite plant (Figure 24.3). Design criteria for such a plant are based on process conditions varying between

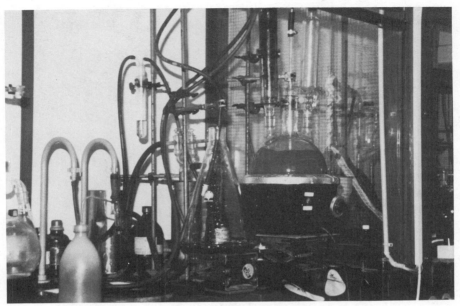

Figure 24.1. Chemical product development at laboratory scale.

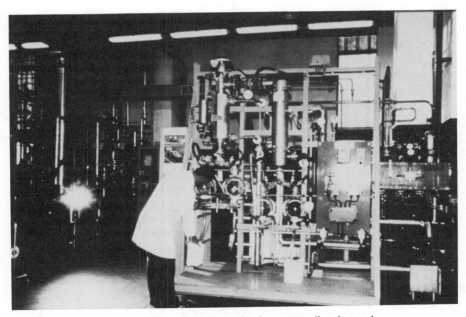

Figure 24.2. Product and process development at pilot-plant scale.

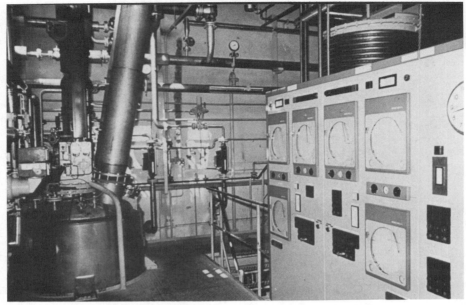

Figure 24.3. Production at full-plant scale.

certain limits. These conditions are considered optimal. Situations such as starting-up or shutdown procedures are situations deviating from the normal, but are still acceptable situations. In a risk-assessment study, conditions deviating from the normal are being recognized (such as internal high pressure, high or extreme temperatures) and their consequences are being studied. Also, such extreme situations as an external fire are taken into account. All these considerations lead to a safe design concept.

The means for transporting dangerous goods up until the present were not based on a total-safety design concept. Roughly, a tank is placed in or on a means of transport. In that case, no systematic analysis is made of the functions that have to be performed in all circumstances as a integrated safety system. The dynamic aspects of the transport process and situations deviating from normal transport conditions, (e.g., possibilities for safe recovery after a turnover of a tank car) are not considered. Therefore, an enumeration will be given of the factors that have to be taken into account in the design of a totally safe means of transport. The design of the confinement is determined by the properties of the substance. The means of transport and confinement have to be integrated in such a way that consideration is given to the dynamic situations during transport and possible (traffic) accidents (see Figures 24.4, 24.5, and 24.6). Up until now, this has only been done based on practical deliberations or experiences.

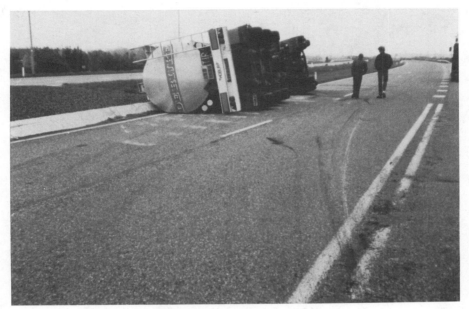

Figure 24.4. Road tank vehicle on its side.

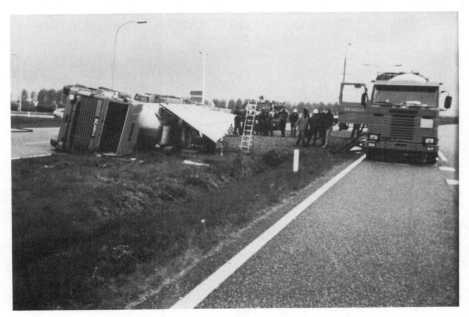

Figure 24.5. Discharging of the tank as much as possible.

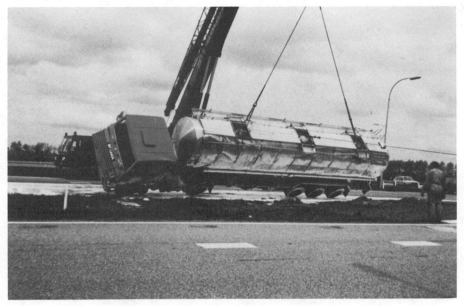

Figure 24.6. Hoisting of the road tank combination on its tank covers tie bolts, for which they are not designed.

ANALYSIS OF THE TRANSSHIPMENT AND THE TRANSPORT PROCESS

An approach similar to that taken for chemical plants has a more principled nature. As a matter of course, the regulations contain safety requirements, but there are remarkable differences in the level of elaboration in the different modes.

This chapter will give the principal approach to the problem of the safe transport and handling of dangerous goods. While doing this, one comes across items that already have been covered in one mode of transport but not in others. In the following paragraphs, subjects are not fully elaborated upon, but examples are given to illustrate the approach.

For the application of a confinement for transport, consideration has to be given to:

The specific properties of the dangerous substance(s)

The typical characteristics of the mode(s) of transport

Operation and handling with the confinement; filling and discharging of the substance

The most important phases in the transhipment process are shown in Figure 24.7.

For each part of the transhipment and the transport process, consideration must be given to safety through:

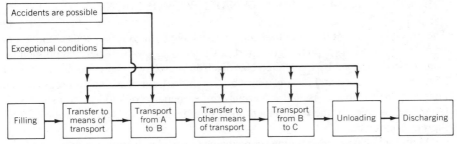

Figure 24.7. Review of the transshipment and transport process.

Construction and operational requirements offering a level of safety under normal conditions

Constructional and safety requirements to cope with operational or transport conditions that deviate from the normal conditions

Additional constructional requirements to cope with extreme situations due to conditions appearing in the vicinity or to accidents

The summing up of basic points of consideration is not exhaustive. The multimodal tank container is the most elaborate example of the advocated approach. The investigatory nature of this chapter leads to a superficial treatment of items. A complete risk analysis for each mode of transport pinpoints weak spots in the design of a means of transport, particularly in accident situations.

While developing starting points for design, we also have to consider combinations of means of transport; that is, the carrying of road and rail vehicles on seagoing vessels and of tractor-trailers on railroad cars ("piggy-back"). This combined transport makes additional requirements necessary to the confinement-carrying vehicle.

An example of the adaptation of vehicles as meant here has been given by Capt. G. T. H. Nicol.[1] The vehicle or container has to be adapted to the specific risks of the other means of transport. Therefore, we have to consider possible combinations of modes of transport that are important when starting points of design for the container and the transport unit have to be set. (See Figure 24.8.)

Mode of Transport	Packagings and IBC's	Tank Containers	Bulk Transport	Ro-Ro	"Piggy-back"
sea	x	x	x	x x	
inland waterways	x	x	x		
rail	x	x	x	x	x
road	x	x	x	x	x
air	x				

Figure 24.8. Means for transport of dangerous goods and practical combinations thereof.

THE REGULATORY BASIS FOR SAFETY PROVISIONS

The provisions for multimodal transport of (packaged) dangerous goods are given in the "Recommendations on the Transport of Dangerous Goods.[2] These recommendations were developed by the United Nations Committee of Experts on the Transport of Dangerous Goods and its subsidiary bodies in the light of technical progress, the advent of new substances and materials, the exigencies of modern transport systems, and, above all, the requirement to ensure the safety of people, property, and the environment.

Applying the recommendations contributes to worldwide harominization of regulations. On the one hand, the recommendations provide a basic scheme when revising or developing regulations in which all particularities of the modes are dealt with in a uniform fashion. On the other hand, they are flexible enough to be brought into correspondence with special requirements of a certain mode of transport; as in air transport, where more stringent requirements may apply.

From the nature of the recommendations, it is obvious that they recommend provisions to be adopted by the regulatory bodies for the different modes of transport. The specific requirements are given in the respective regulations for each mode and/or by governmental bodies. The regulatory international bodies for each mode of transport in Europe are shown in Figure 24.9.

It may be evident that the provisions for packaging, IBCs, and tank containers should be multimodal, and they should give consideration to the particular requirements of each mode of transport.

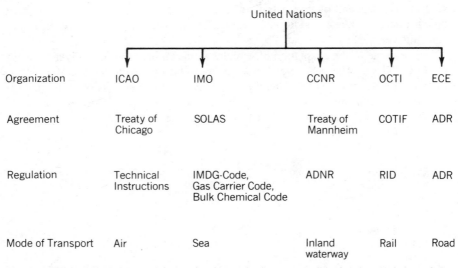

United Nations				
Organization				
ICAO	IMO	CCNR	OCTI	ECE
Agreement				
Treaty of Chicago	SOLAS	Treaty of Mannheim	COTIF	ADR
Regulation				
Technical Instructions	IMDG-Code, Gas Carrier Code, Bulk Chemical Code	ADNR	RID	ADR
Mode of Transport				
Air	Sea	Inland waterway	Rail	Road

Figure 24.9. United Nations and international organizations responsible for the regulation of the transport of dangerous goods.

THE ORIGIN OF DANGERS IN DANGEROUS GOODS

Dangerous goods are classified in nine classes and their respective divisions. Appendix 24.1 covers the nature of the dangers, the conditions according to which these substances can be accepted for transport, and the possibilities and means for handling the dangerous properties in a controlled manner.

Dangerous goods have to be offered for transport in an appropriate container. During handling and transport, the substance in its confinement can be exposed to conditions that can lead to loss of confinement. To cope with these situations, emergency or contingency plans are to be developed. For sea transport, this already has been done.

WHAT ARE CONSIDERED "NORMAL CONDITIONS OF TRANSPORT"?

During transport, packages or means of transport are subjected to so-called normal conditions of transport, operation, and handling activities, but also to conditions deviating from the normal, and even accident situations. In the aforementioned recommendations, the following climatological and physical transport conditions can be recognized:

Temperatures from - 40°C to 55 or 65°C

Radiation from the sun (e.g., ultraviolet-radiation resistance as prescribed for plastics material)

Relative humidity (e.g., for testing paper bags, 65 percent at 20°C)

Impacts liable to occur during transport or handling

Vibrations related to the modes of transport

Electromagnetic radiation at all relevant frequencies (maximum intensity 100 W/m.^{2})

Static electricity.

Examples of specific normal conditions in the various modes of transport are:

Air: In general, packagings can be subjected to a reduction of pressure of 68 kPa. Venting devices on packages are prohibited; there are limited possibilites for the crew to act when leakage occurs. Vibration has to be taken into account. Accelerations up to 8 *g* are possible (*g* = constant of gravitation).

Sea: The marine environment makes it necessary to pay special attention to corrosion in general. Special care has to be given to aluminum as a construction material because of its behavior in fires and its corrosion sensitivity. Also, the crew of a vessel has limited possibilities to handle problems with dangerous goods. They have to be dealt with independently; that is, without help from elsewhere.

Rail: Accelerations of 4 g; for tank containers, 2 g are acceptable due to the fact that tank-container-carrying cars (wagons) are equipped with a hydraulic system to suppress the effect of the acceleration.

Road: Accelerations of 2 g.

As provisions for normal operating conditions, one can consider:

The properties of the product(s) to be transported (this has consequences for the choice of materials for construction and for equipment such as valves, measuring equipment, insulation, temperature conditioning, bottom openings, etc.).

Provisions for safe filling and discharging (e.g., filling temperature and discharging by gravity, pumping, or under gas pressure).

The lifting and tie-down attachments for horizontal or vertical movements.

Normal conditions during transport (e.g., accelerations, vibrations, sloops).

As operational conditions deviating form normal conditions, one has to deal with:

Minimum/maximum temperature during filling or discharging.

Minimum/maximum pressure (dependent on possible bulk temperatures, overfilling).

Situations deviating from the normal transport conditions, such as an extreme deceleration in a collision, a heavy swell, glazed frost (blockage of safety devices), and tropical conditions.

Conditions during transport, that are usually not considered normal can be recognized:

Accident situations such as collision and/or turnover (e.g., a road tank vehicle on it side or upside down)

Complete fire engulfment

Being flooded

Being hit by projectiles, falling objects, or lightning

As a matter of fact, experiences with means of confinement and means of transport for dangerous goods have led to provisions to avoid as much as possible the loss of confinement caused by accidents. This so-called "accident resistance" of a package, a tank, or a means of transport is introduced in the recommendations as practicable measures of a preventive nature. A systematic analysis of the risks involved in handling, operation, and transport can improve the accident resistancy of means of transport that are to be developed in the future.

Handling and operating activities are as a matter of course part of the normal transport process. Therefore, there are several requirements concerning these activities that have to be incorporated into the principal design, as well as measuring equipment to control the condition of the contents of a container during transport or to avoid overfilling (including signaling and/or alarm devices).

Safe filling and discharging are also of concern with regard to chemical plant safety. Therefore, provisions as to the means of transport and those in the chemical plant should be attuned to each other.

DEVELOPMENT OF STARTING POINTS FOR DESIGN

The above-mentioned items have addressed some starting points for design and provisions for safe transport. Having indicated the nature of the dangers of the goods itself, the particularities of the modes of transport, and the possibilities of accidents, it has to be shown what the consequences of this all might be and these consequences formulated as starting points for the design of packaging and IBCs, tank containers, and means of transport.

This can be done along two lines:

Using existing provisions, for example, for packaging, tank containers, and means of transport

Via lessons learned from risk-analysis studies.

For packagings in the past, design criteria were given. These have proved confusing and less practicable because of possible differences in interpretation of the provisions.

Packaging and IBCs for dangerous goods now are subjected to performance tests as given in Chapters 9 and 16 of the recommendations. UN design-type tested packaging has met a performance standard. Packaging made according to the type tested is considered to be ble to withstand normal conditions of transport, and even some incidents. Some design criteria for packaging are listed in Appendix 24.2.

Packages can be stowed on a pallet and provided with a strong covering or can be overpacked in a freight container. A freight container gives packaged goods and IBCs additional protection in accident situations, such as when a steel container is completely engulfed by fire. But the stowing together of packaged thermal sensitive goods has a disadvantage, as pointed out by Perbal, and colleagues.[3] Because regular means of packaging only withstand normal conditions of transport, it is necessary to prescribe pressure vessels for some substances.

For tank containers, starting points for design are given in a general form in Appendix 24.3. They originate from IMO. The text as given is based on the afore-mentioned recommendations. Tank containers are built to a design in which considerable concern is dedicated to safety. Two items are worth special attention.

The tank and the frame of tank containers should be capable of withstanding the most severe combination of static and dynamic stresses in handling and transport conditions (see Figures 24.10 and 24.11). This means that tank containers and their fastenings should be capable of withstanding the following separately applied forces based on:

1. Twice the total mass acting in the direction of travel of the tank simultaneous with the weight of the tank.

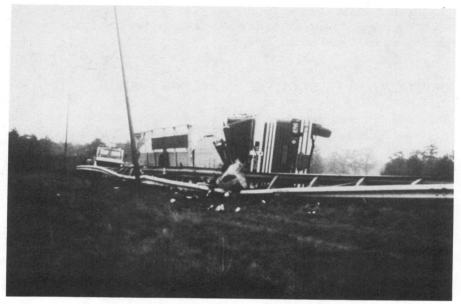

Figure 24.10. Tank container transport vehicle in the crash barrier.

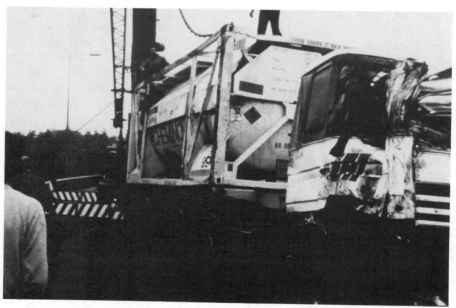

Figure 24.11. The tank container transport unit hoisted back on its wheels on the fastenings of the container.

2. The total mass acting horizontally at right angles to the direction of travel of the tank (where the direction of travel is not clearly determined, twice the total mass should be used) with the weight of the tank.

3. The total mass acting vertically upwards.

4. Twice the total mass acting vertically downward.

Under each of these loads, the safety factors to be observed should be as follows:

1. For metals having a clearly defined yield point, a safety factor of 1.5 in relation to the determined yield stress.

2. For metals with no clearly defined yield point, a safety factor of 1.5 in relation to the guaranteed 0.2 percent proof stress (1.0 percent proof stress for austenitic steels).

These forces and the safety factor are considered necessary to guarantee a level of safety during normal conditions of transport and handling of the tank container.

Also, the provisions for multimodal tank containers deal with conditions deviating from normal, that is, extreme conditions during transport. In the following, some (existing and not yet existing) provisions will be given, because these items clearly have everything to do with a certain built-in accident resistance.

As a design criterion to cope with accidental situations, it is required that tank containers be adequately protected against lateral and longitudinal impact and against overturning. If the tanks and the service equipment are so constructed as to withstand impact or overturning, they need not be protected in this way.

Examples of protection of shells against collision:

Protection against lateral impact may consist, for example, of longitudinal bars protecting the tank on both sides at the level of the median line.

Protection of tank containers against overturning may consist, for example, of reinforcement rings or bars fixed across the frame.

Protection against rear impact may consist of a bumper or frame.

External fittings should be designed or protected so as to preclude the release of contents upon impact or overturning of the tank upon the fittings. (Blokker and Kooyman[4] show the value of such a provision in case the accident resistance of a tank container is tested. A similar property is highlighted by Schulz-Forberg[5] for chlorine tanks).

A tank container can be subjected to an accident in which it lands on its side or upside down. In these situations, no loss of contents may occur, so release valve settings should be set at least at the level of the hydraulic pressure. It may be necessary to unload the tank. This has to be done in a safe manner and provisions have to be made to achieve this.

A tank container can be provided with thermal insulation in order to maintain a certain temperature of the contents. Insulation can also be applied in order to avoid nearly immediate unwanted physical effects from the contents of the tank container in a complete fire and to gain time for fire-fighting action. For tank containers for peroxides, for example, there is the provision that, even after an accidental failure of 1 percent of the insulation, during a period of one hour of complete fire engulfment [i.e., a heat load for design of 10.9 W/cm^2 (2.60 gcal/cm^2 · sec = 34.500 Btu/sq. ft. hr.),] no dangerous effects can occur.

For a means of transport, provisions for transport and handling can be given in the same way as for tank containers. For the sea mode, the idea of provisions to guarantee a level of accident resistance is, for example, given in the Gas Carrier Code. For vessels carrying liquefied gases in bulk, conditions that deviate from the normal and extreme situations were taken into account when developing the code. This was done in order to minimize the risk to the vessel, its crew, and the environment with regard to the nature of the products involved.

The code recognizes that severe collisions or stranding could lead to cargo tank damage, resulting in the uncontrolled release of the product. The requirements in the Gas Carrier Code are intended to minimize this risk of release, evaporation, and dispersion of the product, and to minimize the possibility of losing the integrity of the vessel, for instance, by brittle fracture of the ship's hull.

The code not only deals with ship design and equipment, but takes the whole transport system into account (training, operational procedures, etc.), including safe filling and discharging of the tanks. This, among other things, is done to cope with extreme situations by:

> Requirements for protection from damage in the case of collision or stranding by locating the tanks at specified minimum distances inboard from the ship's shell plating.
>
> Survival requirements in case of the flooding of the ship.
>
> Tank supports that are able to withstand a certain collision force acting on the tank.
>
> In principle, not to use materials with a melting point below 925°C for piping outside the cargo tank (because of possible external fire).
>
> The requirement that when a cargo pump is not accessible for repair with the tanks in service, two independent means to transfer cargo from each cargo tank should be provided.
>
> Requirements to override the normal pressure-relieving system in fire conditions (98–104°C).
>
> Requirements for fire protection and fire extinguishing.
>
> Requirements for personnel protection against the effects of a "major cargo release."

THE BENEFIT OF RISK ANALYSIS

For road tank vehicles, rail tank cars (wagons) and inland waterway tankers, the executed designs still show the traces of the concept of putting a tank on or in a means of transport. The results of such a concept and, in particular, the level of accident resistance of these means of transport, become evident when risk-analysis studies are executed.

Studies on the risk of liquefied petroleum gas (LPG) have evinced the following items, which are useful as examples of starting points for design. This summing up of possible preventive measures is not exhaustive but is illustrative of the approach to be followed.

For LPG-road tank vehicles, the following starting points for design are recognized:

There are no adequate safe means built into the piping system to empty the tank vehicle in case of overturning.

The piping should not be placed at the rear end of the truck but at the side or be completely protected. The rear end is vulnerable to head-tail collisions.

The tank should be equipped with internal valves to be closed in case of emergency shutdown of the plant where the tanks are filled or discharged.

Relief valves should not be placed at the top of the front end of the tank, which is the first place to be hit while passing under bridges, etc.

It is important to protect the tank against heat from fuel tanks or tires that catch fire, and also against heat from the exhaust system (by thermal insulation or shielding).

The use of material in constructing the tank that do not take into account the ability to withstand mechanical impact can lead to tanks of high-tensile-strength materials with relatively thin walls, strong enough for the loads during normal transport conditions but with little survival capability against external loads resulting from accidents.

When a road tank vehicle or rail tank car (wagon), as well as a tank container, falls on its side, it is necessary to bring it to an upright position. Therefore, it is necessary to equip these means of transport with hoisting facilities strong enough to hoist the whole transport unit even when the tank is loaded.

From risk analysis and accidents with rail tank cars (wagons) it has been learned that:

The central couplings that are used in the United States can penetrate relatively easily into the adjacent rail tank car (wagon).

Without relief valves, the overfilling of rail tank cars (wagons) can lead to excessive rise of internal pressure and eventually to the failure of the tank.

Thermal insulation of a road tank vehicle or a rail tank car (wagon) diminishes the probability of a boiling-liquid expanding vapor cloud explosion in case of external heat input into the tank, particularly when the tank is not equipped with pressure-relief devices.

This also diminishes the probability of so-called domino effects when a train of more than one tank car is involved in an accident.

From risk analysis on inland waterway vessels, the following have been shown to be important.

To maintain a residual floating ability so that the vessel can be towed from populated areas or to a place that does not block the waterway.

To install the piping for cargo operations as close to the centerline of the ship as possible, as this is safest place in case of collision.

To apply internal valves or valves that are tightly connected to the strong tank domes, thus diminishing the probability of pipe rupture in case of a collision.

To minimize the possibility of the tank's being hit by parts of the ship's structure by removing sharp elements from the vicinity of the tank.

To maximize the possibility of energy absorption in case of a collision by, for instance, special hull construction (see Figure 24.12) or in the case of pressure vessels, preventing the possibility of a rapid penetration by a part of the ship's construction.

For combined transport on ships and road tank vehicles or railway tank cars (wagons) the specific requirements for the sea mode have to be incorporated into the design of the road vehicle or railway car (wagon).

The study by Captain Nicol[12] is a good example of this. This chapter deals with the forces in the lashings. The forces on the lashed object are another matter. But are these forces taken into account in the design of a road tank vehicle or a rail tank car (wagon)?

The same type of problem occurs when a road tank vehicle is put on a railway car (wagon). Is the road tanker secure enough for even accidental conditions such as derailments?

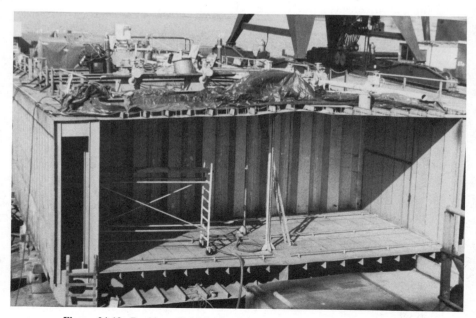

Figure 24.12. Double-walled inland waterway tanker with stainless-steel tank.

ARE SAFETY MEASURES WORTH CONSIDERATION?

In the transport of dangerous goods, valuable goods as well as valuable means of transport are involved. The tool of risk analysis has been developed to such an extent that a design of a new tank container, road tanker, rail tank car (wagon), inland waterway vessel, or seagoing ship can incorporate the latest preventive measures. By doing so, a higher standard of safety and protection of the environment can be achieved. The inclusion of preventive measures is a much better investment than spending money for recovery and cleaning up after an accident.

To illustrate that preventive measures are worthwhile, the following examples are given:

For the sea mode, aluminum is, in principle, only acceptable as a material of construction if it is insulated to prevent significant loss of physical properties when it is subjected to a heat load.

The design reference temperature for calculation of the maximum allowable working pressure for a nonrefrigerated, pressure liquifiable gas tank with a diameter of more than 1.5 meters is set at 60°C for a tank without insulation or sun shield; with a sun shield, it can be set at 55°C and with insulation at 50°C.

CONCLUDING REMARKS

Multimodal door-to-door transport of dangerous goods involves the consideration of an integral-safety concept with regard to the means for accomplishing this. From this chapter, the conclusion can be drawn that for the transport of dangerous goods by sea and air, a start on such a concept has been made; for transport by road, rail, and inland waterways, a lot of safety measures still can be introduced in the design concept, especially where Ro-Ro and "piggy-back" transport is concerned.

The concept of integral safety implies that items have to be considered that do not strictly concern the responsibility of the modes of transport. The authors are of the opinion that safety in filling and discharging, the transfer of the means of transport, safety in case of accident (i.e., prevention of leakage or spills or possible worsening of a situation during fire), and safety of repressive activities need to be integrated into the design concept of the means of transport, and consequently into the regulations for each mode. Transport of dangerous goods is involved, and therefore, they must also be included in the international transport regulations. There is also the "reciprocity" of requirements as far as RoRo and piggy-back transport is concerned. Requirements specific for the sea mode have to adapted to the road tank vehicle or the railway tank car (wagon). The same is true for a road tank vehicle to be transported on a railway car (wagon): the fastening has to be designed to account for the forces working on both means of transport.

From a more complete analysis, more fundamental questions will arise, such as: can a fire around a tank containing a substance that can release toxic gasses be extinguished safely, and is insulation necessary for tanks with these substances?

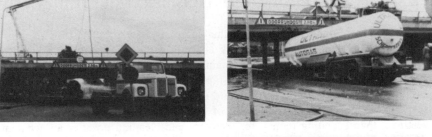

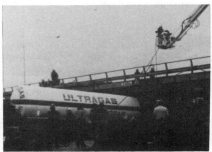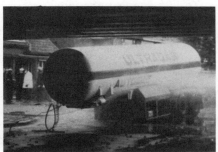

Figure 24.13. This LPG tank car was too high to pass under the bridge.

What is gained by a higher level of safety is the saving if valuable products, limitation of damage to goods and the environment, and greater safety and efficiency in all situations. Safety can save money. This chapter is intended to initiate a discussion on the merits of a integral-safety concept for means of transport of dangerous goods.

EPILOGUE

The authors have taken a more fundamental approach to the safe handling and transport of dangerous goods. However, even when the more principled approach is put into practice, there will be accidents because it is still a human being who makes errors or wrong judgments (see Figure 24.13) or is the source of an unwanted event or loss of confinement of a dangerous substance. We expect that the physical effects will be less dramatic when we can reach an equivalent level of safety for all modes and all means of transporting dangerous goods.

REFERENCES

1. *Recommendations on the Transport of Dangerous Goods,* 4th rev. ed., United Nations Publication, ST/SG/AC.10/1/Rev. 4. ISBN 92-1-139022-2.

2. G. T. H. Nicol, "Restraint of Vehicles, Containers and Unit Loads on Board Roll-on Roll-off Ships, the New Zealand Experience," *Proceedings, 7th International Symposium on the Transport of Dangerous Goods by Sea and Inland Waterways,* Vancouver, Sept. 27–30, 1982. vol. 1, pp. 219–235.

3. R. Perbal, A. H. Heemskerk, and Th. M. Groothuizen, "The Influence of Temperature Piling on the Self-ignition Behaviour of Unstable Substances During Transport in ISO Containers," *Proceedings, 9th International Symposium on the Transport of Dangerous Goods by Sea and Inland Waterways,* Rotterdam, April 13–17, 1987.

4. E. F. Blokker and W. P. Kooyman, "Safety Regulations for the Transhipment of Dangerous goods as General Cargo in the Port of Rotterdam," *Ibid.*

5. B. Schulz-Forberg, "Chlorine Tanks in Simulated Accidents," *Ibid.*

Appendix 24.1: Risks, Properties, and Means of Control of Dangerous Goods

Application of dangerous goods introduces the risk of:

Explosion with blast and/or projections (intense light or heat; loud noise)

Fire (heat radiation, smoke)

Exposure to radioactivity

Poisoning (oral, dermal, or by inhalation; affecting only human or animals)

Environmental effects

Whether a substance is dangerous or not is a matter of definition. The principles, starting points, and classification criteria are given in Ref. 1.

Some substances or articles are too dangerous to be transported because:

They have intrinsic properties that pose risk (e.g., excessively sensitive explosives, like some azides, or highly reactive substances, unless appropriately packed).

They cannot be accepted in the amount in which they are offered to be transported (e.g., for some organic peroxide formulations, specific packing is required or only packages containing not more than a certain net mass are accepted; also, bulk transport of aluminium borohydride is prohibited).

They are accepted for transport only with special authorization of a competent authority of a state with specific requirements (e.g., aqueous solutions with more than 20 percent hydrocyanic acid, perchloric acid in a concentration of more than 72 percent, or symmetrical-dichlorodimethylether, nitrogen trioxide, methyl-nitrite).

They can only be generally accepted under specific requirements as (proven) chemical stability (e.g., the addition of the word "inhibited" or "stabilized," or mercury can only be transported by air when packaging meets the Packing Group I requirements).

Remarks: Some substances are classified as dangerous for one mode only (e.g., for air—calcium oxide, copper chloride, and sodium aluminate; for sea transport—fish meal, stabilized). Also, some substances, when packaged in limited quantities can be exempted from regulation.

Substances' dangers can arise from their intrinsic properties or their physical state. Both factors are important in choosing the proper packaging.

Dangerous chemical properties of substances caused by inherent instability that can be set off by heat, (auto-)catalytic action, or contact with acids or heavy metal compounds, amine friction, or impact are:

Thermal sensitivity (exothermic instability)

Sensitivity to ignition

Sensitivity to mechanical stimuli

Polymerization (with evolution of heat)

Self-reactivity (e.g., alphatic azo compounds, aromatic sulphahydrazides, N-nitroso compounds, or diazonium salts and sponge blowing agents)

Exothermic decomposition

There are also compounds that contain one or more nondangerous constituents or small amounts of dangerous substances that on impact combine to react chemically (such as the safety device in the steering wheels of cars that consists of a bag blown up by gas envolved by chemical reaction or a device to make T-joints in a existing piping system).

Dangers arising from the physical state or property of the good or the packaging as offered for transportor:

Radioactivity (more than 70 kBq/kg)

High pressure (caused by vapor pressure or thermal liquid expansion)

High or low temperature

Exposed free area (e.g., amorphous state, particle size, precipitation on a carrier)

Crystallization

Separation of phases in mixtures, leading to dangerous concentrations

Electrostatic properties (see the need for grounding the confinement during filling or discharging of flammable liquids with a low flash point, powders liable to dust explosion)

Properties may become apparent when the substance comes into contact with the environment (oxygen, humidity, or water):

Pyrophoricity (e.g. aluminium alkyls, white phosphorus)

Self-heating properties (e.g., direct reduced iron, ferrous metal borings, shavings)

Emission of flammable vapors of gasses, including upon autoignition (e.g., ferrosilicon);

Emission of poisonous vapors or gases (e.g., chlorosilanes)

Fortunately, these dangerous properties can be controlled. Possible methods include the following.

1. The packing method:

   a. When test results prove that the substance as packaged for transport no longer possesses the dangerous property (e.g., methyl ethyl ketone peroxide with not more than 52 percent in solution with more than 10 percent oxygen; maximum contents of whole package 50 kg)

   b. Limitations of contents of packaging

   c. Specific or stringent requirements on packaging (e.g., venting devices for peroxy acetic acid—intermediate and outer packaging of rubber or rubberized textile bags filled with water and antifreeze agent is required for some explosive substances and even pressure vessels for methyl- and ethyl isocyanate)

   d. Maximum degree of filling at 55°C—95 percent or 98 percent

   e. Limited period of use for plastic packaging

   (For some peroxides, any extra confinement can introduce a significant risk of explosion for these particular substances.)

2. Dilution

   a. With water; here measures have to be taken to prevent freezing—for example, the refrigeration temperature for peroxides may be lower than the control temperature but should be selected so as to avoid dangerous separation of phases

   b. With other solvents (e.g., solutions of pyrophoric substances)

3. Desensitization or phlegmatization adding organic liquids or solids or inorganic solids or water (pastes). (The effect of adding desensitizing substances has to be proved; e.g., the addition of water to technically pure disuccinic acid peroxide will decrease its thermal stability.)

4. Stabilization or addition of an inhibitor.

5. Coating or immersion of a solid substance (e.g., hexamine and asbestos).

6. A specific production method that leads to suppression of a dangerous property (e.g., dibasic lead phosphite or phthalic anhydride with not more than 0.05 percent of maleic anhydride through which this substance is considered as nondangerous, or castor bean products that have undergone sufficient heat treatment to render them nondangerous).

7. Granulation (e.g., hafnium, titanium, and zirconium powder: carriage of these substances is prohibited in the dry state when mechanically produced in a particle size less than 10 microns. These substances are considered nondangerous when produced in particle sizes of, respectively, more than 53 and 840 microns).

8. Prescribing a preventive measure as temperature control during transport or keeping the substance in a cool and well-ventilated place, away from all sources of heat, or a construction of a receptacle so that internal pressure is relieved.

Also, by definition substances can be considered dangerous or nondangerous. Examples of exclusions are:

As substances indicated by name (e.g. ferro- and ferricyanides, sodium carbonate peroxyhydrate)

When the concentration is below a certain limit (e.g., aqueous solutions containing not more than 24 percent ethanol by volume, hydrogen peroxide aqueous solutions with less than 8 percent of hydrogen peroxide)

Dilution can lead to differentiation in danger levels, for example, hypochlorite solutions with:

Not less than 16 percent available chlorine should be placed in Packing Group II

More than 5 percent but less than 16 percent available chlorine should be placed in Packing Group III

With less than 5 percent available chlorine, it is considered nondangerous

Appendix 24.2: Some Starting Points for Packaging Design

Starting points for designing packaging mainly involve the following items.

Materials used should be of good quality and free from any defect that could impair the strength of the material.

Plastic packaging should be resistant against degradation by ultraviolet radiation, against permeation of the substance to be carried, sensibility to stress, and no significant weakening of the material after a certain time of storage is required.

Packaging may be provided with a venting device. This type of packaging is prohibited for air transport.

Breakage, leakage, or puncturing (e.g., by nails or staples) or attack of unprotected closure or venting device should be prevented during transport.

Any leakage of the contents of inner packaging should not substantially impair the protective properties of cushioning material or of the outer packaging.

For design-type-tested packaging, a quality-assurance program is necessary.

Appendix 24.3: Design Criteria for Tank Containers

In addition to the provisions given in the following paragraphs, the applicable requirements of the International Convention for Safe Containers (CSC) have to be fulfilled by any multimodal tank container. Tank-container frameworks intended to be lifted or secured by their corner castings should be subjected to internationally accepted special tests, for example, the ISO system.

Tank containers should be manufactured to a recognized technical code, such as a pressure vessel code. The shell should have a minimum wall thickness, depending on the dimensions and the material of construction. The body, service equipment lining, gaskets, fittings, and pipework should be immune to attack by the substance(s) to be carried and resistant to brittle fracture and to fissuring corrosion under tensile stress at temperatures of −30 or −20°C to design reference temperature, resistant to galvanic action due to the juxtaposition of dissimilar metals, have compatible thermal expansion characteristics, and when necessary should be passivated or neutralized.

A tank for liquids should withstand a minimum test pressure of 1.5, 2.65, 4, or 6 bar. Even tanks for liquids, which have virtually no vapor pressure, should be built as a pressure vessel. The tank has to withstand thermal loads due to possible loading temperatures of the substance to be carried.

The tank and frame should be capable of withstanding the most severe combination of static and dynamic stresses in handling and transport conditions. This means that tank containers and their fastenings should be capable of withstanding the following separately applied forces based on:

1. Twice the total mass acting in the direction of travel of the tank simultaneous with the weight of the tank
2. The total mass acting horizontally at right angles to the direction of travel of the tank (where the direction of travel is not clearly determined, twice the total mass should be used) simultaneously with the weight of the tank
3. The total mass acting vertically upward
4. Twice the total mass acting vertically downward

Under each of these loads, the following safety factors are to be observed:

1. For metals having a clearly defined yield point, a safety factor of 1.5 in relation to the determined yield stress,
2. For metals with no clearly defined yield point, a safety factor of 1.5 in relation to the guaranteed 0.2 percent proof stress (1.0 percent proof stress for austenitic steels)

If the connection between the frame and the tank shell allows relative movement as between subassemblies, the equipment should be so fastened as to permit such movement without risk of damage to working parts.

Suitable lifting, tie-down attachments should be capable of withstanding forces equal to those of twice the total mass; fork-lift pockets at least the forces equal to the total maximum mass.

Filling and discharge valves, piping, fittings, closures, venting and vacuum devices, flame traps, devices needed for safe testing, for heating or cooling, for gaging or measuring, and secondary means of sealing should be so positioned that they are readily apparent but also protected against risk of being wrenched off or damaged during transport and handling.

Service equipment should be secured from opening due to vibrations or impact.

Large tank containers for liquids should be divided into compartments by partitions provided with openings large enough to enable the compartments to be inspected.

Tank containers for the transport of flammable liquids or gases should be capable of being electrically grounded. For these liquids, precautions should be taken against frictional or percussive contact (e.g., aluminum and unprotected steel liable to rust).

The design of tank mountings (e.g., cradles and frameworks) and tank lifting and tie-down attachments should not cause undue concentration of stresses in any portion of the tank. The combined stresses include those caused by tank mountings and portion of the tank. In the design of supports and frameworks, due regard should be paid to the effects of environmental corrosion such as in the marine environment, and in calculations for all structural members not constructed of corrosion-resistant materials a minimum corrosion allowance should be added.

For pressure-relief devices, a number of requirements are given in the regulations. They concern such items as capacity (for liquids and gases enough to release the vapor pressure of the contents after complete fire engulfment for 30 minutes), setting, type and construction, siting, connections, number, and application of frangible disks. The same is true of other service equipment items. It is beyond the scope of this chapter to deal with this in further detail.

Testing, quality assurance, servicing, and maintenance all are important for the safety of means for transport of dangerous goods. Further elaboration is also beyond the scope of this chapter.

To avoid loss of contents in accidental situations, tank containers should be adequately protected against lateral and longitudinal impact and against overturning. If the tanks and the service equipment are so constructed as to withstand the impact of overturning, they need to be protected in this way.

Examples of protection of shells against collision:

Protection against lateral impact may consist, for example, of longitudinal bars protecting the tank on both sides at the level of the median line.

Protection of tank containers against overturning may consist, for example, of reinforcement rings or bars fixed across the frame.

Protection against rear impact may consist of a bumper or frame.

External fittings should be designed or protected so as to preclude the release of contents upon impact or overturning of the tank upon the fittings.

It is advised that, in order to avoid a worsening of the situation during fire in the vicinity of a tank containing toxic or unstable substances, the tank should be insulated. The jacketed insulation should remain effective at all temperatures up to 650°C and should be designed to a heat load of 10.9 W/cm^2 (2.60 gcal/cm$^2 \cdot$ sec = 34.500 Btu/sq. ft. hr.) for a period of at least 30 minutes. Insulation is also of importance for the capcity of relief devices. It should be protected so as to prevent the ingress of moisture; if the protection is to be gastight, any dangerous pressure should be prevented from developing. Insulating materials should not deteriorate unduly in service. Tanks for refrigerated gases and organic peroxides already are required to be insulated.

Appendix 24.4: Explanation of Abbreviations

IMO	International Maritime Organization
OCTI	Office Central des Transports Internationaux par Chemins de Fer
ECE	Economic Commision for Europe
CCNR	Commission Centrale Pour la Navigation du Rhin
ICAO	International Civil Aviation Organization
SOLAS	Safety of Life at Sea
COTIF	Convention Relative aux Transports Internationaux Ferroviaires
ADR	Accord Européen Relatif au Transport International des Marchandises Dangereuses par Route
IMDG Code	International Maritime Dangerous Goods—Code
RID	Règlement Concernant le Transport International Ferroviaire des Marchandises Dangereuses
ADNR	Règlement pour le Transport des Matières Dangereuses sur le Rhin
IBC	Intermediate bulk container

25
Data and Training Resources

Howard H. Fawcett

AAOHN (American Association of Occupational Health Nurses), 50 Lenox Pointe N.E., Atlanta, GA 30324   (404) 262-1162

AAOM (American Acadaemy of Occupational Medicine), 2340 S. Arlington Heights, IL 60005   (312) 228-6850

AAOS (American Association of Suicidology), 2459 South Ash St., Denver, CO 80222   (303) 692-0985

ACGIH (American Conference of Governmental Industrial Hygienists), Bldg. D-5, 6500 Glenway Ave., Cincinnati, OH 45211

ACS (American Chemical Society), 1155 16th St. N.W., Washington, DC 20036   (202) 872-4511, 4509, 4515, or 6000

DCHAL—Division of Chemistry and The Law, P.O. Box 395, Palo Alto, CA 94302, or c/o Ms. Shirley B. Radding, 2994 Cottonwood Ct., Santa Clara, CA 95051

DCHAS—Division of Chemical Health and Safety, c/o Dr. James Kaufman, Chemistry Dept., Curry College, Milton, MA 02186   (617) 333 0500, ext. 220; or 237 13335

ACTI (Asbestos Control Technology), P.O. Box 183, Maple Shade, NJ 08052 (800) 221-1911

ADAMA (National Clearinghouse for Alcohol Information), P.O. Box 2345, Rockville, MD 20852   (301) 468-2600

AFL-CIO (American Federation of Labor and Congress of Industrial Organizations), Department of Health, Safety, and Social Security, 815 16th St. N.W., Washington, DC 20006

AHCM (Academy of Hazard Control Management), 5010A Nicholson Lane, Rockville, MD 20852   (301) 984-8969

AIA (American Insurance Association), 85 John St., New York, NY 10038   (212) 669-0400

AIC (American Institute of Chemists), 7315 Wisconsin Ave., Suite 525E, Bethesda, MD 20814-9990 (202) 652-2447

AIDS NATIONAL INFORMATION SERVICE (800) 342-AIDS (800-342-2437)

AIF (Atomic Industrial Forum, Inc.,) 7101 Wisconsin Ave., Bethesda, MD 20814-4891 (301) 654-9260

AIHA (American Industrial Hygiene Foundation), 475 Wolf Ledges Parkway, Akron, OH 44311 (216) 762-7294

AIHC (American Industrial Health Council), 1075 Central Park Ave., Scarsdale, NY 10583

ALA (American Lung Association), 1740 Broadway, New York, NY 10019 (212) 315-8700

ANSI (American National Standards Institute), 1430 Broadway, New York, NY 10018 (212) 354-3300

AOMA (American Occupational Medicine Association), 2340 S. Arlington Road, Arlington Heights, IL 60005

APA (American Psychiatric Association), 1400 K St. N.W., Washington, DC 20005 (202) 682-6020, or 6158

APHA (American Public Health Association), 1015 15th St. N.W., Washington, DC 20005 (202) 789-5600

API (American Petroleum Institute), 1220 L St. N.W., Wshington, DC 20005 (202) 682-8319

ASSE (American Society of Safety Engineers), 850 Busse Highway, Park Ridge, IL 60068 (312) 6920-4121

Batelle Software Products Center, 655 Metro Place South, Dublin, OH 43017 (614) 761-7300 (mainframe, minis)

BOM (Bureau of Mines, U.S. Dept. of the Interior), 2401 E St. N.W., Washington, DC 20041 (202) 343-1100 or 634-1004, or Bruceton, PA facility (412) 892-6622

BRS Information Technologies, 1200 Route 7, Latham, NY 12110 (518) 783-1161 (on-line service)

Carlton Industries, Inc., P.O. Box 280, LaGrange, TX 78945 (800) 231-5988

CARS (Center for Atomic Radiation Studies), P.O. Box 72, Acton, MA 01720 (617) 635-0045

CGA (Compressed Gas Association), 1235 Jefferson Davis Highway, Arlington, VA 22202 (703) 979-0900

Chem Service, Inc., P.O. Box 3108, West Chester, PA 19381 (215) 692-3026 (MSDS Data System on Disks)

CHEMTREC (Chemical Transportation Emergency Response Center) (800) 424-9300

CIS (Cancer Information Service) (800) 4-CANCER (800-422-6237) or (800) 492-6600

CIS (Chemical Information Systems, Inc.), 7215 York Road, Baltimore, MD 21212   (800) 247-8737

CIS Abstracts, International Occupational Safety and Health Information Office, BIT, 1211 Geneva, Switzerland, or 1750 New York Ave. N.W., Washington, DC 20006   (202) 376-2315

Clean Water Action, 317 Pennsylvania Ave. S.E., Washington, DC 20003   (202) 547-1196

CMA (Chemical Manufacturers Association), 2501 M St. N.W., Washington, DC 20037   (202) 887-1100; or Chemical Referral Center, (800) 262-8200; or transportation emergencies, CHEMTREC, (800) 424-9300

COH (Center for Occupational Hazards), 5 Beekman St., New York, NY 10038   (212) 227-6220 (Specializes in health hazards encountered by artists)

COPPE (Council on Plastics and Packaging in the Environment), 1275 K St. N.W., Suite 400, Washington, DC 20005

CPSC (Consumer Products Safety Commission), 5401 Westbard Ave., Bethesda, MD   (800) 638-2772

CSMA (Chemical Specialties Manufacturers Assocation), 1001 Connecticut Ave. N.W., Washington, DC 20036   (202) 872-8110

DIALOG Information Systems, 3460 Hillview Ave., Palo Alto, CA 94304   (800) 227-1960

Digital Equipment Corp., Medical Systems Group, Two Iron Way, P.O. Box 1003, Marlboro, MA 01752   (617) 467-2369

DOT (U.S. Department of Transportation), 400 7th St. S.W., Washington, DC 20590   (202) 366-4488, or (800) 752-6367

EPA (U.S. Environmental Protection Agency), Public Information Center, 401 M St. S.W., Washington, D.C. 20460   (202) 382-2080), or Press Office (202) 382-2981

ERM Computer Services, 999 West Chester Pike, West Chester, PA 19382   (215) 696-9110 (micro)

Fawcett Consultations, Inc., P.O. Box 9444, Wheaton, MD 20906   (301) 933-2521 (chemical health and safety)

FDA (Food and Drug Administration), 5600 Fishers Lane, Rockville, MD 20857   (301) 443-3170 for foods; (301) 295-8012 for drugs

First System, 134 Middle Neck Rd., Great Neck, NY 11021   (516) 829-5858 (OHM-TADS and CHRIS Systems for IBM or compatible computers)

Fisher Scientific Co., 711 Forbes Ave., Pittsburgh, PA 15219   (412) 562-8468 (micro)

Flow General, Inc. 7655 Old Springhouse Road, McLean, VA 22102   (703) 893-5915

FICOE (Federal Interagency Committee on Explosives), Department of the Treasury, Bureau of Alcohol, Tobacco and Firearms, Washington, DC 20226   (202) 566-7777

Health and Energy Institute, 236 Massachusetts Ave. N.E., Suite 506, Washington, DC 20002   (202) 543-1070 (health and environmental effects of radiation exposure)

HESIS (Hazard Evaluation System), State of California, 2151 Berkeley Way, Berkeley, CA 94704

HM Health and Safety at Work Commission (Act of 1974), 1 Chepstow Place, Westbourne Grove, London W2, United Kingdom   (01-229-3456)

IARC (International Agency for Research on Cancer), Lyon, France; IARC publications available from WHO-USA Publications, 49 Sheridan Ave., Albany, NY 12210   (518) 436-9686

ICF, Inc., 9300 Lee Highway, Fairfax, VA 22031-1207   (703) 934-3000.

IHF (Industrial Health Foundation), 34 Penn Circle W., Pittsburgh, PA 15206   (412) 363-6600

ILO (International Labour Organization), BIT, CH-1211 Geneva, 22 Switzerland; U.S. office, 1750 New York Ave., Washington, DC 20006   (202) 376-2315

Institute of Makers of Explosives, 1575 I St. N.W., Washington, DC 20036   (202) 789-0310

Institution of Chemical Engineers, 165-171 Railway Terrace, Rugby CV21 3HQ, United Kingdom (Bernard M. Hancock, Manager, Safety and Loss Prevention)

International Association of Fire Chiefs, 1329 18th St. N.W., Washington, DC 20036   (202) 833-3420

International Association of Fire Fighters, 1750 New York Ave. N.W., Washington, D.C. 20006   (202) 737-8484

ICWU (International Chemical Workers Union—AFL-CIO), 1126 16th St. N.W., Washington, DC 20036   (202) 659-3747; or WLM Bldg., 1655 W. Market St., Akron, OH 44313   (216) 867-2444

ILO (International Labour Organization) (Georg Kliesch, Director, Occupational Safety and Health Branch; Georges Coppe, M.D., Head, Medical Branch,) ILO-BIT, CH-1211, Geneva, Switzerland

IOM (Institute of Medicine), c/o National Academy of Sciences, 2101 Constitution Ave. N.W., Washington, DC 20418   (202) 334-2169 or 2138

LEF (Life Extension Foundation), 1185 Avenue of the Americas, New York, NY 10036

MHIDAS (Major Hazard Incident Data Service), Major Hazards Assessment Unit of the Health and Safety Executive, United Kingdom Atomic Energy Authority, Wigshaw Lane, Culcheth, Warrington, Cheshire WA3 4NE, United Kingdom

MIOT (Maritime Institute of Technology and Graduate Studies), 5700 Hammonds Ferry Rd., Lithicum Heights, MD 21090   (301) 859-5700

NCI (National Cancer Institute), IARC Data Base (202) 496-7403, and NIEHS National Toxicology Program (919) 541-3991; for general inquiries, (800) 4-CANCER or (800) 422-6237

NEHA (National Environmental Health Association), 1200 Lincoln St., Suite 704, Denver, CO 80203

NEMA (National Electrical Manufacturers Association), 2101 L St. N.W., Suite 300, Washington, DC 20037   (202) 457-8400

NETC (National Emergency Training Center, Federal Fire Academy), 16825 South Seton Ave., Emmitsburg, MD 21727-8995   (301) 447-1000

NIEHS (National Institute for Environmental Health Sciences), Douglas Walters, P.O. Box 12233, Research Triangle Park, NC 27709   (919) 541-3355

NLM (National Library of Medicine), MEDLARS Management Section, 8600 Rockville Pike, Bethesda, MD 20209   (800) 638-8480)

NIOSH (National Institute for Occupational Safety and Health), Robert A. Taft Laboratories, 4676 Columbia Parkway, Cincinnati, OH 45226   (513) 684-8326

NP&CA (NATIONAL PAINT AND COATINGS ASSOCIATION), 1500 Rhode Island Ave., N.W. Washington, DC 20036   (202) 462-6272

NTSB (National Transportation Safety Board), 800 Independence Ave. S.W., Washington, DC 20594   (202) 382-6600 or 6735

NWF (National Wildlife Foundation), 1412 16th St. N.W., Washington, DC 20036   (202) 797-6800

OCAW (Oil, Chemical and Atomic Workers Union—AFL-CIO), 255 Union Blvd., Lakewood, CO 80228, or P.O. Box 2812, Denver, CO 80201   (303) 987-2229

OHI (Occupational Health Institute), 2340 S. Arlington Heights Road, Arlington Heights, IL 60005

OSHA (Occupational Safety and Health Administration), 200 Constitution Ave. N.W., Washington, DC 20210 (Technical Data Center, D. Marsick)   (202) 523-9700

Power Technologies, Inc., Technology Assessment Group, P.O. Box 1058, 1482 Erie Blvd., Schenectady, NY 12301-1058   (518) 374-1220

RMA (Rubber Manufacturers Association), 1901 Pennsylvania Ave. N.W., Washington, DC   (202) 785-2602

SOCMA (Synthetic Organic Chemical Manufacturers Association), 1075 Central Park Ave., Scarsdale, NY 10583

SOEH (Society for Occupational and Environmental Health), 2021 K St. N.W., Washington, DC 20006

UNESCO International Centre for Chemical Studies, Edvard Kardelj University, P.O. Box 18/L, Vegova 4, 61001 Ljubljana, Yugoslavia

WOHRC (Women's Occupational Health Resource Center), School of Public Health, 21 Audubon Ave., Columbia University, New York, NY 10032

World Wildlife Fund and Conservation Foundation, 1250 24th St. N.W., Washington, DC 20037   (202) 293-4800

Young, Jay, 12916 Allerton Lane, Silver Spring, MD 20904   (301) 384-1768 (chemical health and safety consultant)

PUBLICATION AND TRAINING AIDS SOURCES

AAR (Association of American Railroads), Mechanical Division, Publications Section, 50 F St. N.W., Washington, DC 20001   (202) 639-2232

AIHA *(American Industrial Hygiene Association Journal),* 475 Wolf Ledges Parkway, Akron, OH 44311

AJOE *(American Journal of Epidemiology),* Society for Epidemiologic Research, 550 N. Broadway, Suite 201, Baltimore, MD 21205

AJPH *(American Journal of Public Health),* American Public Health Association, 1015 15th St. N.W., Washington, DC 20005

American Institute of Chemical Engineers, 345 E. 47th St., New York, NY 10017   (212) 705-7338 *(Chemical Engineering Progress* published monthly, also Division of Safety and Health)

Annals of Occupational Hygiene, Pergamon Press, Maxwell House, Fairview Park, Elmsford, NY 10523

Archives of Dermatology, American Medical Association, 535 N. Dearborn, Chicago, IL 60610

Art Hazard News, Center for Occupational Hazards, 5 Beekman St., New York, N.Y. 10038

ASB Asbestos Information Service, Programme de Recherche sur L'Amiante de L'Universite der Sherbrooke (PRAUS), University of Sherbrooke, Sherbrooke, Quebec, Canada J1K 231

Biosciences Information Service, 2100 Arch St., Philadelphia, PA 19103   (215) 587-4800

BNA (Bureau of National Affairs), 1231 25th St. N.W., Washington, DC 20037   (202) 452-4200

Bioengineering News (weekly), P.O. Box 1210, Port Angeles, WA 98362   (800) 541-3377

Canada—Dangerous Goods Regulations and Bulletins, Regulations Branch, Transport of Dangerous Goods Directorate, Tower "A," Place de Ville, Ottawa, Ontario K1A ON5, Canada

CHAS Newsletter, Division of Chemical Health and Safety, American Chemical Society (M. Renfrew, Editor), 1271 Walenta, Moscow, Idaho 83843   (208) 882-5947

Chemical Health and Safety—An International Periodical, (L. Jewel Nicholls, Editor), Chemistry Dept., University of Illinois, P.O. Box 4348, Chicago, IL 60680   (312) 996 4439

Chemical Processing (monthly), Putman Publishing Co., 301 E. Ohio St., Chicago, IL 60611

Chief Fire Executive (bi-monthly; Alan J. Saly, Managing Editor), Firehouse Communications, 33 Irving Place, New York, NY 10003   (212) 475-5400

Dupont (E. I. Du Pont de Nemours & Co., Inc.), P19-1105 P.O. Box 4500, Greenville, DE 19807   (800) 532-SAFE or (302) 999-6990

Environmental Policy and Law (monthly; international journal), Elsevier Science Publishers, P.O. Box 1991, 1000 BZ Amsterdam, the Netherlands; or Elsevier Science Publishers, Journal Information Center, 52 Vanderbilt Ave., New York, NY 10017 (USA and Canada)

ERIC Oryx Press, 2214 N. Central, Phoenix, AZ 85004   (602) 254-6156

Federal Register (daily; legal notices of government), 1100 L St. N.W., Room 8301, Washington, DC 20408   (202) 523-5227

FEMA (Federal Emergency Management Agency), Office of Printing and Publications, Washington, DC 20472; also Federal Fire Academy of FEMA, 16825 South Seton Ave., Emmitsburg, MD 21727-8995   (301) 447-1000

HCB Hazardous Cargo Bulletins, 38 Tavistock St., London WC2E 7PB, United Kingdom

Hazardous Materials Control (bi-monthly), Hazardous Materials Control Research Institute, 9300 Columbia Blvd., Silver Spring, MD 20910-1702

Hazardous Waste and Hazardous Materials (journal; N. Beecher, Editor), Mary Ann Liebert, Inc., 1651 Third Ave., New York, NY 10128

Hseline (Laboratory Hazards Bulletin), Pergamon Infoline, Inc., 1340 Old Chain Bridge Road, McLean, VA 22101   (800) 336-7575

Industrial Training Systems, 20 W. Stow Road, Marlton, NJ 08053-9990   (609) 983-7300 (videos and other training materials)

Information Handling Services (material safety data sheets), 15 Inverness Way East, Englewood, CO 80150   (800) 525-7052, ext. 700

Journal of Hazardous Materials (G. F. Bennett and R. E. Britter, Editors), Elsevier, Amsterdam, the Netherlands

Journal of the American College of Toxicity (M. S. Christian, Editor), Mary Ann Liebert, Inc., 1651 Third Ave., New York, NY 10128

LFC (London Food Commission), 88 Old St., London EC1 V9AR, United Kingdom   (01) 253-9513, ext. 45

NBS Fire Research Publications, National Technical Information Service, Springfield, VA 22161

NFPA (National Fire Protection Association), Batterymarch Park, Quincy, MA 02269   (800) 344-3555

NIH (National Institutes of Health), 9000 Rockville Pike, Bethesda, MD 20892   (301) 496-4000

NSC (National Safety Council), 444 N. Michigan Ave., Chicago, IL 60611   (312) 527-4800 (chemical and R&D sections)

NSTA (National Science Teachers Association), 1742 Connecticut Ave. N.W., Washington, DC 20009   (202) 328-5800

Occupational Hazards (monthly; Ivan L. Weinstock, Publisher), Penton Publishing Co., 1100 Superior Ave., Cleveland, OH 44114

OH&S (Occupational Health and Safety) *Monthly,* Medical Publications, Inc., 225 N. New Road, Waco, TX 76710   (817) 776-9000

OMEC International, Inc., 727 15th St. N.W., Washington, DC 20005 (202) 639-890 (biotechnology and related biological aspects)

OSU-DRC (Ohio State University Disaster Research Center), 128 Derby Hall, 154 North Oval Mall, Columbus, OH 43210 (614) 422-5916

Pollution Engineering (monthly), Pudvan Publishing Co., 1935 Shermer Rd., Northbrook, IL 60062

Recombinant DNA Technical Bulletin (monthly, NIH Publication No. 87-99), Public Health Service—National Institutes of Health, Office of recombinant DNA Activities, Bethesda, MD 20892

Research and Development Monthly, P.O. Box 1030, Barrington, IL 60010 (312) 381-1840

Shell Chemical Safety Guide (101 pages), Shell Chemical Company, 2001 Kirby Rd., Houston, TX 77019 (713) 526-4631

Sierra Club Books, 730 Polk St., San Francisco, CA 94109 (415) 776-2211

Small Chem Biz Newsletter (Kenneth W. Greenlee, Editor), Division of ACS Small Chemical Businesses, Box 14373, Columbus, OH 43214 (614) 268-2976

UL (Underwriters Laboratories), 333 Pfingsten Rd., Northbrook, IL 60062 (312) 272-8800

Worldwatch Institute, 1776 Massachusetts Ave. N.W., Washington, DC 20036 (202) 452-1999

Z-88 American National Standard on Respiratory Protection (Robert de Rosa, Chair), Lawrence Livermore Laboratory, Livermore, CA 94550 (414) 422-5228

26

Scenarios of Mock Trials to Train Lawyers

James M. Brown

The growing interest in the legal as well as economic and ethical aspects of hazardous materials has inspired increased attention to the exposures of people that produce injuries. This "toxic tort" potential liability has given lawyers a relatively new field of operation, and is reflected in "mock trials," such as the ones currently in operation as training aids at the George Washington University National Law Center in Washington, D.C. Typical mock trials are included to train the students in the complex problems associated with such actions. Examples of recent "trials" are described in the following.

EPISODE: PCB SPILLS FROM TRANSFORMER ON TRUCK (1986)

One of the renovation contracts between the U.S. Navy and Marine Lift, Inc., involved, as one component of the work done on a floating power generator, the replacement of several electrical transformers. These transformers and other debris and wreckage were in the way of operations and scheduled for removal to various salvage yards, smelting plants, incinerators, and landfills. On August 10, 1984, Harry Foreman, yard superintendant for Marine Lift, began feeling the pinch for space and asked his subordinate, Marie Decker, to find the hauler who was supposed to get the trash and debris cleaned out. Marie reported that the contract hauler had suffered a breakdown on his low-boy transport and would not be able to pick up any bulky items for at least 10 days. "Then get me someone else," Harry growled. "I've got to get the transformers out of the way by the end of next week. I have to have that space. Be sure you get somebody with a big-enough rig. Those things are heavy, and the gunk they have in their innards ain't exactly what people serve for breakfast." Marie called around trying to locate a hauler who could give prompt service, but, as she reported to Harry, for short-notice single-trip contracts, they are "few and far between." Harry said: "Keep trying until you find somebody—anybody, Marie. But get me somebody. I've got to get rid of those transformers. I can't even swing a fork-lift around them in Charlie Bay with those monsters sitting there. Keep trying until you get somebody."

Marie had no luck until 4 P.M., when she reached Jerbill Trucking and Transport dispatcher Morgan Ready. Morgan wanted all the information she had on the transformers, particularly their size, manufacturer, serial number, date of manufacture, weight, overall dimensions, and condition, etc. In exasperation Marie finally said: "Hey look, buddy, I only work here. These things aren't being put out to stud—they're going to the junkyard. What is it with all this pedigree stuff, anyway?"

Morgan answered: "Listen, sister, those things are hotter than you ever dreamed of being. Just give me the information. You get paid until quitting time, don't you?" After he got his information, he put Marie on hold and worked up his proposal. When he came back on the line, he said: "Well, here you are, Sis. We'll have to handle the disposition of the load as well as haul it. If you want to ride along, maybe it will warm you up a little. Anyway, the gig will cost your boss 44 big bills."

Marie was used to being "taken" on emergency hauling jobs, but this was "something else." "O.K., wise guy, let me tell you what you can do with your bid. You can ice it. Then you ought to feel real comfortable sitting on it. Like, forever." She slammed down the phone just as Harry walked into the office. "Any luck?" he asked. "I just hung up on the only bid I've had so far," Marie snarled. "This guy was gross." Harry did a double take and said, "We can't be too sensitive at four o'clock and no bites yet, Marie. How gross was he anyway?" "He was 44,000 good old American dollars worth of 'gross,' snapped Marie. "Like my mother always said," Harry responded, "get yourself a good sensitive female assistant and you'll go far in this work. Thank goodness you always get feisty at 3:59 P.M. So keep pluggin'." Marie grinned in spite of herself. "Don't give up yet, boss. I'm warming to the task." That remark, of course, left Harry cold.

Working on down through her list of "call-backs," Marie again tried Equipment Distributers, Inc., of Long Beach. When they told her they just could not help her, Marie began to feel desperate. "Oh, please, you've got to help me," she pleaded. "My boss is going to kill me!" The voice on the other end of the line sounded sympathetic. "Maybe I can find someone else who could help you out, lady," it said. "Hold the line while I get on the other phone a minute." After a bit, he came back on and said, "Yeh, they got a heavy-duty low-boy. And they haul transformers. They haul *anything*. But I need to give them some information. They are on the other line. What do they weigh, how high are they, and what outside dimensions?" Marie gave him the information and asked: "What else do you need to know?" After a pause, he asked: "Do they haul them to your dump or to theirs?" "To theirs, of course," Marie answered politely, crossing her fingers as she did so. "By next week?," the voice queried. "Yes, and with no ands, ifs, or buts," replied Marie.

"O.K., lady, for six grand apiece, I've got an outfit on line who will take all five of them, and move 'em out this Friday." Marie could have kissed him! "Who are they?" Marie asked. "Kinkus Stamp Fluid and Waste Disposal Co." said the voice. "Mister, you've got a deal," Marie crooned. "Feisty and foxy," Harry commented when she reported the good news. "You can come to work again tomorrow. I'm going home and write your mother a thank-you letter."

As it turned out, the Kinkus rig was big enough to also make a couple of other pickups, and, as driver Ben Jones grumbled: "If they had tried to route me all over town, they couldn't have done better." Then he had to go another six miles in the wrong direction to pick up his girl friend, Betty, whom he had invited along for the ride because they could stop at their favorite Mexican restaurant in Palmdale on the return run from Mojave. Betty wasn't ready and he had to park out in front for nearly an hour before she came down. As she walked around the back of the rig, she noticed a puddle. "Hey, Ben, you got another leak in that radiator? I don't want to get stalled out in the desert again." "Naw," Ben answered, "I saw that puddle. It's one of them transformers leakin'. Truck's all right."

Ben delivered the five transformers to the Rolling Reduction Co. smelter in Mojave, hosed down the bed of his low-boy, where apparently at least two transformers had been leaking, and headed for Palmdale and their favorite restaurant. In the meantime, someone else had noticed the leaks, back in Los Angeles. "The spot was slick and had a 'funny smell.' " The city fire department was called and sent out a pumper truck to hose down the spot. When it was learned that the transformers had been on the low-boy, they called in the county health department. It was ascertained that the truck had been leaking since it left the Marine Lift establishment. It was also established that the leaking product was a once-popular coolant that no longer is used in such units, namely, PCB (polychlorinated biphenyl), which is known to cause cancer and liver disease in animals.

After performing a costly cleanup within the city, the City of Los Angeles filed a civil suit against Marine Lift, Equipment Distributors, Rolling Reduction Smelting Co., and Kinkus, for "unlawful storage, transportation and disposal of five electrical transformers containing PCBs." Criminal charges were also filed against the companies and their managing officers. The City Attorney told reporters that the suit could result in fines of $14 million, and in 279 years of jail time for some of the top executives charged. The City of Los Angeles had incurred major cleanup expenses. The county was still cleaning up, and there was a question as to whether the disposition at the smelter was properly done or that activity had spread contamination through large parts of Antelope Valley. After consulting with the city and county officials, the governor's office agreed to "stay out of it as long as you people are sure you can handle it," but agreed to "come in if needed."

For the mock trial, students were asked to play various roles representing the several persons and organizations identified in the script, in addition to the City Attorney of Los Angeles, the County Attorney, the EPA, the Department of Justice, the Department of Defense, and Ben Jones.

EPISODE: FOAM INSULATION/FORMALDEHYDE (1986)

The energy conservation movement of the 1970s stimulated the development of various thermal insulation products for the home. One product that has been used in over 500,000 houses nationwide is foam insulation. This insulating material, composed of a liquid resin, a foaming agent, and compressed gas, is pumped as a foam into the exterior walls of a building. After several days, the foam solidifies, forming a highly effective heat barrier.

The majority of foam-insulation manufacturers have used formaldehyde as a chemical binding agent in the liquid resin component of the foam. Formaldehyde, a colorless gas, is widely used as a chemical adhesive in the manufacture of numerous household products, including plywood, particleboard, paneling, and carpeting. Formaldehyde is also an ingredient found in some shampoos, toothpastes, cosmetics, and clothing containing synthetic fibers.

During the late 1970s, a number of studies began to link certain health problems with formaldehyde. Homeowners whose homes had been insulated with urea-formaldehyde foam insulation (UFFI) began to complain of irritating odors in the home. Many of these homeowners also experienced eye, nose, and throat irritation, respiratory problems, skin irritation, nausea, and headaches following the installation of UFFI. Examination of the houses containing UFFI revealed that over a period of months following foam installation, the solidified foam decomposes, and a process of "off-gassing" occurs, whereby formaldehyde is released from the insulation into the surrounding air.

In 1982, the Consumer Product Safety Commission (CPSC) issued a final rule banning UFFI in residences and schools. The rule followed a finding by the CPSC that formaldehyde foam insulation posed an unreasonable risk of injury from skin and eye irritation. This rule was subsequently vacated in Gulf South Insulation v. CPSC, 701 F. 2d 1137 (5th Cir. 1983).

Hundreds of lawsuits seeking recovery of damages for personal injury and property damage have been instituted by homeowners against formaldehyde-foam-insulation manufacturers and installers. It is likely that the number of suits will increase as more evidence accumulates concerning the adverse health effects caused by formaldehyde. However, plaintiff homeowners face several obstacles to recovery from the UFFI industry. First, given the fact that formaldehyde is present in many household products, it is difficult for plaintiffs to demonstrate that the source of the injury-producing formaldehyde is merely UFFI. Second, the majority of insulation manufacturers are small companies that are not adequately capitalized or insured. The major UFFI manufacturer, Energy Conseration, Inc., filed for bankruptcy in 1982. Therefore, even if plaintiffs can demonstrate causation, the defendant foam manufacturers may be judgment-proof. A discussion of the formaldehyde insulation health problems and related litigation considerations appears in Dworkin and Mallor, "Liability for Formaldehyde-Contaminated Housing Materials: Toxic Torts in the Home," 21 *Am. Bus. L.J.* 307 (1983).

Rapco Foam Inc. (RAPFINC) is a California corporation based in Los Angeles. The company manufactures a variety of products designed to conserve energy.

Included among its products are solar heating systems [its subsidiary, Sol-Powered Homes Inc. (Robert Goodridge), builds solar-powered homes in the Antelope Valley, insulated exterior siding, and foam insulation]. The foam RAPFINC manufactures is sold under the name Tripolymer. Although Tripolymer foam is not a UFFI, and is not manufactured with formaldehyde, recent studies have revealed that formaldehyde can be released from Tripolymer foam several months after installation. RAPFINC was aware that the UFFI had the potential for releasing harmful formaldehyde. The ingredients composing Tripolymer foam have a molecular structure quite similar to formaldehyde, and it is theorized that during decomposition of the foam, formaldehyde is actually formed and off-gassed at certain temperature and humidity levels.

Kuffi Insulation Co. (KII) is a California corporation based in Los Angeles. KII provides various insulation services to homeowners and businesses throughout the Los Angeles area. One portion of KII's business is to install foam insulation manufactured by companies such as RAPFINC.

During a typical installation, KII will send a team of several installers to a work site. These workers will drill 1-inch holes in specified patterns through the exterior and into the wall cavities of the building to be insulated. The installers will then combine the various foam components (resin, foaming agent, gas) and will inject the foam mixture through the 1-inch holes into the wall cavities of the building. After installation, the holes are sealed, and the walls, windows, and ceilings are examined for leaks caused by the foam.

In 1978, RAPFINC and KII entered into a contract whereby RAPFINC agreed to sell Tripolymer foam to KII. In addition to agreeing to pay the contract price for the Tripolymer foam, KII agreed to allow RAPFINC to inspect any installation performed by KII, to ensure that the RAPFINC foaming procedures were followed. RAPFINC retained the right, under the contract, to terminate the agreement if KII installation procedures were deemed by RAPFINC to be inadequate.

Under the contract, RAPFINC specified that Tripolymer foam would provide sufficient insulating value for residential use throughout California. No representations or warranties were made by RAPFINC with respect to the commercial use of the product, which had only been used for residences before the 1978 contract.

James Woodson (age 38), his wife, Clara (age 36), and their daughter, Janie (age 12), live in the outskirts of Lancaster, Calif., where they operate the family business, Woodson's Wholesome Farm Products. They advertise that their product is bought only from producers who use natural pesticide control. They assure the same with respect to products they raise on their 20 acres. For the most part, their production is limited to tomatoes. They have amazing yields of large, succulent tomatoes, thanks to being able to trade some of their production to John D. R. Mowgli, in exchange for sufficient quantities of Krilium Soil Conditioner, a product he doles out to them with the understanding that (1) it is perfectly safe for the uses they are making of it, and (2) they will not disclose their source, because he bought up the entire remaining stock when the company he worked for as a chemist went out of business several years back, and there is no more when that is gone, except for what he can manufactuer with his pilot plant in his barn.

In 1981, the Woodsons entered into a contract with Kuffi for the installation of Tripolymer foam in the Woodson's residence at a cost of $1200. Jim and Carla Woodson entered into a second contract with KII for the installation of Tripolymer foam in the Woodson's newly constructed aluminum warehouse building. For 10 years, the Woodsons have operated their vegetable and fruit wholesaling operation under the name "Woodson's Wholesale Food Products." They buy produce from selected, reliable "organic" farmers in the Antelope Valley area and the San Jaoquin Valley. They resell to "natural foods" retailers in the Los Angeles area. Their business has steadily expanded, and in 1980 they decided to construct an additional storage facility for their product. Since constant temperature is essential for the storage of produce, the Woodsons contacted several insulation companies for the purpose of obtaining adequate thermal insulation for their new warehouse.

Sandifer Kosar, president of Kuffi, met with the Woodsons and assured them that KII could satisfy their insulation needs for both the residence and the 10,000-square-foot produce warehouse. On the strength of Kosar's representation, the Woodsons agreed to pay KII $8700 for the installation of Tripolymer foam in the warehouse, in addition to the earlier-mentioned home installation contract. In June 1981, KII installed Tripolymer foam in both buildings as per contract.

Within a few weeks of the installation of foam by KII, the Woodson family began to notice unusual odors in their house. Each family member also began to experience severe headaches and nausea. They were examined by a physician, who was unable to determine the cause of their symptoms. A month after the foam installation, Carla Woodson began to experience respiratory problems.

About this time, Jim Woodson read an article in a local newspaper regarding the link between certain health problems and home products, including formaldehyde insulation. He immediately arranged for tests to be performed inside his house by a local industrial toxicologist, Dr. Winter. The tests revealed the presence of formaldehyde gas in the ambient air of the Woodson home in quantities approximately 28 percent higher than of the average house. Dr. Winter took a sample of the foam installed in the Woodson's exterior walls and conducted laboratory tests on it. The sample produced small quantities of formaldehyde gas. On the basis of these tests, however, Dr. Winter was unable to determine with certainty that the foam insulation was the predominant source of formaldehyde within the house.

During the summer of 1981, southern California experienced above-average temperatures. The Woodsons attempted to maintain low temperatures in their warehouse, but their efforts failed and the produce stored in their new warehouse spoiled. An examination of the warehouse walls revealed large gaps in the foam. As a result of the spoilage of the produce, the Woodsons lost approximately $80,000 in inventory. Based on average sales over the past five years, this amount of inventory would have netted them a $10,000 profit. The loss of the inventory and consequential default on delivery promises also diminished Woodson's reputation as a wholesaler. The word got out about his "contaminated house," and soon the rumor about contamination included his warehouse and its products.

To top off their rash of problems, John D. R. Mowgli experienced an infestation of ground insects that began eating at the leaves of his guayule plants. He hired

Crop Dusters of Antelope Valley to spray his fields. Something the sole proprietor of that business called Dieldrin was used, and in making his passes over Mowgli's fields, the owner/proprietor/pilot failed to consider adequately the strength of the wind, and also sprayed the Woodson tomato fields. Mowgli treated the complaint lightly, saying: "You just got some free protection for your garden, Jimmy. I'm not going to charge you for it, so don't worry." But Woodson no longer had tomatoes that were free from chemical pesticides.

Jim Woodson also tried to call, and then wrote to, Kosar of KII, but he received no response, in spite of repeated efforts to make contact. He finally decided it was time to seek legal advice, and came to "our" firm. There may be causes of action for breach of contract, negligence, strict liability in tort, nuisance, and misrepresentation inherent in the situation.

SCENARIO: CADILLAC/FAIRFIELD TORRENCE SITE ACQUISITION (1986)

In the early 1940s, the U.S. government released a report to the effect that, because of the war, its requirements for rubber and rubber products were rising drastically. In response to this, it purchased several properties that were appropriate for rubber-processing facilities and synthetic rubber plants. One of these was located at Del Amo Boulevard and Vermont Avenue (Torrence site).

The government set up the Defense Plant Corporation to manage these facilities. In 1942, it leased a part of the Torrence site to the Now Chemical Company of Middletown, Mich. Now Chemical operated the facility until 1962 as a synthetic rubber plant. It no longer has offices or plants in California but makes sales in that state on a regular basis. As a part of its Torrence operations, it periodically disposed of benzene, ethylbenzene, aluminum chloride, sodium hydroxide, sodium chloride, dichlorobutane, and dichlorobutene, among other products, all such dispositions being made within the Torrence site.

From time to time, Now Chemical allowed other companies to dump their chemicals in Now's fenced-in disposal area. One local resident clearly remembers seeing trucks labeled "Specialties Products Co." pulling into the site on a regular basis. Specialties manufactures a unique form of brake oil that is used only in airplane manufacturing and operations. The process uses a great deal of organic solvents, such as benzene and trichloroethylene, which must be disposed of regularly.

In addition, an ex-employee recalls seeing some "beat-up" tank trucks that came by the plant regularly and dumped their contents on the back lot "way over by the fence." She is not certain, but thinks that some of these trucks bore the name "Kinkus Disposal" on the side of their tanks. Kinkus, a California corporation, originally produced and marketed in bulk a fluid composed basically of 1,1,1-trichloroethane for use in detecting water-mark identification signs on stamps. It subsequently entered the industrial-waste-disposal business and concentrated primarily on that type of operation from 1955 through 1970. Since 1970, it has been trying to make a go of recycling used oils at a facility in Fresno, and in hauling toxic and hazardous wastes to various disposal sites, including the Rolling Reduction Smelting Co. plant in Mojave, Calif.

In 1960, Now Chemical Co. let its lease on the Torrence site expire. By then, the Defense Plant Corporation had ceased to exist and the General Services Administration (GSA) had taken over all of its property-management duties. GSA held the property until 1972, when it sold it to Torrence Investers Limited Partnership (TILP). TILP's general partner was Sam Gogetter, a local real-estate developer. The limited partners were John Larson, a national television personality; Merwin Biggs, a successful northern California attorney; John Derbakey, a well-known brain surgeon; and Sally B. Gogetter, Sam's wife. TILP paid "top dollar" for the Torrence site, which it thought would serve as an ideal site for a family resort park. (The rubber plant had been torn down in the early 1960s.) TILP spent a lot of money on preliminary site plans, but never performed a detailed site analysis. Because of the 1973–1974 recession, TILP did not build on the property.

In 1980, TILP listed the Torrence site property for sale, at four times what it cost TILP. After much negotiation, Cadillac/Fairfield Development Corp. bought the property for about 3½ times TILP's purchase price. TILP conveyed to Cadillac/Fairfield by a general waarranty deed. At no time during the negotiations did TILP mention any of the uses to which the property had been put prior to TILP's purchase.

In January 1982, after several slow years, TILP liquidated its remaining assets and distributed the proceeds to the partners. Sam Gogetter received 30 percent ($300,000) of the assets. He has since put this into other real-estate ventures in the area. Larson's business manager has reinvested his proceeds ($75,000) in an oil and gas venture in central Kansas. Biggs and Derbakey put their $75,000 shares into a joint trust to fund cancer research. Sally Burns (the former Mrs. Gogetter) has not been heard from in three years.

In February 1982, Cadillac/Fairfield hired an engineering firm, TST Associates, to do a preliminary site analysis. It planned to build a low-density office complex on the property.

Cordladdie Park, a residential subdivision, is located less than 400 yards from the Torrence site property. Cordladdie Park derives its drinking water from a privately owned water company, R. P. Drinking Systems, Inc. (RPDSI). RPDSI draws all of its water from wells in and near the Cordladdie Park subdivision. These wells tap an aquifer some 50 feet below the surface, which flows roughly west at 10–70 feet per year.

Cordladdie Park Citizens' Association became frustrated over the seeming inability to get meaningful action with respect to the cleanup of the Cadillac/Fairfield site on Del Amo Blvd. The members then received another fright. The Los Angeles Regional Water Quality Control Board issued an order to R. P. Water Co., which holds the franchise for supplying potable water to the Cordladdie Park neighborhood, directing it to stop distributing water from its supply wells nos. 2, 3, and 5 until it has eliminated the toxic-waste residues found therein on the last tests conducted by the board's chemists. As a consequence of this order, R. P. Water Co. had to notify the Cordladdie Park residents that for the time being it would truck in water to their area, and would provide Lister bags at 200-foot intervals from which residents could draw water for drinking and cooking purposes. It advised that as soon as alternative piping could be completed and a state inspection held, it would again distribute water through its piping system. It stated in its notification that it did not believe its water had been contaminated, but that since the water quality board had found trace levels of some potentially toxic products in the untreated well water at the point where it tapped the 70-foot aquifer, it had appropriately issued the order to cut those wells out of the system until it could be determined without question that they were safe.

One of the residents obtained an official copy of a letter sent by TST Associates, an engineering firm, to Cadillac/Fairfield, advising that in conducting soil tests on the site, it had found the following chemicals:

Benzene	50 ppm
Aluminum chloride	traces
Dichlorobutane	traces
Naphthalene	traces
Formaldehyde	30 ppm
1,1,1-trichloroethane	70 ppm
Dioxin	1–20 ppb

The report indicated that it was just preliminary, but with such chemicals listed, lay members of the association were quick to associate the higher-than-normal incidence of illness, malaise, irritability, and respiratory problems, that had plagued the neighborhood since Cadillac/Fairfield had disturbed the soil of the Del Amo site. They concluded that since the EPA, having reportedly made an inspection of the site, refused to disclose whether it had done so, and also refused to divulge any information concerning toxics at the site, and reticence thus exhibited was in itself a warning that things were not as they should be. They recalled the EPA's move into Times Beach, Mo., after months of silence, to take over and shut down the town as being too dangerous to permit continued occupancy, the main contaminant being dioxin. One of the children in the Cordladdie Park subdivision had recently been diagnosed as having leukemia. Now this water scare had surfaced, and it seemed obvious that the chemicals had seeped from the ground at the Cadillac/Fairfield site, leaching down into the water table, and contaminating the aquifer from which their water came.

We had advised the association members who had been delegated to consult with us that at that time it seemed futile to initiate suit against Cadillac/Fairfield or against EPA. Now they want us to bring suit against the R. P. Water Co., contending that it knowingly sold and delivered to the Cordladdie Park customers water that was dangerous and unhealthy to drink and had imposed emotional distress and physical illness upon the customers in the process (not to mention the present inconvenience). Association members also felt that they were entitled to damages for the company's breach of its water-supply contracts and for its negligence in operating its business, to the damage of the plaintiffs.

SCENARIO: CATCHER CHEMICAL/CATCHER RECYCLING EPA INVESTIGATION (1986)

After looking into the complaints that had been forwarded to it, noting the deep concern of Governor Deukmejian, and accepting the state of California's sense of urgency as sincere and well founded, EPA decided to conduct its own inspection of the Catcher Chemical Co./Catcher Recycling Co. waste-treatment and disposition site in the Antelope Valley, Los Angeles County, adjacent to the Armagosa Creek in the northwestern half of the southwestern fourth of section 15, Twp. 7 north, Rge. 12 west of the San Bernardino meridian.

The EPA investigation revealed contamination not only of the soil but of the groundwater at the site. It was determined that Catcher Recycling had used the site for bulk storage and deposit, and also had, for a period of two years, operated an incinerator on the site for the destruction of hazardous wastes. The incinerator site had become contaminated, and Catcher Recycling had shut it down under threat that if it continued in operation, the state would close it down. Catcher Recycling ceased recycling and other waste operations and disposition and treatment activities, removed all its equipment from the site, including three above-ground storage tanks, and has been exploring other activities that it could pursue.

EPA has chosen a "pump and treat" remedy estimated to cost $20 million. EPA was prepared to expend Superfund dollars to accomplish the remedy when Catcher Recycling president Frank Catcher found a set of records identifying what parties had shipped waste materials to Catcher for incineration.

EPA's review of these records has revealed the following generators of waste.

Company	Subtance	Amount
Catcher Chemical Co.	solvents	150,000 gal.
Pac. Gas & Elect. Co., Windpower Division	contaminated oil	125,000 gal.
Kinkus Stamp Fluid	solvents	250,000 gal.
Vintage Properties, Inc.	sludge	150 gal.
Belgian Paint Girl Co.	off-spec. paint	40,000 gal.
Smell Oil Co.	solvents	180,000 gal.
Marine Lift, Inc.	solvents	6,700 gal.
Now Chemical Co.	sludge	3,500 gal.
Equipment Dist. Co.	solvents	17,500 gal.
Specialties Products Co.	solvents and mixed waste	50,000 gal.

Company	Subtance	Amount
Crop Dusters of A.V.	mixed pesticides	550 gal.
A.V. Country Club	HTH	10 drums
Burger Queen of A.V.	#6 fuel oil	750 gal.
U.S. Coast Guard	bilge oil	10,000 gal.
Energy Conservation Co.	off-spec. foam insul.	750 drums
Lockheed Aircraft Co.	solvents	10,000 gal.
U.S. Air Force (plant 42)	jet fuel and sand	2,500 gal.
Velco Dept. Store	bottom sludge/water	3,000 gal.
Harbor Services	contaminated water	15,000 gal.
Zamco Distributors	solvents	2,000 drums

The following information is not known to EPA

1. Catcher Chemical, Burger Queen, Specialties Products, and Zamco received certificates of incineration.

2. Pacific Gas and Electric, Windpower Division, shipped oil contaminated with PCBs to Catcher Recycling Co.

3. Kinkus Stamp Fluid and Waste Disposal Co. pumped solvents out of a lagoon at Safeway, Inc., in Lancaster, hauling it to Rolling Reduction Smelting Co. in Mojave, and arranged for Catcher Recycling Co. to pick up the waste at the Rolling Reduction Smelting Co. site. Catcher Recycling invoiced Kinkus, and Kinkus thereupon invoiced Safeway, Inc., in the same amount.

4. Victor Vinson called the state Department of Environmental Protection after his home heating oil truck sprung a leak and ran into his swimming pool. He was referred to Catcher Recycling, which pumped out his pool.

5. Harbor Services, Inc., called Catcher Recycling Co. for Marine Lift, Inc., to have it pump sludge from an abandoned barge that was in the way of operations at Marine Lift, Inc. Catcher Recycling invoiced Harbor Services, which, in turn, forwarded the bill to Marine Lift, Inc.

6. Burger Queen's heating oil tank, which Catcher Recycling had pumped out and cleaned, frequently clogged. Burger Queen had, from time to time, added various types of solvents in an attempt to solve the problem before calling Catcher Recycling.

SCENARIO: KINKUS DISPOSAL CO. (1986)

Kinkus Disposal Co. is a small recycler of industrial wastes. From 1955 through 1984, the activity of transporting and disposing of or recycling hazardous industrial wastes accounted for the major share of its gross profits.

Kinkus, a California corporation, originated as a business dedicated to the production and marketing in bulk of a fluid consisting principally of 1,1,1-trichloroethane for use in detecting water-mark identification signs on postage stamps. After unsatisfactorily struggling with the need to dispose of its own waste products, it concluded that it was best served by creating the capacity to handle such disposition itself. Initially as an accommodation, it sometimes provided this service for other firms. After a time, it decided to expand its capacity and to market that service, which it performed for a numer of years as a very profitable operation. Ultimately it took action to officially include the words "and Waste Disposal" in its corporate name.

Although the stamp fluid side of its business is still producing a tolerable profit, Kinkus finds itself on the verge of bankruptcy as a consequence of difficulties experienced in complying with all applicable state and federal statutes and regulations controlling the hazardous-waste transport, disposition, and recycling end of its business. Since 1982, Kinkus has subcontracted with Specialties Products Co. to obtain 1,1,1-trichlorothane for its stamp fluid division, and also has contracted with that firm on occasion to dispose of accumulating quantities of that product, which, as a consequence of Kinkus's bottling operation, intermittently become contaminated with impurities that stamp fluid customers would complain about. Kinkus has fallen further and further in arrears in meeting its payment obligations to Specialties Products, which, on July 10, 1984, notified Kinkus that it would no longer transport or dispose of any Kinkus waste products or supply it with chemicals until its account was paid. A similar situation has been developing with respect to the Rolling Reduction Co. of Mojave as to payments for services rendered. However, Rolling Reduction has not cut Kinkus off, but has put it on a "cash on delivery" basis until Kinkus substantially reduces its arrears.

On July 15, 1984, Kinkus advised its employees that unless operating costs were cut substantially within the next two quarters, it would have to retrench, and its first major cut would be with respect to the night shift. That shift is the one that does the bulk of the pickup, transport, and disposal of waste products. Since that time, on two or three evenings a week, day-shift driver Ben Jones has come in late from the day shift and has logged on as overtime a night-shift stint. Unknown to anyone but Kinkus's night-shift operations foreman, Bart Vigorito, who devised the scheme with Ben Jones over beer and pretzels at a bar. Ben has been loading most of the more treacherous liquid-waste products into a tanker truck, which he and Bart have rigged so that Ben can open the drainage valve from the cab as he drives down the road. Selecting little-used country roads, often in the foothills, including most of the roads between the Pearblossom Highway exit from the Antelope Valley Freeway (one of which was the Elizabeth Lake Road and its unpaved "tributaries") and the exit to Mojave, Ben has cruised his nightly run and returned before dawn with an empty rig. Last week Ben told Bart that he was going to have to stop working nights because even though the overtime pay was great, his girl friend was getting angry because she didn't get to see him as often as she liked. Ben said that he would keep on a little longer because he wanted to save enough to buy a new car, but that would be it.

Anticipating the possible ultimate need to file for voluntary bankruptcy, Kinkus's accountants were attempting to consolidate all outstanding accounts. In the process, they came across an old purchase order from Catcher Chemical Co., which they sent to you as the Kinkus Company attorney, because they were aware of the worries that the Kinkus management team was experiencing over possible liability for the company's past disposal practices.

SCENARIO: ON-SITE LOW-LEVEL RADIOACTIVE WASTE STORAGE (SAN ONOFRE NUCLEAR GENERATING STATION)

In 1963, Congress, through the passage of PL 88-82, 77 Stat. 115, authorized the Secretary of the Navy to grant an easement over a portion of Camp Pendleton, Calif., "for the construction, operation, maintenance, and use of a nuclear electric generating station, consisting of one or more generating units, and appurtenances thereto." Following the grant of the authorized easement, executed on May 12, 1964, three generating plants, with a combined capacity of 2650 megawatts, were constructed on the easement site. The easement was for a 60-year term, grantees being the Southern California Edison Company (a majority interest), the San Diego Gas and Electric Co., and cities of Riverside and Anaheim (minority interests) as cotenants in common, upon "87 acres of Camp Pendleton's northern shorefront." An additional 387 acres surrounding the easement site was made subject to the creation of an "exclusion area" within which the San Onofre Nuclear Generating Station (SONGS) had the right to exclude or remove personnel and property in order to protect the public health and safety.

On March 29, 1982, the Department of the Navy executed a lease of a separate but nearby parcel consisting of 49.10 acres, desired by Southern California Edison for "the provision of maintenance, repair, support, and emergency services to the San Onofre Nuclear Power Station. . ."

In 1980, Congress enacted the Low-Level Radioactive Waste Policy Act, partly in response to the growing resistance arising in the states of Nevada, South Carolina, and Washington to continued status as the disposal sites for all of the nation's nuclear waste. Low-level waste from SONGS was consigned to the Richland, Wash., facility. Under the 1980 Act, states were given five years to provide a facility for long-term storage of low-level radioactive waste (LORAD waste) within their own state, or through an interstate compact, within an abutting state. California proposed to enter into such a compact with Arizona. However, California "dragged its feet" and Arizona was lethargic. It soon became apparent to the Nuclear Regulatory Commission (NRC) [which had displaced the old Atomic Energy Commission (AEC)] that California and a number of other states would not meet the deadline set by the 1980 Act. The NRC thus found itself obliged to relax its own restrictions on onsite storage of LORAD waste and to establish standards for such temporary on-site storage. This was accomplished through the issuance, on November 10, 1981, to "all holders of and applicants for operating licenses and construction permits" of "Generic Letter 81-83," which begins: "Subject: Storage of

Low-Level Radioactive Waste at Power Plant Sites." Under the 1980 Act, after the last day of 1985, the three present recipient states would no longer be obliged to accept LORAD waste from any out-of-state power-plant operator. All three announced their intent to take full advantage of this right of denial.

With the necessary legislation in place, it will take an estimated four years or more of construction time to build a functioning LORAD-waste-disposal facility, Following issuance of the 1981 NRC letter, which, inter alia, set forth specific criteria governing the construction and operation of an on-site interim storage facility, the owners of the SONGS facility decided to build a concrete warehouse (wall thickness of 2 feet or more) for such interim storage. When this decision was reached, it provoked a question as to "whether use of the facility for the storage of low-level nuclear waste on the Camp Pendleton easement property is prohibited by 10 U.S.C. sec. 1692, enacted in 1984." Southern California Edison received a memo of law dated May, 31, 1985, prepared for it by outside counsel, Orrick, Herrington & Sutcliffe, which concludes that "section 2692 does not apply to construction of an interim LORAD waste storage facility at SONGS." That memo agreed with in-house counsel's conclusions.

Ideally, you would prefer that this facility be built on the leasehold you have at Pendleton, but you can accommodate it on the easement ground if that becomes necessary. You should be certain that geographically and geologically you could do so, in anticipation of the probability that the Pendleton commander and superiors do not want your waste storage anywhere within the camp area. It should be noted that, on February 7, 1985, a bill was introduced (H.R. 1083, 99th Congress, 1st Session) seeking to amend the Low-Level Radioactive Waste Policy Act for the purpose, inter alia, of extending the time during which the three existing LORAD waste-storage states must continue to accept LORAD waste from out-of-state generators.

Appendix **A**

Extremely Hazardous Substances and Their Threshold Planning Quantities (Section 302 of SARA)

CAS No.	Chemical name	Notes	Reportable quantity* (pounds)	Threshold planning quantity (pounds)
75–86–5	Acetone Cyanohydrin		10	1,000
1752–30–3	Acetone Thiosemicarbazide	e	1	1,000/10,000
107–02–8	Acrolein		1	500
79–06–1	Acrylamide	d, l	5,000	1,000/10,000
107–13–1	Acrylonitrile	d, l	100	10,000
814–68–6	Acrylyl Chloride	e, h	1	100
111–69–3	Adiponitrile	e, l	1	1,000
116–06–3	Aldicarb	c	1	100/10,000
309–00–2	Aldrin	d	1	500/10,000
107–18–6	Allyl Alcohol		100	1,000
107–11–9	Allylamine	e	1	500
20859–73–8	Aluminum Phosphide	b	100	500
54–62–6	Aminopterin	e	1	500/10,000
78–53–5	Amiton	e	1	500
3734–97–2	Amiton Oxalate	l	1	100/10,000
7664–41–7	Ammonia		100	500
16919–58–7	Ammonium Chloroplatinate	a, e	1	10,000
300–62–9	Amphetamine	e	1	1,000
62–53–3	Aniline	d, l	5,000	1,000
88–05–1	Aniline, 2,4,6-Trimethyl-	e	1	500
7783–70–2	Antimony Pentafluoride	e	1	500
1397–94–0	Antimycin A	c, e	1	1,000/10,000
86–88–4	ANTU		100	500/10,000
1303–28–2	Arsenic Pentoxide	d	5,000	100/10,000
1327–53–3	Arsenous Oxide	d, h	5,000	100/10,000
7784–34–1	Arsenous Trichloride	d	5,000	500
7784–42–1	Arsine	e	1	100
2642–71–9	Azinphos-Ethyl	e	1	100/10,000
86–50–0	Azinphos-Methyl		1	10/10,000
1405–87–4	Bacitracin	a, e	1	10,000
98–87–3	Benzal Chloride	d	5,000	500
98–16–8	Benzenamine, 3-(Trifluoromethyl)-	e	1	500
100–14–1	Benzene, 1-(Chloromethyl)-4-Nitro-	e	1	500/10,000
98–05–5	Benzenearsonic Acid	e	1	10/10,000
98–09–9	Benzenesulfonyl Chloride	a	100	10,000
3615–21–2	Benzimidazole, 4,5-Dichloro-2-(Trifluoromethyl)-	e, g	1	500/10,000
98–07–7	Benzotrichloride	d	1	100
100–44–7	Benzyl Chloride	d	100	500
140–29–4	Benzyl Cyanide	e, h	1	500
15271–41–7	Bicyclo[2.2.1]Heptane-2-Carbonitrile, 5-Chloro-6-((((Methylamino)Carbonyl)Oxy)Imino)-, (1s-(1-alpha, 2-beta, 4-alpha, 5-alpha, 6E))-.	e	1	500/10,000
534–07–6	Bis(Chloromethyl) Ketone	e	1	10/10,000
4044–65–9	Bitoscanate	e	1	500/10,000
10294–34–5	Boron Trichloride	e	1	500
7637–07–2	Boron Trifluoride	e	1	500
353–42–4	Boron Trifluoride Compound With Methyl Ether (1:1)	e	1	1,000
28772–56–7	Bromadiolone	e	1	100/10,000

Source: Federal Register, **52,** No. 7 (April 22, 1987), pp. 13397–13403.

CAS No.	Chemical name	Notes	Reportable quantity* (pounds)	Threshold planning quantity (pounds)
7726-95-6	Bromine	e, l	1	500
106-99-0	Butadiene	a, e	1	10,000
109-19-3	Butyl Isovalerate	a, e	1	10,000
111-34-2	Butyl Vinyl Ether	a, e	1	10,000
1306-19-0	Cadmium Oxide	e	1	100/10,000
2223-93-0	Cadmium Stearate	c, e	1	1,000/10,000
7778-44-1	Calcium Arsenate	d	1,000	500/10,000
8001-35-2	Camphechlor	d	1	500/10,000
56-25-7	Cantharidin	e	1	100/10,000
51-83-2	Carbachol Chloride	e	1	500/10,000
26419-73-8	Carbamic Acid, Methyl-, 0-(((2,4-Dimethyl-1, 3-Dithiolan-2-yl)Methylene)Amino)-	e	1	100/10,000
1563-66-2	Carbofuran		10	10/10,000
75-15-0	Carbon Disulfide	l	100	10,000
786-19-6	Carbophenothion	e	1	500
2244-16-8	Carvone	a, e	1	10,000
57-74-9	Chlordane	d	1	1,000
470-90-6	Chlorfenvinfos	e	1	500
7782-50-5	Chlorine		10	100
24934-91-6	Chlormephos	e	1	500
999-81-5	Chlormequat Chloride	e, h	1	100/10,000
107-20-0	Chloroacetaldehyde	a	1,000	10,000
79-11-8	Chloroacetic Acid	e	1	100/10,000
107-07-3	Chloroethanol	e	1	500
627-11-2	Chloroethyl Chloroformate	e	1	1,000
67-66-3	Chloroform	d, l	5,000	10,000
542-88-1	Chloromethyl Ether	d, h	1	100
107-30-2	Chloromethyl Methyl Ether	c, d	1	100
3691-35-8	Chlorophacinone	e	1	100/10,000
1982-47-4	Chloroxuron	e	1	500/10,000
21923-23-9	Chlorthiophos	e, h	1	500
10025-73-7	Chromic Chloride	e	1	1/10,000
7440-48-4	Cobalt	a, e	1	10,000
62207-76-5	Cobalt, ((2,2'-(1,2-Ethanediylbis (Nitrilomethylidyne))Bis(6-Fluorophenolato))(2-)-N,N',O,O')-,	e	1	100/10,000
10210-68-1	Cobalt Carbonyl	e, h	1	10/10,000
64-86-8	Colchicine	e, h	1	10/10,000
117-52-2	Coumafuryl	a, e	1	10,000
56-72-4	Coumaphos		10	100/10,000
5836-29-3	Coumatetralyl	e	1	500/10,000
95-48-7	Cresol, o-	d	1,000	1,000/10,000
535-89-7	Crimidine	e	1	100/10,000
4170-30-3	Crotonaldehyde		100	1,000
123-73-9	Crotonaldehyde, (E)-		100	1,000
506-68-3	Cyanogen Bromide		1,000	500/10,000
506-78-5	Cyanogen Iodide	e	1	1,000/10,000
2636-26-2	Cyanophos	e	1	1,000
675-14-9	Cyanuric Fluoride	e	1	100
66-81-9	Cycloheximide	e	1	100/10,000
108-91-8	Cyclohexylamine	e, l	1	10,000
287-92-3	Cyclopentane	a, e	1	10,000
633-03-4	C. I. Basic Green 1	a, e	1	10,000
17702-41-9	Decaborane(14)	e	1	500/10,000
8065-48-3	Demeton	e	1	500
919-86-8	Demeton-S-Methyl	e	1	500
10311-84-9	Dialifor	e	1	100/10,000
19287-45-7	Diborane	e	1	100
84-74-2	Dibutyl Phthalate	a	10	10,000
8023-53-8	Dichlorobenzalkonium Chloride	a, e	1	10,000
111-44-4	Dichloroethyl Ether	d	1	10,000
149-74-6	Dichloromethylphenylsilane	e	1	1,000
62-73-7	Dichlorvos		10	1,000
141-66-2	Dicrotophos	e	1	100
1464-53-5	Diepoxybutane	d	1	500
814-49-3	Diethyl Chlorophosphate	e, h	1	500
1642-54-2	Diethylcarbamazine Citrate	e	1	100/10,000
93-05-0	Diethyl-p-Phenylenediamine	a, e	1	10,000
71-63-6	Digitoxin	c, e	1	100/10,000
2238-07-5	Diglycidyl Ether	e	1	1,000
20830-75-5	Digoxin	e, h	1	10/10,000
115-26-4	Dimefox	e	1	500
60-51-5	Dimethoate		10	500/10,000
2524-03-0	Dimethyl Phosphorochloridothioate	e	1	500
131-11-3	Dimethyl Phthalate	a	5,000	10,000
77-78-1	Dimethyl Sulfate	d	1	500
75-18-3	Dimethyl Sulfide	d	1	100
75-78-5	Dimethyldichlorosilane	e, h	1	500
57-14-7	Dimethylhydrazine	d	1	1,000
99-98-9	Dimethyl-p-Phenylenediamine	e	1	10/10,000
644-64-4	Dimetilan	e	1	500/10,000
534-52-1	Dinitrocresol		10	10/10,000
88-85-7	Dinoseb		1,000	100/10,000
1420-07-1	Dinoterb	e	1	500/10,000
117-84-0	Dioctyl Phthalate	a, e	5,000	10,000
78-34-2	Dioxathion	e	1	500
646-06-0	Dioxolane	a, e	1	10,000
82-66-6	Diphacinone	e	1	10/10,000
152-16-9	Diphosphoramide, Octamethyl-		100	100
298-04-4	Disulfoton		1	500

CAS No.	Chemical name	Notes	Reportable quantity* (pounds)	Threshold planning quantity (pounds)
514–73–8	Dithiazanine Iodide	e	1	500/10,000
541–53–7	Dithiobiuret		100	100/10,000
316–42–7	Emetine, Dihydrochloride	e, h	1	1/10,000
115–29–7	Endosulfan		1	10/10,000
2778–04–3	Endothion	e	1	500/10,000
72–20–8	Endrin		1	500/10,000
106–89–8	Epichlorohydrin	d, l	1,000	1,000
2104–64–5	EPN	e	1	100/10,000
50–14–6	Ergocalciferol	c, e	1	1,000/10,000
379–79–3	Ergotamine Tartrate	e	1	500/10,000
1622–32–8	Ethanesulfonyl Chloride, 2-Chloro-	e	1	500
10140–87–1	Ethanol, 1,2-Dichloro-, Acetate	e	1	1,000
563–12–2	Ethion		10	1,000
13194–48–4	Ethoprophos	e	1	1,000
538–07–8	Ethylbis(2-Chloroethyl)Amine	e, h	1	500
371–62–0	Ethylene Fluorohydrin	c, e, h	1	10
75–21–8	Ethylene Oxide	d, l	1	1,000
107–15–3	Ethylenediamine		5,000	10,000
151–56–4	Ethyleneimine	d	1	500
2235–25–8	Ethylmercuric Phosphate	a, e	1	10,000
542–90–5	Ethylthiocyanate	e	1	10,000
22224–92–6	Fenamiphos	e	1	10/10,000
122–14–5	Fenitrothion	e	1	500
115–90–2	Fensulfothion	e, h	1	500
4301–50–2	Fluenetil	e	1	100/10,000
7782–41–4	Fluorine	k	10	500
640–19–7	Fluoroacetamide	j	100	100/10,000
144–49–0	Fluoroacetic Acid		1	10/10,000
359–06–8	Fluoroacetyl Chloride	c, e	1	10
51–21–8	Fluorouracil	e	1	500/10,000
944–22–9	Fonofos	e	1	500
50–00–0	Formaldehyde	d,l	1,000	500
107–16–4	Formaldehyde Cyanohydrin	e, h	1	1,000
23422–53–9	Formetanate Hydrochloride	e,h	1	500/10,000
2540–82–1	Formothion	e	1	100
17702–57–7	Formparanate	e	1	100/10,000
21548–32–3	Fosthietan	e	1	500
3878–19–1	Fuberidazole	e	1	100/10,000
110–00–9	Furan		100	500
13450–90–3	Gallium Trichloride	e	1	500/10,000
77–47–4	Hexachlorocyclopentadiene	d, h	1	100
1335–87–1	Hexachloronaphthalene	a, e	1	10,000
4835–11–4	Hexamethylenediamine, N,N'-Dibutyl-	e	1	500
302–01–2	Hydrazine	d	1	1,000
74–90–8	Hydrocyanic Acid		10	100
7647–01–0	Hydrogen Chloride (Gas Only)	e, l	1	500
7664–39–3	Hydrogen Fluoride		100	100
7722–84–1	Hydrogen Peroxide (Conc >52%)	e, l	1	1,000
7783–07–5	Hydrogen Selenide	e	1	10
7783–06–4	Hydrogen Sulfide	l	100	500
123–31–9	Hydroquinone	l	1	500/10,000
53–86–1	Indomethacin	a, e	1	10,000
10025–97–5	Iridium Tetrachloride	a, e	1	10,000
13463–40–6	Iron, Pentacarbonyl-	e	1	100
297–78–9	Isobenzan	e	1	100/10,000
78–82–0	Isobutyronitrile	e, h	1	1,000
102–36–3	Isocyanic Acid, 3,4-Dichlorophenyl Ester	e	1	500/10,000
465–73–6	Isodrin		1	100/10,000
55–91–4	Isofluorphate	c	100	100
4098–71–9	Isophorone Diisocyanate	b, e	1	100
108–23–6	Isopropyl Chloroformate	e	1	1,000
625–55–8	Isopropyl Formate	e	1	500
119–38–0	Isopropylmethylpyrazolyl Dimethylcarbamate	e	1	500
78–97–7	Lactonitrile	e	1	1,000
21609–90–5	Leptophos	e	1	500/10,000
541–25–3	Lewisite	c, e, h	1	10
58–89–9	Lindane	d	1	1,000/10,000
7580–67–8	Lithium Hydride	b, e	1	100
109–77–3	Malononitrile		1,000	500/10,000
12108–13–3	Manganese, Tricarbonyl Methylcyclopentadienyl	e, h	1	100
51–75–2	Mechlorethamine	c, e	1	10
950–10–7	Mephosfolan	e	1	500
1600–27–7	Mercuric Acetate	e	1	500/10,000
7487–94–7	Mercuric Chloride	e	1	500/10,000
21908–53–2	Mercuric Oxide	e	1	500/10,000
108–67–8	Mesitylene	a, e	1	10,000
10476–95–6	Methacrolein Diacetate	e	1	1,000
760–93–0	Methacrylic Anhydride	e	1	500
126–98–7	Methacrylonitrile	h	1	500
920–46–7	Methacryloyl Chloride	e	1	100
30674–80–7	Methacryloyloxyethyl Isocyanate	e, h	1	100
10265–92–6	Methamidophos	e	1	100/10,000
558–25–8	Methanesulfonyl Fluoride	e	1	1,000
950–37–8	Methidathion	e	1	500/10,000
2032–65–7	Methiocarb		10	500/10,000
16752–77–5	Methomyl	h	100	500/10,000

CAS No.	Chemical name	Notes	Reportable quantity* (pounds)	Threshold planning quantity (pounds)
151–38–2	Methoxyethylmercuric Acetate	e	1	500/10,000
80–63–7	Methyl 2-Chloroacrylate	e	1	500
74–83–9	Methyl Bromide	l	1,000	1,000
79–22–1	Methyl Chloroformate	d, h	1,000	500
624–92–0	Methyl Disulfide	e	1	100
60–34–4	Methyl Hydrazine		10	500
624–83–9	Methyl Isocyanate	f	1	500
556–61–6	Methyl Isothiocyanate	b, e	1	500
74–93–1	Methyl Mercaptan		100	500
3735–23–7	Methyl Phenkapton	e	1	500
676–97–1	Methyl Phosphonic Dichloride	b, e	1	100
556–64–9	Methyl Thiocyanate	e	1	10,000
78–94–4	Methyl Vinyl Ketone	e	1	10
502–39–6	Methylmercuric Dicyanamide	e	1	500/10,000
75–79–6	Methyltrichlorosilane	e, h	1	500
1129–41–5	Metolcarb	e	1	100/10,000
7786–34–7	Mevinphos		10	500
315–18–4	Mexacarbate		1,000	500/10,000
50–07–7	Mitomycin C	d	1	500/10,000
6923–22–4	Monocrotophos	e	1	10/10,000
2763–96–4	Muscimol	a, h	1,000	10,000
505–60–2	Mustard Gas	e, h	1	500
7440–02–0	Nickel	a, d	1	10,000
13463–39–3	Nickel Carbonyl	d	1	1
54–11–5	Nicotine	c	100	100
65–30–5	Nicotine Sulfate	e	1	100/10,000
7697–37–2	Nitric Acid		1,000	1,000
10102–43–9	Nitric Oxide	c	10	100
98–95–3	Nitrobenzene	l	1,000	10,000
1122–60–7	Nitrocyclohexane	e	1	500
10102–44–0	Nitrogen Dioxide		10	100
62–75–9	Nitrosodimethylamine	d, h	1	1,000
991–42–4	Norbormide	e	1	100/10,000
0	Organorhodium Complex (PMN–82–147)	e	1	10/10,000
65–86–1	Orotic Acid	a, e	1	10,000
20816–12–0	Osmium Tetroxide	a	1,000	10,000
630–60–4	Ouabain	c, e	1	100/10,000
23135–22–0	Oxamyl	e	1	100/10,000
78–71–7	Oxetane, 3,3-Bis(Chloromethyl)-	l	e	500
2497–07–6	Oxydisulfoton	e, h	1	500
10028–15–6	Ozone	e	1	100
1910–42–5	Paraquat	e	·1	10/10,000
2074–50–2	Paraquat Methosulfate	e	1	10/10,000
56–38–2	Parathion	c, d	1	100
298–00–0	Parathion-Methyl	c	100	100/10,000
12002–03–8	Paris Green	d	100	500/10,000
19624–22–7	Pentaborane	e	1	500
76–01–7	Pentachloroethane	a, d	1	10,000
87–86–5	Pentachlorophenol	a, d	10	10,000
2570–26–5	Pentadecylamine	e	1	100/10,000
79–21–0	Peracetic Acid	e	1	500
594–42–3	Perchloromethylmercaptan		100	500
108–95–2	Phenol		1,000	500/10,000
97–18–7	Phenol, 2,2'-Thiobis(4,6-Dichloro-	e	1	100/10,000
4418–66–0	Phenol, 2,2'-Thiobis(4-Chloro-6-Methyl-Phenol, 2,2'-Thiobis (4-Chloro-6-Methyl)-	e	1	100/10,000
64–00–6	Phenol, 3-(1-Methylethyl)-, Methylcarbamate	e	1	500/10,000
58–36–6	Phenoxarsine, 10,10'-Oxydi-	e	1	500/10,000
696–28–6	Phenyl Dichloroarsine	d, h	1	500
59–88–1	Phenylhydrazine Hydrochloride	e	1	1,000/10,000
62–38–4	Phenylmercury Acetate		100	500/10,000
2097–19–0	Phenylsilatrane	e, h	1	100/10,000
103–85–5	Phenylthiourea		100	100/10,000
298–02–2	Phorate		10	10
4104–14–7	Phosacetim	e	1	100/10,000
947–02–4	Phosfolan	e	1	100/10,000
75–44–5	Phosgene	l	10	10
732–11–6	Phosmet	e	1	10/10,000
13171–21–6	Phosphamidon	e	1	100
7803–51–2	Phosphine		100	500
2703–13–1	Phosphonothioic Acid, Methyl-, O-Ethyl O-(4-(Methylthio)Phenyl Ester	e	1	500
50782–69–9	Phosphonothioic Acid, Methyl-, S-(2-(Bis(1-Methylethyl)Amino)Ethyl O-Ethyl Ester	e	1	100
2665–30–7	Phosphonothioic Acid, Methyl-, O-(4-Nitrophenyl) O-Phenyl Ester	e	1	500
3254–63–5	Phosphoric Acid, Dimethyl 4-(Methylthio) Phenyl Ester	e	1	500
2587–90–8	Phosphorothioic Acid, O,O-Dimethyl-S-(2-Methylthio) Ethyl Ester	c, e, g	1	500
7723–14–0	Phosphorus	b, h	1	100
10025–87–3	Phosphorus Oxychloride	d	1,000	500
10026–13–8	Phosphorus Pentachloride	b, e	1	500
1314–56–3	Phosphorus Pentoxide	b, e	1	10
7719–12–2	Phosphorus Trichloride		1,000	1,000
84–80–0	Phylloquinone	a, e	1	10,000
57–47–6	Physostigmine	e	1	100/10,000
57–64–7	Physostigmine, Salicylate (1:1)	e	1	100/10,000
124–87–8	Picrotoxin	e	1	500/10,000
110–89–4	Piperidine	e	1	1,000
5281–13–0	Piprotal	e	1	100/10,000
23505–41–1	Pirimifos-Ethyl	e	1	1,000
10025–65–7	Platinous Chloride	a, e	1	10,000

CAS No.	Chemical name	Notes	Reportable quantity* (pounds)	Threshold planning quantity (pounds)
13454-96-1	Platinum Tetrachloride	a, e	1	10,000
10124-50-2	Potassium Arsenite	d	1,000	500/10,000
151-50-8	Potassium Cyanide	b	10	100
506-61-6	Potassium Silver Cyanide	b	1	500
2631-37-0	Promecarb	e, h	1	500/10,000
106-96-7	Propargyl Bromide	e	1	10
57-57-8	Propiolactone, Beta-	e	1	500
107-12-0	Propionitrile		10	500
542-76-7	Propionitrile, 3-Chloro-		1,000	1,000
70-69-9	Propiophenone, 4-Amino-	e, g	1	100/10,000
109-61-5	Propyl Chloroformate	e	1	500
1331-17-5	Propylene Glycol, Allyl Ether	a, e	1	10,000
75-56-9	Propylene Oxide	l	100	10,000
75-55-8	Propyleneimine	d	1	10,000
2275-18-5	Prothoate	e	1	100/10,000
95-63-6	Pseudocumene	a, e	1	10,000
129-00-0	Pyrene	c	5,000	1,000/10,000
140-76-1	Pyridine, 2-Methyl-5-Vinyl-	e	1	500
504-24-5	Pyridine, 4-Amino-	h	1,000	500/10,000
1124-33-0	Pyridine, 4-Nitro-, 1-Oxide	e, h	1	500/10,000
53558-25-1	Pyriminil	a, e	1	100/10,000
10049-07-7	Rhodium Trichloride	e	1	10,000
14167-18-1	Salcomine	e	1	500/10,000
107-44-8	Sarin	e, h	10	10
7783-00-8	Selenious Acid	e, h	10	1,000/10,000
7791-23-3	Selenium Oxychloride	e	1	500
563-41-7	Semicarbazide Hydrochloride	e	1	1,000/10,000
3037-72-7	Silane, (4-Aminobutyl)Diethoxymethyl-	e	1	1,000
128-56-3	Sodium Anthraquinone-1-Sulfonate	a, e	1	10,000
7631-89-2	Sodium Arsenate	d	1,000	1,000/10,000
7784-46-5	Sodium Arsenite	d	1,000	500/10,000
26628-22-8	Sodium Azide (Na(N3))	b	1,000	500
124-65-2	Sodium Cacodylate	e	1	100/10,000
143-33-9	Sodium Cyanide (Na(CN))	b	10	100
62-74-8	Sodium Fluoroacetate		10	10/10,000
131-52-2	Sodium Pentachlorophenate	e	1	100/10,000
13410-01-0	Sodium Selenate	e	1	100/10,000
10102-18-8	Sodium Selenite	h	100	100/10,000
10102-20-2	Sodium Tellurite	e	1	500/10,000
900-95-8	Stannane, Acetoxytriphenyl-	e, g	1	500/10,000
57-24-9	Strychnine	c	10	100/10,000
60-41-3	Strychnine, Sulfate	e	1	100/10,000
3689-24-5	Sulfotep		100	500
3569-57-1	Sulfoxide, 3-Chloropropyl Octyl	e	1	500
7446-09-5	Sulfur Dioxide	e, l	1	500
7783-60-0	Sulfur Tetrafluoride	e	1	100
7446-11-9	Sulfur Trioxide	b, e	1	100
7664-93-9	Sulfuric Acid		1,000	1,000
77-81-6	Tabun	c, e, h	10	10
13494-80-9	Tellurium	e	1	500/10,000
7783-80-4	Tellurium Hexafluoride	e, k	10	100
107-49-3	TEPP		10	100
13071-79-9	Terbufos	e, h	1	100
78-00-2	Tetraethyllead	c, d	10	100
597-64-8	Tetraethyltin	c, e	1	100
75-74-1	Tetramethyllead	c, e, l	10	100
509-14-8	Tetranitromethane		10	500
1314-32-5	Thallic Oxide	a	100	10,000
10031-59-1	Thallium Sulfate	h	100	100/10,000
6533-73-9	Thallous Carbonate	c, h	100	100/10,000
7791-12-0	Thallous Chloride	c, h	100	100/10,000
2757-18-8	Thallous Malonate	c, e, h	100	100/10,000
7446-18-6	Thallous Sulfate		100	100/10,000
2231-57-4	Thiocarbazide	e	1	1,000/10,000
21564-17-0	Thiocyanic Acid, 2-(Benzothiazolylthio)Methyl Ester	a, e	1	10,000
39196-18-4	Thiofanox		100	100/10,000
640-15-3	Thiometon	a, e	1	10,000
297-97-2	Thionazin		100	500
108-98-5	Thiophenol		100	500
79-19-6	Thiosemicarbazide		100	100/10,000
5344-82-1	Thiourea, (2-Chlorophenyl)-		100	100/10,000
614-78-8	Thiourea, (2-Methylphenyl)-	e	1	500/10,000
7550-45-0	Titanium Tetrachloride	e	1	100
584-84-9	Toluene 2,4-Diisocyanate		100	500
91-08-7	Toluene 2,6-Diisocyanate		100	100
110-57-6	Trans-1,4-Dichlorobutene	e	1	500
1031-47-6	Triamiphos	e	1	500/10,000
24017-47-8	Triazofos	e	1	500
76-02-8	Trichloroacety Chloride	e	1	500
115-21-9	Trichloroethylsilane	e, h	1	500
327-98-0	Trichloronate	e, k	1	500
98-13-5	Trichlorophenylsilane	e, h	1	500
52-68-6	Trichlorophon	a	100	10,000
1558-25-4	Trichloro(Chloromethyl)Silane	e	1	100
27137-85-5	Trichloro(Dichlorophenyl)Silane	e	1	500

CAS No.	Chemical name	Notes	Reportable quantity* (pounds)	Threshold planning quantity (pounds)
998–30–1	Triethoxysilane	e	1	500
75–77–4	Trimethylchlorosilane	e	1	1,000
824–11–3	Trimethylolpropane Phosphite	e, h	1	100/10,000
1066–45–1	Trimethyltin Chloride	e	1	500/10,000
639–58–7	Triphenyltin Chloride	e	1	500/10,000
555–77–1	Tris(2-Chloroethyl)Amine	e, h	1	100
2001–95–8	Valinomycin	c, e	1	1,000/10,000
1314–62–1	Vanadium Pentoxide		1,000	100/10,000
108–05–4	Vinyl Acetate Monomer	d, l	5,000	1,000
3048–64–4	Vinylnorbornene	a, e	1	10,000
81–81–2	Warfarin		100	500/10,000
129–06–6	Warfarin Sodium	e, h	1	100/10,000
28347–13–9	Xylylene Dichloride	e	1	100/10,000
58270–08–9	Zinc, Dichloro(4,4-Dimethyl-5((((Methylamino) Carbonyl)Oxy)Imino)Pentanenitrile)-,(T-4)-..	e	1	100/10,000
1314–84–7	Zinc Phosphide	b	100	500

*Only the statutory or final RQ is shown. For more information, see 40 CFR Table 302.4

Notes:
a This chemical does not meet acute toxicity criteria. Its TPQ is set at 10,000 pounds.
b This material is a reactive solid. The TPQ does not default to 10,000 pounds for non-powder, non-molten, non-solution form.
c The calculated TPQ changed after technical review as described in the technical support document.
d Indicates that the RQ is subject to change when the assessment of potential carcinogenicity and/or other toxicity is completed.
e Statutory reportable quantity for purposes of notification under SARA sect 304(a)(2).
f The statutory 1 pound reportable quantity for methyl isocyanate may be adjusted in a future rulemaking action.
g New chemicals added that were not part of the original list of 402 substances.
h Revised TPQ based on new or re-evaluated toxicity data.
j TPQ is revised to its calculated value and does not change due to technical review as in proposed rule.
k The TPQ was revised after proposal due to calculation error.
l Chemicals on the original list that do not meet toxicity criteria but because of their high production volume and recognized toxicity are considered chemicals of concern ("Other chemicals").

Note: The 40 chemicals which are marked with an l have been deleted by the Administration of EPA on January 22, 1988.

Acutely Toxic Chemicals (CEPP) with CAS Numbers

Common Name	CAS Number
Acetone cyanohydrin	00075-86-5
* Acetone thiosemicarbazide	01752-30-3
Acrolein	00107-02-8
Acrylyl chloride	00814-68-6
Aldicarb	00116-06-3
Aldrin	00309-00-2
Allyl alcohol	00107-18-6
Allylamine	00107-11-9
Aluminum phosphide	20859-73-8
* Aminopterin	00054-62-6
* Amiton	00078-53-5
* Amiton oxalate	03734-97-2
Ammonium chloroplatinate	16919-58-7
* Amphetamine	00300-62-9
* Aniline, 2,4,6-trimethyl-	00088-05-1
Antimony pentafluoride	07783-70-2
* Antimycin A	01397-94-0
Antu	00086-88-4
* Arsenic pentoxide	01303-28-2
Arsenous oxide	01327-53-3
Arsenous trichloride	07784-34-1
Arsine	07784-42-1
* Azinphos-ethyl	02642-71-9
Azinphos-methyl	00086-50-0
* Bacitracin	01405-87-4
Benzal chloride	0098-87-3
Benzenamine, 3-(trifluoromethyl)-	00098-16-8
Benzene, 1-(chloromethyl)-4-nitro-	00100-14-1

Source: Federal Register, **52,** No. 107 (June 4, 1987).

Common Name	CAS Number
* Benzenearsonic acid	00098-05-5
Benzenesulfonyl chloride	00098-09-9
Benzotrichloride	00098-07-7
Benzyl chloride	00100-44-7
Benzyl cyanide	0140-29-4
* Bicyclo [2.2.1]heptane-2-carbontrile, 5-chloro . . .	15271-41-7
* Bis(chloromethyl) ketone	00534-07-6
* Bitoscanate	04044-65-9
Boron trichloride	10294-34-5
Boron trifluoride	07637-07-2
Boron trifluoride compound with methyl ether (1:1)	00353-42-4
Bromadiolone	28772-56-7
Butadiene	00106-99-0
Butyl isovalerate	00109-19-3
Butyl vinyl ether	00111-34-2
C.I. basic green 1	00633-03-4
Cadmium oxide	01306-19-0
Cadmium stearate	02223-93-0
Calcium arsenate	07778-44-1
Camphechlor	08001-35-2
* Cantharidin	00056-25-7
* Carbachol chloride	00051-83-2
* Carbamic acid, methyl-, O-[[(2,4-dimethyl . . .	26419-73-8
Carbofuran	01563-66-2
Carbophenothion	00786-19-6
Carvone	02244-16-8
* Chlordane	00057-74-9
Chlorfenvinfos	00470-90-6
Chlorine	07782-50-5
* Chlormephos	24934-91-6
Chlormequat chloride	00999-81-5
Chloroacetaldehyde	00107-20-0
Chloroacetic acid	00079-11-8
Chloroethanol	00107-07-3
* Chloroethyl chloroformate	00627-11-2
Chloromethyl ether	00542-88-1
* Chloromethyl methyl ether	00107-30-2
Chlorophacinone	03691-35-8
* Chloroxuron	01982-47-4
* Chlorthiophos	21923-23-9
Chromic chloride	10025-73-7
Cobalt	07440-48-4
Cobalt carbonyl	10210-68-1
* Cobalt, [[2,2'-[1,2-ethanediylbis(nitrilomethy . . .	62207-76-5
* Colchicine	00064-86-8
Coumafuryl	00117-52-2
Coumaphos	00056-72-4
* Coumatetralyl	05836-29-3

Common Name	CAS Number
Cresylic acid	00095-48-7
* Crimidine	00535-89-7
Crotonaldehyde	00123-73-9
Crotonaldehyde	04170-30-3
Cyanogen bromide	00506-68-3
Cyanogen iodide	00506-78-5
* Cyanophos	02636-26-2
Cyanuric fluoride	00675-14-9
Cycloheximide	00066-81-9
Cyclopentane	00287-92-3
Decaborane(14)	17702-41-9
Demeton	08065-48-3
* Demeton-S-methyl	00919-86-8
* Dialifos	10311-84-9
Diborane	19287-45-7
Dibutyl phthalate	00084-74-2
Dichlorobenzalkonium chloride	08023-53-8
Dichloroethyl ether	00111-44-4
Dichloromethylphenylsilane	00149-74-6
Dichlorvos	00062-73-7
Dicrotophos	00141-66-2
Diepoxybutane	01464-53-5
Diethyl chlorophosphate	00814-49-3
Diethyl-p-phenylenediamine	00093-05-0
* Diethylcarbamazine citrate	01642-54-2
* Digitoxin	00071-63-6
Diglycidyl ether	02238-07-5
* Digoxin	20830-75-5
* Dimefox	00115-26-4
Dimethoate	00060-51-5
Dimethyl phosphorochloridothioate	02524-03-0
Dimethyl phthalate	00131-11-3
Dimethyl sulfate	00077-78-1
Dimethyl sulfide	00075-18-3
Dimethyl-p-phenylenediamine	00099-98-9
Dimethyldichlorosilane	00075-78-5
* Dimethylhydrazine	00057-14-7
Dimetilan	00644-64-4
Dinitrocresol	00534-52-1
* Dinoseb	00088-85-7
Dinoterb	01420-07-1
Dioctyl phthalate	00117-84-0
Dioxathion	00078-34-2
Dioxolane	00646-06-0
Diphacinone	00082-66-6
Diphosphoramide, octamethyl-	00152-16-9
Disulfoton	00298-04-4
* Dithiazanine iodide	00514-73-8

Common Name	CAS Number
Dithiobiuret	00541-53-7
* EPN	02104-64-5
Emetine, dihydrochloride	00316-42-7
* Endosulfan	00115-29-7
Endothion	02778-04-3
* Endrin	00072-20-8
* Ergocalciferol	00050-14-6
* Ergotamine tartrate	00379-79-3
* Ethanesulfonyl chloride, 2-chloro-	01622-32-8
Ethanol, 1,2-dichloro-, acetate	10140-87-1
Ethion	00563-12-2
* Ethoprophos	13194-48-4
* Ethyl thiocyanate	00542-90-5
* Ethylbis (2-chloroethyl)amine	00538-07-8
Ethylene fluorohydrin	00371-62-0
Ethylenediamine	00107-15-3
* Ethyleneimine	00151-56-4
Ethylmercuric phosphate	02235-25-8
Fenamiphos	22224-92-6
Fenitrothion	00122-14-5
* Fensulfothion	00115-90-2
Fluenetil	04301-50-2
Fluorine	07782-41-4
* Fluoroacetamide	00640-19-7
* Fluoroacetic acid	00144-49-0
Fluoroacetyl chloride	00359-06-8
* Fluorouracil	00051-21-8
Fonofos	00944-22-9
Formaldehyde cyanohydrin	00107-16-4
* Formetanate	23422-53-9
* Formothion	02540-82-1
* Formparanate	17702-57-7
* Fosthietan	21548-32-3
* Fuberidazole	03878-19-1
Furan	00110-00-9
Gallium trichloride	13450-90-3
Hexachlorocyclopentadiene	00077-47-4
* Hexachloronaphthalene	01335-87-1
Hexamethylenediamine, N,N',-dibutyl-	04835-11-4
Hydrazine	00302-01-2
Hydrocyanic acid	00074-90-8
Hydrogen fluoride	07664-39-3
Hydrogen selenide	07783-07-5
* Indomethacin	00053-86-1
Iridium tetrachloride	10025-97-5
Iron, pentacarbonyl-	13463-40-6
* Isobenzan	00297-78-9
Isobutyronitrile	00078-82-0

Common Name	CAS Number
Isocyanic acid, 3,4-dichlorophenyl ester	00102-36-3
* Isodrin	00465-73-6
* Isofluorphate	00055-91-4
Isophorone diisocyanate	04098-71-9
Isopropyl chloroformate	00108-23-6
* Isopropyl formate	00625-55-8
* Isopropylmethylpyrazolyl dimethylcarbamate	00119-38-0
Lactonitrile	00078-97-7
* Leptophos	21609-90-5
* Lewisite	00541-25-3
* Lindane	00058-89-9
Lithium hydride	07580-67-8
Malononitrile	00109-77-3
Manganese, tricarbonyl methylcyclopentadienyl	12108-13-3
* Mechlorethamine	00051-75-2
* Mephosfolan	00950-10-7
Mercuric acetate	01600-27-7
Mercuric chloride	07487-94-7
Mercuric oxide	21908-53-2
Mesitylene	00108-67-8
* Methacrolein diacetate	10476-95-6
* Methacrylic anhydride	00760-93-0
Methacyrlonitrile	00126-98-7
Methacryloyl chloride	00920-46-7
Methacryloyloxyethyl isocyanate	30674-80-7
Methamidophos	10265-92-6
* Methanesulfonyl fluoride	00558-25-8
* Methidathion	00950-37-8
Methiocarb	02032-65-7
Methomyl	16752-77-5
* Methoxyethylmercuric acetate	00151-38-2
Methyl 2-chloroacrylate	00080-63-7
Methyl chloroformate	00079-22-1
Methyl disulfide	00624-92-0
Methyl isocyanate	00624-83-9
* Methyl isothiocyanate	00556-61-6
Methyl mercaptan	00074-93-1
* Methyl phenkapton	03735-23-7
Methyl phosphonic dichloride	00676-97-1
* Methyl thiocyanate	00556-64-9
Methyl vinyl ketone	00078-94-4
Methylhydrazine	00060-34-4
* Methylmercuric dicyanamide	00502-39-6
Methyltrichlorosilane	00075-79-6
* Metolcarb	01129-41-5
* Mevinphos	07786-34-7
* Mexacarbate	00315-18-4
* Mitomycin C	00050-07-7

Common Name	CAS Number
Monocrotophos	06923-22-4
* Muscimol	02763-96-4
* Mustard gas	00505-60-2
Nickel	07440-02-0
Nickel carbonyl	13463-39-3
Nicotine	00054-11-5
* Nicotine sulfate	00065-30-5
Nitric acid	07697-37-2
Nitric oxide	10102-43-9
* Nitrocyclohexane	01122-60-7
Nitrogen dioxide	10102-44-0
Nitrosodimethylamine	00062-75-9
* Norbormide	00991-42-4
* Organorhodium complex	PMN-82-147
* Orotic acid	00065-86-1
Osmium tetroxide	20816-12-0
* Ouabain	00630-60-4
Oxamyl	23135-22-0
Oxetane, 3,3-bis(chloromethyl)	00078-71-7
* Oxydisulfoton	02497-07-6
Ozone	10028-15-6
Paraquat	01910-42-5
* Paraquat methosulfate	02074-50-2
Parathion	00056-38-2
Parathion-methyl	00298-00-0
Paris green	12002-03-8
* Pentaborane	19624-22-7
Pentachloroethane	00076-01-7
Pentachlorophenol	00087-86-5
* Pentadecylamine	02570-26-5
Peracetic acid	00079-21-0
Perchloromethylmercapton	00594-42-3
* Phenoxarsine, 10, 10'-oxdi	00058-36-6
Phenol	00108-95-2
* Phenol, 2,2'-thiobis(4-chloro-6-methyl-	04418-66-0
Phenol, 2,2'-thiobis[4,6-dichloro-	00097-18-7
* Phenol, 3-(1-methylethyl)-, methylcarbamate	00064-00-6
* Phenyl dichloroarsine	00696-28-6
Phenylhydrazine hydrochloride	00059-88-1
Phenylmercury acetate	00062-38-4
Phenylsilatrane	02097-19-0
* Phenylthiourea	00103-85-5
Phorate	00298-02-2
* Phosacetim	04104-14-7
* Phosfolan	00947-02-4
Phosmet	00732-11-6
Phosphamidon	13171-21-6
Phosphine	07803-51-2

Common Name	CAS Number
* Phosphonothioic acid, methyl-, O-(4-nitrophenyl . . .	02665-30-7
* Phosphonothioic acid, methyl-, O-ethyl O-[4- . . .	02703-13-1
* Phosphonothioic acid, methyl-, S-[2-[bis . . .	50782-69-9
* Phosphoric acid, dimethyl 4-(methylthio)phenyl . . .	03254-63-5
Phosphorous trichloride	07719-12-2
Phosphorous	07723-14-0
Phosphorous oxychloride	10025-87-3
Phosphorous pentachloride	10026-13-8
Phosphorous pentoxide	01314-56-3
* Phylloquinone	00084-80-0
* Physostigmine	00057-47-6
* Physostigmine, salicylate (1 : 1)	00057-64-7
* Picrotoxin	00124-87-8
Piperidine	00110-89-4
* Piprotal	05281-13-0
* Pirimifos-ethyl	23505-41-1
Platinous chloride	10025-65-7
Platinum tetrachloride	13454-96-1
* Potassium arsenite	10124-50-2
Potassium cyanide	00151-50-8
Potassium silver cyanide	00506-61-6
* Promecarb	02631-37-0
Propargyl bromide	00106-96-7
Propiolactone, .beta.-	00057-57-8
Propionitrile	00107-12-0
* Propionitrile, 3-chloro-	00542-76-7
Propyl chloroformate	00109-61-5
Propylene glycol, allyl ether	01331-17-5
Propyleneimine	0075-55-8
* Prothoate	02275-18-5
Pseudocumene	00095-63-6
Pyrene	00129-00-0
Pyridine, 2-methyl-5-vinyl-	00140-76-1
Pyridine, 4-amino-	00504-24-5
* Pyridine, 4-nitro-, 1-oxide	01124-33-0
* Pyriminil	53558-25-1
Rhodium trichloride	10049-07-7
* Salcomine	14167-18-1
* Sarin	00107-44-8
* Selenium oxychloride	07791-23-3
Selenous acid	07783-00-8
Semicarbazide hydrochloride	00563-41-7
Silane, (4-aminobutyl)diethoxymethyl-	03037-72-7
* Sodium anthraquinone-1-sulfonate	00128-56-3
Sodium arsenate	07631-89-2
Sodium arsenite	07784-46-5
Sodium azide (Na(N3))	26628-22-8
Sodium cacodylate	00124-65-2

Common Name	CAS Number
Sodium cyanide (Na(CN))	00143-33-9
Sodium fluoroacetate	00062-74-8
Sodium pentachlorophenate	00131-52-2
* Sodium selenate	13410-01-0
Sodium selenite	10102-18-8
* Sodium tellurite	10102-20-2
Strychnine	00057-24-9
Strychnine, sulfate	00060-41-3
Sulfotep	03689-24-5
* Sulfoxide, 3-chloropropyl octyl	03569-57-1
Sulfur tetrafluoride	07783-60-0
Sulfur trioxide	07446-11-9
Sulfuric acid	07664-93-9
* TEPP	00107-49-3
* Tabun	00077-81-6
Tellurium	13494-80-9
Tellurium hexafluoride	07783-80-4
Terbufos	13071-79-9
Tetraethyllead	00078-00-2
* Tetraethyltin	00597-64-8
Tetranitromethane	00509-14-8
Thallic oxide	01314-32-5
* Thallous carbonate	06533-73-9
Thallous chloride	07791-12-0
* Thallous malonate	02757-18-8
* Thallous sulfate	07446-18-6
* Thallous sulfate	10031-59-1
* Thiocarbazide	02231-57-4
Thiocyanic acid, (2-benzothiazolylthio)methyl . . .	21564-17-0
* Thiofanox	39196-18-4
* Thiometon	00640-15-3
* Thionazin	00297-97-2
Thiophenol	00108-98-5
Thiosemicarbazide	00079-19-6
* Thiourea, (2-chlorophenyl)-	05344-82-1
* Thiourea, (2-methylphenyl)-	00614-78-8
Titanium tetrachloride	07550-45-0
Toluene, 2,4-diisocyanate	00584-84-9
Toluene, 2,6-diisocyanate	00091-08-7
* Triamiphos	01031-47-6
* Triazofos	24017-47-8
Trichloro(chloromethyl)silane	01558-25-4
Trichloro(dichlorophenyl)silane	27137-85-5
Trichloroacetyl chloride	00076-02-8
Trichloroethylsilane	00115-21-9
* Trichloronate	00327-98-0
Trichlorophenylsilane	00098-13-5
Trichlorphon	00052-68-6
Triethyoxysilane	00998-30-1

Common Name	CAS Number
Trimethylchlorosilane	00075-77-4
* Trimethylolpropane phosphite	00824-11-3
Trimethyltin chloride	01066-45-1
Trimethyltin chloride	00639-58-7
* Tris(2-chloroethyl)amine	00555-77-1
Valinomycin	02001-95-8
Vanadium pentoxide	01314-62-1
Vinylnorbornene	03048-64-4
Warfarin	00081-81-2
Warfarin sodium	00129-06-6
Xylylene dichloride	28347-13-9
Zinc phosphide	01314-84-7
* Zinc, dichloro [4,4-dimethyl-5-[[[(methylamino) . . .	58270-08-9
trans-1,4-Dichlorobutene	00110-57-6

Other Chemicals	CAS Number
Acrylamide	79-06-1
Acrylonitrile	107-13-1
Adiponitrile	111-69-3
Ammonia*	7664-41-7
Aniline	62-53-3
Bromine	7726-95-6
Carbon disulfide	75-15-0
Chloroform	67-66-3
Cumene**	98-82-8
Cyclohexylamine	108-91-8
Epichlorohydrin	106-89-8
Ethylene oxide	75-21-8
Formaldehyde	50-00-0
Hydrochloric acid	7647-01-0
Hydrogen peroxide	7722-84-1
Hydrogen sulfide	7783-06-4
Hydroquinone	123-31-9
Isopropanol**	67-63-0
Methanol**	67-56-1
Methyl bromide	74-83-9
Nitrobenzene	98-95-3
Phosgene	75-44-5
Propylene oxide*	75-56-9
Sulfur dioxide*	7446-09-5
Tetramethyl lead	75-74-1
Vinyl acetate monomer*	108-05-4

*These chemicals do not have acute toxicity measures that strictly meet the criteria for listing as "Other Chemicals." However, based on production capacity, toxicity, and known danger, these chemicals remain listed as "Other Chemicals." Only the reason for listing is changed.

**These chemicals are removed from the list based on their relatively lesser toxicity compared to all of the acutely toxic chemicals listed.

Appendix **C**

Emergency Response Commissions in the Fifty States

One part of the new SARA (PL 99-499) law is Title III, the Emergency Planning and Community Right-to-Know Act of 1986. Title III establishes requirements for federal, state, and local governments and industry regarding emergency planning and community "right-to-know" reporting on hazardous and toxic chemicals. This legislation builds upon EPA's Chemical Emergency Preparedness Program (CEPP) and numerous state and local programs aimed at helping communities to better meet their responsibilities in regard to potential chemical emergencies. The community right-to-know provisions of Title III will help to increase the public's knowledge and access to information on the presence of hazardous chemicals in their communities and releases of these chemicals into the environment.

Under section 301-303, each state governor is required to designate a state emergency commission which, in turn, must designate local emergency planning districts by July 17, 1987 and appoint local emergency planning committees within one month after a district is designated. The local committee's primary responsibility will be to develop an emergency response plan by October 17, 1988. In developing this plan, the local committee will evaluate available resources for preparing for and responding to a potential chemical accident.

As of April 17, 1987, the deadline for appointment of the state emergency response commissions, the following state-by-state data was available:

ALABAMA

Alabama Emergency Response Commission
Mr. Leigh Pegues, Co-chair (Notification and Data)
Director, Alabama Department of Environmental Management
1751 Federal Drive, Montgomery, Alabama 36109
(205) 271-7700   Contact: E. John Williford
Mr. J. Danny Cooper, Co-chair (Planning and Emergencies)
Director, Alabama Emergency Management Agency
520 South Court Street, Montgomery, Alabama 36130
(205) 834-1375   Contact: Dave White

ALASKA

Amy Kyle, Chair
Alaska State Emergency Response Commission
P.O. Box O, Juneau, Alaska 99811
(907) 465-2600

ARIZONA

Carl F. Funk
Arizona State Emergency Response Commission
Division of Emergency Service
5636 E. McDowell Road, Phoenix, Arizona 85008
(602) 244-0504

ARKANSAS

Dr. Phyllis Moore, Chair
Arkansas Hazardous Materials Emergency Response Commission
Director, Arkansas Department of Pollution Control and Ecology
P.O. Box 9583, 8001 National Drive, Little Rock, Arkansas 72219
(501) 562-7444

CALIFORNIA

William Medigovich, Chair
California Emergency Response Commission
Director, Office of Emergency Services
2800 Meadowview Road, Sacramento, California 95832
(916) 427-4201

COLORADO

J. Pat Byrne, Chair
Colorado Emergency Planning & Community Right-to-Know Commission
Division of Disaster Emergency Services
Camp George West, 1500 Golden Road, Golden, Colorado 80401
Additional address: Colorado Department of Health
Division of Hazardous Materials and Waste
4210 East 11th Avenue, Denver, Colorado 80220

CONNECTICUT

Christopher Cooper
Connecticut Emergency Response Commission
State Office Building, Room 161
165 Capitol Avenue, Hartford, CT 06106
(203) 566-4017

DELAWARE

Edward Steiner
Delaware Commission on Hazardous Materials and Emergency Response
Department of Public Safety, Administrative Center
P.O. Box 818, Dover, Delaware 19901
(302) 834-4531 and (302) 736-4321

DISTRICT OF COLUMBIA

Joseph P. Yeldell
Office of Emergency Preparedness
2000 14th Street, N.W., 8th Floor, Washington, D.C. 20009
(202) 727-6161

FLORIDA

Thomas G. Pelham, Chair
Florida Emergency Response Commission
Secretary, Florida Department of Community Affairs
2571 Executive Center Circle East, Tallahassee, Florida 32399
(904) 487-4915   Contact: Kevin Bloom

GEORGIA

J. Leonard Ledbetter, Chair
Georgia Emergency Response Commission
Commissioner, Georgia Department of Natural Resources
205 Butler Street S.E., Floyd Towers East, Atlanta, Georgia 30334
(404) 656-4713   Contact: Jim Setser

HAWAII

Bruce S. Anderson
Hawaii Emergency Response Commission
Hawaii Department of Health, Environmental Epidemiology Program
P.O. Box 3378, Honolulu, Hawaii 96801
(808) 548-2076 or (808) 548-5832

IDAHO

Jack Peterson, Chair
Jenny Davey, Staff Coordinator
Idaho Emergency Response Commission
Department of Health and Welfare
State House, Boise, Idaho 83720
(208) 334-5898

ILLINOIS

Oran Robinson
Illinois Emergency Response Commission
Illinois Emergency Service and Disaster Agency, attn: Hazmat Section
110 E. Adams Street, Springfield, Illinois 62706
(217) 782-4694

INDIANA

Skip Powers
Indiana Department of Environmental Management
Emergency Response Branch
5500 West Bradbury Street, Indianapolis, Indiana 46241
(317) 243-5176

IOWA

Ellen Gordon, Chair
Iowa Emergency Response Commission
Iowa Office of Disaster Services
Hoover Building, Room A-29, Des Moines, Iowa 50319
(515) 281-6175

KANSAS

Karl Birns
State Emergency Response Commission
Kansas Department of Health and Management
Forbes Field, Building 728, P.O. Box C-300, Topeka, Kansas 66601-0300
Planning & Training under Section 302-304
Colonel Retired Mahlon G. Weed
Deputy Director, Division of Emergency Preparedness
Office of Adjutant General
P.O. Box C-300
Topeka, Kansas 66601-0300

KENTUCKY

Colonel James H. "Mike" Molloy, Chair
Kentucky Emergency Response Commission
Executive Director, Kentucky Disaster and Emergency Services
Boone National Guard Center, Frankfort, KY 40601
(502) 564-8682   Contact: Mike Molloy or Tom Little

LOUISIANA

Wiley McCormick, Coordinator

Louisiana Emergency Response Commission
Department of Public Safety and Correction
P.O. Box 66614, Baton Rouge, Louisiana 70896
(504) 925-6117

MAINE

James H. McGowan, Director
Bureau of Labor Standards, Attn. SARA
State Office Building, Station 82, Augusta, Maine 04333
(207) 289-4291

MARYLAND

Charles Meagher
Governor's Management Advisory Council
Maryland Emergency Management and Civil Defense
2 Sudbrook Lane East, East Pikesville, MD 21208
(301) 486-4422

MASSACHUSETTS

Mr. Arnold Sarpenter
Title III Emergency Response Commission
Department of Environmental Quality Engineering
1 Winter Street, Boston, Massachusetts 02108

MICHIGAN

Lynelle Marolx
Michigan Department of Natural Resources
Environmental Response Division, Title III Notification
P.O. Box 30028, Lansing, Michigan 48909
(517) 373-9893

MINNESOTA

Minnesota Emergency Response Commission
Division of Emergency Services
Room B-5, State Capitol, St. Paul, Minnesota 55155

MISSISSIPPI

J. E. Maher, Chair
Mississippi Emergency Response Commission
Director, Mississippi Emergency Management Agency
P.O. Box 4501, Fondren Station, Jackson, Mississippi 39216-0501
(601) 352-9100

MISSOURI

Dean Martin, Chair; Fred Brunner, Director
Missouri Emergency Response Commission
Missouri Department of Natural Resources
Box 176, Jefferson City, Missouri 65102
(314) 751-7929

MONTANA

Thomas Ellenhoff, Co-chair
Montana Emergency Response Commission
Environmental Sciences Division
Department of Health and Environmental Sciences
Cogswell Building, A-107, Helena, Montana 59620
(406) 444-3948

NEBRASKA

Clark Smith, Coordinator
Nebraska Emergency Response Commission
Nebraska Department of Environmental Control, attn: Technical Services Section
P.O. Box 94877, State House Station, Lincoln, Nebraska 68509
(402) 471-4230

NEVADA

Gaylen Ozawa
Nevada Division of Emergency Management
2525 S. Carson Street, Carson City, Nevada 89710
(702) 885-4240 or 885-5300

NEW HAMPSHIRE

Richard Strome, Director
New Hampshire Emergency Management Agency
State Office Park South, 107 Pleasant Street, Concord, New Hampshire 03301
(603) 271-2231

NEW JERSEY

New Jersey Emergency Response Commission
SARA Title III Project
Department of Environmental Protection
Division of Environmental Quality, CN-402
Trenton, New Jersey 08625
(609) 633-7289
Also New Jersey Department of Environmental Protection
401 East State Street, Trenton, New Jersey 08625

NEW MEXICO

Maryann Walz, Coordinator
New Mexico Emergency Response Commission
New Mexico State Police
Hazardous Materials Bureau
P.O. Box 1628, Santa Fe, New Mexico 87504-1628
(505) 827-9226

NEW YORK

New York Emergency Response Commission
New York State Department of Environmental Conservation
Bureau of Spill Prevention and Response
50 Wolf Road, Room 326, Albany, New York 12233-3510
(518) 457-9949
Also New York Department of Health
Tower Building, Empire State Plaza, Albany, New York 12237

NORTH CAROLINA

Joseph Myers, Chair
North Carolina Emergency Response Commission
Director, Division of Emergency Management
Secretary, North Carolina Department of Crime Control and Public Safety
116 W. Jones Street, Raleigh, North Carolina 27611
(919) 733-2126   Contact: Vance Kee

NORTH DAKOTA

Dana Mount
North Dakota Emergency Response Commission
1200 Missouri Avenue, P.O.Box 5520, Bismarck, North Dakota 58502-5520
(701) 224-2370

OHIO

Ken Schultz, SARA Title III Coordinator
Ohio Emergency Response Commission
Ohio Environmental Protection Agency
Office of Emergency Response
P.O. Box 1049, Columbus, Ohio 43266-0149
(614) 481-4300

OKLAHOMA

Jack Muse, Coordinator
Emergency Response Commission
Office of Civil Defense
P.O. Box 53365, Oklahoma City, Oklahoma 73152-53365

OREGON

Michael Wang
Oregon Emergency Response Commission
c/o State Fire Marshall
3000 N.E. Market Street, Suite 534, Salem, Oregon 97310
(503) 378-2885

PENNSYLVANIA

Sanders Courtner
Pennsylvania Emergency Response Commission
SARA Title III Officer, PEMA Response and Recovery
P.O. Box 3321, Harrisburg, Pennsylvania 17105-3321
(717) 783-8150 or 783-8193

PUERTO RICO

Santos Rohena, Chair
Puerto Rico Emergency Response Commission
Environmental Quality Board
P.O. Box 11488, Santurce, Puerto Rico
(809) 722-1175 or 722-2173

RHODE ISLAND

Joseph A. Demarco, Executive Director
Rhode Island Emergency Response Commission
Rhode Island Emergency Management Agency
State House M-27, Providence, Rhode Island 02903
(401) 421-7333

SOUTH CAROLINA

Stan M. McKinney, Chair
South Carolina Emergency Response Commission
Division of Public Safety Programs
Office of the Governor
1205 Pendleton Street, Columbia South Carolina 29201
(803) 734-0424   Contact: Stan McKinney or Purdy McLeod

SOUTH DAKOTA

Joel Smith
South Dakota Response Commission
Department of Water and Natural Resources
Joe Foss Building, 523 East Capitol, Pierre, South Dakota 57501-3181
(605) 773-3151

TENNESSEE

Lacy Suiter, Chair
Tennessee Emergency Response Commission
Director, Tennessee Emergency Management Agency
3041 Sidco Drive, Nashville, Tennessee 37204
(615) 252-3300 or (800) 258-3300   Contact: Lacy Suiter or Tom Durham

TEXAS

Mike Scott, Coordinator
Texas Emergency Response Commission
Division of Emergency Management
P.O. Box 4087, Austin, Texas 78773-0001
(512) 465-2138

UTAH

Neil Taylor (311-313 Reporting)
Utah Hazardous Chemical Emergency Response Commission
Department of Health
288 N. 1460 West, P.O. Box 16690, Salt Lake City, Utah 84116-0690
Lorayne Tempest-Frank (302-304 Planning)
Comprehensive Emergency Management
P.O. Box 8100, Salt Lake City, Utah 84108
(801) 533-5271

VERMONT

Jeanne VanVlandren, Commissioner
Department of Labor and Industry
120 State Street, Montpelier, Vermont 05002
(802) 828-2286

VIRGINIA

Cynthia V. Bailey, Chair
Virginia Emergency Response Council
Department of Waste Management
James Monroe Building, 11th Floor, 101 N. 14th Street, Richmond, VA 23219
(804) 225-2999

WASHINGTON (STATE)

Hugh Fowler, Chair
Washington Emergency Response Commission
Division of Emergency Management
4220 East Martin Way, Mail Stop PT-11, Olympia, Washington 98504
(206) 753-5255

WEST VIRGINIA

Ron R. Potesta
Director, Department of Natural Resources
West Virginia Emergency Response Commission
Capitol Building, Room 669
1800 Washington Street East, Charleston, West Virginia 25305
(304) 348-2758

WISCONSIN

Richard I. Braund
Division of Emergency Government
4802 Sheboygan Avenue, P.O. Box 7865, Madison, Wisconsin 53707
(608) 266-3232

WYOMING

Ed Usui, Coordinator
Wyoming Emergency Management Agency
Wyoming State Emergency Response Commission
Comprehensive Emergency Management
5500 Bishop Boulevard, P.O. Box 1709, Cheyenne, Wyoming 82003
(307) 777-7566

Chemicals to Be Reported to State Commissions Under Section 372.45 of SARA by Facilities in Standard Industrial Classification Codes 20 through 39

Chemical name	CAS No.	Generic classification code	Effective date
Acetaldehyde	75-07-0	C07	01/01/87
Acetamide	60-35-5	C09	01/01/87
Acetone	67-64-1	C07	01/01/87
Acetonitrile	75-05-8	C11	01/01/87
2-Acetylaminofluorene	53-96-3	C10	01/01/87
Acrolein	107-02-8	C07	01/01/87
Acrylamide	79-06-1	C09	01/01/87
Acrylic acid	79-10-7	C08	01/01/87
Acrylonitrile	107-13-1	C11	01/01/87
Aldrin [1,4:5,8-Dimethanonaphthalene,1,2,3,4,10,10-hexachloro-1,4,4a, 5,8,8a-hexahydro-(1.alpha.,4.alpha.,4a.beta.,5.alpha.,8.alpha.,8a.beta.)-]	309-00-2	C03	01/01/87
Allyl chloride	107-05-1	C03	01/01/87
Aluminum (fume or dust)	7429-90-5	C15	01/01/87
Aluminum oxide	1344-28-1	C15	01/01/87
2-Aminoanthraquinone	117-79-3	C10	01/01/87
4-Aminoazobenzene	60-09-3	C10	01/01/87
4-Aminobiphenyl	92-67-1	C10	01/01/87
1-Amino-2-methylanthraquinone	82-28-0	C10	01/01/87
Ammonia	7664-41-7	C16	01/01/87
Ammonium nitrate (solution)	6484-52-2	C16	01/01/87
Ammonium sulfate (solution)	7783-20-2	C16	01/01/87
Aniline	62-53-3	C10	01/01/87
o-Anisidine	90-04-0	C10	01/01/87
p-Anisidine	104-94-9	C10	01/01/87
o-Anisidine hydrochloride	134-29-2	C10	01/01/87
Anthracene	120-12-7	C01	01/01/87
Antimony	7440-36-0	C15	01/01/87
Arsenic	7440-38-2	C15	01/01/87
Asbestos (friable)	1332-21-4	C16	01/01/87
Auramine [Benzeneamine, 4,4'-carbonimidoylbis[N,N-dimethyl-]	492-80-8	C10	01/01/87
Barium	7440-39-3	C15	01/01/87
Benzal chloride	98-87-3	C02	01/01/87
Benzamide	55-21-0	C09	01/01/87
Benzene	71-43-2	C01	01/01/87
Benzidine	92-87-5	C10	01/01/87
Benzoic trichlorides (Benzotrichloride)	98-07-7	C02	01/01/87
Benzoyl chloride	98-88-4	C09	01/01/87
Benzoyl peroxide	94-36-0	C09	01/01/87
Benzyl chloride	100-44-7	C02	01/01/87
Beryllium	7440-41-7	C15	01/01/87

Source: Federal Register, **52,** No. 107 (June 4, 1987), pp. 21168–21173.

Chemical name	CAS No.	Generic classification code	Effective date
Biphenyl	92-52-4	C01	01/01/87
Bis(2-chloroethyl) ether	111-44-4	C06	01/01/87
Bis(chloromethyl) ether	542-88-1	C06	01/01/87
Bis(2-chloro-1-methylethyl) ether	108-60-1	C06	01/01/87
Bis(2-ethylhexyl) adipate	103-23-1	C08	01/01/87
Bromoform (Tribromomethane)	75-25-2	C02	01/01/87
Bromomethane (Methyl bromide)	74-83-9	C02	01/01/87
1,3-Butadiene	106-99-0	C01	01/01/87
Butyl acrylate	141-32-2	C08	01/01/87
n-Butyl alcohol	71-36-3	C05	01/01/87
sec-Butyl alcohol	78-92-2	C05	01/01/87
tert-Butyl alcohol	75-65-0	C05	01/01/87
Butyl benzyl phthalate	85-68-7	C08	01/01/87
1,2-Butylene oxide	106-88-7	C06	01/01/87
Butyraldehyde	123-72-8	C07	01/01/87
C.I. Acid Blue 9, diammonium salt	2650-18-2	C13	01/01/87
C.I. Acid Blue 9, disodium salt	3844-45-9	C13	01/01/87
C.I. Acid Green 3	4680-78-8	C13	01/01/87
C.I. Basic Green 4	569-64-2	C10	01/01/87
C.I. Basic Red 1	989-38-8	C10	01/01/87
C.I. Disperse Yellow 3	2832-40-8	C14	01/01/87
C.I. Food Red 5	3761-53-3	C14	01/01/87
C.I. Food Red 15	81-88-9	C10	01/01/87
C.I. Solvent Orange 7	3118-97-6	C14	01/01/87
C.I. Solvent Yellow 3	97-56-3	C14	01/01/87
C.I. Solvent Yellow 14	842-07-9	C14	01/01/87
C.I. Vat Yellow 4	128-66-5	C07	01/01/87
Cadmium	7440-43-9	C15	01/01/87
Calcium cyanamide	156-62-7	C11	01/01/87
Captan [1H-Isoindole-1,3(2H)-dione,3a,4,7,7a-tetrahydro-2- [(trichloromethyl)thio]-]	133-06-2	C13	01/01/87
Carbaryl [1-Naphthalenol,methylcarbamate]	63-25-2	C09	01/01/87
Carbon disulfide	75-15-0	C13	01/01/87
Carbon tetrachloride	56-23-5	C02	01/01/87
Carbonyl sulfide	463-58-1	C13	01/01/87
Catechol	120-80-9	C05	01/01/87
Chloramben [Benzoic acid, 5-amino-2,5-dichloro-]	133-90-4	C11	01/01/87
Chlordane [4,7-Methanoindan, 1,2,4,5,6,7,8,8-octachloro-2,3,3a,4,7,7a- hexahydro-]	57-74-9	C03	01/01/87
Chlorinated fluorocarbon (Freon 113)[Ethane, 1,1,2-trichloro-1,2, 2-trifluoro-]	76-13-1	C02	01/01/87
Chlorine	7782-50-5	C16	01/01/87
Chlorine dioxide	10049-04-4	C16	01/01/87
Chloroacetic acid	79-11-8	C08	01/01/87
2-Chloroacetophenone	532-27-4	C07	01/01/87
Chlorobenzene	108-90-7	C04	01/01/87
Chlorobenzilate [Benzeneacetic acid, 4-chloro-.alpha.-(4-chlorophenyl)-.alpha.-hydroxy-, ethyl ester]	510-15-6	C08	01/01/87
Chloroethane (Ethyl chloride)	75-00-3	C02	01/01/87
Chloroform	67-66-3	C02	01/01/87
Chloromethane (Methyl chloride)	74-87-3	C02	01/01/87
Chloromethyl methyl ether	107-30-2	C06	01/01/87
Chloroprene	126-99-8	C03	01/01/87
Chlorothalonil [1,3-Benzenedicarbonitrile,2,4,5,6-tetrachloro-]	1897-45-6	C09	01/01/87
Chromium	7440-47-3	C15	01/01/87
Cobalt	7440-48-4	C15	01/01/87
Copper	7440-50-8	C15	01/01/87
p-Cresidine	120-71-8	C06	01/01/87
Cresol (mixed isomers)	1319-77-3	C05	01/01/87
m-Cresol	108-39-4	C05	01/01/87
o-Cresol	95-48-7	C05	01/01/87
p-Cresol	106-44-5	C05	01/01/87
Cumene	98-82-8	C01	01/01/87
Cumene hydroperoxide	80-15-9	C05	01/01/87
Cupferron [Benzeneamine, N-hydroxy-N-nitroso, ammonium salt]	135-20-6	C12	01/01/87
Cyanide compounds	57-12-5	C16	01/01/87
Cyclohexane	110-82-7	C01	01/01/87
2,4-D [Acetic acid, (2,4-dichloro-phenoxy)-]	94-75-7	C08	01/01/87
Decabromodiphenyl oxide	1163-19-5	C04	01/01/87
Diallate [Carbamothioic acid, bis(1-methylethyl)-, S-(2,3- dichloro-2-propenyl) ester]	2303-16-4	C13	01/01/87
2,4-Diaminoanisole	615-05-4	C10	01/01/87
2,4-Diaminoanisole sulfate	39156-41-7	C10	01/01/87
4,4'-Diaminodiphenyl ether	101-80-4	C10	01/01/87
Diaminotoluene (mixed isomers)	25376-45-8	C10	01/01/87
2,4-Diaminotoluene	95-80-7	C10	01/01/87
Diazomethane	334-88-3	C11	01/01/87
Dibenzofuran	132-64-9	C06	01/01/87
1,2-Dibromo-3-chloropropane (DBCP)	96-12-8	C02	01/01/87
1,2-Dibromoethane (Ethylene dibromide)	106-93-4	C02	01/01/87
Dibutyl phthalate	84-74-2	C08	01/01/87
Dichlorobenzene (mixed isomers)	25321-22-6	C04	01/01/87
1,2-Dichlorobenzene	95-50-1	C04	01/01/87
1,3-Dichlorobenzene	541-73-1	C04	01/01/87
1,4-Dichlorobenzene	106-46-7	C04	01/01/87
3,3'-Dichlorobenzidine	91-94-1	C10	01/01/87
Dichlorobromomethane	75-27-4	C02	01/01/87
1,2-Dichloroethane (Ethylene dichloride)	107-06-2	C02	01/01/87
1,2-Dichloroethylene	540-59-0	C03	01/01/87
Dichloromethane (Methylene chloride)	75-09-2	C02	01/01/87
2,4-Dichlorophenol	120-83-2	C05	01/01/87
1,2-Dichloropropane	78-87-5	C02	01/01/87
1,3-Dichloropropylene	542-75-6	C03	01/01/87
Dichlorvos [Phosphoric acid, 2,2-dichloroethenyl dimethyl ester]	62-73-7	C13	01/01/87
Dicofol [Benzenemethanol, 4-chloro-.alpha.-(4-chlorophenyl).alpha.-(trichloromethyl)-]	115-52-2	C04	01/01/87
Diepoxybutane	1464-53-5	C06	01/01/87
Diethanolamine	111-42-2	C10	01/01/87

504

Chemical name	CAS No.	Generic classification code	Effective date
Di-(2-ethylhexyl) phthalate (DEHP)	117-81-7	C08	01/01/87
Diethyl phthalate	84-66-2	C08	01/01/87
Diethyl sulfate	64-67-5	C13	01/01/87
3,3'-Dimethoxybenzidine	119-90-4	C10	01/01/87
4-Dimethylaminoazobenzene	60-11-7	C10	01/01/87
3,3'-Dimethylbenzidine(o-Tolidine)	119-93-7	C10	01/01/87
Dimethylcarbamyl chloride	79-44-7	C09	01/01/87
1,1-Dimethyl hydrazine	57-14-7	C11	01/01/87
2,4-Dimethylphenol	105-67-9	C05	01/01/87
Dimethyl phthalate	131-11-3	C08	01/01/87
Dimethyl sulfate	77-78-1	C13	01/01/87
4,6-Dinitro-o-cresol	534-52-1	C12	01/01/87
2,4-Dinitrophenol	51-28-5	C12	01/01/87
2,4-Dinitrotoluene	121-14-2	C12	01/01/87
2,6-Dinitrotoluene	606-20-2	C12	01/01/87
n-Dioctyl phthalate	117-84-0	C08	01/01/87
1,4-Dioxane	123-91-1	C06	01/01/87
1,2-Diphenylhydrazine(Hydrazobenzene)	122-66-7	C11	01/01/87
Direct Black 38	1937-37-7	C14	01/01/87
Direct Blue 6	2602-46-2	C14	01/01/87
Direct Brown 95	16071-86-6	C14	01/01/87
Epichlorohydrin	106-89-8	C06	01/01/87
2-Ethoxyethanol	110-80-5	C06	01/01/87
Ethyl acrylate	140-88-5	C08	01/01/87
Ethylbenzene	100-41-4	C01	01/01/87
Ethyl chloroformate	541-41-3	C09	01/01/87
Ethylene	74-85-1	C01	01/01/87
Ethylene glycol	107-21-1	C05	01/01/87
Ethyleneimine (Aziridine)	151-56-4	C11	01/01/87
Ethylene oxide	75-21-8	C06	01/01/87
Ethylene thiourea	96-45-7	C13	01/01/87
Fluometuron [Urea, N,N-dimethyl-N'-[3-(trifluoromethyl)phenyl]-]	2164-17-2	C09	01/01/87
Formaldehyde	50-00-0	C07	01/01/87
Heptachlor [1,4,5,6,7,8,8-Heptachloro-3a,4,7,7a-tetrahydro-4,7- methano-1H-indene]	76-44-8	C03	01/01/87
Hexachlorobenzene	118-74-1	C04	01/01/87
Hexachloro 1,3-butadiene	87-68-3	C03	01/01/87
Hexachlorocyclopentadiene	77-47-4	C03	01/01/87
Hexachloroethane	67-72-1	C02	01/01/87
Hexachloronaphthalene	1335-87-1	C04	01/01/87
Hexamethylphosphoramide	680-31-9	C13	01/01/87
Hydrazine	302-01-2	C11	01/01/87
Hydrazine sulfate	10034-93-2	C11	01/01/87
Hydrochloric acid	764-01-07	C16	01/01/87
Hydrogen cyanide	74-90-8	C16	01/01/87
Hydrogen fluoride	7664-39-3	C16	01/01/87
Hydroquinone	123-31-9	C07	01/01/87
Isobutyraldehyde	78-84-2	C07	01/01/87
Isopropyl alcohol (mfg.—strong acid processes)	67-63-0	C05	01/01/87
4,4'-Isopropylidenediphenol	80-05-7	C05	01/01/87
Lead	7439-92-1	C15	01/01/87
Lindane [Cyclohexane, 1,2,3,4,5,6-hexachloro-,(1.alpha.,2.alpha., 3.beta. 4.alpha.,5.alpha.,6.beta.)-]	58-89-9	C02	01/01/87
Maleic anhydride	108-31-6	C08	01/01/87
Maneb [Carbamodithioic acid, 1,2-ethanediylbis-, manganese complex]	12427-38-2	C16	01/01/87
Manganese	7439-96-5	C15	01/01/87
Melamine	108-78-1	C10	01/01/87
Mercury	7439-97-6	C15	01/01/87
Methanol	67-56-1	C05	01/01/87
Methoxychlor [Benzene, 1,1'-(2,2 2-trichloroethylidene)bis[4-methoxy-]	72-43-5	C03	01/01/87
2-Methoxyethanol	109-86-4	C06	01/01/87
Methyl acrylate	96-33-3	C08	01/01/87
Methyl tert-butyl ether	1634-04-4	C06	01/01/87
4,4'-Meth lenebis(2-chloro aniline) (MBOCA)	101-14-4	C10	01/01/87
4,4'-Methylenebis(N N-dimethyl) benzenamine	101-61-1	C10	01/01/87
Methylenebis(phenylisocyanate) (MBI)	101-68-8	C11	01/01/87
Methylene bromide	74-95-3	C02	01/01/87
4,4'-Methylenedianiline	101-77-9	C10	01/01/87
Methyl ethyl ketone	78-93-3	C07	01/01/87
Methyl hydrazine	60-34-4	C11	01/01/87
Methyl iodide	74-88-4	C02	01/01/87
Methyl isobutyl ketone	108-10-1	C07	01/01/87
Methyl isocyanate	624-85-9	C11	01/01/87
Methyl methacrylate	80-62-6	C08	01/01/87
Michler's ketone	90-94-8	C07	01/01/87
Molybdenum trioxide	1313-27-5	C15	01/01/87
Mustard gas [Ethane, 1,1'-thiobis[2-chloro-]	505-60-2	C13	01/01/87
Naphthalene	91-20-3	C01	01/01/87
alpha-Naphthylamine	134-32-7	C10	01/01/87
beta-Naphthylamine	91-59-8	C10	01/01/87
Nickel	7440-02-0	C15	01/01/87
Nitric acid	7697-37-2	C16	01/01/87
Nitrilotriacetic acid	139-13-9	C08	01/01/87
5-Nitro-o-anisidine	99-59-2	C12	01/01/87
Nitrobenzene	98-95-3	C12	01/01/87
4-Nitrobiphenyl	92-93-3	C12	01/01/87
Nitrofen [Benzene, 2,4-dichloro-1-(4-nitrophenoxy)-]	1836-75-5	C15	01/01/87
Nitrogen mustard [2-Chloro-N-(2-chloroethyl)-N-methylethanamine]	51-75-2	C10	01/01/87
Nitroglycerin	55-63-0	C12	01/01/87
2-Nitrophenol	88-75-5	C12	01/01/87
4-Nitrophenol	100-02-7	C12	01/01/87
2-Nitropropane	79-46-9	C12	01/01/87
p Nitrosodiphenylamine	156-10-5	C12	01/01/87

505

Chemical name	CAS No.	Generic classification code	Effective date
N,N-Dimethylaniline	121-69-7	C10	01/01/87
N-Nitrosodi-n-butylamine	924-16-3	C12	01/01/87
N-Nitrosodiethylamine	55-18-5	C12	01/01/87
N-Nitrosodimethylamine	62-75-9	C12	01/01/87
N-Nitrosodiphenylamine	86-30-6	C12	01/01/87
N-Nitrosodi-n-propylamine	621-64-7	C12	01/01/87
N-Nitrosomethylvinylamine	4549-40-0	C12	01/01/87
N-Nitrosomorpholine	59-89-2	C12	01/01/87
N-Nitroso-N-ethylurea	759-73-9	C12	01/01/87
N-Nitroso-N-methylurea	684-93-5	C12	01/01/87
N-Nitrosonornicotine	16543-55-8	C12	01/01/87
N-Nitrosopiperidine	100-75-4	C12	01/01/87
Octachloronaphthalene	2234-13-1	C04	01/01/87
Osmium tetroxide	20816-12-0	C15	01/01/87
Parathion [Phosphorothioic acid, 0,0-dieth 1-0-(4-nitrophenyl)ester]	56-38-2	C13	01/01/87
Pentachlorophenol (PCP)	87-86-5	C04	01/01/87
Peracetic acid	79-21-0	C09	01/01/87
Phenol	108-95-2	C05	01/01/87
p-Phenylenediamine	106-50-3	C10	01/01/87
2-Phenylphenol	90-43-7	C05	01/01/87
Phosgene	75-44-5	C09	01/01/87
Phosphoric acid	7664-38-2	C16	01/01/87
Phosphorus (yellow or white)	7723-14-0	C16	01/01/87
Phthalic anhydride	85-44-9	C08	01/01/87
Picric acid	88-89-1	C08	01/01/87
Polychlorinated biphenyls (PCBs)	1336-36-3	C04	01/01/87
Propane sultone	1120-71-4	C13	01/01/87
beta-Propiolactone	57-57-8	C08	01/01/87
Propionaldehyde	123-38-6	C07	01/01/87
Propoxur [Phenol, 2-(1-methylethoxy)-,methylcarbamate]	114-26-1	C09	01/01/87
Propylene (Propene)	115-07-1	C01	01/01/87
Propyleneimine	75-55-8	C11	01/01/87
Propylene oxide	75-56-9	C06	01/01/87
Pyridine	110-86-1	C11	01/01/87
Quinoline	91-22-5	C11	01/01/87
Quinone	106-51-4	C07	01/01/87
Quintozene [Benzene, pentachloronitro-]	82-68-8	C12	01/01/87
Saccharin (manufacturing) [1,2-Benzisothiazol-3(2H)-one,1,1-dioxide]	81-07-2	C09	01/01/87
Safrole	94-59-7	C06	01/01/87
Selenium	7782-49-2	C16	01/01/87
Silver and compounds	7440-22-4	C15	01/01/87
Sodium hydroxide (solution)	1310-73-2	C16	01/01/87
Sodium sulfate (solution)	7757-82-6	C16	01/01/87
Styrene	100-42-5	C01	01/01/87
Styrene oxide	96-09-3	C06	01/01/87
Sulfuric acid	7664-93-9	C16	01/01/87
Terephthalic acid	100-21-0	C08	01/01/87
1,1,2,2-Tetrachloroethane	79-34-5	C02	01/01/87
Tetrachloroethylene (Perchloroethylene)	127-18-4	C03	01/01/87
Tetrachlorvinphos [Phosphoric acid, 2-chloro-1-(2,4,5-trichlorophenyl)ethenyl dimethyl ester]	961-11-5	C13	01/01/87
Thallium	7440-28-0	C15	01/01/87
Thioacetamide	62-55-5	C13	01/01/87
4,4'-Thiodianiline	139-65-1	C13	01/01/87
Thiourea	62-56-6	C13	01/01/87
Thorium dioxide	1314-20-1	C15	01/01/87
Titanium dioxide	13463-67-7	C15	01/01/87
Titanium tetrachloride	7550-45-0	C15	01/01/87
Toluene	108-88-3	C01	01/01/87
Toluene 2,4 diisocyanate	584-84-9	C11	01/01/87
Toluene-2,6-diisocyanate	91-08-7	C11	01/01/87
o-Toluidine	95-53-4	C10	01/01/87
o-Toluidine hydrochloride	636-21-5	C10	01/01/87
Toxaphene	8001-35-2	C02	01/01/87
Triaziquone [2,5-Cyclohexadiene-1,4-dione,2,3,5-tris(1-aziridinyl)-]	68-76-8	C11	01/01/87
Trichlorfon [Phosphonic acid, (2,2,2-trichloro-1-hydroxyethyl)-,dimethyl ester]	52-68-6	C13	01/01/87
1,2,4-Trichlorobenzene	120-82-1	C04	01/01/87
1,1,1-Trichloroethane (Methyl chloroform)	71-55-6	C02	01/01/87
1,1,2-Trichloroethane	79-00-5	C02	01/01/87
Trichloroethylene	79-01-6	C03	01/01/87
2,4,5-Trichlorophenol	95-95-4	C04	01/01/87
2,4,6 Trichlorophenol	88-06-2	C04	01/01/87
Trifluralin [Benzeneamine, 2,6-dinitro-N,N-dipropyl-4-(trifluoromethyl)-]	1582-09-8	C12	01/01/87*
1,2,4-Trimethylbenzene	95-63-6	C01	01/01/87
Tris(2,3-dibromopropyl) phosphate	126-72-7	C13	01/01/87
Urethane (Ethyl carbamate)	51-79-6	C09	01/01/87
Vanadium (fume or dust)	7440-62-2	C15	01/01/87
Vinyl acetate	108-05-4	C08	01/01/87
Vinyl bromide	593-60-2	C03	01/01/87
Vinyl chloride	75-01-4	C03	01/01/87
Vinylidene chloride	75-35-4	C03	01/01/87
Xylene (mixed isomers)	1330-20-7	C01	01/01/87
m-Xylene	108-38-3	C01	01/01/87
o-Xylene	95-47-6	C01	01/01/87
p-Xylene	106-42-3	C01	01/01/87
2,6-Xylidine	87-62-7	C10	01/01/87
Zinc (fume or dust)	7440-66-6	C15	01/01/87
Zineb [Carbamodithioic acid, 1,2-ethanediylbis-, zinc complex]	12122-67-7	C15	01/01/87

Appendix E

Toxic Pollutant Effluent Limitations and Standards for Direct Discharge Point Sources that Use End-of-Pipe Biological Treatment

	Effluent Limitations (BAT and NSPS)*	
Effluent Characteristics	Maximum for Any One Day	Maximum for Monthly Average
Acenaphthene	59	22
Acrylonitrile	242	96
Benzene	136	37
Carbon Tetrachloride	38	18
Chlorobenzene	28	15
1,2,4-Trichlorobenzene	140	68
Hexachlorobenzene	28	15
1,2-Dichloroethane	211	68
1,1,1-Trichloroethane	54	21
Hexachloroethane	54	21
1,2-Dichloroethane	59	22
Chloroethane	268	104
Chloroform	46	21
2-Chlorophenol	98	31
1,2-Dichlorobenzene	163	77
1,3-Dichlorobenzene	44	31
1,4-Dichlorobenzene	28	15
1,1-Dichloroethylene	25	16
1,2-trans-Dichloroethylene	54	21
2,4-Dichlorophenol	112	39

Source: Federal Register, **52,** No. 214 (November 5, 1987), p. 42581.

Effluent Characteristics	Effluent Limitations (BAT and NSPS)*	
	Maximum for Any One Day	Maximum for Monthly Average
1,2-Dichloropropane	230	153
1,3-Dichloropropylene	44	29
2,4-Dimethylphenol	36	18
2,4-Dinitrotoluene	285	113
2,6-Dinitrotoluene	641	255
Ethylbenzene	108	32
Fluoranthene	68	25
Bis(2-Chloroisopropyl) ether	757	301
Methylene Chloride	89	40
Methyl Chloride	190	86
Hexachlorobutadiene	49	20
Naphthalene	59	22
Nitrobenzene	68	27
2-Nitrophenol	69	41
4-Nitrophenol	124	72
2,4-Dinitrophenol	123	71
4,6-Dinitro-o-cresol	277	71
Phenol	26	15
Bis(2-ethylhexyl) phthalate	279	103
Di-n-butyl phthalate	57	27
Diethyl phthalate	203	81
Dimethyl phthalate	47	19
Benzo(a)anthracene	59	22
Benzo(a)pyrene	61	23
3,4-Benzofluoranthene	61	23
Benzo(k)fluoranthene	59	22
Chrysene	59	22
Acenaphthylene	59	22
Anthracene	59	22
Fluorene	59	22
Phenanthrene	59	22
Pyrene	67	25
Tetrachloroethylene	56	22
Toluene	80	26
Trichloroethylene	54	21
Vinyl Chloride	268	104
Total Chromium	2,770	1,110
Total Copper	3,380	1,450
Total Cyanide	1,200	420
Total Lead	690	320
Total Nickel	3,980	1,690
Total Zinc	2,610	1,050

Note: All units are micrograms per liter. BAT means best available technology economically achievable. NSPS means new source performance standards.

*In addition to the above, pH, BOD (biological oxygen demand) and TSS (total suspended solids) must be controlled and monitored within specified limits.

Index